MW01275435

Lectures On Surgical Pathology

LECTURES

on

SURGICAL PATHOLOGY.

LECTURES

ON

SURGICAL PATHOLOGY,

DELIVERED AT THE

ROYAL COLLEGE OF SURGEONS OF ENGLAND,

BY

JAMES PAGET, F.R.S.,

LATELY PROFESSOR OF ANATOMY AND SURGERY TO THE COLLEGE; ASSISTANT SURGEON AND
LECTURER ON PHYSIOLOGY AT ST. BARTHOLOMEW'S HOSPITAL.

SECOND AMERICAN EDITION.

HYPERTROPHY: ATROPHY: REPAIR: INFLAMMATION: MORTIFICATION:
SPECIFIC DISEASES: AND TUMORS.

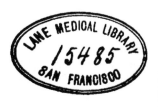

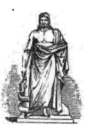

PHILADELPHIA:
LINDSAY & BLAKISTON.
1860.

HENRY B. ASHMEAD, BOOK AND JOB PRINTER,
Sansom Street above Eleventh.

TO

P. M. LATHAM, M. D.,

AND

GEORGE BURROWS, M. D.,

WHOSE SKILL HAS BEEN PERMITTED TWICE TO SAVE MY LIFE,

WHOSE FRIENDSHIP ADDS LARGELY TO MY HAPPINESS,

AND TO WHOSE TEACHING

I SHALL ATTRIBUTE MUCH OF WHATEVER GOOD MY WORK MAY DO,

I DEDICATE THIS VOLUME,

WITH GRATITUDE, AFFECTION, AND RESPECT.

PREFACE.

NEARLY all these Lectures were delivered at the Royal College of Surgeons, during the six years, from 1847 to 1852, in which I held the office of Professor of Anatomy and Surgery to the College. So many listened favorably to them, that I venture to hope I am not wrong in thus enabling many more to read them. But, in offering them to this larger class, some explanation of their scope and plan seems necessary.

The circumstances of my election to the professorship indicated the Pathological Museum of the College as the appropriate subject of the Lectures; and the first portion of the Museum, devoted to the illustration of General Pathology, seemed to offer the best plan by which the knowledge acquired in a long study of the whole collection might be communicated.

The modes were many in which such a subject might be treated in lectures; but, as circumstances had decided the subject, it seemed well to let them determine, also, the method, and to adopt that which was most natural to one engaged in the simultaneous practice of surgery and teaching in physiology. Thus guided, I designed to give lectures which might illustrate the general pathology of the principal surgical diseases, in conformity with the larger and more exact doctrines of physiology; and the plan seemed the more reasonable, because it was in accordance with the constant design of the great founder of the Museum.

The Museum limited, while it indicated, the subjects of the Lectures. They were, therefore, not constructed to form a system of surgical pathology: several subjects, which might fill considerable places in such a system, were scarcely alluded to in them; and, although I have added some lectures, which could not be conveniently included in any of the courses, yet I have not gone beyond the range of such pathology as a Museum may illustrate.

The wood-engravings are, for the most part, copied from the same specimens and drawings as were the diagrams used in the Lectures; and I wish them to be regarded as intended for only the same purpose as such diagrams may serve; viz., that of assisting the more difficult parts of the descriptions of the objects to which they refer.

I have endeavored to make the Lectures less incomplete, and more correct, by the aid of numerous facts ascertained since they were delivered, and have added to them many things which time, or their inaptness for oral delivery, obliged me to omit. Among these are the references to specimens and illustrations; as well as to numerous authors who could not, in speaking, be conveniently quoted, but whom I am now glad to acknowledge as instructors. And I will here offer my thanks to some, to whom my debts are more than would be expressed, even by referring to all the occasions on which their works have aided me in the composition of the Lectures. Such acknowledgments are due, especially, to Mr. Lawrence, Mr. Stanley, Professor Owen, and Dr. Carpenter, from whom, during many years of valued friendship, I have derived, at every interview, either knowledge, or guidance in observing and thinking. I am deeply obliged, also, to all my colleagues on the staff of St. Bartholomew's, from whom the constant help that I receive adds daily to the debt of gratitude incurred during my pupilage. And there are many friends besides, to whom it is my happiness to be indebted for knowledge used in these Lectures, and whom I thank collectively, not because I owe them little, but because I cannot name them all, and cannot thank some without appearing ungrateful to the rest.

The lectures after the twentieth, and especially those on Cancers, are enlarged far beyond their original extent, by the addition of cases, statistical tables, and various statements which may be worth reading, but of which the recital could not be made agreeable to an audience. In making these additions, I have endeavored to adduce sufficient evidence for the general conclusions I have drawn, without encumbering the book with such a mass of details as would be repulsive to the majority of readers. I can hardly imagine, that a full relation of so many cases as I have referred to would be acceptable to any besides those who are engaged in the especial study of the subjects of the Lectures. To all who are so occupied, I will very gladly give whatever further information my manuscript records of cases can supply.

It is an unavoidable defect in lectures on general pathology, that they cannot be conveniently used in the study of the diseases of particular organs. I have endeavored to amend this, in some measure, by a full index, referring, under the title of each organ, to the descriptions of the tumors of which it is most apt to be the seat.

I desire, in conclusion, to express my acknowledgments to the Members of the Council of the College, both for the repeated honor they conferred on me by so often electing me to the Professorship, and for the kindness with which many of them devoted their valuable time to attendance at the Lectures. The encouragement they thus afforded me, makes me hope, that the labor with which I strive to justify their choice, may have some success in the promotion of scientific surgery.

HENRIETTA STREET, CAVENDISH SQUARE.

TITLES OF THE LECTURES.

LIST OF ILLUSTRATIONS.

LECTURES

on

SURGICAL PATHOLOGY.

LECTURE I.

NUTRITION—ITS NATURE, PURPOSE, AND CONDITIONS.

MR. PRESIDENT AND GENTLEMEN:—I believe that I owe the honor of being elected Professor of Anatomy and Surgery to the College, chiefly to my having been long engaged in the study of the pathological department of the Museum, while arranging and describing it, under the superintendence of Mr. Stanley, for the new catalogue. I may, therefore, fairly suppose it to be the wish of the Council that, as the Museum is open to the examination of the members and pupils of the College, and men of scientific pursuit, so should be the knowledge and conditions which it has supplied or suggested to those who have had occasion to study it most deeply. For, indeed, to what thus grows out of the study of the Museum, the College has, in some measure, the right which the proprietor has to the produce of the cultivated soil. And when, through a long time past, your most learned Hunterian Professor Owen has every year brought in, from every source, so large a store of deep and wide-extending knowledge, of sagacious interpretation, and acute suggestion of the ways of Nature, I scarcely wonder that some return should be looked for from an inferior laborer in the field.

The subjects on which I shall first beg your favorable hearing are those to the general illustration of which the first two series of preparations in the Pathological Museum are devoted—namely, hypertrophy and and atrophy; the simple excess, and the simple deficiency, of nutrition in parts. But let me previously speak of the healthy nutrition of the tissues, and, herein especially, of the formative process which maintains them by assimilation.

In the natural course of life, the formative process manifests itself in three modes, which, though they bear different names, and are sometimes described as if they were wholly different things, yet, probably, are only three expressions of one law, three effects of the same force operating in different conditions. The three, enumerating them in the order of their time, are development, growth, and assimilation or maintenance.

By development, we mean, generally, the process by which a tissue or organ is first formed; or by which one, as yet imperfectly formed, is so changed in shape or composition as to be fitted for a higher function, or, finally, is advanced to the state in which it exists in the most perfect condition of the species.

We must carefully distinguish development from mere increase: it is the acquiring, not of greater bulk, but of new forms and structures, which are adapted to higher conditions of existence. For example, when, in the embryo, groups of nucleated cells are changed into bundles of muscular fibrils, there is not, necessarily, an increase of size; or, if there be, there is something more; there is a change of texture, and an acquirement of power adapted to a higher state of existence: these constitute development. So, when, from the simple cavity and walls of the embryonic digestive system, the stomach, intestines, liver, pancreas, and other organs are produced, these are developed; there is increase, but, at the same time, something more than mere increase.

The distinction between development and increase, or growth, is well shown in this,—that, sometimes, even in instances in which they usually concur, the one proceeds without the other. I might quote many examples of this. I will choose two or three, which at the same time, may illustrate some other striking facts. Among the malformations in the Museum of St. Bartholomew's Hospital (Series A, 121 and 123), are the brains of two adult idiots. They are equally diminutive, and of nearly equal size: but in one, so far as we can see, there is a due proportion of the several parts; it is only too small: in the other, the parts are not well proportioned; the posterior parts of the cerebrum do not half cover the cerebellum; indeed, no posterior cerebral lobes appear to be formed. Herein we recognize something more than a checked growth; for this truncation of the cerebrum indicates an arrest of its development at the time when its hinder lobes—the parts last produced, and peculiarly characteristic of the human brain—were only just beginning to be formed. Our explanation of this most interesting specimen must be, that, when the brain had attained that degree of development which, according to Professor Retzius,* is proper to the human fœtus about the beginning of the fifth month, and corresponds with the completed development of the brain of lower mammalia, then its development ceased. But though in form it is like the fœtal brain in the fifth month, yet, in all its dimensions, it is larger; so that, although its development had ceased, its growth continued, and was not checked till the brain had

* Arch d'Anat. et de Physiol., Jan. 1846.

attained the size of that of a mature fœtus. In this brain, therefore, we find at once defective development and defective growth; but in the other the development proceeded, and the growth alone was checked.

Again, for examples in which development was checked and growth proceeded even beyond its normal limits, we may examine some of the numerous malformed hearts in the Museum. One among them presents only a single cavity; no partition has been developed between its auricles or its ventricles; it is, in respect of its development, like the heart of a fœtus in the second month : but, though its development was checked thus early, its growth continued, and it has more than the average size of the hearts of children of the same age. In another, development was arrested at a later period, when the septum of the ventricles was incompletely formed; the patient lived eleven years after birth; the development made no further progress, but the growth passed its ordinary bounds.

And, once more, for instances in which the development was normal and growth abnormal, you may examine such skeletons as those of O'Byrne, the giant, and of Mdlle. Cracimi, the dwarf, in the Physiological Museum. The one is eight feet high, the other is only twenty inches : but if you compare these with the model skeletons which stand beside them, you will not find in the one a defect, nor in the other an excess, of development; the dwarf has not less than all the characteristic human forms, the giant has no more; but the one is defective, the other is excessive, in its bulk; the growth alone has been erroneous in both.

It is, then, in the change to a higher state of form or composition, that development differs from growth, the second mode of the formative process. In mere growth, no change of form or composition occurs; parts only increase in weight, and usually, in size. In growth, there is an addition of quantity, but no improvement in the quality, of a part; the power of the growing part increases with the growth, but is only more of the same power ; so, in the attainment of manhood, the heart of the boy, having all its necessary parts, and all well-formed, acquires perfection by acquiring greater bulk, and, therewith, greater power.

Lastly, in the formative process, as it is normally manifested in the adult, i. e., in ordinary assimilation or maintenance, parts only preserve their *status*. No perceptible change of size or weight ensues, no change of form or composition; sameness is maintained through the regular formation of new parts in the place of those which, in the ordinary course of life, are impaired, or die.

Such are the methods of the formative process in the nutrition of organs. I shall have to show in future lectures, that some of the terms just used are, in a measure, conventional and arbitrary; that some instances of what we call development, e. g., that of cartilage into bone, are not in every sense justly so named; and that the sameness, which is maintained in the adult body, fades into a gradual degeneration. But, for the present, the terms that I have used may suffice. It is convenient, also, to think of the three methods of formation, as if each might be separately manifested; yet, probably, they are always concurrent; the maintenance of the whole organs being achieved only by the constant development and growth of new elemental structures in the place of those that are outworn.

Now, for the elucidation of this maintenance of parts by the constant mutation of their elemental structures, let me speak—

1st. Of the sources of impairment, or, if I may so say, of the wear and tear, to which every part of the body appears to be subject.

2dly. Of the conditions necessary for the healthy state of the process of nutrition by which the results of the wear and tear are repaired.

3dly. Of the formative process itself.

First, then, the deterioration of the body may be traced to two principal sources; namely, the wearing-out of parts by exercise, and the natural deterioration or death of the elemental structures of every part or organ, independent of the decay or death of the whole body, after a certain period of existence.

From the first of these, the wearing-out of parts by exercise, it is probable that no tissue or part enjoys immunity. For although, in all the passive apparatus of the body—the joints, bones, ligaments, elastic vessels, and the like—much of the beauty of their construction consists in the means applied to diminish the effects of the friction, and the various pressures and stretchings to which they are subject, yet, in enduring these at all, they must be impaired, and, in the course of years, must need renewal. Doubtless, however, the waste of these parts by exercise is much less than that of the more active organs, such as the muscles, and, perhaps, the nervous system. With regard to the muscles, it is clear that chemical decomposition and consumption of their substance attend their continued action. Such action is always followed by the increased discharge of urea, carbonic acid, and water. The researches of Helmoltz* show, that the muscles themselves, after long repeated contractions, are changed in chemical composition; and those of G. Liebig,† have detected and measured the formation of carbonic acid in them during similar contractions.

We have nearly similar evidence of the impairment of the nervous system by prolonged exertion of its power. We have, indeed, no proof that the simple conduction of an impression through a nervous cord can affect in any way its composition or its structure; but the abundance of phosphates occasionally discharged with the urine, after great mental exertion, shows that the various acts of the mind impair the brain through which they are manifested. To this point tend, also, the researches of

* Müller's Archiv. 1845, p. 72.
†Ibid. 1850, p. 393.

Dr. Bence Jones,* who has shown that the excretion by the kidneys of a large quantity of phosphate of salts is usual in acute inflammation of the brain. And to this conclusion, that mental exercise, whether perceptive or active, impairs the structure of the brain, we might be led by our sensations and by our knowledge of the nature of the mind. For to the principle, the immaterial thing, we cannot ascribe a weariness; it cannot be obnoxious to waste or to decay: mental fatigue is only what the Mind feels of an impaired state of the brain, and the recovery from what we call a weary mind is the restoration, not of the Mind itself, but of the organs which it feels, which connect it with the external world, and in which, during tranquil sleep, the reparative nutrition goes on undisturbed.

It is further probable that no part of the body is exempt from the second source of impairment; that, namely, which consists in the natural death or deterioration of the parts (independent of the death or decay of the whole body) after a certain period of their life. It may be proved, partly by demonstration, and partly by analogy, that each integral or elemental part of the body is formed for a certain natural period of existence in the ordinary condition of active life, at the end of which period, if not previously destroyed by outward force or exercise, it degenerates and is absorbed, or dies and is cast out; needing, in either case, to be replaced for the maintenance of health.†

The simplest examples that I can adduce of this are in the hair and teeth; and in the process which I shall describe, and illustrate with a diagram (on p. 22), we seem to have an image in which are plainly marked, though, as it were, in rough outline, all the great features of the process by which tissues are maintained.

An eyelash which naturally falls, or which can be drawn out without pain, is one that has lived its natural time, and has died, and been separated from the living parts. In its bulb such an one will be found very different from those that are still living in any period of their age. In the early period of the growth of a dark eyelash, we find its outer end almost uniformly dark, marked only with darker short linear streaks, and exhibiting no distinction of cortical and medullary substance. Not far from its end, however, this distinction is plainly marked; dark as the cortical part may be, the medullary appears like an interior cylinder of much darker granular substance: and in a young hair this condition is continued down to its deepest part, where it enlarges to form the bulb. (Fig. 1. A.) Now this enlargement, which is of nearly cup-like form, appears to depend on the accumulation of round and plump nucleated

* Med. Chir. Trans., vol. xxx., p. 20.

† Hunter (Works, vol. iii., p. 495), and Treviranus (Biologie, B. iii. 482), may be thought to have had some insight into this important law; but the merit of having first maintained in terms nearly similar to the above, and as more than an hypothesis, that "each part of the organism has an individual life of its own," and "a limited period of existence," belongs to Dr. Carpenter.—Principles of Human Physiology, 3d edit., p. 623.

cells, which, according to their position, are either, by narrowing and elongation, to form the dry fibro-cells of the outer part of the growing

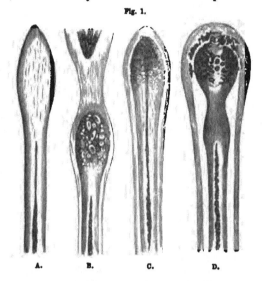

Fig. 1.

A.   B.   C.   D.

and further protruding shaft, or are to be transformed into the air-holding cells of the medullary portion. At this time of most active growth, both cells and nuclei contain abundant pigment-matter, and the whole bulb looks nearly black. The sources of the material out of which the cells form themselves are, at least, two; namely, the inner surface of the sheath or capsule, which dips into the skin, enveloping the hair, and the surface of the vascular pulp, which fits in a conical cavity in the bottom of the hair-bulb.

Such is the state of parts so long as the growing hair is all dark. But, as it approaches the end of its existence, it seems to give tokens of advancing age, by becoming gray. (Fig. 1, B, C.) Instead of the almost sudden enlargement at its bulb, the hair only swells a little, and then tapers nearly to a point; the conical cavity in its base is contracted, and hardly demonstrable, and the cells produced on the inner surface of the capsule contain no particle of pigment. Still for some time it continues thus to live, and grow, and we find that the vigor of the conical pulp lasts rather longer than that of the sheath or capsule; for it continues to produce pigment matter some time after the cortical substance of the hair has been entirely white, and it is still distinct, because of the pig-ment-cells covering its surface.

At length the pulp can be no longer discerned, and uncolored cells alone are produced, and maintain the latest growth of the hair. With these it appears to grow yet some further distance, for we see traces of their elongation into fibres or fibro-cells, in lines running from the inner surface of the capsule inwards and along the surface of the hair; and we can always observe that the dark column of medullary air-containing substance ceases at some distance above the lower end of the contracted hair-bulb. (C, D.)

The end of all is the complete closure of the conical cavity in which the hair-pulp was lodged; the cessation of the production of new cells; and the consequent detachment of the hair as a dead part, which now falls by the first accident; falls, sometimes, quite bare and smooth on the whole surface of its white bulb, but sometimes bringing with it a layer of cells detached from the inner surface of the capsule. (D.)

Such is the life of a hair, and such its death; which death, you see, is natural, spontaneous, independent of exercise, or of any mechanical external force, the natural termination of a certain period of life. Yet, before it dies, provision is made for its successor; for when its growth is failing, you often find, just below the base of the old hair, a dark spot, the germ or young pulp of the new one; it is covered with cells containing pigment, and often connected by a series of pigment-cells with the old pulp or capsule. (Fig. 1, c.) And this appears to be the product, as it were an offshoot, from some portion of the capsule of the old hair; for though it may sometimes appear only in the form of a conical pulp, yet more often, I think, it shows signs of connection with the capsule, and the cone is only more evident than the rest because of its covering of dark cells.*

I believe that we may assume in intimate analogy between the process of successive life and death, and life communicated to a successor, which is here shown, and that which is believed to maintain the ordinary nutrition of a part. It may be objected, indeed, that the death and casting out of the hair cannot be imitated in internal parts; but we are not without an example in which the absorption of a worn out internal particle is exactly imitated in larger organs, at the end of their appointed period of life. I adduce the instance of the deciduous or milk-teeth.

We trace each of these developed from its germ, and in the course of its own development, separating a portion of its capsule for the germ of its successor: then each, having gained its due perfection, retains for a time its perfect state, and still lives, though it does not grow. But at length, as the new tooth comes, the deciduous tooth dies, coincidently, not consequently; or rather, the crown of the old tooth dies, and is cast out like a dead hair; while its fang, with the bony sheathing, and the

---

* This account of the change of the hair is confirmed by the much more minute description of Kölliker (Mikrosk. Anatomie, B. ii., p. 141.) His observations were made chiefly in the young child, mine in the adult; but, doubtless, his account of the complete continuity of the sheath of the new hair with that of the old one, of the gradual extrusion of the old hair, and of most of the details of the process, might be added to what I have described.

vascular and nervous pulp, degenerate, and are absorbed. It is here especially to be observed, that the degeneration is accompanied by some spontaneous transformation of the fang; for it could not be absorbed unless it were first so changed as to be soluble. And it is degeneration, not death, which precedes its removal; for when a tooth-fang really dies as that of the second tooth does in old age, then it is not absorbed, but is cast out entire, as a dead part.

Such, or nearly such, it seems almost certain, is the process of nutrition everywhere: these may be taken as types of what occurs in other parts; for these are parts of complex organic structure and composition, and the teeth-pulps, which are absorbed as well as the fangs, are very vascular and sensitive, and therefore, we may be nearly sure, are conformed to only the same laws as prevail in all equally organized parts.

Nor are these the only instances that might be adduced. We see the like development, persistence for a time in the perfect state, death, and discharge, in all the varieties of cuticles, with which, also, we may connect the example of the gland cells; and in the epidermis we have, as in the teeth, an evidence of chemical change in the old cells, in the very different influence which acetic acid and potash exercise on them and on the younger cells, making these transparent, but leaving them scarcely changed.

These things, then, seem to show that the ordinary course of each elementary organ in the body, after the attainment of its perfect state by development and growth, is, to remain in that state for a time; then, independently of the death or decay of the whole body, and, at least in a great measure, independently of its own exercise or exposure to external violence, to die or to degenerate; and then, being cast out or absorbed, to make way for its successor.

It appears moreover very probable, that the length of life which each part is to enjoy is fixed and determinate, though of course in some degree, subject to accidents, which may shorten it, as sickness may prevent death through mere old age; and subject to the expenditure of life in the exercise of function. I do not mean that we can assign, as it is popularly supposed we can, the time that all our parts will last; nor is it likely that all parts are made to last an equal time, and then to be changed. The bones, for instance, when once completely formed, must last longer than the muscles and other softer tissues. But, when we see that the life of certain parts is of determined length, whether they be used or not, we may assume, from analogy, the same of nearly all.

For instance, the deciduous human teeth have an appointed duration of life: not, indeed, exactly the same in all persons, yet, on the whole, fixed and determinate. So have the deciduous teeth of other animals. And, in all those numerous instances of periodical moulting, of shedding of the antlers, of the entire desquamation of serpents, and of the change of plumage in birds, and of the hair in mammalia; what means all this, but that these organs live their severally appointed times, degenerate, die, are cast away, and in due time are replaced by others; which, in their turn, are to be developed to perfection, to live their life in the mature state, and to be cast off? We may discern the same laws of life in some elementary structures; for example, in the blood-corpuscles, of which a first set, formed from embryo-cells, disappear at a certain period in the life of the embryo, being replaced and superseded by a second set formed from lymph-corpuscles. And in these, also, we may see an example of the length of life of elemental parts being determined, in some measure, by their activity in function; for if the development of the tadpole be retarded, by keeping it in a cold, dark place, and if, in this condition, the function of the first set of blood-corpuscles be slowly and imperfectly discharged, they will remain unchanged for even many weeks longer than usual: their individual life will be thus prolonged, and the development of the corpuscles of the second set will be, for the same time postponed.*

The force of these facts is increased by the consideration of the exact analogy, the almost identity, of the processes of secretion and nutrition; for in no instance is the fact of this limited life of individual parts more clearly shown than in the gland-cells, by which periodical secretions are elaborated. The connecting link between such gland-cells and the most highly organized parts, as well as a manifest instance of determinate length of life and natural death, is found in the history of the ova. These attain their maturity in fixed successive periods of days: they are separated (as the materials of several secretions are) while yet living, and with a marvellous capacity of development, if only they be impregnated during the few days of life that remain to them after separation; but, if these days pass, and impregnation is not effected, they die, and are cast out, as impotent as the merest epithelial cell.

Now from these cases it is not by a far-fetched analogy that we assume the like mortality in all other tissues; and that this is the principal source of impairment, and of change for the worse, which every part of the body has within itself, even in the most perfect state, and in the conditions most favorable to life. And I may anticipate a future subject of consideration, by saying that the application of these truths is of some importance in practical pathology; inasmuch as the results of this degeneration of parts, at the close of their natural term of life, may be mingled with the effects of all the morbid processes by which the natural nutrition of a part is hindered or perverted. Hence, at least in part, the long-continuing or permanent loss of power in an organ (say a muscle) which has been disused, or has been the seat of inflammation. This loss is not wholly due to a primary disease of the fibre; in part, it is because the inflammatory process and the organization of the morbid exudation exclude the ordinary process of nutrition; and the muscular fibres, which

* See Kirkes's Physiology, pp. 65 and 290.

now, in the ordinary course of life, degenerate, are not replaced, or are imperfectly repaired.

Of the results of these natural and unrepaired degenerations of tissues I shall speak more hereafter. Let me now consider the conditions under which the repair of parts thus deteriorated is effected; for it is against the effects of these natural deteriorations that the process of nutrition in the adult is chiefly directed; and it appears to be by the disturbance or removal of certain necessary conditions, more often than by any suspension or perversion of itself, that error is engendered in the process of formation. And, in speaking of these conditions of healthy nutrition, I shall take leave occasionally to diverge, even very far, into the consideration of certain points of interest in the general physiology of the process.

Doubtless the conditions necessary to the normal nutrition of parts are very many: but the chief of them are these four:—

1. A right state and composition of the blood or other nutritive material.

2. A regular and not far distant supply of such blood.

3. (At least in most cases) a certain influence of the nervous system.

4. A natural state of the part to be maintained.

And, first, of the right state of the blood, I may observe that I use the expression "right state" rather than "purity," because, if the latter be used, it seems to imply that there is some standard of composition to which all blood might be referred, and the attainment of which is essential to health; whereas the truth seems rather to be, that, from birth onwards, the blood and tissues of each creature are adapted to one another, and to the necessary external circumstances of life, and that the maintenance of health depends on the maintenance and continual readjustment of the peculiarities on which this exact adaptation depends.

The necessity for this right or appropriate state of the blood, as a condition of healthy nutrition, involves of course the necessity for the due performance of the blood-making and blood-purifying functions; it requires healthy digestion, healthy respiration, healthy excretion. Any one of these being disturbed, the formative process in a part or in the whole body may be faulty, for want of the appropriate material. But, important as these are, we must not let the consideration of them lead us to forget that there is something in the blood itself, which is at least as essential to the continuance of its right and healthy state as these are, and which is, indeed, often occupied in correcting the errors to which these, more than itself, are subject; I mean the power of assimilation or maintenance which the blood possesses, in and for itself, as perfectly and at least as independently as any of the tissues. By this it is, that notwithstanding the diversity of materials put into the blood, and the diversity of conditions in which the functions ministering to its formation are discharged, yet the blood throughout life retains, in each person, certain characters as peculiar as those of his outer features for the continual renewal of which it provides appropriate materials.   And by this assimilative power of the blood is it that the tissues are continually guarded ; for by it many noxious substances introduced into the blood are changed and made harmless before they come to the tissues ; nor can any substance, introduced from without, produce disease in an organ, unless it be such an one as can escape the assimilative and excretory power of the blood itself.

In this maintenance is the chief manifestation of the life of the adult-blood ; a life, in all essential things, parallel and concurrent with that of the tissues.   For in the blood we may trace all those which we recognise as signs and parts of life in the solids : we watch its development, its growth, its maintenance by the assimilation of things unlike itself ; we find it constituting an adapted purposive part of the organism ; possessing organic structures ; capable of disease and of recovery ; prone to degeneration and to death.   In all these things, we have to study the life of the blood as we do that of the solid tissues ; the life, not only of the structures of the blood, but of its liquid also ; and as, in first development, the blood and tissues are made, of similar materials, in exact conformity with one another, so, through later life, the normal changes of each concur to maintain a like conformity and mutual adaptation.   I cannot now dwell on these points ;* but they will be frequently illustrated in the following lectures, and some of them at once, in what I have to say of the precision of adjustment in which the "right state" of the blood consists.

Notwithstanding its possession of the capacity of maintenance, the blood is subject to various diseases, in consequence of which the nutrition of one or more tissues is disordered.   The researches of modern chemistry have detected some of these changes; finding excesses or deficiencies of some of the chief constituents of the blood, and detecting in it some of the materials introduced from without.   But a far greater number of the morbid conditions of the blood consist in changes from the discovery of which the acutest chemistry seems yet far distant, and for the illustration and discussion of which we cannot adopt the facts, though we may adopt the language and the analogies, of chemistry.   It is in such diseases as these that we can best discern how nice is that refinement of mutual influence, how exact and constant that adaptation, between the blood and tissues, on which health depends.

I know no instance so well adapted to illustrate this as the examples of symmetrical diseases.   The uniform character of such diseases is, that a certain morbid change of structure on one side of the body is repeated in the exactly corresponding part on the other side.   In the lion's pelvis, for example, which is sketched in the annexed diagram from a specimen, (No. 3030,) in the College Museum, multiform as the

* They formed the subject of the course of Lectures delivered at the College in 1848, an abstract of a part of which is given by Dr. Kirkes in his "Handbook of Physiology," p. 64, ed. 2.

pattern is in which the new bone, the product of some disease comparable with a human rheumatism, is deposited—a pattern more complex
and irregular than the spots upon a map—there is not one spot or line
on one side which is not represented, as exactly as it would be in a mirror,
on the other. The likeness has more than Daguerreotype exactness, and
was observable in numerous pairs of the bones similarly diseased.

I need not describe many examples of such diseases. Any out-patients'
room will furnish abundant instances of exact symmetry in the eruptions
of eczema, lepra, and psoriasis; in the deformities of chronic rheumatism,
the paralyses from lead; in the eruptions excited by iodide of potassium
or copaiba. And any large museum will contain examples of equal
symmetry in syphilitic ulcerations of the skull; in rheumatic and syphilitic deposits on the tibiæ and other bones; in all the effects of chronic
rheumatic arthritis, whether in the bones, the ligaments, or the cartilages; in the fatty and earthy deposits in the coats of arteries.

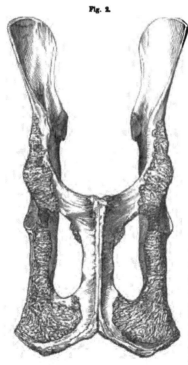

Fig. 1.

Now, these facts supply excellent evidence of the refinement of
the affinities which are concerned
in the formative process. Excluding, perhaps, the cases of congenital defects that are symmetrical, and a few which seem to
depend on morbid influence of the
nervous system, it may be stated,
generally, that all symmetrical
diseases depend on some morbid
material in the blood. You may
find the proof of this position in
papers written simultaneously by
Dr. William Budd and myself;*
and in Dr. Budd's essay you may
find it nearly demonstrated, by a
masterly discussion of the subject,
that, in most of these cases, the
morbid material enters into combination with the tissue which is
diseased, or with the organized
product of the morbid process.
Now the evident and applicable
truth in all these cases is, that the
morbid substance in the blood, be
it what it may, acts upon and
changes only certain portions of what we might suppose to be all the
very same tissue. Such a substance fastens on certain islands on the

† Medico-Chirurg. Trans. vol. xxv.

surfaces of two bones, or of two parts of the skin, and leaves the rest unscathed; and these islands are the exactly corresponding pieces upon opposite sides of the body. The conclusion is unavoidable, that these are the only two pieces that are exactly alike; that there was less affinity between the morbid material and the osseous tissue, or the skin, or the cartilage, close by; else, it also would have been similarly diseased. Manifestly, when two substances display different relations to a third, their composition cannot be identical; so that though we may speak of all bone or of all skin as if it were all alike, yet there are differences of intimate composition; and in all the body the only parts which are exactly like each other, in their mutual relation with the blood, are those which are symmetrically placed upon the opposite sides. No power of artificial chemistry can, indeed, detect the difference; but a morbid material can: it tests out the parts to which it has the greatest affinity, unites with these, and passes by the rest.*

I might magnify the wonder of this truth by showing how exceedingly small, in some of these cases, must be the quantity of the morbid material existing in the blood. But I prefer to illustrate a fact which singularly corroborates the evidence, afforded by symmetrical diseases, of the refinement of the operations of the affinities, if we may so call them, between the blood and the tissues. The fact is that of certain blood-diseases having "seats of election." For example, in another lion's pelvis, No. 3024, diseased like that sketched above, not only is the morbid product just as symmetrical, but its arrangement is exactly similar: hardly a spot appears on one pelvis which is not imitated on the.other. And these are only examples of a large class of cases of syphilis, rheumatism, and various skin-diseases, of which the general character is, that the disease is much more apt to affect one certain portion of a bone, or of the skin, or of some other tissue, than to attack any other portion. We are all in the habit of using the fact as an aid in diagnosis; but we may have overlooked its bearing on the physiology of nutrition. It proves, on the one hand, as the cases of symmetrical diseases do, that the composition of the several portions of what we call the same tissue is not absolutely identical: if it were, these diseases should affect one part of a bone or other tissue as often as another part, or should affect all parts alike.

* Some of the differences here noticed are not permanent, but may seem to depend on the several parts of a bone, or of the skin, of a limb (for example), being in different stages of development or degeneration. The symmetrical parts of the tissue, being exactly alike, may be simultaneously and equally affected by a disease, while other parts of the same remain unaffected, till, in the course of time, they attain, by development or degeneration, the very same condition as the parts first affected. Then, if the morbid material still exist in the blood, these parts also become diseased: and so in succession may nearly the whole of a tissue. This view agrees very well with the fact that symmetrical diseases often spread, and so prove that a part which, in one week or month, is not susceptible of the influence of a morbid material, may, in the next, become as susceptible as that which was first affected. This susceptibility, however, may be due not to normal changes, but to the influence which the diseased portion of the tissue exercises on those around it.

And it proves, on the other hand, a constant similarity, even an identity, of the morbid material on which each of these diseases depends, though it be produced in different individuals; so that we may venture to predict, that whenever chemistry shall discover the composition of these materials, it will be found as constant and as definite as the composition of those inorganic substances which the science has most successfully scrutinized.

Moreover, Dr. William Budd has proved that, next to the parts which are symmetrically placed, none are so nearly identical in composition as those which are homologous. For example, the backs of the hands and of the feet, or the palms and soles, are often not only symmetrically, but similarly, affected with psoriasis. So are the elbows and the knees; and similar portions of the thighs and the arms may be found affected with icthyosis. Sometimes, also, specimens of fatty and earthy deposits in the arteries occur, in which exact similarity is shown in the plan, though not in the degree, with which the disease affects severally the humeral and femoral, the radial and peroneal, the ulnar and posterior tibial, arteries.

To conclude, these symmetrical diseases with seats of election, prove—

1st. That in the same person the only parts of any tissue which are identical in composition are, or may be, first, those which occupy symmetrical positions on the opposite sides of the body; and next, those which are in serial homology.

2dly. That the portions of the bodies of different individuals which are identical, or most nearly so, in composition, are those in exactly corresponding positions..

3dly. That even in different individuals the specific morbid materials, on which many of the diseases of the blood depend, are of identical composition.

It would be foreign to my purpose to enter now upon all the subjects of interest which are illustrated by these cases. I may refer you again to the papers already mentioned, especially to Dr. Budd's. For the present it will be sufficient if I have proved (without pretending to explain or describe) the perfect and most minute exactness of the adaptation which, in health, exists between the blood and all the tissues; and that certain inconceivably slight disturbances of this adaptation may be sources of disease. If this be proved, I shall not fear to be met with an objection against too great refinement in what I shall next say concerning some of the means by which that right state of the blood, which is appropriate to the healthy nutrition of all the parts, is attained and preserved.

LECTURE II.

THE CONDITIONS NECESSARY TO HEALTHY NUTRITION.

I NEED not dwell on the physiology of the processes of digestion, absorption, excretion, and others, which, on the large scale, serve in the development and maintenance of the blood. The admitted doctrines concerning these I must assume to be well known, while I proceed with the consideration of those minuter relations, in which the blood and the several tissues exercise their mutual influence, and by which each is maintained in its right state. And first, let me endeavor to develop a principle, the germ of which is in the writings of Treviranus. His sentence is, that "each single part of the body, in respect of its nutrition, stands to the whole body in the relation of an excreted substance."* In other words, every part of the body, by taking from the blood the peculiar substances which it needs for its own putrition, does thereby act as an excretory organ, inasmuch as it removes from the blood that which, if retained in it, would be injurious to the nutrition of the rest of the body. Thus, he says, the polypiferous zoophytes all excrete large quantities of calcareous and siliceous earths. In those which have no stony skeleton these earths are absolutely and utterly excreted; but in those in which they form the skeleton, they are, though retained within the body, yet as truly excreted from the nutritive fluid and all the other parts, as if they had been thrown out and washed away. So the phosphates which are deposited in our bones are as effectually excreted from the blood and the other tissues, as those which are discharged with the urine.

But Trevirance seems not to have apprehended the full importance of the principle which he thus clearly, though so briefly stated; for it admits, I think, of far extension and very interesting application.

Its influence may be considered in a large class of outgrowing tissues. The hair, for example, in its constant growth, serves, not only local purposes, but for the advantage of the whole body, in that, as it grows, it removes from the blood the various constituents of its substance, which are thus excreted from the body. And this excretion office appears, in some instances, to be the only one by which the hair serves the purpose of the individual; as, for example, in the foetus. Thus, in the

* Die Erschein, und Gesetze des organischen Lebens, B. I, p. 401.

foetus of the seals that take the water as soon as they are born, and, I believe, in many of those other mammals, though they are removed from all those conditions against which hair protects, yet a perfect coat of hair is formed within the uterus, and before, or very shortly after birth, this is shed, and is replaced by another coat of wholly different color, the growth of which began with the uterus. Surely, in these cases, it is only as an excretion, or chiefly as such, that this first growth of hair serves to the advantage of the individual. The *lanugo* of the human foetus is an homologous production, and must, I think, similarly serve in the economy by removing from the blood, as so much excreted matter, the materials of which it is composed.

Further, I think, we may carry this principle to the apprehension of the true import of the hair which exists, in a kind of rudimental state, on the general surface of our bodies, and to that of many other permanently rudimental organs, such as the mammary glands of the male, and others. For these rudimental organs certainly do not serve, in a lower degree, the same purposes as are served by the homologous parts which are completely developed in other species, or in the other sex. To say they are useless, is contrary to all we know of the absolute perfection and all-pervading purpose of creation ; to say they exist merely for the sake of conformity with a general type of structure, seems unphilosophical, while the law of the unity of organic types is, in larger instances, not observed, except when its observance contributes to the advantage of the individual. Rather, all these rudimental organs must, as they grow, be as excretions, serving a definite purpose in the economy by removing their appropriate materials from the blood, and leaving it fitter for the nutrition of other parts, or by adjusting the balance which might else be disturbed by the formation of some other part. Thus they minister to the self-interest of the individual, while, as if for the sake of wonder, beauty, and perfect order, they are conformed with the great law of the unity of organic types, and concur with the universal plan observed in the construction of organic beings.

And again,—the principle that each organ, while it nourishes itself, serves the purpose of an excretion, has an application of peculiar interest in the history of development. For if it be influential when all the organs are already formed, and are only growing or maintaining themselves, much more will it be so when the several organs are successively forming. At this time, as each nascent organ takes from the nutritive material its appropriate constituents, it will co-operate with the gradual self-development of the blood, to induce in it that condition which is essential, or most favorable, to the formation of the organs next in order to be developed.

The importance of this principle will the more appear, if we connect with it another, equally characteristic of the minuteness of the relation between the blood and the tissues, namely, that the existence of certain materials in the blood may determine the formation of structures in which they may be incorporated.

This seems to be established, as a general law in pathology, by the cases in which diseased structures evidently incorporate materials that had their origin or previous existence in the blood. Such are most of those inoculable and other blood diseases in which morbid organisms are produced; as vaccina, variola, chancre, glanders, &c. The same law may be made very probable in physiology also. For example, when one kidney is destroyed, the other often becomes much larger, does double work, as it is said; and the patient does not suffer from the retention of urine in the blood: the full meaning of which (a well known fact, and not without parallel) may be thus expressed :—The principal constituents of the urine are, we know, ready formed in the blood, and are separated through the kidneys by the development, growth, and discharge of the renal cells in which they are, for a time, incorporated. Now, when one kidney is destroyed, there must for a time be an excess of the constituents of urine in the blood; for since the separation of urine is not mere filtration, the other kidney cannot at once, and without change of size, discharge a double quantity. What, then, happens? The kidney grows; more renal cells develop, and discharge, and renew themselves; in other words, the existence of the constituents of the urine in the blood that is carried to every part determines the formation of the appropriate renal organs in the one appropriate part of the body.

An analogous fact is furnished by the increased formation of adipose tissues in consequence of the existence of abundant hydro-carbon principles in the blood. Another, bearing on the same point, though not admitting of definite description, is the influence exercised by various diets in favoring the especial growth of certain tissues; as the muscles, the bones, the hair, or the wool. Similar facts are yet more evident in the cultivation of vegetables, to which various materials are supplied, in the assurance that certain corresponding tissues will be consequently formed. And an evident illustration of the same principle is in the abundant formation of fruit on a branch in which the matured sap has been made to accumulate by *ringing*.

I add again, on this point, as on a former one, that the case as concerning nutrition is remarkably corroborated by the observation of similar facts in instances of secretions. Thus, the excesses of albuminous materials taken in food, if they be not incorporated in the more highly organised tissues, are excreted; that is, they, or the materials into which they are transformed, enter into the construction of the transient tissue of the kidney or some excretory organ. The constituents of food, plainly as they influence the quantity and quality of milk, do so only by affecting, after their admission into the blood, the formation of the transient parts of the mammary gland-tissue. Medicines, such as diuretics, that are

3

separated from the body by only certain organs, are, for a time, we must believe, incorporated in the tissues of those organs.

These facts seem enough to make highly probable the principle I mentioned—namely, that the existence of certain materials in the blood may determine the formation of structures into the composition of which those materials may enter. At any rate we make it nearly certain for the more lowly organized tissues, and for the products of disease; and hence, by analogy, we may assume it for the other tissues. Even for the very highest, we may safely hold that a necessary condition of their formation is this previous existence of the peculiarly appropriate materials in the blood.

Now, if we combine these two principles—first, that the blood is definitely altered by the abstraction of every material necessary for the nutrition of a part, and secondly, that the existence of certain materials in the blood induces the formation of corresponding tissues, we may derive from them some very probable conclusions bearing on the questions before us. First, we may conclude that the order in which the several organs of the body appear in the course of development, while it is conformable with the law of imitation of the parent, and with the law of progressive ascent towards the higher grade of being, is yet in part, and in this more directly, the result of necessary and successive consequences: the formation of one organ, or series of organs, inducing, or supplying a necessary condition for, the formation of others, by the changes successively produced in the composition of the blood or other nutritive material. In other words, we may hold, in accordance with these principles, that the development of each organ or system, co-operating with the self-development of the blood, prepares it for the formation of some other organ or system; till, by the successive changes thus produced, and by its own development and increase, the blood is fitted for the maintenance and nutrition of the completed organism.

Secondly, I think that these principles may be applied to individual instances. They may suggest that certain organs stand, in their nutrition, in a complemental relation to each other; so that neither of them can be duly formed, or maintained in healthy structure, unless the right condition of the blood be induced and preserved by the formation of the other.

It is, of course, very difficult, or even impossible, to find instances by which this theory of complemental nutrition can be proved; while, really, we neither know exactly what materials are necessary for the formation of any organ, nor have the means of detecting the presence of more than a very few of them in the blood. It is very well for the discussion of certain parts of physiology to say, for instance, that a muscle mainly consists of a material like fibrin; but when we are considering the physiology of the formation of organs, we must remember that in every muscular fibre there are at least three different compounds—those of the sarcolemma, of the nucleus, and of the fibril; that these are all equally essential to the formation of the fibre; and that we know not the composition of any one of them, nor could detect the absence of any one of them from the blood, though the result of that absence might be to render the formation of a muscular fibre impossible.

But, though it may lack direct evidence, the theory seems, in itself, probable; and there are many facts which we can explain by it so well, that they become evidence for it:—which facts, moreover, are fair subjects for theoretical explanation, since, I believe, they are admitted to be as yet wholly unexplained.

Among these is the general fact that a great change in nutrition rarely takes place in one organ at a time, but usually affects simultaneously two or more parts, between whose nutrition there is a manifest and constant connection, although there is little or no relation between their external functions. Such, to take an instance from a large class, is the connection between the growth of various appendages of the integuments, and the development or maintenance of the genital organs. This appears to be a general rule. The growth of the beard at the period of puberty in man, with which we are so familiar, is more instructively represented in many animals: especially in birds. In these, as you know, at the approach of every breeding time, the genital organs begin to develop themselves for the season, as in man they do for the whole time of vigorous life. And, commensurately with this development, the plumage (especially in the male bird) becomes brighter and more deeply colored, both by the growth of new feathers, and by the addition of color to the old ones. The height and perfection of the plumage are coincident with the full development and activity of the reproductive organs; but as in man, when the development of the genital organs is prevented, the development of the beard and all the other external sexual characters, is, as a consequence, hindered, so, in the birds, when the breeding season ends, and the sexual organs pass gradually into their periodic atrophy, at once the plumage begins to assume the paler and more sober colors which characterize the barrenness of winter.

So it is, also, at least in certain instances, in the mammalia, of which we have interesting evidence in the history of specimens presented to the museum of the College by Sir Philip Egerton. These show that if a buck be castrated while his antlers are growing and still covered with the velt, their growth is checked, they remain as if truncated, and irregular nodules of bone project from their surfaces. Or, if the castration be performed when the antlers are full-grown, these, contrary to what Redi said, are shed nearly as usual, at the end of the season; but in the next season, only a kind of low conical stumps are formed in the place of antlers.*

* This formation of imperfect antlers may depend on the accessory organs of reproduction being developed; for these would not necessarily fail to be developed because the testicles

I need not multiply examples: it is a general fact, that the development and activity of the reproductive organs have, as a consequence, or as a necessary coincidence, a peculiar development and active growth or nutrition of certain other structures; which structures, therefore, form the external sexual characters, though their external functions stand in no apparent, often in no conceivable, connection with the generation of the species. The fact is not hitherto explained; it is explicable on the theory of complemental nutrition, by believing that the materials which, in the formation of these organs of external sexual character, are removed from the blood, leave or maintain the blood in the state necessary for the further development, growth, and active function of the proper sexual or reproductive organs. In other words, I would say, that where two or more organs are thus manifestly connected in nutrition, and not connected in the exercise of any external office, their connection is because each of them is partly formed of materials left in the blood on the formation of the other; and each, at the same time that it discharges its own proper and external office, maintains the blood in the condition most favorable to the formation of the other.

If this theory be admissible, we may find through it the meaning of the commensurate development and nutrition of many other organs, which in their external functions appear unconnected. Such are the concurrent development and activity of the thymus gland and the air-breathing organs, during the body's growth; of the thyroid gland and the brain (instances of commensurate development cited by Mr. Simon);* of the spleen and pancreas (as pointed out by Professor Owen); and, I would add, of the embryo and the mammary gland; for the same theory may hold true concerning the formation of certain organs which are, finally, connected in their external functions.

In these, and other like cases, I think it will be hereafter proved that the several organs are, in their nutrition, complemental; that the formation of each leads to the production of some material necessary for the construction of the other; and that, as we may be sure of Treviranus' law, in general—that each organ of the body, while it nourishes itself, is in the character of an excretion towards all the rest,—so, we may believe, more particularly, that certain organs are, mutually, as excretions from each other.

But, thirdly, if there be any probability in the principles I have endeavored to illustrate, they must deserve careful consideration in the pathology of the blood. I shall have to illustrate them in this view in future lectures. At present I will only suggest, that if each part, in its normal nutrition, is as an excreting organ to the rest, then the cessation or per-

---

were extirpated. And that the difference caused by castration is not due to the disturbance of nervous sympathies, is proved by the absence of any similar effect when the testes arc only transplanted. See Berthold in Müller's Archiv., 1849, p. 42.

* Essay on the Thymus Gland; and Philosophical Transactions, 1844, Part 2.

version of nutrition in one must, by no vague sympathy, but through definite change in the condition of the blood, affect the nutrition of the rest, and be thus the source of "constitutional disturbance." If, in health, there be such a thing as complemental nutrition, it must, in disease, be the source of many sympathies in nutrition between parts which are not specially connected through the nervous system. If the condition of the blood can, in favorable circumstances, determine the formation of organisms incorporating its materials, we may study the characteristic structures of specific diseases as the evidences of corresponding conditions of the blood, and as organs which, by removing specific materials from the blood, affect its whole constitution, and either restore its health, or produce in it secondary morbid changes.

The extent of application that these principles admit of will, I trust, justify the distance to which I may seem to have diverged from my starting-point. Let me now return to it, and remind you that this long discussion grew out of the consideration of the first condition necessary for healthy nutrition,—namely, the right state of the blood; a state not to be described merely as purity, but as one of exact adaptation to the peculiar structure and composition of the individual: an adaptation so exact that it may be disturbed by the imperfect nutrition of a single organ, and that for the maintenance of it, against all the disturbing forces of the outer life of the body, nothing can suffice except continual readjustment by the assimilative power of the blood itself.

The second condition of which I spoke as essential to the healthy process of nutrition, is—

A regular supply of appropriate blood in or near the part to be nourished.

The proofs of the necessity of this condition must be familiar to all. Instances will at once occur to your minds, in which too little blood being sent to a part, it has suffered atrophy: others, in which the supply being wholly cut off, mortification has ensued: others, in which the blood being stagnant in a part, has not efficiently contributed to its nutrition.

If I can give interest to this part of the subject at all, it is only by adducing interesting examples of the fact. Reserving for future lectures the examples of merely diminished and of perverted nutrition, I will mention now only some of the specimens in the Museums I have chiefly studied, which illustrate how the process of nutrition is wholly stopped by the absence or deficiency of fresh blood.

One of Mr. Swan's donations to the College Museum (No. 1821), is the larynx of a man who, while in low health, cut his throat, and suffered so great a loss of blood that the nutrition became impossible in one of those parts to which blood is most difficultly sent; and before he died, his nose sloughed.

The case is like one which, you may remember, is recorded by Sir

Benjamin Brodie.* A medical man wished to be bled, in a fit of exceeding drunkenness; and some one bled him,—bled him to three pints. He became very ill, and next day both his feet were mortified, from the extremities of the toes to the instep.

A specimen (No. 141), presented by Mr. Guthrie, exhibits a mortified, *i. e.*, a completely unnourished leg, from a case in which the femoral artery was obliterated near the groin through disease of its coats. The leg was amputated by Mr. Guthrie with justifying success; for the stump, though cut at some distance below the obliteration of the artery, did not slough; the collateral circulation was sufficient for its nutrition; and the patient, an elderly lady, died only of exhaustion.

For a similar, and very rare, example of sloughing after the obliteration of a main artery, I may refer to the case, described by Mr. Vincent, of a large slough in the very substance of one of the hemispheres of the cerebrum, in consequence of a wound of the supplying common carotid, —a wound made by a tobacco-pipe thrust into the bifurcation of the carotid, and nearly closing its channel.†

A specimen in the Museum of St. Bartholomew's Hospital (Series i. 134) exhibits an instance of dry gangrene occurring in very unusual circumstances. A woman, 48 years old, died, under the care of Mr. Earle, having received some injury of the femur eighteen months before death. Whether it were a fracture, or, indeed, what it was, cannot now be said; but the injury was followed by enlargement of that portion of the wall of the femur with which the artery and vein are nearly in contact, as they pass in the sheath of the triceps adductor muscle. At this part, then, the vein is compressed, and the artery, though not distinctly compressed, appears to have been hindered from enlarging. The consequence was dry gangrene of the leg, which slowly destroyed life, and which had no other apparent cause than this.

And, lastly, let me refer to two specimens, which are as interesting in the history of surgery as in pathology. One is a tibia and fibula, the lower ends of which, together with the whole foot, perished in consequence of the obstruction of the circulation by an aneurism in the ham. It is a Hunterian specimen in the College Museum (No. 710); and surely we may imagine that sometimes Mr. Hunter would contemplate it with pride, to think how rare such things would be in after times; for here is a strong contrast: the limb of a man who once had an aneurism, like the one which in the former case was so destructive, and on whom Hunter was permitted to confer fifty years of healthy life by his operation of tying the artery at a distance from the diseased part. The Museum of St. Bartholomew's owes this rare specimen and most interessing relic to the zeal of my colleague, Mr. Wormald. The patient was the fourth on whom Mr. Hunter performed his operation. He was 36 years old at the

---

* Lectures on Pathology and Surgery, p. 350.

† Medico-Chirurgical Transactions, vol. xxix., p. 38.

time; and though the tumor was not large, yet the whole leg was swollen, the veins were turgid, and he was exhausted, and in such bad health, that the case seemed desperate; but he recovered, and lived, as I have said, fifty years. The artery was tied in the sheath of the triceps muscle; and in this operation, for the first time, Mr. Hunter did not include the vein in the ligature. He thus diminished exceedingly the danger of the defective supply of arterial blood. The preparation shows the whole length of the artery obliterated from the origin of the profunda, to that of the anterior tibial, and the aneurismal sac, even after fifty years, not yet removed, but remaining as a hard mass like an olive.*

Now, the supply of appropriate blood, of which these specimens prove the necessity, must be in or near the part to be nourished. We cannot exactly say how near it must be, but, probably, all that is necessary is, that the nutritive material should admit of being imbibed in sufficient quantity into the substance of the part. For imbibition must be regarded as the means by which all parts supply themselves with nutritive matter: thus deriving it from the nearest blood-vessels, and the blood-vessels themselves being only the channels by which the materials are brought near. The blood-vessels thus serve alike for the nutrition of the vascular, and, as we call them, the non-vascular, parts, the difference between which parts, in this regard, is really very little. For the vascular, the nutritive food is carried in streams into their interior; for the other it flows on one surface: but in both alike, the parts to be nourished have to imbibe the nutritive fluid; and though the passage through the walls of the blood-vessels may effect some unknown change in the materials, yet all the business of formation is, in both alike, outside the vessels. Thus, in muscular tissue, the fibrils in the very centre of the fibre nourish themselves; yet these are distant from all blood-vessels, and can only by imbibition receive their nutriment. So, in bones, the spaces between the blood-vessels are wider than in muscle; yet the parts in the spaces nourish themselves, imbibing materials from the nearest source. And the non-vascular epidermis, though no vessels pass into its substance, similarly imbibes nutritive matter from those of the immediately subjacent cutis, and maintains itself, and grows. The instances of the cornea, the vitreous humor, and the peripheral part of the umbilical cord, are stronger, yet similar.

There is, therefore, no real difference as to the mode in which these tissues obtain their nutriment: and, sometimes, even the same tissue is in one case vascular, in the other not; as the osseous tissue, which, usually, when it is in masses or thick layers, has blood-vessels running into it; but when it is in thin layers, as in the lachrymal and turbinated bones, has not. These thin bones subsist on materials from the blood

---

* The preparation is in Ser. 13, Sub-Ser. F. No. 4. The case is in the "Transactions of a Society for the Improvement of Medical and Surgical Knowledge," vol. i., p. 138; and in Hunter's Works, vol. iii., p. 604.

flowing in the minute vessels of the mucous membrane, from which, on the same plan, the epithelium derives nutriment on one side, the bone on the other, and the tissue of the membrane itself on every side.

It is worth while to remember this, else we cannot understand how the non-vascular tissues, such as the cornea, the hair, the articular cartilages, and the various cuticles, should be liable to diseases proper to themselves, primarily and independently. And, except by thus considering the subject, we shall not be clear of the error and confusion which result from speaking of the "action of vessels;" as if the vessels really made and unmade the parts. We have no knowledge of the vessels as anything but carriers of the materials of nutrition to and fro. These materials may, indeed, undergo some change as they pass through the vessels' walls; but that change is not an assuming of definite shape; the vessels only convey and emit the "raw material;" it is made up in the parts, and in each after its proper fashion. The real process of formation of tissues is altogether extra-vascular, even, sometimes, very far extra-vascular; and its issue depends in all cases chiefly, and in some entirely, on the affinities (if we may so call them) between the part to be nourished and the nutritive fluid.

The third condition essential to the healthy nutrition of parts, is a certain influence of the nervous system. It may be held, I think, that, in the higher vertebrata, some nervous force is habitually exercised in the nutrition of all the parts in or near which nerves are distributed; and that it is exercised not merely in affecting or regulating the size of the blood-vessels of the part, but, with a more direct agency, as being one of the forces that concur in the formative process.

Of late years, a current of opinion has run against the belief of this; and, of those who admit some influence of the nervous system upon the nutrition of parts, many do it, as it were, grudgingly and doubtfully. They hold that at most the influence is exercised only indirectly, through the power which the nervous system has of affecting the size of the blood-vessels; or that the nervous system influences only the degree, without affecting at all the mode of nutrition in a part.

One chief argument against the belief that the nervous force has a direct and habitual influence in the nutritive processes is, that in plants and the early embryo, and in the lowest animals in which no nervous system is developed, all nutrition goes on well without it. But this is no proof that in animals which have a nervous system, nutrition is independent of it; rather, even if we had no positive evidence, we might assume that in ascending development, as one system after another is added or increased, so the highest, and, highest of all, the nervous system, would be inserted and blended in a more and more intimate relation with all the rest. This would, indeed, be only according to the general law, that the interdependence of parts augments with their development: for high organisation consists not in mere multiplication or diversity of independent parts, but in the intimate combination of many parts in mutual maintenance.

Another argument implies that the nervous force can manifest itself in nothing but impressions on the mind, and muscular contraction-force. So limited a view of the convertibility of nervous force, is such an one as the older electricians would have held, had they maintained that the only possible manifestations of electricity were the attractions and repulsions of light bodies, or that the electric force could never be made to appear in the form of magnetism, of chemical action, or of heat. We are too much shackled with these narrow dogmas of negation. The evidence of the correlation and mutual convertibility of the physical forces might lead us to anticipate a like variety of modes of manifestations for the nervous and other forces exercised in the living body.* We might anticipate, too, that, as the nervous force has its origin in the acts of nutrition by which the nerve substance is formed, so, by reciprocal action, its exercise might affect the nutritive parts. As (for illustration sake) the completed blood affects all the processes by which itself was formed, so, we might suppose, would the nervous force be able to affect all the acts of which itself is the highest product.

But we need not be content with these probable deductions concerning the direct influence of the nervous force on the nutritive process. The facts bearing on the question seem sufficient for the proof.

A first class of them are such as show the influence of the mind upon nutrition. Various conditions of the mind, acting through the nervous system, and by nervous force, variously affect the formative processes in the whole body. There is scarcely an organ of nutrition of which may not be thus effected by the mind. It is hardly necessary to adduce examples of a fact so often illustrated; yet I may mention this one:—Mr. Lawrence removed, several years ago, a fatty tumor from a woman's shoulder; and, when all was healed, she took it into her head that it was a cancer, and would return. Accordingly, when by accident I saw her some months afterwards, she was in a workhouse, and had a large and firm painful tumor in her breast, which, I believe, would have been removed, but that its nature was obscure, and her general health was not good. Again, some months afterwards, she became my patient at the Finsbury Dispensary: her health was much improved, but the hard lump in her breast existed still, as large as an egg, and just like a portion of indurated mammary gland. Having heard all the account of it, and how her mind constantly dwelt in fear of cancer, I made bold to assure her, by all that was certain, that the cancer, as she supposed it, would go away: and it did become very much smaller without any help from medicine. As it had come under the influence of fear, so it very nearly

* See Carpenter on the Mutual Relation of the Vital and the Physical Forces, Phil. Trans., 1850, and General Physiology, p. 34.

disappeared under that of confidence.   But I lost sight of her before the removal of the tumor was complete.

The other classes of cases are those in which the influence of the nervous system alone, independent of the Mind, is shown.   Of course, such cases can only be drawn from those of abstraction or perversion of the nervous influence ; and the effects of these are most plainly expressed in the nutrition of parts exposed to external agencies, as the integuments generally, the extremities, and other external parts; but we may fully believe, that what is observed in these, occurs also, in corresponding measure, in more deeply-seated parts.

Now, for the result of the abstraction or diminution of nervous force, I cite the following from among many similar facts :—In the Museum of St. Bertholomew's (Ser. 9, No. 9) is an example of central penetrating ulceration of the cornea, in consequence of destruction of the trunk of the trigeminal nerve, by the pressure of a tumor near the pons.*   The whole nutrition of the corresponding side of the face was impaired ; the patient had repeated attacks of erysipelatous inflammation, bleeding from the nose, and, at length, destructive inflammation of the tunics of the eye, and this ulceration of the cornea.

In the College museum (No. 2177) is the hand of a man, whose case is related by Mr. Swan, the donor of the preparation.   The median nerve, where it passes under the annular ligament, is enlarged, with adhesion to all the adjacent tissues, and induration of both it and them.   A cord had been drawn very tight round this man's wrist seven years before the amputation of the arm.   At this time, it is probable, the median and other nerves suffered injury ; for he had constant pain in the hand after the accident, impairment of the touch, contraction of the fingers, (and which bears most on the present question,) constantly repeated ulcerations at the back of the hand.

Mr. Hilton has told me this case :—A man was at Guy's Hospital, who, in consequence of a fracture of the lower end of the radius, repaired by an excessive quantity of new bone, suffered compression of the median nerve.   He had ulceration of the thumb and fore and middle fingers, which resisted various treatment, and was cured only by so binding the wrist that, the parts on the palmar aspect being relaxed, the pressure on the nerve was removed.   So long as this was done, the ulcers became and remained well ; but as soon as the man was allowed to use his hand, the pressure on the nerves was renewed, and the ulceration of the parts supplied by them returned.

Mr. Travers† mentions a case in which a man had paraplegia after fracture of the lumbar vertebræ.   He fractured at the same time his humerus and his tibia.   The former, in due time, united: the latter did not.

* The case is related by Mr. Stanley in the Medical Gazette, vol. i. 531.
† Further Inquiry concerning Constitutional Irritation, p. 436.

Mr. De Morgan* has related a similar case. A man fractured his twelfth dorsal vertebra, and crushed the cord; dislocated his left humerus, and fractured fourteen ribs and his left ankle. He lived eighteen days, during which the reparative process was active at the injuries above the damage of the cord, but seemed to be wholly wanting at those below it.

Sir B. C. Brodie mentions having seen mortification of the ankle begin within twenty-four hours after an injury of the spine.†

It would be easy to multiply facts of this kind, without adducing instances of experiments on lower animals, which, though they be corroborative, cannot be fairly applied here. I will only refer in general to the numerous recorded examples of the little power which paralyzed parts have of resisting the influence of heat; of the sloughing after injury of the spinal cord; of the slower repair and reproduction of parts whose nerves are paralyzed or divided; all which facts alike contribute to prove, that the integrity of the nervous centres and trunks which are in anatomical relation with a part, is essential to its due nutrition, or, to its capacity of maintaining itself against the influence of external forces, which capacity is itself an expression of the formative power.

Lastly, for cases illustrating the effects produced in nutrition by disturbances of the nervous force, I must refer to the Lectures on Inflammation. At present, I can only allude to the cases of inflammation of the conjunctiva excited by stimulus of the retina; or inflammation of the testicle in consequence of mechanical irritation of the urethra; of the vascular congestion which is instantly produced around a killed or intensely irritated part, or in and around a part in which paroxysms of neuralgia are felt; of the inflammations whose range seems to be determined by the course or distribution of nerves, as in Herpes Zona. In all these cases, I know no explanation for the disturbance of nutrition, except that it is the consequence of the nervous force in the part being directly, or by reflection disturbed.

The value of all these facts is strengthened by the consideration of the manifold and distinct influences of the nervous force upon secretion; for the process of secretion is so essentially similar to that of nutrition, that whatever can be proved of the method of one might be inferred for that of the other. And I think the proof of the direct influence of the nervous force upon the formative process would be thus beyond question, if it were not for the inconstancy of the results of injury of the spinal cord and nerves. Even in the warm-blooded animals the division of the cord does not always retard the healing of injuries in the paralyzed limbs; sometimes it scarcely affects any part of their nutrition; and even in man, healing may be effected in paralyzed limbs after injuries, though they be produced by such trivial causes as would not have dis-

* London Medical and Surgical Journal, January 4th, 1834.
† Lectures on Pathology and Surgery, p. 309.

turbed the nutrition of sound limbs. I remember a man with nearly complete paraplegia and distorted feet, the consequence of injuries of the spine, in whom some tendons were subcutaneously divided, and appeared to be healing; but a bandage being applied rather tightly, sloughing ensued at the insteps, on which the chief pressure fell, and extended widely and deeply to the ankle joints. Both the dorsal arteries were laid open when the sloughs separated, and both the ankle joints, and the case presented a most striking example of the defective self-maintenance of paralyzed parts. But granulations formed after the separation of the sloughs, and the healing process went on slowly, but uninterruptedly, till all was covered in with a well-formed scar. In another case, a girl, with softening of the brain, had sloughs on nearly every part of the body that was subject to even slight pressure: for instance, on the back of her head resting on the pillow, on her elbows and heels; and yet, while several of these sloughs were extending with fearful rapidity, an ulcer, which had remained after the separation of a slough over the patella, healed perfectly.

Such cases as these seem incongruous in their several parts, and irreconcilable with the general rules which I previously illustrated: I cannot attempt to explain them; but neither can I think that they materially invalidate the rule.

Let me add, further, that no tissue seems to be wholly exempt from the influence of the nervous force on its nutrition. In the cuticle it is manifest; and, for its influence in acting even through a considerable distance, I may mention a case, which is also in near relation to those in which the hair grows quickly gray in mental anguish. A lady, who is subject to attacks of what are called nervous headaches, always finds in the morning after such an one, that some patches of her hair are white, as if powdered with starch. The change is effected in a night, and in a few days after, the hairs gradually regain their dark brownish color.

If, now, we may hold this influence of the nervous system to be proved, we may consider the question,—through what class of nerves is the nutritive process influenced?

Indirectly, it is certain that the motor or centrifugal nerves may influence it; for when these are paralyzed, the muscles they supply will be inactive, and atrophy will ensue, first, in these muscles: then, in the bones (if a limb be the seat of the paralysis), for the bones, in their nutrition, observe the example of their muscles: and, finally, the want of energy in the circulation, which is in some measure dependent on muscular action, will bring about the atrophy of the other tissues of the part. Hence, after a time, the evidences of paralysis of the facial nerve may be observed in nearly all the tissues of the face.

But the effects of destruction of the trigeminal nerve, while the motor nerves of the parts which it supplies are unimpaired, prove that a more direct influence is exercised through sensitive or sympathetic nerves.

The olfactory, optic, third, fourth, sixth, and facial nerves, may be one and all destroyed, yet no disturbance of the nutrition of the nose or eye may ensue. After destruction of the facial, indeed, there may be inflammation of the eye from irritants, which the paralyzed orbicularis palbebrarum cannot shut out or help to remove ; but neither this nor any other injury of these nerves is comparable with the consequences of the destruction of the trigeminal : consequences which in the rabbit are manifest, and may be very grave, within a day of the destruction of the nerve, and may be completely destructive of the eye within three days.

In many of these cases it is difficult to say whether the influence on nutrition is exercised through sensitive nerve fibres of the cerebro-spinal system, or through sympathetic (ganglionic) nerve-fibres; and I think it is probable that it may be exercised through either.

On the one side we have the fact that the destruction of the eye ensues more quickly after division of the trigeminal nerve in front of the Casserian ganglion, than when the division is made between the ganglion and the brain. This may imply that filaments derived from the ganglion, or passing through it from the sympathetic nerve, are those through which the influence on nutrition is exercised. And their sufficiency is supported by the fact that great disturbance in the nutrition of the eye is an ordinary consequence of the extirpation of the superior cervical ganglion of the sympathetic, even when the trigeminal nerve is unaffected.

But, on the other side, we have the facts of the destruction of the eye when the trigeminal nerve is spoiled near its origin, the sympathetic nerve being sound (as in the case by Mr. Stanley); and of the defective nutrition in consequence of injuries of the spinal cord, when also the sympathetic centres are uninjured; as in the cases by Sir B. C. Brodie and Mr. Travers. For this view, also, is the occurrence of general atrophy in consequences of diseases of the brain.

Finally, when defective nutrition follows injury of the spinal cord, it appears to be directly due to the injury of the sensitive, rather than the motor, nerve-fibres. Sloughing of the bladder and other parts occurs, I believe, in such cases earlier and more extensively when sensation, than when motion alone, is lost. And Mr. Curling has recorded this case :*— Two men were, at nearly the same time, taken to the London Hospital with injury of the spine ; one had lost only the power of motion in the lower extremities ; the other had lost both motion and sensation ; and at the end of four months the atrophy of the lower extremities in this last was far more advanced than in the first.

None of these cases, however, enable us to say whether the influence on nutrition is exercised through sensitive fibres of the cranio-spinal system, or through sympathetic fibres ; nor do I think this question can be yet determined.

* Medico.Chir. Trans. vol. xx. p. 342.

The last condition which I mentioned as essential to healthy nutrition, is a healthy state of the part to be nourished.

This is, indeed, involved in the very idea of the assimilation which is accomplished in the formative process, wherein the materials are supposed to be made like to the structures among which they are deposited: for unless the type be good, the anti-type cannot be.

In a part which was originally well formed, and with which the three conditions of nutrition already illustrated have been always present, this fourth condition will probably be never wanting; for the part will not of itself deflect from the normal state. But when any part, or any constituent of the blood has been injured or diseased, its unhealthy state will interfere with its nutrition long after the immediate effects of the injury or disease have passed away. Just, as in healthy parts, the formative process exactly assimilates the new materials to the old, so does it in diseased parts: the new-formed blood and tissues take the likeness of the old ones in all their peculiarities whether normal or abnormal; and hence the healthy state of the part to be nourished may be said to be essential to the healthy process of nutrition.

The exactness of assimilation accomplished by the formative process in healthy parts has been already, in some measure, illustrated, as preserving through life, certain characteristic differences, even in the several parts of one organ; preserving, also, all those peculiarities of structure and of action, which form the proper features, and indicate the temperament, of the individual. In these, and in a thousand similar instances, the precision of assimilation in the formative process is perfect and absolute, except in so far as it admits of a very gradual alteration of the parts, in conformity with the law of change in advancing years.

Nor is there less of exactness in the assimilation of which a part that has been diseased is the seat. For, after any injury or disease, by which the structure of a part is impaired, we find the altered structure,—whether an induration, a cicatrix, or any other,—as it were, perpetuated by assimilation. It is not that an unhealthy process continues: the result is due to the process of exact assimilation operating in a part of which the structure has been changed: the same process which once preserved the healthy state, maintains now the diseased one. Thus, a scar or a diseased spot may grow and assimilate as its healthy neighbors do. The scar of the child, when once completely formed, commonly grows as the body does, at the same rate, and according to the same general rule; so that a scar which the child might have said was as long as his own forefinger, will still be as long as his forefinger when he grows to be a man.

Yet though this increase and persistence of the morbid structure be the general and larger rule, another within it is to be remembered; namely, that in these structures there is usually (especially in youth) a tendency towards the healthy state. Hence, cicatrices, after long endurance, and even much increase, may, as it is said, wear out; and thickenings and indurations of parts may give way, and all become again pliant and elastic.

The maintenance of morbid structures is so familiar a fact, that not only its wonder, but its significance, seem to be too much overlooked. What we see in scars and thickenings of parts appears to be only an example of a very large class of cases; for this exactness by which the formative process in a part maintains the change once produced by disease, offers a reasonable explanation of the fact that certain diseases usually occur only once in the same body. The poison of small-pox, or of scarlet fever, being, for example, once inserted, soon, by multiplication or otherwise, affects the whole of the blood; alters its whole composition; the disease, in a definite form and order, pursues its course; and, finally, the blood recovers, to all appearance, its former state. Yet it is not as it was: for now the same material, the same variolous poison, will not produce the same effect upon it; and the alteration thus made in the blood or the tissues is made once for all: for, commonly, through all after life, the formative process assimilates, and never deviates from, the altered type, but reproduces materials exactly like those altered by the disease; the new ones, therefore, like the old, are incapable of alteration by the same poison, and the individual is safe from the danger of infection.

So it must be, I think, with all diseases which, as a general rule, attack the body only once. The most remarkable instance, perhaps, is that of the vaccine virus. Inserted once in almost infinitely small quantity: yet, by multiplying itself, or otherwise, affecting all the blood, it may alter it once for all. For, unsearchable as the changes it affects may be; inconceivably minute as the difference must be between the blood before, and the blood after, vaccination; yet, in some instances, that difference is perpetuated; in nearly all it is long retained; by assimilation, the altered model is precisely imitated, and all the blood thereafter formed is insusceptible of the action of the vaccine matter.

In another set of diseases we see an opposite, yet not a contradictory, result. In these, a part once diseased, is, more than it was before, liable to be affected by the same disease; and the liability to recurrence of the disease becomes greater every time, although in the intervals between the successive attacks the part may have appeared quite healthy. Such is the case with gout, with common inflammation of a part, as the eye, and many others, in which people become, as they say, every year more and more subject to the disease.

I do not pretend to determine the essential difference between the two classes of disease in these respects, in which they are antipodal; but in reference to the physiology of the formative process, they both prove the same thing, viz., that an alteration once produced in a tissue, whether by external influence, or by morbid material in the blood, is likely to be perpetuated by the exactness of assimilation observed in the formative process, *i. e.* by the constant reproduction of parts in every respect precisely like their immediate predecessors.

But it will be said, the rule fails in every case (and they are not rare) in which a disease that usually occurs but once in the same body, occurs twice or more; and in every case of the second class in which liability to disease is overcome. Nay, but these are examples of the operation of that inner, yet not less certain, law,—that after a part has been changed by disease, it tends naturally, to regain a perfect state. Most often the complete return is not effected; but sometimes it is, and the part, at length, becomes what it would have been if disease had never changed it.

I will here refer again to what was said in the first lecture concerning the blood's own assimilative power. After the vaccine and other infectious or inoculable diseases, it is, most probably, not the tissues alone, but the blood as much or much more than they, in which the altered state is maintained; and in many cases it would seem that, whatever materials are added to the blood, the stamp once impressed by one of these specific diseases is retained; the blood, by its own formative power, exactly assimilating to itself, its altered self, the materials derived from the food.

And this, surely, must be the explanation of many of the most inveterate diseases; that they persist because of the assimilative formation of the blood. Syphilis, lepra, eczema, gout, and many more, seem thus to be perpetuated: in some form or other, and in every varying quantity, whether it manifests itself externally or not, the material they depend on is still in the blood; because the blood constantly makes it afresh out of the materials that are added to it, let those materials be almost what they may. The tissues once affected may (and often do) in these cases recover; they may have gained their right or perfect composition; but the blood, by assimilation, still retains its taint, though it may have in it not one of the particles on which the taint first passed: and, hence, after many years of seeming health, the disease may break out again from the blood, and affect a part which was never before diseased. And this appears to be the natural course of these diseases, unless the morbid material be (as we may suppose) decomposed by some specific; or be excreted in the gradual tendency of the blood (like the tissues) to regain a normal state: or, finally, be, if I may so speak, starved by the abstraction from the food of all such things as it can possibly be made from.

In all these things, as in the phenomena of symmetrical disease, we have proofs of the surpassing precision of the formative process, a precision so exact that, as we may say, a mark once made upon a particle of blood, or tissue, is not for years effaced from its successors. And this seems to be a truth of widest application; and I can hardly doubt that herein is the solution of what has been made a hinderance to the reception of the whole truth concerning the connection of an immaterial

Mind with the brain. When the brain is said to be essential, as the organ or instrument of the Mind in its relations with the external world, not only to the perception of sentence, but to the subsequent intellectual acts, and, especially, to the memory of the things which have been the objects of sense,—it is asked, how can the brain be the organ of memory when you suppose its substance to be ever changing? or, how is it that your assumed nutritive change of all the particles of the brain is not as destructive of all memory and knowledge of sensuous things as the sudden destruction by some great injury is? The answer is,—because of the exactness of assimilation accomplished in the formative process: the effect once produced by an impression upon the brain, whether in perception or in intellectual act, is fixed and there retained; because the part, be it what it may, which has been thereby changed, is exactly represented in the part which, in the course of nutrition, succeeds to it. Thus, in the recollection of sensuous things, the Mind refers to a brain, in which are retained the effects, or, rather, the likenesses, of changes that past impressions and intellectual acts had made. As in some way passing far our knowledge, the Mind perceived, and took cognizance of, the change made by the first impression of an object acting through the sense-organs on the brain; so afterwards, it perceives and recognizes the likeness of that change in the parts inserted in the process of nutrition.

Yet here also the tendency to revert to the former condition or to change with advancing years, may interfere. The impress may be gradually lost or superseded, and the Mind, in its own immortal nature unchanged, and immutable by anything of earth, no longer finds in the brain the traces of the past.

LECTURE III.

THE FORMATIVE PROCESS: GROWTH.

HAVING now considered the sources of the impairment to which the completely formed blood and tissues are prone, and the chief conditions necessary for the perfection of the formative process by which, notwithstanding this impairment, they are maintained almost unchanged, I propose to speak of the process itself.

You may remember that I referred to the impairment, or wear and tear, of the body to two principal sources—namely, the deterioration which every part suffers in the exercise of its function; and the natural degeneration or death to which every part is subject after a certain period of existence, independently of the death or degeneration of the whole body, and, in some measure, independently of the exercise of function.

The first question, therefore, in the consideration of the nutritive process, may be,—what becomes of the old particle, the one for the replacement of which the process of formation is required? In answer, we must probably draw a distinction, though we can hardly define it, between the parts which die, and those which only degenerate, when they have finished their course; those which die are cast out entire: those which degenerate are disintegrated or dissolved, and absorbed. We seem to have a good example of this difference in the fangs of the two sets of teeth. Those of the deciduous ones degenerate, are transformed so as to become soluble, and are absorbed; those of what are called permanent,—more properly, those of teeth which are not to be succeeded by others deriving germs from themselves—die, and are cast out entire. And we may probably hold it as generally true, that, as Mr. Hunter was aware, living parts alone are absorbed in the tissues: dead parts, it is most probable, however small, are usually separated and cast out; and, as the phenomena of necrosis show, this must be accomplished, not by the absorption of the dead part themselves, or their borders, but by the absorption or retirement of the adjacent borders or surfaces of the living parts.

External, merely integumental, parts appear thus to die, and to be cast out entire from the body; but we have no certain knowledge of the changes they may undergo before they die. And with regard to the changes which take place in the degeneration that precedes absorption of the old particles, we have, again, but little knowledge. Chemistry has, indeed, revealed much concerning the final disposal of the old materials; finding their elements in the excretions; and proving that the process is one of descent towards simplicity of organic chemical composition; one of approximation towards inorganic character; and, perhaps always, one accomplished by the agency of oxygen. It has, also, we may safely believe, found in the muscles some of the substances into which the natural constituents of the tissues are transformed, before they assume the composition in which they are finally excreted. Kreatine and kreatinine are, most probably, examples of such transitional compounds, intermediate between some of the proper constituents of muscle, and urea or uric acid. And I think the frequency with which fatty matter is found in degenerate parts is an indication that it is an usual product of similar transformation preparatory to absorption, and to the more complete combination with oxygen in the formation of carbonic and water for excretion. However, while we have so little knowledge of these intermediate or transitional substances, we can only hold it as generally probable, that the components of the degenerate and out-worn tissues pass through a series of chemical transformations, which begin in their natural degeneration before absorption, till they are completed by the oxidation in the blood which brings the materials to the state appropriate for excretion.

With regard to the formative portion of the process,—that by which the old particle, however disposed of, is to be replaced,—it is probably always a process of development; a renewal, for each particle, of the process which was in nearly simultaneous operation for the whole mass in the original development of the tissue. The fibril, for example, which is to be formed anew in a muscle, passes, most probably, through the same stages of development as those did which were first formed in the embryo. We are led to this conclusion, not only by the evident probability of the case, but, first, by the analogy of the hair, the teeth, the epidermis, and all the tissues we can watch; in all, the process of repair or replacement is effected through development of the new parts: and, secondly, by the existence of nuclei or cytoblasts in, I think, all parts which are the seats of active nutrition. For these nuclei (such as are seen so abundantly in strong, active muscles), are not the loitering impotent remnants of the embryonic tissue, but apparatus of power for new formation. Their abundance is, I think, directly proportionate to the activity of growth. They are always abundant in the fœtal tissues, and those of the young animal; so they are in many quickly growing tissues; and they are more plentiful in the muscles and the brain than, so far as I know, any other non-secreting tissue of the adult. It is interesting, too, and significant in this regard, to notice their absence or infrequency in the nerve-fibres of the adult, which in so many points are comparable with the muscular fibres. And I think I may add that their disappearance from a part in which they usually exist is a sure accompaniment and sign of degeneration.

A subject of very interesting inquiry is involved in the difference which we may perceive between what may be called nutritive reproduction and nutritive repetition. I may illustrate my meaning by reference again to the teeth. In our own case, as the deciduous tooth is being developed, a part of its productive capsule is detached, and serves as a germ for the formation of the second tooth; in which second tooth, therefore, the first may be said to be reproduced, in the same sense as that in which we speak of the organs by which new individuals are formed, as the reproductive organs. But in the shark, in which we see row after row of teeth succeeding each other, the row behind is not formed from germs derived from the row before: the front row is simply repeated in the second one, the second in the third, and so on.

It is the same in the blood. The new blood-corpuscles, that are being constantly formed for the renovation of the blood, are not developed from germs given off from the old ones; neither are they formed by any assimilative force exercised by the old ones. By watching the stages of their construction, we may see that the development of each is an independent repetition of the process by which the first were formed. And so with the successive developments of ova and epithelial cells, and many others; each is developed independently of the rest, and each repeats the changes through which its predecessor passed.

Probably we shall find hereafter an analogy in this respect between tissues and whole animals; and that, as in the latter, the capacity of regeneration of lost parts is in direct proportion to the degree in which the members of the body are only repetitions one of another, so in the tissues, much of the difference in the degree of repair they severally undergo, after injuries or diseases, is connected with the ordinary mode of nutrition by repetition or by reproduction. When the whole cuticle of a part is removed, it may be again formed by repetition; but when a portion of muscle is removed, its germs are taken with it, and it is not reproduced.

Whether by repetition or reproduction, let it be observed that each new elementary structure is made, in successive stages, like what the old one was, not like what it is: as we see in the young hair following the course of the old one, or as the child is made like, not what his father is now, but what he was at his age. The new particle is, therefore, not made after a present model.

If, now, we turn from the consideration of the method of the formative process in the maintenance of the tissues, and from that of the conditions under which it is exercised, to inquire into the nature of the forces which actuate it; if we try to answer why any structure just new-formed has assumed nearly the same form as the old structure had which it replaces; we may find suggestions for an answer in the three classes of facts last mentioned. Among these facts we find (1), as detailed in p. 46, that a structure already formed exercises a certain assimilative influence on organic materials brought into contact or near proximity with it; (2), as in pp. 22–23, that, in many cases, certain parts of perfect structures are, as it were, set apart to be or contain the germs of the next succeeding similar structures, so that, in succession as in likeness, the new-formed structure may be called a reproduction of the older; and (3) that in many cases, as cited in p. 51, and yet more clearly in instances of repair and reproduction of injured and lost parts, the replacing structures are formed entirely anew, and independently of both these conditions. In these cases, no model structure is present to which the new-forming one may be assimilated; no tissue-germ which, by its development, may imitate the structure from which itself was derived; the new structure seems as if its own inherent properties had determined the form that it should take.

Resting on the first two classes of facts, it seems to some a sufficient explanation of the process of maintenance, to say that each structure in the body has the power of taking from the blood, by a kind of elective affinity, certain appropriate materials, and of so influencing them that they assimilate themselves to it; i. e., that they adopt or receive its form and properties, and incorporate themselves with it. By others, it is held that each cell or structural element of a part, while developing itself into some higher form, leaves behind or produces tissue-germs, or off-shoots, which, of course, pass through the same development as itself, and in due time succeed to its place and office.

Now, without doubt, the existence of these things is justly assumed, and we may, by reference to them, express correctly a part of the processes by which the maintenance of the body is accomplished. Still it is, I think, clear that they are not sufficient for the maintenance of the body in its perfection. For, in explanation of all the facts of the third class cited above, a theory of maintenance of the tissues by assimilation, or by the development of successive tissue-germs or cytoblasts, is inapplicable,—not merely insufficient, but inapplicable; for a postulate of this theory is the existence of a present model or germ for the construction of the forming part; and in all these cases no such germ or model can be found. Therefore, finding, in these cases, that the formative process is accomplished in the maintenance of certain parts, without either assimilation or a succession of germs, we may assume, I think, that even where either of these conditions is present, it is only as an auxiliary of some more constant and sufficient force.

Of this force, by whatever name we designate it, whether as the formative, or the plastic, or, more explicitly, as the force by which organic matter, in appropriate conditions, is shaped and arranged into organic structure; of this force, and of those that co-operate with it, we can, I think, only apprehend that they are, in the completed organism, the same with those which actuated the formation of the original tissues, in the development of the germ and of the embryo. As we have seen that the new formation of elemental structures in the maintenance of tissues is a repetition of the process observed in their first development, so we may assume that the forces operative are the same in both processes.*

Thus, then, for explanation of the maintenance of tissues by the constant formation of nearly similar elemental structures, we are referred back to the history of their first formation: and we might be content to rest in the belief that the mystery of the development of a germ is wholly inscrutable. We can discern in its method only this; that the materials of which the impregnated germ first consists, and all that it

---

* Concerning the very nature of such forces, and their correlations, I must refer to the admirable essays of Mr. Grove (The Correlation of Physical Forces), and Dr. Carpenter (On the Mutual Relations of the Vital and Physical Forces). "In speaking of *forces* as possessing an absolute existence, it is not intended," says Dr. Carpenter, "on the one hand to imply that they are anything else than 'affections of matter;' nor, on the other, to regard them in any other light than as the direct operation of the Primal All-sustaining Cause. We can form no conception of matter except as possessing *properties*, which, when in action, give rise to *powers* or *forces;* whilst on the other hand, we cannot think of forces, except as operating through some form of matter, of whose properties they are the manifestation. The existence of matter, and the action of forces to which material phenomena (whether physical or vital) are attributable, are alike the expressions of the Divine Will; and our aim must be limited to the discovery of the plan, according to which it has pleased the Creator to develop and maintain the existing condition of the universe we inhabit."— (General Physiology, p. 36.)

appropriates, are developed according to the same method as was observed in its progenitors, so that at every stage it is like what they were at the same stage. It is in conformity with the same law of formation according to the example of progenitors, that when the general development of the body is completed, each of its parts is still maintained or gradually changed. In each period of life, the offspring resembles the parents at the corresponding periods of their life; and, especially, in those degenerative changes which ensue in old age, we can discern no other method, or law, than still the same; that the parental form, and properties, and life, are imitated or reproduced in the offspring.

Now, can we trace anything further back than this fact? Probably not: but we may express it in other terms, which may be more conveniently used in our further inquiries, by saying that each germ derives from its parents such material properties that, being placed in the conditions necessary for the operation of the formative and other vital forces, it will imitate in all the phases of the life of each of its parts, the changes through which the corresponding parts passed in the parents. It is convenient, and probably right, while we assume the operation of a formative force, still to refer the method of its peculiar manifestations to the material properties of the substance in which it acts. In the case before us, we may accordingly assume, that peculiar and typical properties are transmitted from its parents to the materials of each impregnated germ; that these determine, under the operation of the formative force, the construction of corresponding peculiar and typical forms; that they are also communicated to whatever materials capable of organization are brought within the sphere of the developing germ, so that these also determine the same, or some definitely related, method of construction; and that thenceforward, throughout life, by similar communication or induction of specific properties in the forming of blood or other nutritive fluid, the same method of formation is maintained in all the tissues.

Unless we thus assume a dependence of form upon composition, of organic structure upon organic constitution, I think we cannot understand, or even clearly speak, of many of the deflections from the normal formative process which are due to injury or disease; deflections which, as we have seen, are maintained in the blood and tissues, and the tendency to which is, in hereditary diseases, transmitted from parent to offspring with the other properties of the germ.

The sum, then, of the hypothesis concerning the formative processes in the maintenance of the tissues is as follows:—It is assumed, 1st, that a certain vital formative, or plastic, or constructing force, is in constant operation; 2dly, that the forms assumed, under its influence, depend primarily, and in greatest measure, on the specific composition and other properties of the organizable materials taken from the blood; and, 3dly, these properties, transmitted in the first instance from the parent to the germ, are thenceforward communicated to all the nutritive materials;

subject, however, to certain progressive changes corresponding to the development and degenerations of the tissues.

It is assumed, further, that the taking of materials from the blood, by each part for its own maintenance, depends, as to quality, on certain definite relations, or "organic affinities" between the blood and the part; and as to quantity, on the waste of the part. As to the influence of an assimilative force, exercised by the tissues already formed, upon the nutritive materials placed in them, it is probable that this is not a plastic or constructive force, but chiefly such an one as, like the assumed catalytic force, or that of a ferment, affects first the composition of the materials not yet organized, and thus indirectly affects the form that they assume in organizing.

I fear I may have seemed to have engaged in a very useless discussion, and to have been talking of words more than of things; but the charge will not be made by one who knows the utility of being clear in the expressions used for the ground-work of teaching; or who will consider the importance in pathology of the principle that specific organic structures correspond with, and are determined by, specific organic compositions.

I propose now to consider, but as yet only generally, the second method of the formative process, Growth, in health and in disease.

It consists in the increase of a part, or of the whole body, by addition of new material like that already existing. The essential characters of each organ or tissue are maintained, but its quantity is increased, and thus it is enabled to discharge more of its usual function.

For a general expression of the course of events, we may say that the development and the growth of the body go on together till all the natural structures are attained; and that then development ceases, and growth goes on alone, till the full stature, and the full proportion of each part to the rest, are gained. But this is only generally true; for we cannot say that all development ceases at a determinate period, since some organs may go on to be developed when many others are complete. Neither can we assign the period of terminated growth; since, not only is the period, even stated generally, very various in different persons, but, some parts, unless placed in unfavorable conditions of disease, continue growing to the latest period of life. M. Bizot and Dr. Clendinning have proved, of the heart and arteries, that their average size regularly increases, though with a decreasing ratio of increase, from childhood to old age, provided only the old age be a lusty one.* And this is a real growth; for the heart not only enlarges with advancing years, but its weight augments, and the thickness of its walls increases; so that we may believe it acquires power in the same proportion as it acquires bulk —the more readily, since the increased power is necessary for the

Croonian Lectures by Dr. Clendenning, Medical Gazette for 1837–8, vol. xxii., p. 450.

increasing difficulties put in the way of the circulation by the increasing rigidity of the parts.

It may be that the same is true of some other parts. This certainly is true—that any part, after it has attained its ordinary dimensions, according to the time of life, may grow larger if it be more exercised: in other words, every part has, throughout life, the power of growing, according to its particular needs, in correspondence with the degree in which its function is discharged.

Now, when such growth as this is the result of the natural, though almost excessive, exercise of a part (as of the limbs, for instance, during hard work), we regard it only as an indication of health, and its result is admitted to be a desirable accession of strength. But, when such growth in one part is the consequence of disease in another, it is commonly described as a disease; it bears the alarming name of Hypertrophy; and it comes to be a subject of consideration in Morbid Anatomy.

But in both these cases the process of growth is the same, and is according to the same rules; and the tendency of the process of genuine hypertrophy in disease, like that of healthy growth in active exercise, is always conservative. I say genuine hypertrophy, meaning, under that term, to include only the cases in which the enlargement of a part is effected with development or increase of its natural tissue, with retention of its natural form, and with increase of power. To include all enlargements under the name of hypertrophy is too apt to lead to misunderstanding.

The rule, then, concerning hypertrophy is, that so long as all conditions remain the same, each part of the body after the attainment of the average size, merely retains its state, or, at most, grows at a certain determinate slow rate; but when the conditions alter, so that a part is more than usually exercised in its office, then it manifests a power of renewing or accelerating its growth. It is as if each healthy part had a reserve power of growth and development which it puts forth in the time of emergency. And the converse is equally true: when a part is less than usually exercised, it suffers atrophy; so that the rule may be that each part nourishes itself according to the amount of function which it discharges.

We may constantly see this rule in many more examples than I need refer to. The simplest case that can be cited is that of the epidermis. In its original formation, even before it has come into relation with the external world, it is formed on the several parts of the body—take, for example, the back and the palm of the hand—in different quantity and kind, adapted to the several degrees in which the cutis It is to protect will be exposed to pressure, friction, and the influence of other external forces. And, not only are its original quantity and construction on those parts different, but its rate of growth is so; for, though the back of the hand loses comparatively little by friction or otherwise, yet its epidermis does not grow thick; and though the palm loses more, yet its epidermis does not grow thin. So, then, both in original construction, and in rate of formation, the epidermis is thus adapted to the amount of function it has to discharge; that is, to the amount of protection it has to afford. But suppose now, that, by some new handicraft, the amount of exercise of the epidermis is increased; its rate of waste is increased in the same proportion, yet it does not grow thin; nay, it grows thicker, till it is completely adapted to protect the cutis from the greater sources of injury to which it is now exposed: it puts forth, as it were, a reserve-power, which is enough not only to repair all amount of waste within certain limits, but, further than this, to increase the quantity of the tissue to the amount required for the discharge of its increased functions.

What we can see in this case of the cuticle, we may be sure of for other tissues; for example, in a muscle; as in a heart, when, by disease of the valves, an obstacle is put in the way of the circulating blood, and the heart, or one of its cavities, acts with additional force to drive it on. But, as we know, the more of action in a muscle, the more the consumption of the tissue, so we might now expect a diminution of the heart. On the contrary, it enlarges; it is hypertrophied: the formative process not only meets the immediate exigencies of the increased consumption of muscular tissue, but produces enough to act with the additional power required by the increased difficulty of the circulation.

Such are the effects of growth in examples of hypertrophy. But, to meet the increasing difficulties of these and the like cases, a part may do more than grow; it may develop itself; it may acquire new structures, or it may improve those of which it is already composed, so as to become fit for higher functions and the exercise of greater power. For example, in the most ordinary hypertrophy of the heart, the muscular tissue is developed to more robustness: its fibres become not only larger, or more numerous, but firmer, more highly colored, and stronger. In the pregnant uterus, such fibres are formed as are not seen in the unimpregnated state: they are, indeed, not a new kind of fibre, but they are so different in size and shape, and so much more powerful than those which existed before, that we may justly speak of them as developed. And this change by development, which in pregnancy is natural, is often imitated in disease, when, by the growth of fibrous tumors in it, the uterus attains the size, the structure, and even the full capacity of action, of the pregnant organ. In several of such cases the uterus has at length imitated the course of labor, and delivered itself of the tumor by its contractile power.

A similar change, by development and growth of muscular fibres, may occur in the gall-bladder, the ureter, and, probably, in any other part that has the smooth muscular fibro-cells.

We have an example of development of a secreting structure in the bursa, which, as Hunter displayed it, is produced under a corn. The corn itself is the result of a kind of hypertrophy, tending to shield the cutis from unnatural pressure; but, itself becoming a source of greater trouble than that against which it was directed, it gives rise to the development of a bursa beneath it, which may, for a time, more effectually protect the joint beneath, by diffusing the pressure over a wider extent of surface.

All these are examples that this hypertrophy, as we call it, though it happens in circumstances of disease, is yet in general, so far as itself is concerned, a process of full and vigorous health, serving to remedy or keep back the ill effects that would ensue from disease in some other part. It is, in a less degree than the repair of a fracture or other mechanical injury, an instance of the truth that we are provided for accidents and emergencies; framed not merely to live in peace and sameness, but to bear disturbances; to meet, and balance, and resist them, and, sometimes at least, to counteract them.

The amplified healthiness of the formative process exercised in hypertrophy is testified by its requiring a full measure of all the conditions of ordinary nutrition. It needs healthy and appropriate blood; and one of the most interesting studies is to watch the hindering influence of disease on the occurrence and progress of hypertrophy, especially that of the heart. In some of these cases to which I shall have again to refer, death seems clearly to be the consequence of impairment of the blood, which can no longer maintain in the heart the exceeding growth required for its increased functions.

We find, moreover, very constantly, that, as if to insure sufficient blood to the grown or growing part, the main arteries and veins belonging to it are enlarged. This is usually well shown in the enlarged coronary arteries of the hypertrophied heart; an instance analogous to the enlargement of the arteries of the pregnant uterus, and the growing antlers of the deer, and many others. According to all analogy, we must consider this increase of the blood-vessels to be secondary. As in the embryo, parts form without vessels, till, for their further nutrition as their structure becomes more complex, the passage of blood into their interior becomes necessary, so, we may be sure, it is here. It is, indeed, strange that a part should have the power, as it seems, of determining in some measure the rate at which blood shall flow into it and through it; but so it is, and nearly all examples of hypertrophy are examples of the fact; though, as I shall presently have to mention, there are instances in which hypertrophy is the consequence, not the cause or precedent, of increased supply of blood.

With the increased supply of blood proportioned to the increased nutrition of the growing part, the nerves may also increase; as in the pregnant uterus and the hypertrophied heart. So, at least, I believe; but probably I need not apologize for evading the discussion of this matter.

The conditions which give rise to hypertrophy are chiefly or only three, namely—

1. The increased exercise of a part in its healthy functions.

2. An increased accumulation in the blood of the particular materials which a part appropriates to its nutrition or in secretion.

3. An increased afflux of healthy blood.

Of hypertrophy as the consequence of the increased exercise of a part, I have already spoken generally; and we need no better examples of it than the muscles of a strong man's arm, fitted for the very exercise in which they acquired bulk and power, or the great robust heart of a man who has suffered some disease producing obstacle to the movement of the blood. Both alike are the results of vigorous healthy growth, brought about by exercise of the part in its proper function.

In a former lecture (page 33) I spoke of the increased growth of the kidney, and of the adipose and other tissues, when the chief constituents of their structure exist in excess in the blood. To these I may refer again as examples of the second kind of hypertrophy. And I just now mentioned, that although in most cases an increased circulation of blood is the consequence of hypertrophy, yet there are cases in which the course of events is inverted. The increased flow of healthy blood through a part, if it be not interfered with by local disease, will give rise to hypertrophy of the part, or, at least, of some of its tissues.

This fact is shown very well in a specimen (No. 6) in the Museum, which Mr. Hunter described as "a sore which had continued inflamed a long time, where the increased action has made the hair grow." The integuments, for about an inch round the ulcer, where probably there was simply increased supply of blood, are covered with thick-set, long, and rather coarse, dark hairs: while on the more distant parts of the integuments, the hair is paler, more slender, and more widely scattered.

Similar examples of overgrowth of the hair through increased supply of blood, assisted probably by more than usual external warmth and moisture, are frequently seen near the ends of stumps which have remained long inflamed, and about old diseased joints; not, indeed, at the very seat of inflammation, but at some little distance from it, where the parts share the increased supply of blood, but not the disease of inflammation. Such cases are often observed on limbs in which fractures have occurred. I remember one very striking case in the thigh of a child about five years old. The femur had been fractured near the middle: the case did not proceed favorably; and union was not accomplished without much distortion. When I saw the child, I was at once struck with a dark appearance on the thigh: it was all covered with dark hair, like that of a strong coarse-skinned man; yet, on the rest of the body, the hair had all the fineness and softness which are proper to it in early life.

Similar facts are presented by some cases of transplantation. When the spur of a cock, for example, is transplanted from the leg to the comb, which abounds in blood, its growth is marvellously augmented, and it increases to a long, strange-looking mass of horny matter, such as is shown in two preparations in the Museum of the College. In one (54) the spur has grown in a spiral fashion, till it is six inches long; in the other (52) it is like a horn curved forwards and downwards, and its end needed to be often cut to enable the bird to bring its beak to the ground in feeding, and to prevent injurious pressure on the side of the neck.

It is worth observing, that these excessive growths have taken place on the combs without any corresponding diminution in the growth of the spurs in their proper places. The legs of these cocks are amply spurred, though the spur thus reproduced is not so long as that which had not been interfered with. In one instance, moreover (No. 53), there is an excessive production of the horny scales upon the legs, while the horny spur was also excessively growing on the comb.

I shall have occasion presently to mention cases which make it very probable that the more complex and vascular tissues, such as the muscles, integuments, and bones of a limb, can be thus hypertrophied by excess of blood. I will now only suggest the probability that the cases of congenital or spontaneous hypertrophy of a hand, or a foot, or of one or more fingers, have their origin in some excessive formation of the vessels, permitting the blood to flow more abundantly through the part. An enlargement of the radial artery has been observed by Dr. John Reid* in a case of such hypertrophy of the thumb and forefinger; but there is no evidence to determine whether in this case the enlargement of the artery was previous or subsequent to the excessive growth of the part.

Whatever be the case in these instances of enlargement, the fact, which the others show, that well-organized tissue, like hair and horn, is produced in consequence of simply increased supply of blood, stands in interesting contrast with the phenomena of inflammation, where no tissue, or only the most lowly organized, is ever formed. No fact can better show how far the mere enlargement of the bloodvessels is from constituting the essential part of inflammation.

Through cases of hypertrophy, such as these, the transition is made to those which, though they appear to consist in simple increase of natural texture of the parts, we yet must regard as morbid, while we do not know that they are adapted to any exigency of the economy. Such are the simple enlargements of the thyroid, thymus, and prostate glands, of the spleen, and tonsils: such too are some examples of mucous polypi, and of cutaneous outgrowths, and warty growths of the skin. These all present an increase of natural textures; and they may be instances of purposive growth, adapted and conservative: but till it is more manifest that they are so, we must be content, I think, to regard them as occupying a kind of middle ground between the genuine hypertrophies of

* London and Edinburg Monthly Journal of Medical Science, 1843, and in a collection by Mr. Curling in the Medico-Chirurg. Trans. vol. xxviii.

which I have been speaking, and the thoroughly morbid outgrowths of which a part of the class of tumors is composed.

On the other side, there are cases intermediate between hypertrophies and the results of inflammation, and no line of distinction can be drawn among them, if we rely on their anatomical characters alone; for, in the lowest degrees of inflammation, the exuded material may be organized into a very near likeness to the natural tissues, and may thus seem to increase their quantity. If these inflammatory hypertrophies, as they have been called, can be distinguished from true one, it is only by their being unattended with increase of functional power, or fitness for the part's relations.

LECTURE IV.

HYPERTROPHY.

LET me now further illustrate the general physiology of Hypertrophy, by adducing some of the specimens in the Museum which exhibit it in the principal tissues.

The first specimen in the Pathological division of the Museum is an urinary bladder hypertrophied in consequence of stricture of the urethra. It affords an admirable instance of genuine unmixed hypertrophy; for every part of the bladder is grown large; it is not contracted as if it had been morbidly irritable; and its mucous membrane, without induration or any similar morbid change, is increased, apparently by simple growth, to a thickness proportionate to that of the muscular coat.

I adduce this especially as an example of hypertrophy of muscular tissue, concerning which, instead of adding to what was said in the last lecture, I will quote Mr. Hunter's account. Referring, perhaps, to this very specimen, he says, in a passage which I have inserted in the catalogue: * "The bladder, in such cases (of obstruction to the passage of urine), having more to do than common, is almost in a constant state of irritation and action; by which, according to a property in all muscles, it becomes stronger and stronger in its muscular coats; and I suspect that this disposition to become stronger from repeated action is greater in the involuntary muscles than the voluntary; and the reason why it should be so is, I think, very evident: for, in the involuntary muscles, the power should be in all cases capable of overcoming the resistance, as the power is always performing some natural and necessary action; for whenever a disease produces an uncommon resistance in the

* Vol. i. p. 3; and Hunter's Works, ii. 299.

involuntary parts, if the power is not proportionally increased the disease becomes very formidable; whereas in the voluntary muscles there is not that necessity, because the will can stop whenever the muscles cannot follow; and if the will is so diseased as not to stop, the power in voluntary muscles should not increase in proportion."

Nothing, surely, could more appositely, or more exactly, express the truth concerning hypertrophy of muscle; and it may be observed, from what he says in a note, that Mr. Hunter appears to have been the first who rightly apprehended the nature of this growth of the bladder. He says, "This appearance was long supposed to have arisen from a disease of this viscus; but, upon examination, I found that the muscular parts were sound and distinct, that they were only increased in bulk in proportion to the power they had to exert, and that it was not a consequence of inflammation, for in that case parts are blended into one indistinct mass."

What this specimen shows in the urinary bladder is an example of the change which ensues in all involuntary muscles under the same circumstances. They all grow and acquire strength adapted to the new and extraordinary emergencies of their case. Thus, the œsophagus, the stomach, the intestinal canal, as often as any portion is the seat of stricture, display hypertrophy of the muscular coat above the stricture. The enormous enlargements of the intestinal canal, which gradually ensue above nearly impassable strictures of the rectum, are not mere dilatations, but growths of the intestinal walls; the muscular coat augmenting in power, to overcome, if it may, the increased hindrance of the propulsion of the contents, and even the glands and other textures of the mucous membrane simultaneously increasing.

In a great majority of cases, the hypertrophy of muscles, whether voluntary or involuntary, is the consequence of an increased obstacle to their ordinary action. Against this obstacle they exert extraordinary force, and this induces, indirectly, extraordinary formation of their tissue. Frequent action of muscles, unless it be also forcible, does not produce hypertrophy. As Mr. Humphry* says, the heart, though it may act with unusual frequency for years, yet does not in these cases grow larger; and the muscles of the hands are not generally so large in mechanics who use great celerity of action, as in those who work with great force. But action of muscles, if it be at once frequent and forcible, may produce hypertrophy, even though the action be unhealthy. This appears to be the case with the bladders of some children, who suffer with frequent and very painful micturition, and nearly all the signs of calculus, but in whom no calculus exists. The bladder in such children is found, after death, exceedingly hypertrophied, and there may be no other disease whatever of the urinary organs. Dr. Golding Bird has

* Lectures on Surgery, in Prov. Med. and Surg. Journal; Reprint, p. 108.

shown that phymosis, by obstructing the free exit of urine, may give rise to these signs, and to extreme hypertrophy of the bladder; but in some cases it appears certain that hypertrophy may occur without either phymosis, calculus, stricture, or any similar obstruction. It was so in a case illustrated in the Museum of St. Bartholomew's (xxvii. 14), in a child four years old, who had suffered intensely with signs of stone in the bladder, but in whom no stone existed; no disease of the urinary organs could be found, except this hypertrophy of the muscular coat of the bladder. An exactly similar case has been recently under Mr. Stanley's care, in which, after exceeding irritability of the bladder, the enlargement of its muscular coat appeared the only change.

In such cases, the too frequent and strong action of the bladder, though irritable and unhealthy, seems alone to give rise to hypertrophy of the fibres. It is, however, possible that the change may be due to narrowing of the uretha by muscular action. If, for example, the compressors of the uretha, instead of relaxing when the muscular coat of the bladder and the abdominal muscles are contracting, were to contract with them, the obstacle they would produce in the uretha would soon engender hypertrophy of the bladder.

Hunter, whose ingenuity was ever tempting on his intellect and industry, asked himself whether the hypertrophy of the heart were accomplished by the addition of new fibres, or by the enlargement of those that already exist. This question could hardly be determined without more microscopic aid than Hunter had at his command. But if we may believe (and there can be no doubt we may) that hypertrophy is, in this respect also, exactly similar to common growth, the question set by Hunter has been answered by Harting,* with whom, on this point, Kölliker† agrees. He has shown that, in the growth of striped muscles, there is no multiplication, no numerical increase, of the fibres, but an enlargement of them with addition to the number of the fibres.

Hypertrophy of bone presents itself in many interesting cases. It is usually a secondary process, ensuing in consequence of change in a part with which some bone is intimately connected. Just as in their natural development and growth, the bones of the skull are formed in adaptation to the brain, and those of the limbs are framed to fitness for the action of the muscles; so, in disease, they submit in their nutrition to adapt themselves to the more active parts. Thus, the skull enlarges when its contents do; and the bones of the limbs strengthen themselves as the muscles inserted on them become stronger and more active; and they do this in adaptation to the force of the muscles, and not merely because of the movements they are subject to: for no extent or force of passive movement would prevent the bones of a limb whose muscles are paralysed from suffering atrophy.

* Rech. Micrométriques, 1845. p. 62.   † Mikrosk. Anatomie, ii. 255.

In the skull, if in any organ, we might speak of two forms of hypertrophy; eccentric and concentric. When the cranial contents are enlarged, the skull is hypertrophied with corresponding augmentation of its area; and when the cranial contents are diminished, the skull (at least in many cases) is also hypertrophied, but with concentric growth, and diminution of its capacity.

The first, or eccentric form, is usually the consequence of hydrocephalus; wherein, as the fluid collects and distends the dura mater, so the skull grows; still, as it were, striving to attain its purpose, and form a complete envelope for the expanding brain.

The process of enlargement in these cases is often one of simple growth, and that, indeed, to a less extent than it may seem at first sight:

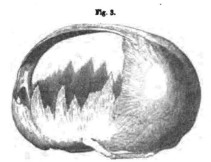

Fig. 3.

for it is very rarely that the due thickness of the skull is attained while its bones are engaged in the extension of their superficial area. Hence, the weight of a hydrocephalic skull is not much, if at all, greater than that of a healthy one; a large parietal bone,* measuring nine inches diagonally, weighs only four ounces, while the weight of an ordinary parietal bone is about three ounces.

It is interesting to observe, in some of these cases, the symmetrical placing of the Wormian bones, by which the extent of the skull is in a measure made up. They show how the formative process, though thus thrown into straits and difficulties, yet conforms, both in growth and development, with the law of symmetry.

It would be yet more interesting if we could certainly trace here something of conformity with the law of unity of organic type, in the mode of insertion of these Wormian intercalary bones, when compared with those of other animals. It cannot be certainly done; and yet, in some of these specimens, there appears (as if in accordance with that law) a tendency to the formation of the Wormian bones at the posterior part of the sagittal suture more than in any other part, as if in imitation of the interparietal bones of Rodents. And in the very rare specimen† sketched in the above diagram, in the midst of great confusion of the other bones, we find a remarkably bony arch, extending from between the two frontals to the occipital bone; occupying, therefore, the place of a large interparietal bone, and reminding us of some of the monkeys, *e.g.*, Cebus and Jacchus. We have a somewhat corroborative

---

* No. 2, in the College Museum.   † No. 3487 in the same Museum.

specimen in the immense hydrocephalic skull of the skeleton from Mr. Liston's Museum (No. 3489), in which the interparietal Wormian bones are larger than any others.

The hypertrophy of the skull, which may be called concentric, is that which attends atrophy with shrinking of the brain, or, perhaps, any disease of the brain in which there is diminution of its bulk. In such a case it usually happens, as was first shown by Dr. Sims,* that the skull becomes very thick.

All the specimens which I have examined show, however, that in these cases the thickening of the skull is not, in itself, a morbid process; it manifests definite purpose; is usually effected by healthy growth; and observes the rules followed in the natural formation of the skull.

Thus, as in first formation, the skull adapts itself to the form and size of the brain, or, rather, of its membranes; only now it does so without representing on its exterior the change which has taken place within. The thickening of the skull is effected by the gradual remodeling of the inner table and diploe of the bones of the vault; so that, although the exterior of the skull may retain its natural form and size, the inner table grows more and more inwards, as if sinking towards the retiring and shrinking brain; not thickening, but simply removing from the outer table, and leaving a wider space filled with healthy diploe.

Again, it is a fact of singular interest, that this thickening, this hypertrophy of the skull, most commonly, if not always, takes place especially and to a greater extent than elsewhere, in the parts of the bones in and about which ossification commenced in the fœtal state: as if, one might say, some of the potency that of old brought the fœtal membrane of these parts first into the development of bone, were always afterwards concentrated in them; or as if a reserve-power of growth had its seat in the same centres where was formerly the originative power of development.

The fact is shown in many of the specimens; especially in one that is represented here (Fig. 4); and we may find some further, though less sure, evidence of the peculiar formative energy of these old cen-

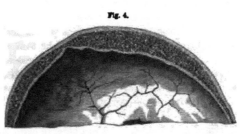

Fig. 4.

tres, in the fact that those diseases of bone which are accompanied with excessive formation, such as morbid thickenings of the skull and tumors, are, in a large majority of cases, seated in or near the centres of ossification; you rarely find them except at the articular ends, or round

* Medico-Chirurgical Transactions, vol. xix., p. 315.

5

the middle of the shaft. The same does not hold of necrosis, rickets, ulceration, or other diseases indicative of depression of the formative power of the bone. Rather, as some specimens (Nos. 390–1–2) of ricketty disease of the skull and femora show, the centres of ossification are remarkably exempt from the change of structure which has extensively affected the latter-formed parts.

This peculiarity of the centres of ossification is the more remarkable when we remember that, in many cases, the thickening of the skull takes place in persons far past the middle period of life; it may happen even in very old age, and may give one more evidence of that precision of assimilation which maintains, throughout life, characteristic distinctions among portions of what we call the same tissue.

Let me, however, remark, that it is not peculiar to old persons: I believe that at whatever age, after the complete closure of the cranial sutures, shrinking of the brain may happen, this hypertrophy of the skull may be its consequence. One specimen, for instance (No. 379), is part of the skull of a suicide, only thirty years old: another (No. 380), from an idiotic woman, has not the characters of an old skull. I once examined a remarkable case, showing the same conditions, in a person less than thirty years old, in whom the thickening of the skull must have begun in early life. She was a lady of remarkable personal attractions, but of slenderly developed intellect, whose head did not, externally, appear below the average female size. Yet her cranial cavity was singularly contracted; the skull had adapted itself to an imperfectly grown brain, by the hypertrophy of its diploe, which was nearly half an inch thick at and near the centres of ossification of the frontal and parietal bones.

Such hypertrophy, however, is not always the mode by which the skull is adapted to the diminished size of the brain. In congenital and very early atrophy of the brain, the skull is proportionally small, and may exactly represent the size and shape of the cerebrum. It does so in the cases of small-skulled idiots, and in a remarkable skull in the Museum of St. Bartholomew's Hospital. The man from whom this skull was taken, received a compound fracture of the left frontal bone when he was only 14 years old. Portions of bone were removed; hernia cerebri ensued, and several pieces of brain were sliced off. But he recovered and lived thirty-three years. The left hemisphere of the cerebrum was altogether small. Where the brain had been sliced off, its surface had sunk in very deep, and had left a cavity filled with a vascular spongy substance containing ill-formed nerve-fibres. You will observe here, that in the modeling of the skull, the left side has become in every part less capacious than the right, adapting itself to the diminished brain without any hypertrophy of the bones.

The cases are very rare in which hypertrophy of any other bones than those of the skull occurs in connection with what is recognized as disease.

For, as I have said, the bulk of most of the other bones is principally determined by the activity of the muscles fixed on them; and a morbidly excessive action of the muscles, sufficiently continued to produce hypertrophy of bones, is seldom, if ever, met with.

But there is a condition of bones so similar to hypertrophy in many respects, and so little different from it in any, that I may well speak of it here; yet not without acknowledging that nearly all I know about it is derived from Mr. Stanley.

When any of the long bones of a person who has not yet attained full stature is the seat of disease attended with unnatural flow of blood in or near it, it may become longer than the other or more healthy bone. For example, a lad, suppose, has necrosis of the femur, it may be of a small portion of it, and he may recover completely from this disease; but for all his life afterwards (as I had constant opportunity, once, of observing in a near relative), he may be lame, and the character of his lameness will show that the limb which was diseased is now too long; so that he is obliged, in walking, to lift the lame leg, almost like a hemiplegic man, lest his toe should trip upon the ground.

Such cases are not uncommon: I once saw, with Mr. Stanley, a member of our profession, in whom this elongation of one femur had taken place to such an extent that he was obliged to wear a very high shoe on the other, that is, the healthy, limb. And this, which he had adapted for himself, affords the only remedy for the inequality of limbs. Nor is the remedy unimportant: for, to say nothing of the unsightly lameness which it produces, the morbid elongation of the limb is apt to be soon complicated by one of two serious consequences. Either the patient, in his endeavors to support himself steadily and upright, will acquire first the habit, and then the malformation, of talipes of the healthy limb; or else, through the habit of always resting on the short, healthy, and stronger limb, he will have lateral curvature of the spine. Cases of both these kinds have occurred in Mr. Stanley's practice; being brought to him for the remedy, not of the elongated femur, but of the consequent deformity of the foot of the spine.

A considerable elongation of the lower extremity almost always depends on the femur being thus effected: another, and very characteristic result ensues from the same kind of hypertrophy when it occurs in the tibia. The femur can grow longer without materially altering its shape or direction, but the tibia is tied by ligaments at its two ends to the fibula; so that when it lengthens, unless the fibula should lengthen to the same extent, it, the tiba, must curve; in no other way, except by the lengthening of the ligaments, which, I believe, never happens to any considerable extent, is elongation of the tibia possible.

Tibiæ thus curved are far from rare; specimens are to be found in nearly every museum; yet I know of none in which the pathology of the disease is clearly shown escept one, in the Museum of St. Bartholomew's (Subser. A, 46), which is here sketched, Fig. 5.

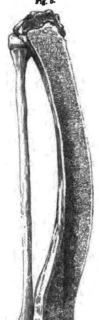

Fig. 5.

In this, the fibula, and the healthy tibia of the opposite limb are preserved with the elongated tibia. The anterior wall of this tibia, measuring it over its curve, is more than two inches longer than that of the healthy one: the posterior wall is not quite so long.

In all such specimens you may observe a characteristic form of the curve, and its distinction from the curvature of rickets. The distinction is established by these particulars: the ricketty tibia is always short; the other is never short, and may be longer than is natural: in the ricketty one the articular ends always enlarge very suddenly, for the shortening is due to the imperfect formation of the ends of the shaft; in the elongated tibia there is usually even less contrast of size between the shaft and epiphyses than is natural, because the elongation of the shaft is commonly attended with some increase of its circumference; but, especially, the ricketty tibia is compressed, usually curved inwards, its shaft is flattened laterally, and its margins are narrow and spinous; while, in the elongated tibia, the curb is usually directed forwards, its margins are broad and round, its surfaces are convex, and the compression or flattening, if there be any, is from before backwards.

The elongation of the bones in these cases may occur, in different instances, in two ways. In some cases it seems due to that change in bone which is analogous to chronic inflammation of soft parts, and which consists in the deposit of the products of inflammation in the interstices of the osseous tissue, their accumulation therein, and the remodeling of the bone around them as they accumulate. Such a change appears to have occurred in the specimen from which the sketch was taken, and would necessarily give rise, in a growing bone, as it does in soft parts, to enlargement in every direction, to elongation as well as increase of circumference.

But, in other cases, the elongation is probably due to the more genuine hypertrophy which follows the increased flow of blood. When, for example, a small portion of bone, as in circumscribed necrosis, is actively diseased, all the adjacent part is more vascular; hence may arise a genuine hypertrophy, such as I have shown in hair under similar circumstances. Or, when an ulcer of the integuments has long existed in a young person, the subjacent bone may share in the increased afflux of blood, and may enlarge and elongate. Even, it appears, when one bone is diseased, another in the same limb may thus be increased in length. A remarkable instance of this kind has lately been observed by Mr. Holden, in a young man, who, in childhood, had necrosis of the left tibia, one of the consequences of which was defective growth of the left leg, with shortening to the extent of more than an inch. Yet the whole limb is not shorter than the other; for without any apparent morbid change of texture, the femur of the same side has grown so as to compensate for the shortening of the tibia.

An interesting example of similar increased growth of one bone, in compensation for the weakness of another, is found sometimes in cases of ill-repaired fractures or diseases of the tibia. The fibula, at the part corresponding with the weak portion of the tibia, is in such cases strengthened sufficiently for the support of the limb. So in a specimen in the Museum of St. Bartholomew's (Ser. 8, 86), taken from a dog ten weeks after a piece of the radius was cut out with its periosteum, while the gap in the radius is filled with only soft tissue, the exactly corresponding portion of the ulna is increased by the formation of new bone beneath its periosteum.

I must not forget to say, that the interest of these cases of inequality of the limbs, by lengthening of one of the bones, is increased by comparison with another class of cases, in which as great or greater inequality of length depends on one limb being anormally short. In these, the short limb has been the seat of atrophy, through paralysis of the muscles dependent on some of the very numerous conditions in which they may be rendered inactive. The complication of the cases, the talipes, and the curvatures of the spine, depending, as they do, on the inequality of the length of the limbs, from whatever cause arising, will be alike in both; and much care may be needed in diagnosis, to tell which of the limbs, the long one or the short one, is in error. The best characters probably are, that when a limb is, through disease or atrophy, too short, it will be found, in comparison with the other, defective in circumference as well as in length; its muscles, partaking of the atrophy, will be weak and flabby, and all its tissues will bear signs of imperfect nutrition. If none of these characters be found in the short limb, the long one may be suspected; and this suspicion will be confirmed, if there be found in it the signs of increased nutrition, such as enlargement, growth of hair, and the rest: or if, in the history of the case, there be evidence of a disease attended with an excess in the supply of blood.

Continuing to select from the Museum only such examples of hypertrophy as may illustrate its general pathology, I pass over many, and take next, those which display the formation of corns; a subject which, while Hunter deemed it worth consideration, we shall not be degraded by discussing. He made many preparations of corns, to show not only the thickening of the cuticle, but the formation of the little sac of fluid, or bursa, between the thickened cuticle and the subjacent articulation. His design appears to have been, mainly, to illustrate the different results of pressure; to show how that which is from without produces thickening: that from within, thinning and absorption of parts. He says, having regard to these specimens, "The cuticle admits of being thickened from pressure in all parts of the body: hence we find that on the soles of the feet of those who walk much the cuticle becomes very thick; also on the hands of laboring men. We find this wherever there is pressure, as on the elbow, upper part of the little toe, ball of the great toe, &c. The immediate and first cause of this thickening, would appear to be the stimulous of necessity given to the cutis by this pressure, the effect of which is an increase of the cuticle to defend the cutis underneath. Not only the cuticle thickens, but the parts underneath, and a sacculus is often formed at the root of the great toe, between the cutis and ligaments of the joint, arising from the same cause, to guard the ligaments below." *

In another place he says, "When from without, pressure rather stimulates than irritates: it shall give signs of strength, and produce an increase of thickening; but, when from within, the same quantity of pressure will produce waste" (as illustrated in Nos. 120 and 121 in the Pathological Museum); "for the first effect of the pressure from without is the disposition to thicken, which is rather an operation of strength; but if it exceeds the stimulus of thickening, then the pressure becomes an irritator, and the power appears to give way to it, and absorption of the parts pressed, takes place, so that Nature very readily takes on those steps which are to get rid of an extraneous body, but appears not only not ready to let extraneous bodies enter the body, but endeavors to exclude them by increasing the thickness of the parts." †

It is evident from these passages that Mr. Hunter was aware that pressure from without might produce atrophy; though he may appear to favor the belief, which, I think, is commonly adopted as on his authority, that the direction of the pressure is that which determines its result. Really, the result seems to depend more on whether the pressure be occasional or constant. Constant extra-pressure on a part always appears to produce atrophy and absorption; occasional pressure may, and usually does, produce hypertrophy and thickening. All the thickenings of the cuticle are the consequence of occasional pressure; as the pressure of shoes in occasional walking, of tools occasionally used with the hand, and the like: for it seems a necessary condition for hypertrophy, in most parts, that they should enjoy intervals in which their nutrition may go on actively. But constant pressure, whether from within or from without, always appears to give rise to unrepaired absorption; and most museums contain interesting examples of its effects.

* Hunter's Works, vol. i., p. 560.   † Ibid., vol. iii., p. 466.

Some vertebræ in the College Museum (121 A.), illustrate very well the results of pressure by aneurisms and tumors. So far as themselves are concerned, the pressure of the aneurism was from without inwards; yet they are atrophied; not ulcerated, but hollowed out, and remodelled in adaptation to the shape of the aneurismal sac: their cancellous tissue is not exposed, but, as in the natural state, is covered by a complete thin external layer of compact tissue.

The pressure of a loose mass of bone in the knee-joint (No. 955 in the same Museum), was from without inwards; but its result was atrophy, as shown in the formation of a deep pit at the lower end of the femur, in which it lay safely and almost tightly lodged.

Again, the effect of constant pressure is shown in the cases in which one of the lower incisor teeth of a rodent animal has continued its growth after the loss of the corresponding upper incisor, and, being no longer worn down by attrition in growing, attains an unnatural length. In such a case, the extremity of the tooth, turning round so as to form nearly a complete circle, has come into contact with the side of the lower jaw, and (like, as they tell, the Fakir's finger-nails growing through the thickness of his clenched hand) it has perforated the whole thickness of the jaw; the absorption consequent on its pressure making way for its onward course.

A yet stranger example was taken from the body of a woman in the dissecting-room of St. Bartholomew's Hospital, and the specimen (Ser. 1, 232) tells all the history that can, or perhaps need, be given. She had an aperture in the hard palate, and for remedy of its annoyance, used to wear a bung, or cork, in it. But the constant pressure of so rough an obturator produced absorption of the edges of the opening, making it constantly larger, and requiring that the cork should be often wound round with tape to fit the widening gap. And thus the remedy went on increasing the disease, till, of all the palatine portions of the upper maxillary and palate bones, nothing but their margin or outer shell remains: the rest is all absorbed. The antrum is on each side obliterated by the apposition of its walls, its inner wall having probably been pushed outwards as the plug was enlarged to fit the enlarging aperture in the palate. Nearly the whole of the vomer also has been destroyed, and the superior ethmoidal cells are laid open.

Lastly, as an instance in which, in the same part, permanent pressure produced atrophy, and occasioned pressure hypertrophy, I may show a Chinese woman's foot. The bandaging, and constant compression in early life, produced this diminished growth; but afterwards, when, with all the miserable doublings-up and crowding of the toes, the foot was used in walking, the parts of pressure became the seats of corns.

We may sometimes observe the same contrast after amputations. A hole may be absorbed in an upper flap where it lies on the end of the bone, and is subject to the constant pressure of its own weight; but, in older stumps, the greater occasional pressure on the artificial limb leads to thickening and hardening of the parts.

These examples, then, may suffice to show, as I have said, that constant pressure on a part produces absorption; occasional pressure (especially if combined with friction) produces thickening or hypertrophy; and that these result whatever be the direction of the pressure. And, yet, let me add, that Mr. Hunter was not far wrong,—he never was; for nearly all pressures from without are occasional and intermittent, and nearly all pressures from within, arising, as they do, from the growth of tumors, the enlargement of abscesses, and the like, are constant.

LECTURE V.

ATROPHY: DEGENERATION.

I PROPOSE now to consider the subject of Atrophy; the very contrary of the hypertrophy which I endeavored to elucidate in the last two lectures.

By atrophy is commonly implied, not the cessation or total privation of the formative process in a part, but its deficiency; and as I limited hypertrophy to the cases in which an increased power is acquired for a part by the growth, or by the development, of healthy tissue; so shall atrophy be here taken to mean only that process by which a part either simply wastes and is reduced in size, with little or no change of texture, or else, gradually and regularly degenerates.

By the terms of this limitation it is implied, that, as there are two modes of hypertrophy, the one with growth, the other with development; so there are two modes of atrophy, the one with simple decrease, the other with degeneration, of tissue. In both, there is a loss of functional power in the part; but in one, this loss is due to the deficient quantity, in the other to the deteriorated quality, of the tissue. But, as in hypertrophy the development and the growth of the affected part usually concur, so, in atrophy, a part which becomes smaller usually also degenerates, and one which degenerates usually becomes smaller. Still, one or other of these, either the decrease or the degeneration, commonly prevails; and we shall see reasons why the distinction is very necessary to be made.

Let me first state, and even at some length, what is to be understood by degeneration, and how its effects may be distinguished from those of disease.

I implied in a former lecture, that the maintenance of a part in its nutrition must not be understood as being the maintenance of an unchanged state: rather, each part may be said to present a series of minute progressive changes, slowly effected, and consistent with that exercise of its functions which is most appropriate to the successive periods of its existence.

Now, after a certain length of life, these changes accumulate into a very noticeable deterioration of all, or nearly all, parts of the body; and they suffer a manifest loss of functional power. Thus changed, we say they are degenerate: these accumulated changes are the signs of decay, the infirmities of age, the senile atrophy. They are the indications of defective formative power, and often speak more plainly of old age than do the years a man may have counted; they testify that the power which prevailed over the waste of the body in childhood and youth, and maintained the balance in vigorous manhood, has now failed: as the tide, after a flood and a period of rest, turns and ebbs down.

All the expressions usually employed about these changes imply that they are not regarded as the results of disease; nor should they be; they are, or may be, completely normal; and were it not that the forces which are efficient in degeneration are, probably, very different from those which actuate the formative processes, we might justly call the degeneration of advanced age another normal method of nutrition. For, to degenerate and die is as normal as to be developed and live: the expansion of growth, and the full strength of manhood, are not more natural than the decay and feebleness of a timely old age; not more natural, because not more in accordance with constant laws, as observed in ordinary conditions. As the development of the whole being, and of every element of its tissues, is according to certain laws, so is the whole process regulated, by which all that has life will, as of its own workings, cease to live. The definition of life that Bichat gave is, in this view, as untrue as it is illogical. Life is so far from being "the sum of the functions that resist death," that it is a constant part of the history of life that its exercise leads naturally to decay, and through decay to death.

Of the manner in which this decay or degeneration of organisms ensues we know but little. Till within the last few years the subject of degenerations was scarcely pursued; and, even of late, the inquiries, which ought to range over the whole field of living nature, have been almost exclusively limited to the human body. The study of development has always had precedence in the choice of all the best workers in physiological science. They who have devoted many years of laborious thought and observation to the study of the changes by which the living being is developed from rudiment to perfection, have given fewer hours to the investigation of those by which, from that perfection, it naturally descends into decay and death. Almost the only essays at a general illustration of the subject have issued in the ridiculous notion that, as the body grows old, so it retrogrades into a lower station in the scale of animal creation. The flattened cornea is supposed to degrade the old man to the level of the fish; while the *arcus senilis*, by a fancied correspondence with an osseous sclerotic ring, maintains him in the eminence of a bird: his dry thick cuticle makes him like the pachydermata; and his shrivelled spleen approximates him to the humility of the mollusk. One can only commend such day-dreams to the modern supporters of the doctrine of transmutation of species; and they might, indeed, form an appropriate supplement to their scheme, if they would maintain that, in these latter days, our species is destined to degenerate into lower and yet lower forms, descending through the grades by which, in bygone times, it ascended to its climax in humanity.

We cannot but wonder at the comparative neglect with which wiser men than these philosophers have treated a study, so full at once of importance and of interest as this, of the natural degeneration of the body. It could not be without interest to watch the changes of the body as life naturally ebbs; changes, by which all is undone that the formative force in development achieved; by which all that was gathered from the inorganic world, impressed with life, and fashioned to organic form, is restored to the masses of dead matter; to trace how life gives back to death the elements on which it has subsisted; the progress of that decay through which, as by a common path, the brutes pass to their annihilation, and man to immortality. Without a knowledge of these things our science of life is very partial, very incomplete. And the study of them would not lack that peculiar interest which appertains to inquiries into final causes. For all the changes of natural decay or degeneration in living beings indicate this design; that, being gradual approximations to the inorganic state of matter, they lead to conditions in which the elements of the body, instead of being on a sudden and with violence dispersed, may be collected into those lower combinations in which they may best rejoin the inorganic world; they are such, that each creature may be said to die through that series of changes which may best fit it, after death, to discharge its share in the economy of the world, either by supplying nutriment to other organisms, or by taking its right part in the adjustment of the balance held between the organic and the inorganic masses.

Nor would the student of the design of these degenerations do well to omit all thought of their adaptation, in our own case, to the highest purposes of our existence. When, in the progress of the "calm decay" of age, the outward senses, and all the faculties to which they minister, grow dim and faint, it may be on purpose that the Spirit may be invigorated and undisturbed in the contemplation of the brightening future; that, with daily renewed strength, it may free itself from the encumbrance of all sensuous things, or may retain only those fragments of thought or intellectual knowledge which, though gathered upon earth, yet bear the marks of truth, and being Truth, may mingle with the

Truth from Heaven, and form part of those things in which Spirits of infinite purity and knowledge may be exercised.

Moreover (and this is in the closest relation to my present subject), the changes of natural degeneration in advanced life have a direct importance in all pathology; because they may guide us to the interpretation of many similar anomalies which, while they occur in earlier life, we are apt to call diseases, but which are only premature degenerations, and are to be considered, therefore, as methods of atrophy; as defects, rather than as perversions, of the nutritive process; or as diseases only in consideration of the time of their occurrence.*

The changes that mark the progress of natural decay or degeneration in old age, and that may, therefore, be regarded as the typical instances of simply defective nutrition, seem to be these:—1. Wasting or withering; the latter term may imply the usually coincident wasting and drying which constitute the emaciation of a tissue. 2. Fatty degeneration, including many of what have been called granular degenerations. 3. Earthy degeneration, or calcification. 4. Pigmental degeneration. 5. Thickening of primary membranes.

Of each of these let me cite one or two examples.

Of *withering*, or wasting and drying, which is perhaps the commonest form of atrophy, we have abundant instances in the emaciation of old age; in which, while some parts are removed by complete absorption, others are only decreased in size, and lose the succulency of earlier life.

The *fatty degeneration* in senility is best shown, as a general occurrence, in the increasing obesity which some present at the onset of old age, and in the general fact that there is more fatty matter in all the tissues, and most evidently in the bones, than there is in earlier life; while, as local senile fatty degenerations, we find the *arcus senilis*, or fatty degeneration of the cornea, and the accumulating fatty or atheromatous degenerations of the arteries.

The *calcareous degeneration* is, in old age, displayed in the gradually increasing proportion of earthy matter in the bones; in the extension of ossification to cartilages, which, in all the period of vigor, had retained their embryonic state; and in the increasing tendency to earthy deposits in the arteries, and other parts.

The *pigmental degeneration* has its best instances in the gradually accumulating black pigment spotting and streaking the lungs; in the slate or ash-color which is commonly seen in the thin mucous membranes of the stomach and intestines of old persons; and in the black spotting

* One can here have in view only the cases in which the degeneration affects the whole, or some considerable part, of an organ; for it is very probable that some of the degenerations which we see en masse in the organs of the old, or in the seats of premature defect of nutrition, are the same as occur naturally in the elementary structures of parts, previous to their being absorbed and replaced, as it were, by one particle at a time, in the regular process of nutrition.

of the arteries of some animals, in which pigments seem to hold the place of the fatty degenerations so usual in our own arteries.

Of the *thickening of primary membranes* we have indications in the usual thickening of the tubules of the testes, and, I think, of some other glands, as their function diminishes in old age; in the opaque white thickening of the primary or inner membrane of nearly all blood-vessels; and in the thickening of the walls of cartilage cells in senile and some other ossifications. To this, also, we have a strong analogy in the thickening of the cells-walls of the heart-wood of plants.

These changes, singly or in various combinations, constitute the most evident degenerations of old age in man. Their combinations give rise to numerous varieties in their appearance; such as, *e. g.*, the increase of both fatty and earthy matter in old bones; the dry, withered, and darkly tinged condition of the epidermis; the coincident fatty and calcareous deposits in the arteries; the thickened walls and fatty contents of the seminal tubes. But, at present, I need not dwell on these; nor on the conditions which determine the occurrence of one rather than another mode of degeneration; for these I cannot tell.

Now, if we observe the conditions in which these senile, and therefore typical, examples of degeneration are imitated in earlier life, they are such as indicate that the changes are still to be ascribed to a defect, not to a perversion, of the conditions of nutrition or of the vital forces.

Thus, these changes are all especially apt to occur in a part of which the functions are abrogated: a motionless limb wastes or becomes fatty as surely as an old one does. They are found ensuing when one or more of the conditions of nutrition are removed, not changed. For example, a fatty degeneration of part of a heart may ensue when, through disease of a coronary artery, its supply of blood is diminished. They often occur in parts that fail to attain the development for which they seemed to be intended. Thus fatty degeneration usually ensues in the cells of unfruitful Graafian vesicles.* In short, all their history, when we can trace it, is that of atrophies.

We may, therefore, safely hold, that, as the changes to which the several tissues are naturally prone in old age are certainly the results of defect, not of perversion, of the nutritive process, so are the corresponding changes when they happen in earlier life; although, through their appearing prematurely, they may bear the features of disease.

The distinction between degeneration and disease is essential, though often it may be obscure. Degeneration, as to its process, is natural, though it may be premature; disease is always unnatural: the one has its origin within, the other without, the body: the one is constant, the other as various as the external conditions in which it may arise: to the one we are prone, to the other only liable.

The general diagnostic characters of degenerations are chiefly these:—

* Reinhardt, in Traube's Beiträge, B. i. p. 145.

1. They are such changes as may be observed naturally occurring, in one or more parts of the body, at the approach of the natural termination of life, or, if not then beginning, yet then regularly increasing.

2. They are changes in which the new material is of lower chemical composition, *i. e.*, is less remote from inorganic matter, than that of which it takes the place. Thus fat is lower than any nitrogenous organic compound, and gelatine lower than albumen, and earthy matter lower than all these.

3. In structure, the degenerate part is less developed than that of which it takes the place: it is either more like inorganic matter, or less advanced beyond the form of the mere granule of the simplest cell. Thus, the approach to crystaline form in the earthy matter of bones, and the crystals in certain old vegetable cells, are characteristic of degeneration; and so are the granules of pigment and many granular degenerations, and the globules of oil that may replace muscular fibres or the contents of gland-cells, and the crystals of cholesterine that are often mingled with the fatty and earthy deposits.

4. In function, the part has less power in its degenerate than in its natural state.

5. In its nutrition, it is the seat of less frequent and less active change, and without capacity of growth or of development.

Such are the characters by which in general we might separate the processes and results of degeneration from those of disease, and of natural nutrition. But we must remember always that the process of degeneration may concur with either of those from which, in its typical examples, it may be so clearly separated. It may mingle with development; or, at least, by a process of degeneration, a part may become adapted to a more developed condition of the system to which it belongs. So it is in the process of ossification. It is usual to speak of a cartilage as being *developed* into bone, and to regard bone as the more developed and more highly organized of the two tissues. But I think it is only in a very limited sense that this mode of expression is just. Professor, Owen, in some admirable remarks* on the cartilaginous state of the endo-skeleton of Chondropterygian fishes, has said—"I know not why a flexible vascular animal substance should be supposed to be raised in the histological scale because it has become impregnated, and, as it were, petrified by the abundant intussusception of earthly salts in its areolar tissue. It is perfectly intelligible that this accelerated progress to the inorganic state may be requisite for some special office of such calcified parts in the individual economy; but not, therefore, that it is an absolute elevation of such parts in the series of animal tissues." Let me add, that all that one sees of the life of cartilage, in the narrow survey of the higher mammalia, is conformable with this view, and would lead us to speak of its change into bone as a degeneration, rather than a development. The change is effected

* Lectures on Comparative Anatomy, vol. ii. p. 146.

not only in the vigor of life, but as constantly, in certain parts, in its decay; and, whenever it is effected, the part that has become bone almost ceases to grow, except by superaddition; the interstitial changes of normal nutrition are reduced to their lowest stage. Cartilage, too, is less frequently and less perfectly repaired after injury than bone is; and its repair is commonly effected by the production of bone; yet it is contrary to all analogy for a lower tissue to be repaired by the formation of a higher one. It may be added that the granular, and in some instances even crystaline, form, in which the earthy matter of bone is deposited, is inconsistent with the supposition that its animal matter has acquired a higher development than it had before in the state of cartilage. So far, therefore, as its position in the series of animal tissues is concerned, bone should be placed below cartilage; as a tissue which has degenerated into a state of less active life, and has acquired characters that approximate it to the more lowly organized and to the inorganic substances. An osseous skeleton is, indeed, proper to the most highly developed state of the individual, and in this relative view bone appears superior to cartilage : but, with as much right, in the same view, the atrophied thymus gland, and the renal capsules almost arrested in their growth, might claim to be regarded as developments from their fœtal state; for these, also, are normal parts of the more perfect organism : they are like the degenerate members of an ennobled society, except in that, in their humiliation, they augment the common weal.

The points of contract, and even of complete fusion, are yet more numerous between degeneration and disease. In many diseases, probably even in the whole class of inflammations, a degeneration of the affected tissue is a constituent part of the morbid process; and in many cases we must still doubt whether the changes of texture that we observe are the results of degeneration or of disease. Among these are the instances of the simple softening of certain organs, such as the brain and spinal cord, and the liquefactions of inflammatory exudations in the suppurative process. If we limit the term degeneration to the changes that imitate the typical examples of old age, these changes cannot be included under it; but they may be, if we consider the conditions in which they occur, and the mere decrease of power which some of them manifest. The softening of the brain and spinal cord, for example, occurs in some cases through mere defect of blood; in some through mere abrogation of function; it is often concurrent with distinct signs of atrophy; and, as I shall describe in the next lecture, it is attended with changes that closely imitate those of fatty degeneration. On the whole, therefore, while admitting the difficulty that must often occur in endeavoring to separate such changes as these from the effects of disease, or of local death, yet I think we should do well to classify them under such a title as that of liquefactive degeneration.

The sum of this discussion respecting degenerations is as follows :—We observe certain changes naturally ensuing in the tissues during advanced age, and we ascribe these to defect, not to disorder, of the formative process : we notice the same or similar changes in earlier life, and we refer them to similar defect, and class them as methods of atrophy : we seem justified in thus regarding them, by the general fact that they often have the same origin, and are concurrent, with the atrophy which is attended with merely defective quantity of tissue ; and lastly, we regard certain changes of texture, such as some forms of softening of organs, as degenerations or atrophies, because, though they are not natural in old age, they occur in nearly the same conditions, and manifest some of the same characters, as the atrophies which imitate those of senility.

Among the degenerations that I have enumerated, only one has been very carefully studied, namely, the fatty degeneration.   This deserves a full description, first, because of its own great importance in pathology, for there is scarcely a natural structure or a product of disease in which it may not occur ; and secondly, for its illustration of the general doctrine of defective nutrition, and for guidance in the study of the degenerations that are at present less understood.   For we may be nearly sure, that general truths, deduced from examples of fatty degeneration, will hold equally of the other forms, and especially of the calcareous and pigmental ; between which and the fatty degenerations there are so many obvious features of close resemblance, that I shall content myself, having . enumerated them, with merely referring to the examples of them that will be described in future lectures.*

The anatomical character of many examples of fatty degeneration will be described in the next and in subsequent lectures.   Their principal general feature is, that in the place of the proper substance of an elemental structure, e. g. in the place of the contents or the nucleus of a cell, or in the very substance of a simple membrane, a blastema, or a fibre, minute particles or granules are seen, which are recognised as consisting of oily or fatty matter, by their peculiar refraction of light, their solubility in ether, their aptness to coalesce into larger oil-drops, and, when they are very abundant, by the greasiness of the whole tissue, its burning with a bright flame, and its yielding to analysis an unusual quantity of fatty manner.   In examining organs in the state of fatty degeneration, we may commonly see the progress of the change in the gradual increase of the fatty particles.   Some cells, for example, may appear quite healthy ; some may deviate from health only in containing two or three shining, black-bordered, oil-particles ; in others, these are increased, and a large part of the cell-cavity is filled with minute oil-particles, or with one or more larger oil-drops ; and in others, the contents of the cell have given place to a single cluster of oil-drops.   In this last

* The index will afford at once a sufficient guide to these examples.

case, the degeneration is nearly complete: the transformed cell is called a "granule cell," or, when, as it often happens, the cell-wall has wasted and disappeared, it is a "granule-mass;" and the last stage of degeneration is that such masses may break up, their constituent molecules may dispart, and the tissue which was an aggregate of nucleated cells may become little more than a mass of molecules or drops of oily matter.

It is probably due in part to such disintegration of degenerate cells, that, in most organs thus degenerate, abundant fatty matter is found free, that is, lying in drops not enclosed, among the proper constituents of the tissue. But this free fat is also derived, in part, from the degeneration of intercellular substances, which is usually concurrent with that ensuing in the cells; and in some cases (as Virchow has observed in the liver) it so follows the arrangement of minute blood-vessels that it may be considered as the residue of a direct deposit or exudation from them.

In most instances the fatty degeneration affects, first and chiefly, as I have described it, the contents of cells or tubules, or the proper substance of membrane or other tissue. And when it thus happens, the nuclei almost always waste, and either shrivel or disappear after gradually fading in their outlines. This may be commonly seen in the fatty degeneration of the renal and hepatic cells, and of the muscular fibres; and it is a fact of some significance, when we remember the constancy and abundance of nuclei in actively growing parts. But, in certain cases, as in fatty degeneration of cartilages, the change appears to begin in the nuclei, which are gradually transformed into granule masses, while the cell-wall may remain unchanged, or may become thickly walled or laminated, or may coalesce with the surrounding tissue.

Such a transformation of a nucleus, while it retains its place and general form, might at once suggest that the fatty matter which collects in these degenerations is not introduced from without into the cells or other elements of the tissues; that it is not placed in them, as it may be in the parts around them, as a morbid deposit, or exudation from the blood-vessels; but rather is one of the products and residues of some chemical transformation which they undergo when the proper nutritive changes are suspended. We might derive the same suggestion from the similarly degenerate muscular fibres; in which we may often find the fat particles arranged in the same manner as the proper constituents of the fibrils, and looking as if there were a gradual transformation of the "sarcous elements" into the little oily particles, which, by clustering, and then by fusion, at length compose the larger oil-drops.

We gain other and better evidence of the fatty matter being derived from chemical changes in the tissue that is degenerate, from many other sources. Such changes are exemplified in the production of fatty matters during the spontaneous decompositions of nitrogenous substances. Many instances* of this are known, but none are so appropriate as the formation of adipocere in muscular tissue. Here, as Dr. Quain discovered, the places of the muscular fibres, blood-vessels, and nerves, are occupied by fatty matter, which could not have existed in them during life, which is far too abundant to have been derived from changes in the fatty matter that they naturally contain, and which, in confused crystals, retains their natural shape, size, and arrangement. And Dr. Quain has completed the evidence of the chemical nature of these degenerative changes, by an artificial imitation of them. He has shown that the textures of hearts (and the same is true of other parts), when placed in very dilute nitric acid, or in diluted spirit, pass into a condition exactly resembling that of the fatty degeneration which I have been describing.† No fact could be more apposite to prove that this form of degeneration is an atrophy for we may be very sure that when imitable chemistry prevails in a part, the forces of life, even those of morbid life, are defective or suspended in it.

The whole history of fatty degenerations concurs to prove that they are the result of defect, not of disease, of the nutritive process; and that they may be therefore classed with the atrophy which we recognize in merely diminished quantity of formation. Let me point out the chief features of this history: for even some repetition of the earlier part of the lecture will be justified by the utility of assigning their right place in pathology to changes of which (as is the case with all these degenerations) we are every year gathering new and very important illustrations.

I have said that the types or standards of degenerations are the changes naturally ensuing in old age. Now, accumulations of fat, which in many parts assume the forms of the fatty degeneration of tissues, are striking characteristics of old age, and especially of the commencement of senile infirmities. The results of senile atrophy are not, indeed, the same in all persons: rather, you find among old people, and you might almost thus arrange them into two classes, the lean and the fat; and these, as you may see them in any asylum for the aged, impersonate the two kinds of atrophy I have spoken of, as the withering and the fatty degenerations.

Some people, as they grow old, seem only to wither and dry up; sharp-featured, shrivelled, spinous old folk, yet withal wiry and tough, clinging to life, and letting death have them, as it were, by small instalments slowly paid. Such are the "lean and slippered pantaloons;" and their "shrunk shanks" declare the pervading atrophy.

* Many are collected by Virchow, in his Archiv., B. i., p. 167; and others by Dr. Quain Med. Chir. Trans., vol. xxxiii., p. 140, et seq. The facts concerning the formation of sugar from nitrogenous compounds in the liver are of the same kind.

† Dr. Quain has candidly referred to many previous observers by whom similar changes were recognized; but the honor of the full proof, and of the right use of it, belongs to himself alone. Respecting the method of the chemical transformations by which the change is accomplished, the best essay is, I think, that of Virchow (Archiv., B. i., p· 152).

Others, women more often than men, as old and as ill-natured as these, yet make a far different appearance. With these the first sign of old age is that they grow fat; and this abides with them till, it may be, in a last illness sharper than old age, they are robbed even of their fat. These, too, when old age sets in, become pursy, short-winded, pot-bellied, pale and flabby; their skin hangs, not in wrinkles, but in rolls; and their voice, instead of rising "towards childish treble," becomes gruff and husky.*

These classes of old people, I repeat, may represent the two chief forms of atrophy; of that with decrease, and that with fatty or other degeneration, of tissues. In those of the first class you find all the tissues healthy, hardly altered from the time of vigor. I examined the muscles of such an one; a woman, 76 years old, very lean, emaciated, and shrivelled. The fibres were rather soft, yet nearly as ruddy and as strongly marked as those of a vigorous man; her skin, too, was tough and dry; her bones, slender indeed, yet hard and clean; her defect was a simple defect of quantity, and of moisture.

But in those that grow fat as they grow old, you find, in all the tissues alike; bulk with imperfect texture; there is fat laid between, and even within, the muscular fibres; fat about and in the fibres of the heart, in the kidneys, and all the vessels; their bones are so greasy that no art can clean them: and they are apt to die through fatty degeneration of some important part, such as the heart, the minute cerebral blood-vessels, or the emphysematous lungs. The defect of all these tissues is the defect of quality.

Now, I do not pretend to account for this great difference in the con-comitants of the other infirmities of old age in different people. The explanation probably lies far among the mysteries of the chemical phy-siology of nutrition, of the formation of fat, and of respiratory excretion; and we may hope to find it when we know why, out of the same diet, and under all the same external conditions, one class of men, even in health and vigor, store up abundant fat, and another class excrete the elements of fat. In relation, however, to the present subject, the main point is, that the similarity of the conditions in which they occur implies similarity in the essential nature of the two changes, and that the defec-tive quantity and the defective quality of the tissues are both atrophies.

The same conclusion may be drawn from the frequent coincidence of the two methods of degeneration in the same part. In the limbs, the most common form of atrophy from disease is manifested in diminution of size, together with increase in the fatty matter combined with the

---

* Mr. Barlow, in some admirably written "General Observations on Fatty Degenera-tion," (Medical Times and Gazette, May 15th, 1852,) has pointed out that the climacteric disease, described by Sir H. Halford, and the "Decline of the Vital Powers in Old Age," described by Dr. Marshall Hall, are probably, in great measure, dependent on such fatty degeneration as these persons extremely exemplify.

muscles and bones. Such is the condition usually displayed by the bones and muscles of paralyzed limbs; in the majority of atrophied stumps after amputation; and in many other similar cases.

In like manner, the fatty degeneration of a part is commonly seen as the consequence of the very causes which, in other instances, give rise to simple wasting or emaciation of the same part. Thus, when the function of a part is abrogated, from whatever cause, the part may in one person shrink, in another degenerate into fat. The emaciation of a paralyzed limb is a familiar object: but in some cases the muscles of paralyzed limbs are hardly reduced in size, but are all transformed into fat. In the College Museum there is a pancreas, with a cancerous tumor pressing on its duct, and all behind the part obliterated is degenerated into fat; and in the Museum of St. Bartholomew's there is also a pancreas, the duct of which was obliterated; but in this, the part behind the obstruction is simply shrivelled, dry, hard, and scarcely lobulated. So, too, among the bones atrophied in different bed-ridden persons, some are exceedingly light, small, and dry: others are not small, but very greasy, full of fatty matter. Either of these results, also, or the two mingled in various proportions, may result from defective supply of blood; as in the cases of atrophy of parts of bones after fractures, as described by Mr. Curling, to which I shall have again to refer. So that from these, and from many other cases hereafter to be mentioned, we may say generally, that nearly all the ordinary causes of atrophy may produce, in any part, in one case reduction of size, in another fatty degeneration, in another a concurrence of the two.

Much yet remains to be said of this important change: but it will be more appropriate to the next and other lectures, in which I shall describe the fatty degenerations of several parts, and of the products of inflammation and other diseases, as well as that remarkable form of the degeneration which ensues, with the rapidity of an acute disease, in the proper textures of some inflamed parts. It seems only necessary, in conclusion, to state that there appears no necessary, or even frequent, connection between the fatty degeneration of any organ in particular, and that general tendency to the formation of fat which constitutes obesity. No doubt, a person, especially an elderly one, who has a natural tendency, even when in health, to become corpulent, will, *cæteris paribus*, be more likely to have fatty degeneration, than to have a wasting atrophy, in any organ which may fall into the conditions in which these changes originate. And, as a general rule, spirit-drinking, and the excessive use of hydro-carbonous articles of food, while favoring a general formation of fat, are apt to give rise to special fatty degeneration in the liver, or some other organ. Yet, on the other hand, one commonly finds the proper elements of the tissues—the heart, the liver, and the rest—quite healthy in men who are very corpulent. The muscular fibres of the heart, or of the voluntary muscles, may be imbedded

in adipose tissue, and yet may be themselves free from the least degeneration. So, also, the hepatic cells may be nearly free from fat within,
though there be much oil around them. Fat accumulated in tissue round
the elements of a part is a very different, probably an essentially different, thing from fat within them; the one is compatible with perfect
strength, the other is always a sign of loss of power. In the muscles of
some fish, such as the eel, it is hard to get a clear sight of the fibres, the
oily matter around them is so abundant: but the fibres are peculiarly
strong, and, in their own texture, make a striking contrast with the fibres
of a degenerate muscle, in which the fat is, in great part, within.

The same essential distinction between general and local fat-formation,
though they may often coincide, is shown in the fact that the local formation very often happens in those whose general condition is that of
emaciation, as in the phthisical and chloritic.

On the whole, therefore, we must conclude that something much more
than a general tendency to form fat, or a general excess of fat in the
blood, is necessary to produce a local fatty degeneration. The general
conditions are favorable, but not essential, to this form of atrophy.

LECTURE VI.

ATROPHY.

THE last lecture was chiefly occupied with a general account of those
changes of texture which are to be regarded as atrophies; and now,
having pointed out what affections may be classed under this term, the
whole subject may be more largely illustrated by particular examples.

First, as to the conditions in which atrophy, whether with decrease or
with degeneration, may ensue. Many of them may be most easily explained as the very contraries of the conditions in which hypertrophy
originates. Thus, as we have seen that when a part is, within certain
limits, over-exercised, it is over-nourished; so, if a part be used less
than is proper, it suffers atrophy. For instance, in the Museum of St.
Bartholomew's (Ser. 12; 57), is the heart of a man fifty years old, who
died with cancer of the stomach in extreme emaciation. It is extremely
small, and weighed only five ounces four drachms; whereas, according to
the estimates of Dr. Clendinning, in a healthy man of the same age the
heart weighs upwards of nine ounces. But, small as it is, this heart was
adapted to the work it had to do; and in this adaptation we have the
purpose of its atrophy. For, because of his cancer, the man had less
blood, and needed less force of the heart to propel it: so that, in direct
opposition to what I described as the course of events in hypertrophy,
here, as the quantity of blood diminished, and the waste of the heart by

exercise in propelling it diminished, so the repair of the waste diminished somewhat more than the waste itself did: and the heart, though less wasted, became smaller, till it was only large enough for the propulsion of the scanty supply of blood.

The same may be said of a heart of which there is a drawing in the same Museum. It was taken from a woman twenty-two years old, who died with diabetes. It weighed only five ounces; yet, doubtless, it was enough for her impoverished supply of blood.

It would be superfluous to describe many instances of atrophy through defective exercise, or abrogated function of parts. The wasted and degenerate limbs of the bed-ridden, the shrunken brains of the aged and the imbecile, the withered overies and uteri of many barren women, are good examples of defective nutrition adapted to defective exercise of function: and so are the atrophied distal parts of nerves whose trunks have been divided, and the atrophied columns of the spinal cord that correspond with inactive portions of the brain. The rapid degeneration and removal of the tissue of the uterus after parturition, and the rapid disappearances of temporary organs of various kinds, are as striking examples of atrophy following the abrogation or completion of office. To some of these examples I shall again refer.

It is in similar contrast with the history of increased growths, that, as an excess of the constituents of which a tissue may form itself produces hypertrophy of that tissue, so may defect of those constituents produce atrophy. Thus, the quantity of adipose tissue diminishes even below what is natural to the several parts, as often as the fat-making constituents are deficient in the food, and therefore in the blood. So, the formation of bones is defective during deficiency of the supply of bone-earths; the mammary glands waste when the materials for the formation of milk are imperfectly supplied; and the whole body wastes in general defect or poverty of blood.

Again, as I showed instances in which the increased flow of healthy blood through a part produced hypertrophy, so are there more numerous examples of merely defective nutrition in consequence of a diminished supply of blood. Some of the most striking of these were first described by Mr. Curling,* in cases of fractured femora and other bones, showing atrophy of that portion which, by the fracture, was cut off from the supply of blood through the great nutritive or medullary artery. The consequence of the withdrawal of so much of the blood from the upper or lower fragment, according to the position of the fracture, is not death; for the anastomosis between the vessels of the wall and those of the medullary tissue of the bone is enough to support life, though not enough to support vigorous nutrition; but the frequent consequence of the fracture is an atrophy of the part thus deprived of a portion of its ready supply of blood.

* Medico-Chirurg. Trans. vol. xx.

Similar instances are seen in the decrease or degeneration of portions of hearts when single branches of a cornary artery are obstructed ;* in the wasting of a portion of kidney when a branch of a renal artery is closed;† and in local softening of the brain, with obliteration of single cerebral arteries.‡

In all these instances we see that conditions contrary to those giving rise to hypertrophy produce atrophy. But there are many other conditions from which atrophy in a part may ensue; defects in quantity, or in the constitution, of the blood; defective or disturbed nervous influence, as through excessive mental exertion; the disturbances of disease or injury, as in inflammations, specific morbid infiltratias, &c. In short, whatever interferes with or interrupts any of those conditions which I enumerated as essential to healthy nutrition, may give rise to atrophy, either general or local. The clinical history of the fatty degeneration of the heart, so largely illustrated by Dr. Ormerod§ and Dr. Quain,‖ may best prove how multiform are the events from which the atrophy of a single organ may arise.

But besides all the instances in which atrophy of a part may arise as a secondary process, there are others in which we are so unable to trace its precedents, that we are tempted to speak of it as primary, or spontaneous, in the same sense as we might so call the natural wasting of the Wolffian bodies, the thymus, and other temporary organs. It is as if an atrophy of old age, instead of affecting all parts simultaneously, took place prematurely in one.

Whatever the true explanation may be, most of the parts of the body appear to be subject to this seemingly spontaneous atrophy; and it generally manifests itself in some form of degeneration. Its most frequent seats are the heart and arteries, the bones, muscles, liver, and kidneys; but it occurs also in the pancreas and the salivary glands, and in the testicle. It is yet more frequent in morbid products, as in the fibrinous deposits on the anterior of arteries, the exudations of inflammation, and tumors of every kind.

The contrast between hypertrophy and atrophy is, thus, nearly as great in the number, as in the kind, of the conditions in which they may severally arise. And, once more, we may contrast them in regard to the mode in which the vessels and nerves adapt themselves. As a part becomes atrophied, its blood-vessels and its nerves are consequently and proportionally changed. In atrophy of the eye, the optic nerve and artery diminish; and, in a case of fatty degeneration of the adductor muscles of the thigh, in consequence of disease of the hip-joint, I found

* Quain, Medico-Chir. Trans. xxxiii. p. 148; Virchow, Archiv. iv. p. 387.
† Simon, Lectures on Pathology, p. 94.
‡ Kirkes, Med.-Chir. Trans. vol. xxxv.
§ Medical Gazette, 1849.
‖ Medico-Chirurgical Trans., vol. xxxiii. 1850.

corresponding atrophy of their nerves. The atrophy of the nerves must have been, in this case, secondary: the course of events being, inaction of the muscles in consequence of the disease of the joint; then, atrophy of them in consequence of their inaction; and, finally, atrophy of the nerves following that of the muscles.

From these general considerations I proceed to speak particularly of Atrophy, as it manifests itself in some of the principal organs and tissues of the body;—and first of the Atrophy of Muscles.

The affection has been well studied in all the three forms of muscular tissue; namely, in the voluntary muscles, in the heart, and in the organic or smooth-fibred muscles; and I will describe it in each of these in order.

The voluntary muscles exhibit, in different conditions, both the chief forms of atrophy; that, namely, with decrease or wasting, and that with fatty degeneration.

In a wasted muscle, such as one sees, for example, in the limbs of those who are only emaciated, the fibres may appear almost perfectly healthy: they are rather paler, indeed, and softer, and more disposed to be tortuous, than in the natural state; for muscles are commonly withered when they are thus reduced in size; yet their transverse striæ, and all their other characteristic features, are well marked.

In the state of fatty degeneration, the whole of a voluntary muscle may appear pale, bleached, or of some yellowish or tawny hue, soft and easily torn. But a more frequent appearance is that in which fasciculi is the healthy state, and others in various degrees of degeneration, lie in parallel bands, and give the whole muscle a streaky appearance, with various hues intermediate between the ruddiness of healthy flesh, and the dull, pale, tawny-yellow, or yellowish-white, of the complete degeneration. In such a case (and this may appear remarkable) healthy primitive fibres may lie among those that are degenerated. Of the latter, some, in place of the transverse striæ, present dark very minute dots arranged in transverse lines; in others, the whole fibre has a dim, pale, granular aspect, with no definite arrangement of the granules; in others, little oil-globules adhere to the interior of the sarcolemma; and in others, such globules are collected more abundantly, and to the proportionally greater exclusion of the proper constituents of the fibres: but the characters of fatty degeneration are rarely, if ever, so well marked in the fibres of voluntary muscles as in those of the heart.

In the examination of different examples of fatty degeneration of the voluntary muscles, you may find much diversity in the tissue between the fibres and fasciculi. In some instances, the interspaces between the fasciculi are filled with cellular tissue, both more abundant and tougher than that in healthy muscle, so that it may be hard to dissect the fibres for the microscope. With this there may be no unusual quantity of fat;

but, in other cases, the quantity of fat between the fibres is very great, and the fibres themselves may seem empty, or wasted, as if overwhelmed by the fat accumulating around them. In such a case, when the accumulating fat has coalesced with that which before surrounded the whole muscle, it may be difficult to find where the muscle was; for the whole of what belonged to it, after its degeneration, may be gone, and in its place there may remain only an obscure trace, if any, of fibrous arrangement, dependent on the position of the principal partitions of the new fatty tissue.

I cannot yet speak positively in explanation of this diversity in the state of parts between the fibres. But, I think, the increase and toughness of the cellular tissue (when it is not the product of organized inflammatory deposit) exist only in atrophied muscles which have had to resist stretching, after the manner of ligaments; as, for example, when their antagonists are not as powerless as themselves. And the increase of fat seems to be found only when a muscle has been very long atrophied, and has remained completely at rest; then, the fibres themselves, after degenerating, may be removed, and give place to a formation of common adipose tissue, which collects in every part that they are leaving, just as it does about shrinking kidneys, some cancers of the breast, old diseased joints, and other parts similarly circumstanced.

In either case, we must distinguish between these formations of fat outside, and those within, the fibres; the former are in no necessary connection with the proper atrophy of the fibres, but generally appear subsequent to it; and when they attain their highest degree, they are not to be regarded as degenerations of the muscular tissue; for they are not, in any sense, formed out of it, though they occupy the place from which it was removed.

The condition in which atrophy of the voluntary muscles most commonly ensues is inaction. Whenever muscles lie long inactive, they either waste or degenerate; and this whether the inactivity depend on paralysis through affection of the nervous centres or fibres, or fixity of the parts they should move, or on any other cause. The degenerative process may be so rapid that, in a fortnight, muscles paralyzed in hemiplegia may present a manifest change of color; but it is commonly a much slower process.

The course of events in these cases appears to be, that the want of exercise of a muscle, whether paralyzed or fixed at its ends, makes its due nutrition impossible; and the atrophy thus brought about is the cause of loss of irritability of the muscle, i. e., of loss of its capacity for contracting. For the experiments of Dr. John Reid* show that loss of contractile power in a paralyzed muscle is due, directly, to its imperfect nutrition, and only indirectly to the loss of connection with the nervous

* Edin. Monthly Jour. of Med. Science, May, 1841. See, also, M. Brown-Sequard, in the Gaz. Médicale, No. 9, 1850.

centres. When he divided the nerves of a frog's hind legs, and left one limb inactive, but gave the muscles of the other frequent exercise, by galvanizing the lower end of its divided nerve, he found (to state the case very briefly) that at the end of two months the exercised muscles retained their weight and texture, and their capacity of contraction; while the inactive ones (though their irratability, it might be said, had not been exhausted by exercise,) had lost half their bulk, were degenerate in texture, and had also lost some of their power of contracting. In other cases, too, he found the loss of proper texture always ensuing in the inactive state, before the power of contraction was lost.

It is doubtless the same in man. A muscle which, by no fault of its own, but through circumstances external to itself, has been prevented from acting, soon becomes incapable of acting even when the external obstacles to action are removed. Hence we may deduce a rule which ought to be acted on in practice. When a person has had hemiplegia, one commonly sees that long after the brain has, to all appearance, recovered its power, or even through all the rest of life, the paralysed limbs remain incapable of action, and as motionless as at the first attack. Now, it is not likely that this abiding paralysis is the consequence of any continuing disease of the brain: rather, we must ascribe it to the imperfect condition into which the muscles and nerve-fibres have fallen during their inaction. So long as the state of the brain makes voluntary action impossible, the cord, nerves, and muscles, are suffering atrophy; then, when the brain recovers, they are not in a state to obey its impulses, because they are degenerate; and thus, their inaction continuing, they degenerate more and more, and all remedy becomes impossible. If this be true, Dr. Reid's experiments suggest the remedy. When muscles are paralysed through affection of the nervous system, we ought to give them artificial exercise: they should be often put in action by electricity or otherwise; their action, though thus artificial, will insure their nutrition; and then, when the nervous system recovers, they may be in a condition ready to act with it.

You will find this suggestion ingeniously supported by my friend Mr. W. F. Barlow, in a paper published by him in the Lancet. In one case, in which I could act upon it, the result was encouraging. A little girl, about eight years old, had angular curvature and complete loss of voluntary movement in the lower extremities. This had existed some weeks, but as I found she had reflex movements, the legs twitching in a very disorderly way as often as the souls were touched, I advised that the limbs should be put in active exercise, for about an hour two or three times a day, by tickling the feet, or in some similar way. The result was, that when, several weeks afterwards, the spinal cord recovered, and she could again direct the effort of the will to the lower limbs, the recovery of strength was speedy and complete; more so, I think, than if, in the paralysed condition, the muscles and nerves had been left to the progress of the atrophy. A similar paralysis, about two years later, occurred again, and was similarly recovered from.

The hindered action of muscles, though the most frequent, is not the only condition from which their atrophy may ensue. They waste, together with all the rest of the body, in most emaciating diseases; as, for example, in phthisis: and they may degenerate into fat, in concert with other tissues, in a generally defective nutrition.

But, besides the general atrophies of muscles, a similar affection occurs sometimes as a primary or spontaneous affection of one or more muscles. We find sometimes one of the muscles of an extremity, or of the back, thoroughly atrophied, while the others are healthy; and no account can be given of its failure.

It is not very unfrequent to find a portion of the lower and posterior part of the recti abdominis muscles in a state of fatty degeneration.

Rokitansky* briefly refers to a spontaneous fatty degeneration of the muscles of the calf attended with extreme pain: and Mr. Mayo† has recorded two cases of apparently spontaneous atrophy of the muscles of the shoulder, in which, in a few weeks after severe pain, but no other sign of acute inflammation, all the muscles about the shoulder became simply, but exceedingly, atrophied.

We name these spontaneous atrophies, and it may be that the defective nutrition is the first event in the abnormal chain; but, I think, we shall hereafter find that, in most of them, the degeneration is a part of some inflammatory process; for, as I shall have to describe in future lectures, there is no tissue in which it is more evident than in the muscles, that a degeneration of the proper elements of an inflamed part is associated with the more obvious effects of inflammation.

Atrophy of the muscular substance of the heart, may, like that of which I have just been speaking, appear in either wasting or degeneration, or in a combination of the two. Of the former, I mentioned examples in the beginning of the lecture, in the heart of a cancerous man 50 years old, which weighed only five ounces four drachms; and that of a diabetic woman, 25 years old, which weighed only five ounces one drachm. Both these had deviated from the general rule of enlargement of the heart with advancing years, in adaptation to the diminished quantity of blood, and the general diminution of the body.

In these cases there is a uniform decrease of the heart: its cavities become small, and its walls proportionally thin; and the fat on its exterior diminishes or is changed into a succulent, œdematous tissue. In other instances the cavities are dilated, without proportionate thickening, or, it may be, even with thinning of their walls. This probably, occurs, chiefly in cases of such increased obstacle to the circulation as might, in

* Pathol. Anat., B. 2, S. 348.
† Outlines of Human Pathology, 1836, p. 117.

other persons, or in other conditions, engender hypertrophy of the heart. Or, the dilatation may be the consequence of wasting in a heart that was once large and strong.

But, an atrophy of the heart much more important than any of these, is that which consists in fatty degeneration.

Extreme instances of fatty degeneration of the heart have been long known. The whole, or the greater part of the heart in such cases, may seem reduced to fat; the degenerate tissue having coalesced with that which lies on the surface, and the degeneration being accompanied by thinning and softening of the walls.

In like manner, the cases have been well known and described for which Dr. Quain proposes the name of "fatty growth," to distinguish them from the "fatty degenerations" of the heart. In these, the adipose tissue accumulates in unusual quantity on those parts of the exterior of the heart in which it naturally exists, and is found, though often emaciated and very soft, even in the thinnest people; viz., along its transverse furrow, the furrows in which the coronary vessels run, and others. From these positions, the fat dipping more and more deeply may nearly displace the fibres, and may lead to a secondary degeneration of them: but, commonly, the heart's fibres are themselves healthy, even when they lie completely imbedded in the overgrown fat.

But these conditions, and their combinations, are too well known to need that I should describe them, or refer particularly to any specimens of them, except to a sheep's heart, which is in the College Museum (No. 1529), and which shows, in an extreme degree, a method of the growth of fat, which is rarely imitated, in even a trivial measure, in the human subject. It exhibits a great accumulation of fat on its surface, and its walls are thin; but the greater part of the cavities of the ventricles and of the left auricle are occupied by large lobulated growths of suet-like fat. The weight of the fat here added to the heart is 25 ounces, and it is said that there was also a large accumulation of fat about the kidneys. But no other history of the case is extant than that the sheep was inactive, and had dyspnœa on exertion.

These cases of extreme fatty growth, or of extreme degeneration, of the heart are much rarer than those of which I have now to speak.

The most common form of fatty degeneration is that in which you find, on opening the heart, that its tissue is in some degree paler and softer than in the natural state, and lacks that robust firmness which belongs to the vigorous heart. But what is most characteristic is, that you may see, especially just under the endocardium, spots, small blotches, or lines, like undulating or zigzag transverse bands, of pale, tawny, buff, or ochre-yellow hue, thickset, so as to give, at a distant view, a mottled appearance. These manifestly depend not on any deposit among the fasciculi, but on some change of their tissue. For, at their borders, you find these spots gradually shaded-off, and merging into the healthy color of the heart; and when you examine portions of such spots with the microscope, you never fail to find the fatty degeneration of the fibre.

The yellow spotting, or transverse marking of the heart, may exist in the walls of all its cavities at once, or may be found in a much greater degree in one than in the others. It may exist in all parts of the thickness of the walls, or may be chiefly evident beneath the endocardium and pericardium. It is far less common in the auricles than in the ventricles; and when it exists simultaneously in all parts it is less advanced in the auricles. It is more common in the left ventricle than in the right; and in the left ventricle it is commonly most advanced on the smooth upper part of the septum, and in the two large prominent fleshy columns. Indeed, it may exist in these columns alone; and when, in such a case, the rest of the heart remains strong, may account for the occasional occurrence of rupture of the columns.

These yellow spottings of the heart, produced by degeneration of scattered portions of its fibres, are, as I have said, the most evident, as well as the most frequent, indications of its degenerative atrophy. But a similar affection may exist in a worse form, though it be less manifest: worse, because the degeneration is more extensive and more uniform; and less manifest, because it is less distinctly visible to the naked eye, and must be recognized by the touch rather than by the unaided sight. The whole heart feels soft, doughy, inelastic, unresisting; it may be moulded and doubled up like a heart beginning to decompose long after death: it seems never to have been in the state of *rigor mortis*. These conditions are more manifest when a section is made through the wall of the left ventricle. Then, if the wall be only partly cut through, the rest of it may be very easily torn, as if with separation of fibres that only stick together; and the cut surface of the wall looks, as it were, lobulated and granular, almost like a piece of soft conglomerate gland, an appearance which is yet more striking when observed with a simple lens of about half an inch focus. In color, the heart has not on its surface, much less on its section, the full ruddy brown of healthy heart, a color approaching that of the strong voluntary muscle; but is, for the most part, of a duller, dirtier, lighter brown, in some parts gradually blending with irregular marks or blotches of a paler fawn, or dead-leaf-color.

These appearances of the degenerate heart may be variously mingled; and they may be variously associated with overgrowths of the external fat, or with previous hypertrophy or other changes of structure in the heart. But, however much the appearances of the affection may be obscured, the general characters of softness, paleness, mottled color, and friability, will be sufficient, if not always to prove, yet always to excite suspicion, that the fatty degeneration of the heart exists: and, if only suspicion is excited, the microscopic examination may be always decisive. The chief microscopic appearances are delineated in the adjoining sketch.

When a portion of the heart's walls, especially if they are very soft, is dissected in the ordinary way, with needles, for the microscope, the fibres are broken into short pieces, some twice, some five or six times, as long as they are broad. The broken ends of these short pieces are usually squared: but some are round, or irregular, or cloven, and broken off lower down. The pieces are almost always completely separated, having no appearance of even cohering at their sides, and they lie scattered disorderly.

Fig. 6.*

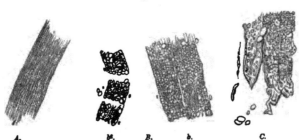

A.   *b².*   *B.*   *b.*   *C.*

In whichever form the degeneration is examined, you may find that, in some pieces, the transverse striæ are still well seen and undisturbed, appearing quite as in health. In more, they are inturrupted or obscured by dark dots, or by glistening particles with shady, black margins, like minute oil-particles scattered without order in the fibres. Where such particles are few, they appear to lie especially, or only, in contact with the interior of the sarcolemma; but, where more numerous, they appear to occupy every part of the fibre, leaving the transverse striæ discernible only at its margins, or even completely obscuring or replacing them, and making the fibre look like a gland-tube filled with dark granules and larger glistening dark-edged fat-particles. Where these particles are very numerous in a fibre, they appear also generally larger, and more generally glistening and black-edged, like larger oil-particles.

There may be no oil-drops floating about; no fat-cells; scarcely even any of the minute particles, which are seen in the fibres, may appear out of them; the field of the microscope may be perfectly clean. In these minor respects, however, many differences exist; though I think it may be stated that the degeneration is very rarely, if ever, accompanied by any morbid product deposited between the fibres; whatever fatty matter may appear between them, is only such as has escaped from them.

As a general rule, the palest parts of the heart are most advanced in

* *A.* Muscular fibres of the healthy human heart.

B. Fatty degeneration of the fibres of the human heart; *b*, early stage; *b²*, more advanced.

C. The same, yet more advanced, all magnified 400 times. From Dr. Quain's plates Med. Chir. Trans., vol. xxxiii., pl. 3.

the disease; but even in microscopic portions some pieces of fibres appear hardly changed, while those all round them are completely granular.

I alluded, in the last lecture, to the defective condition of the nuclei of degenerate elemental structures. This is peculiarly well shown in the degenerate fibres of the heart. When those of a healthy heart are placed in diluted acetic acid, they display a longitudinal series of nuclei, at nearly equal distances apart, and usually lying in the middle of the presenting surface of the fibre. Such nuclei are, so far as I know, peculiar to the heart-fibres. They are large, reddish-yellow, like blood-globules, especially when the heart is very robust: they are elongated, oval, or nearly quadrilateral; and at each of their ends one almost always sees tapering groups of small, isolated, yellowish granules, like particles separated from them, and gradually withering. But in the degenerate fibre, when the change is least advanced, the outlines of the nucleus look dim, and it loses its color: when the change has made further progress, the nucleus cannot be seen at all, though its former place may be indicated by some of the narrw group of granules; and in a yet later stage, when the sarcolemma appears nearly full of fatty particles, all trace is lost alike of the nucleus and of the granules.

I have spoken of fatty degeneration of the heart at this great length, both because there is no better example for illustration of the general pathology of such offections, and because it is extremely important that this condition of the heart should be recognized after death, even when no suspicion could be entertained of it during life. For it often introduces unexpected dangers into the ordinary practice of surgery: it is, I believe, not rarely the cause of sudden death after operations; it is one of the conditions in which chloroform should be administered with more than ordinary caution. They who labor under it may be fit for all the ordinary events of calm and quiet life, but they are unable to resist the storm of a sickness, an accident, or an operation. And let it not be said that one learns little in learning too late the existence of an incurable disease; for very often the death that has come from such a disease has been ascribed to a wrong cause, and has spoiled confidence in good men and their good measures. Nor does the caution seem unnecessary that, serious as the effects of the disease are, the change of structure may escape any but a very careful and practised examiner. For, often, the change is hardly manifest to the eye, though while it affects the whole heart, it may have destroyed life.*

Atrophy of the organic or smooth-fibred muscles doubtless occurs as

---

* When the lecture was delivered, in 1847, I related some cases of sudden death from this affection; and expressed the hope that its whole clinical history would be traced by Dr. Ormerod, who helped me very much in investigating its morbid anatomy. The hope has been fulfilled far beyond my expectation by both him and Dr. R. Quain, who was, at the same time, actively occupied with a similar course of inquiry. I may therefore refer the reader to their essays, in the Medical Gazette for 1849, vol. ii.; and in the Medico-Chirurgical Transactions, vol. xxxiii.: essays, valuable alike for the importance of their facts, and for the thoroughly scientific spirit in which they are conceived.

a simple decrease of them in the thinning of the coats of the intestines, stomach, and other hollow organs, which is sometimes associated with general emaciation, or with diminished function : but the change has not been carefully studied. Of the fatty degeneration of this muscular tissue, examples are described in the muscular coats of the arteries,* which partake in the corresponding change, or atheromatous affection, of their thickened internal coats; in the coats of the urinary bladder ;† and in the uterus.‡ In the latter organ the change has peculiar interest ; taking place, as it does, quickly after the fulfilment of office in parturition ; affecting all the muscular fibro-cells which, during gestation, had been developed to their perfection ; and preceding their absorption and replacement by new-formed fibro-cells, like those which existed in the young and unimpregnated uterus. The series of changes thus traced by Kilian tell a complete history of nutrition, in the succession of development and growth to perfection, of discharge of function, consequent degeneration, absorption, and replacement by new structures that, in their progress, pass through the same phases as their predecessors. The production of fat in the uterine tissue confirms also the probability which I have already mentioned (p. 50), that fat is one of the usual results of the chemical change which takes place in muscular action, and is, in this relation, a substance, like the kreatine, which is also found in the uterine tissue after birth,§ intermediate and transitional between the proper constituents of the tissues and the oxidised materials of excretions. It may be added, that the whole substance of the uterus and its membranes partakes of the degenerative change, and that the removal of the old tissues and the formation of new ones is so total, that, as it has been justly said, a person has a new uterus after each delivery. But the peculiarity of the case is only in that the change is accomplished quickly, manifestly, and simultaneously in a large mass of tissue : in the same sense, though at unknown times, men have often new hearts, new glands, and new brains.

In the bones we may probably consider that a calcareous degeneration occurs as a method of atrophy, in addition to those just described in the muscles : for to such a degeneration we may ascribe the increased proportion of bone-earths in the skeletons of aged persons. The augmentation of earthy constituents is not attended with increased strength of the

---

* Rokitansky, Pathol. Anat., ii. p. 543; Kölliker, Zeitschr. für wissensch. Zoologie, i. p. 81.

† Mr. Hancock, as quoted by Mr. Barlow, Med. Times and Gazette, May 15, 1852.—The change of which I spoke, in this lecture, as a kind of fatty degeneration of the bladder in old people, was not proved to be degeneration of the muscular fibres : neither, I think, has this been yet proved, though it is highly probable, in the muscular coat of the gall-bladder.

‡ Kölliker, l. c. p. 73. Kilion, in Henle und Pfeufer's Keitschr. für rat. Mediciu, vols. viii. and ix.

§ Siegmund, in the Würzburg Verhandlungen, B. iii. H. 1.

bones: rather, they become, in old persons, thin-walled, and more easily broken; the change being commonly associated with both wasting and fatty degeneration, and the whole tissue being rarified. It is through this general want of compactness in their construction that old bones are weak: for, as Dr. Stark's analysis show very well, the strength of bones depends more on their compactness than on the proportion of their constituents.

I am not aware that any analysis of diseased or other bones have shown a calcareous degeneration of them, except in old age: but its frequent occurrence is highly probable. The other modes of atrophy may be more fully illustrated in the two forms already often referred to. The simple wasting of a bone is a common change. Examples have been already adduced in connection with the subject of unequal length of the limbs (p. 69), and with that of the effects of pressure (p. 71), as well as in relation to the general history of atrophies. Among many specimens in the College Museum, the most striking is the skeleton of an hydrocephalic patient from the collection of Mr. Liston (No. 3489). It is the more remarkable, because while all the bones of the trunk and limbs are reduced by atrophy, to exceeding thinness and lightness, the bones of the cranium are as exceedingly enlarged in adaptation to the enormous volume of their contents.

Another interesting specimen is a skull (No. 8) fitted up by Hunter to show the movements of the edentulous lower jaw, as he has described them in his "Natural History of the Teeth." It shows the atrophy not only of the alveolar margins, but of every part of the jaws, and even of their palatine parts, and those of the palate bones, which are quite thin and transparent.

A rare specimen of atrophy of the lower jaw is shown in a case of complete osseous anchylosis of both temporo-maxillary articulations, from Mr. Howship's Museum (No. 966). Similar atrophy of bone in its extreme state is illustrated by an example of anchylosis of the knee (No. 384), from the case described by Mr. Thurnam.* Considerable apertures are formed in the wasted walls of the femur and tibia, and they were covered in by the periosteum alone: the whole thickness of these portions of the walls having been removed in the progress of the atrophy.

In the Museum of St. Bartholomew's is a specimen in which simple atrophy of the femora led to such fracture as, being effected by a slight force, is called spontaneous. The atrophy of these bones occurred coincidently with extreme emaciation of all the other parts, as well as of the skeleton; an emaciation which was to be described, I believe, more to starvation than to anything else. The shafts of the femora are exceedingly small, and their walls are so thin that, although their texture appears healthy, they could not resist the force of the muscles acting on he articular ends. They broke: and the result shows a remarkable example of the capacity for repair of injuries even while the process of ordinary nutrition seems almost suspended: for the fractures were firmly reunited.

I might greatly multiply examples of such simple wasting atrophy of bones; but let this suffice, that I may speak now of fatty degeneration of the bones.

I have already said that it is common, in many atrophied bones, to find an excess of fatty matter; I referred to old bones laden with fat as examples of a form of senile atrophy; and sometimes, in cases of diseased joints, the form of atrophy assumed by the disused bones is that not merely of exceeding thinness of the walls and wasting of the cancelli, but of an accumulation of soft fat filling every interstice and maintaining the size of the bone. But it is now to be added, that the bones, like other organs, are liable to a fatty degeneration, which, because of the obscurity of its origin, we must be content to call spontaneous; and this fatty degeneration of the bones is the disease which most English writers have described as Mollities Ossium.

The Museum of the College has a remarkably rich collection of specimens of this disease: a collection embracing specimens from nearly all the cases with whose histories we are most familiar.

Well-marked examples of the fatty degeneration are shown in No. 400. These are two femora fractured by a slight force, and, in their dried state, light, very greasy, mahogany-brown, and so soft that you may crush many parts of them with the fingers. Their excess of fat is evident.; but no more of their history is known than that they came from an elderly, if not an old man,—an Archbishop of Canterbury.

In No. 398 is a section of a humerus, affected, as many other bones of the same person were, with extreme fatty degeneration; and the Catalogue contains, with its description, a reprint of an essay, by Mr. Hunter, which escaped even the careful research of the editor of his works, Mr. Palmer. His essay is entitled, "Observations on the Case of Mollities Ossium described," &c., by Mr. Goodwin, in the London Medical Journal.* It was communicated in a letter to Dr. Simmons, the editor of that journal, and I will quote one passage, to show both what was the original appearance of the bones, and how completely Mr. Hunter's description confirms the opinion that this Mollities Ossium was really a fatty degeneration of the bones. He says, speaking of this humerus, "The component parts of the bone were totally altered, the structure being very different from other bones, and wholly composed of a new substance, resembling a species of fatty tumor, and giving the appearance of a spongy bone, deprived of its earth, and soaked in soft fat."

Nothing can better express the character of the change, or its simi-

* Vol. vi., 1785.

larity to the fatty degenerations of other organs, in which we find the proper substance of the part gradually changed for fat, and the whole tissue spoiled, while the size and outer form of the part remain unaltered.

The same characters are shown in the often-quoted case by Mr. Howship, of which specimens are preserved in Nos. 401–2–3. The last of these specimens shows what remained of the upper part of a femur after boiling; scarce anything besides a great quantity of white crystaline fatty matter.

It is the same with a femur (No. 403 B) presented to the Museum by Mr. Tamplin, in the examination of which I first obtained, with the microscope, the conviction of the nature of the change which constitutes what we call Mollities Ossium. This has the same characters as the specimens already shown, and the medulla of the bone had the bright yellow, pink, and deep crimson hues, which are so striking in many instances of the disease. But the constituents of this apparently peculiar material were, free oil in great quantity; crystals of margarine, free, or enclosed in fat-cells; a few fat-cells full of oil as in health, but many more, empty, collapsed, and rolled-up in strange and deceptive forms. The pink and crimson colors were owing to the bright tints of a part of the oil-globules, and of the nuclei and granules in the collapsed fat-cells; and there was no appearance whatever of an excess of blood in the bone, or any of its contents.

From this examination, therefore, as well as from all the other facts, I concur entirely in Mr. Curling's opinion respecting this disease.[*] A specimen (No. 403 A) from the case on which he chiefly founded his opinion, and which he has very accurately described, closely resembles those I have referred to. He proposes the name "Eccentric Atrophy of Bone" to express one of the principal characters of the disease; and I would have adopted it, as preferable to "Osteoporosis," under which I think Rokitansky would include these cases, but that it seems desirable to class this affection with others to which it bears the closest analogy, by giving the same generic name in the designation, fatty degeneration of bones.

The cases to which I have now referred include the principal examples of the disease observed and recorded in England under the name of mollities ossium; and to these, I think, may be added the case described by Mr. Solly,[†] for the appearances presented by the femur (No. 403 C) are strikingly similar to those in the specimens already referred to, and the material filling its medully cavity contained abundant fatty matter.

You might ask, then, what is the real Mollities Ossium? or is there such a disease different from what these specimens show? I could not from my own observations answer such a question; for I have never seen a specimen which appeared to fulfil in any degree the general notion of Mollities Ossium, as a disease consisting in the removal of the earthy matter of bone, and the reduction of any part of the skeleton to its cartilaginous, base. I do not doubt the accuracy of what others have written of such an affection: but I am sure, that the cases I have cited are not simple softenings of bone, but fatty degenerations; and that those cases must be very different to which Rokitansky refers under the names of, Osteomalacia, Malakosteon, Knochenerweichung, and Rachitismus adultorum. He gives, as a characteristic of the disease, that it affects the bones of the trunk, or a part of them, much more often, and more severely, than the bones of the extremities, and occurs especially after child-bed. Now, in the cases which I have endeavored to illustrate, the extremities, not the trunk, are the chief seats of the disease; and there is no evidence of the fatty degeneration occurring more often after delivery than in any other period or condition of life. So that, on the whole, I think we may consider there are two diseases included under the name of Mollities Ossium; namely, the fatty degeneration which these specimens show, and which seems to be the more frequent in England; and the simpler softening of bone, or rickets of the adult, to which Rokitansy's description alludes, and in which the bones are flexible rather than brittle, and appear reduced to their cartilaginous state. This affection seems to be more frequent than the fatty degeneration in Germany and France: and I think the only probable, well recorded instance of its occurrence in England, is that related by Mr. Dalrymple,[*] Dr. Bence Jones,[†] and Dr. Macintyre.[‡]

I feel, however, that there is still much doubt respecting the relations of these affections; they are, perhaps, more nearly allied than, at first sight, they may seem; and I think some clue to their alliance may be obtained from the relation which they both have to the rickets of the young subject. The relation is best shown in the bones of the skull, and is illustrated by specimens in the College Museum (Nos. 392 to 396, and 2857 to 2860); but I need not now dwell upon it while wishing to give only a general account of the atrophies of bone.[§]

I can scarcely doubt that future inquiries will ascertain that, in every tissue, changes such as these which I have described in muscle and in bone are the results of simply defective nutrition. But I have neither knowledge nor space for more than a few additional instances. Among these, the degenerations of blood-vessels may be cited. The blood-vessels of an atrophied part, I have already said, decrease in adaptation

---

* Dublin Journal of Med. Science, vol. ii., 1846.
† Philos. Trans., 1848.   ‡ Medico-Chir. Trans., vol. xxxiii.
§ I have minutely described the specimens here referred to, as well as the later changes which the bones undergo, in the Pathological Catalogue of the College Museum, vol. ii. p. 22, and vol. v. p. 7.

to the part: they become less, till they can carry no more blood than is just enough to meet the diminished requirements of nutrition: and this they do, not by such muscular contraction as adapts them to a temporary decrease of function in a part, but (if one may so speak) by a diminishing growth. Moreover, when a part degenerates, its blood-vessels are likely to degenerate in the same manner. There are, I think, instances in which fatty degenerations of blood-vessels have occurred in consequence of similar change in the part that they supply. But the more interesting examples are those of primary degeneration of the blood-vessels. This has been long known in the atheromatous disease, as it was called, of the larger arteries; the true nature of which, as a fatty and calcareous degeneration of the inner, and, consecutively, of the middle, arterial coat, was discovered by Mr. Gulliver.* The descriptions of this affection by him and by Rokitansky have left nothing unsaid that is yet known; but the observations are each year becoming more numerous and interesting of similar changes in the minutest blood-vessels. Such changes are especially observable in the minutest cerebral vessels; and their importance, in relation to apoplexy, of which they seem to be the most frequent precedent, as well as for the general illustration of the minute changes on which the defective nutrition of organs may depend, will justify, I hope, my repeating the description which I wrote from the first instances in which they were observed, and has since, I think, been sufficiently confirmed.†

In the least degree of this affection, the only apparent change of structure is, that minute, shining, black-edged particles, like molecules of oil,‡ are thinly and irregularly scattered beneath the outer surface of the small blood-vessels of the brain. Such a change may be seen in the vessels of portions of the brain that appear quite healthy, as well in the capillaries as in branches of both arteries and veins of all sizes, from 1-150th of an inch in diameter, to those of smallest dimension.

As the disease makes progress, the oil-particles may increase in number till the whole extent of the affected vessels is thick-set with them, and the natural structures, even if not quite wasted, can hardly be discerned. While their number thus increases, there is, also, usually, a considerable increase of the size of many of the oil-particles, and they may be seen of every size, from an immeasurable minuteness to the diameter of 1-2000th of an inch. In other places one sees, instead of this increase of scattered

* Medico-Chirurg. Trans., vol. xxvi. p. 86.   † Medical Gazette, vol. xlv.

‡ Dr. Jenner (Med. Times and Gaz., Jan. 31, 1852) has shown that these appearances of oil-particles are very closely imitated by equally minute particles similarly deposited, but which are proved to be calcareous by their solubility in hydrochloric acid. I think it very probable that what I have here described as fatty or oily matter may often be, at least in part, calcareous: we may reasonably expect this affection of the small vessels to be exactly analogous to the common fatty and calcareous degeneration of the larger arteries, although there is no generality of coincidence between them. I have also seen a pigmental degeneration of small cerebral arteries very similar to the fatty one described above.

oil-particles, or together with it, groups or clusters of similar minute particles, which are conglomerated, sometimes in regular oval or round masses, like large granule-cells, but more often in irregular masses or patches, in the wall of a great part of the circumference of a blood-vessel.

In a single fortunately selected specimen, one may see, in different branches of a vessel, all these degrees or states of the degeneration; the less and the more thickly scattered minute oil-particles, the clusters of such particles in various sizes and shapes, and the larger particles like drops of oil.

When the degeneration has made much progress, changes in the structure, and, not rarely, changed in the shape also, of the affected blood-vessels may be observed. The chief change of structure appears to consist in a gradual wasting of the more developed proper structures of the vessels; growing fainter in, apparently, the same proportion as the disease makes progress, the various nuclei or fibres are at length altogether lost, and blood-vessels of even 1-150th of an inch in diameter appear like tubes of homogeneous pellucid membrane, thick-set with the fatty particles. The structures of the vessels are not merely obscured by the abnormal deposits; they waste and totally disappear.

The changes of shape which the vessels may at the same time undergo are various. Very commonly, the outer layer of the wall is lifted up by one or more clusters of oil-particles, and the outline of the vessel appears uneven, as if it were tuberous or knotted. Sometimes the outer or cellular coat of the vessels is for some distance raised far from the middle coat, as if it were inflated, and the space between them contains numerous particles of oil; (but, perhaps, this raising up of the outer coat is often produced by water being imbibed while preparing the specimen for examination.) Sometimes (but, I think, only in vessels of less than 1-500th of an inch in diameter), partial enlargements, like aneurismal dilatations or pouches of their walls, are found.

The vessels most liable to this disease are, I think, the arteries of about 1-300th of an inch in diameter; but it exists, generally, at the same time, in the veins of the same or of less size. As a general rule (judging from the specimens hitherto examined), the disease decreases in nearly the same proportion as the size of the vessels, and the smallest capillaries are least, if at all, affected. But there are many exceptions to this rule; and it is not rare to find vessels of from 1-2000th to 1-3000th of an inch in diameter, having parts of their walls nearly covered with the abnormal deposits.

The principal and first seat of the deposits is, in arteries, in the more or less developed muscular or transversely fibrous coat; in veins, it is in the corresponding layer, immediately within their external fibro-cellutar nucleated coat: in vessels, whether arteries or veins, whose walls consist of only a simple pellucid membrane bearing nuclei, the substance of this membrane is the first seat of the deposits. In some cases, the outer fibro-cellular coat of both arteries and veins appears to contain abundant fatty matter. But it is seldom that, in an advanced stage of the affection, any of the several coats of a blood-vessel can be assigned as its chief seat; for even in large four-coated arteries they wholly waste, and their remains appear united in a single pellucid layer, of which the whole thickness may be occupied by the deposit.

The figures represent some of the most usual appearances of the degeneration.

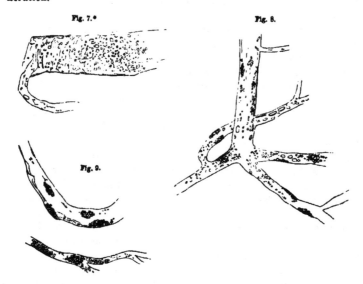

Fig. 7.*

Fig. 8.

Fig. 9.

The cases in which these changes were first observed were cerebral apoplexies in which the hemorrhage appeared certainly due to rupture of the wasted and degenerate blood-vessels. The probability of such an event is evident; as it is, also, that the less sudden effect of this condition of the vessels is likely to be a gradual degeneration of the parts of the brain which they supply. The relation between organs and their blood-vessels must in this respect be mutual; in the same measure, though not in the same way, as atrophy of an organ, whether wasting or degenerative, induces a corresponding atrophy of its blood-vessels, so will the

* Fig. 7. An artery, of 1-300th of an inch in diameter, and a branch given from it, from a softened corpus striatum. Numerous oil-particles of various sizes are scattered in the muscular coat, traces of the tissue of which appear in obscure transverse marks.

Fig. 8. From the same part, a vein 1-600th of an inch in diameter, with branches from 1-1200th to 1-1800th, and portions of capillaries. Scattered oil-particles, and groups like broken irregular granule-cells, are seen in the homogeneous pellucid walls of all the vessels.

Fig. 9. A vessel of 1-600th of an inch in diameter, and another of 1-1800th, with a branch of 1-3000th of an inch. Groups and scattered oil-particles are thick-set in the simple, pellucid, membranous walls.

imperfection of degenerate vessels lead to atrophy of the part in which they are distributed.

I suppose that the minute blood-vessels of many other parts might be often found thus degenerate, if we could examine them as easily as we can those of the brain; but I am not aware that any have been so described except those of the eye, in the case of *arcus senilis*, to which I shall presently refer, and those of the lungs and placenta. In the lungs, Dittrich[*] has traced affections of the arteries which, he says, the account I have given above exactly fits, and the consequences of which, in pulmonary apoplexy, correspond with the cerebral apoplexies due to rupture of the small blood-vessels of the brain.

Many facts of exceeding interest are known concerning the degenerations of nervous tissues, but, as yet, they are rather fragments than a continuous history.

First, in relation to the causes of degeneration, two are chiefly known; namely, defect of blood, and arrested function. Cases of softening of the brain have been long recognized as the consequence of ligature, or obstructive disease, of the carotid or other large arteries; but they have received a new interest from Dr. Kirkes's discovery[†] of their frequency in consequence of the obstruction of healthy cerebral arteries by masses of fibrine carried into them, after being dislodged from the valves of the left side of the heart, or from some part of the arterial system. In these cases, the extent of softening nearly corresponds with the range in which the branches of the obstructed artery are distributed; for, beyond the circle of Willis, the anastomosis among the cerebral arteries, like that among the cardiac, is not sufficient to carry a full supply of blood into a part from which the main stream is hindered, though generally enough to prevent the complete death or sloughing of the part.

Of the atrophy following diminished or abrogated function of nervous parts I have already mentioned examples in the shrinking of the brain in old people, in the wasting of the nerves of paralyzed or fixed muscles, and in that of the optic nerve and tract in cases of blindness. To these may be added the cases observed by Dr. Waller;[‡] who has discovered that when a nerve is divided, its distal part, *i. e.*, the portion between the place of division and the place of distribution, the portion in which the nerve-office can be no longer exercised always suffers atrophy, wasting and degenerating. The same atrophy ensues in the whole length of any spinal nerve whose root is divided; and in any system of nerves through which, after injury of the spinal cord, reflex actions cannot be excited. The change, in divided nerves, begins at the distal extremities of the

* Ueber den Laennecshen Lungen-infarktus. Erlangen, 1850.
† Med.-Chir. Trans., vol. xxxv.
‡ Philos. Trans., 1850, Part 2; and more fully in the London Journal of Medicine, July 1852.

nerve-fibres, and gradually extends upwards in the branches and trunk of the nerve; but is repaired if the divided portions of the nerve be allowed to reunite. I need not say how great interest these facts have in relation to the anatomy and physiology of the nervous system; but it is equalled by those related by Dr. Turck,[*] which may be used for ascertaining the functions of the several columns of the spinal cord, and their relations to the different parts of the brain, in the same manner as, by those of Dr. Waller, knowledge may be gained of the course and distribution, and of the centripetal or centrifugal office, of the several nerves. The main fact discovered by Dr. Turck is, that after diseases of parts of the brain or spinal cord there gradually ensues a softening, as by atrophy, of those tracts or columns of the cerebro-spinal axis through which, in health, impressions were habitually conveyed from the diseased part. The same general truth is illustrated by both these series of observations; namely, that nerve-fibres through which, from whatever cause, nerve-force can be no longer exercised, are gradually atrophied. The atrophy took place very quickly in the frogs that were the subjects of Dr. Waller's experiments: commencing in young frogs, during the summer, in from three to five days, and being completed in from twenty to thirty days. But, in the human subject, the process, reckoned by the observations of Turck, and those in which I have examined nerves atrophied in paralyzed muscles, is much slower. Changes in the spinal cord are not, he says, discernible in less than half a year after the apoplexy or other affection of the brain of which they are the consequence.

The changes in the nerve-fibres thus atrophied are minutely described by Dr. Waller. At first, transverse lines appear in the intratubular substance, indicating its loss of continuity; then it appears as if divided into round or oblong coagulated masses, as if its two component materials were mingled; then these are converted into black granules, resisting the action of acids and alkalies; and, finally, these granules are slowly and imperfectly eliminated.

In the atrophies of the brain and spinal cord, whether from obstructed circulation or from hindered function, the chief changes that are observed are, the liquefaction or softening of the whole substance, the breaking-up of the nerve-fibres, and the production of abundant granule-cells or masses, and free-floating granules. The exact nature of the change on which the softening of the substance depends is not yet known; neither can we be sure of the origin of the granule-cells. They are very like those commonly formed in the granular or fatty degeneration of various cells of both normal and morbid origin: but, produced as they are in parts of the brain and cord in which no cell structures naturally exist (for they may be as abundant in the white substance as in the gray), we have yet, I believe, to trace the source and method of their formation.

---

[*] Ueber secundäre Erkrankung einzelner Rückenmarksstränge. Wien, 1851.

Their likeness to the granule-cells of recognized fatty degenerations might be thought sufficient to justify the arrangement of the softenings of nerve-substance with the rest of that great division of atrophies: but the concurrence of so peculiar a softening of texture, and the similar examples of softening or liquefaction, concurrent with the formation of granule-cells, which are observed in numerous morbid growths, incline me to suggest that, for the present, it will be better to speak of these changes as liquefactive degenerations.

The last example of atrophy of which I will speak is that which is manifested in the arcus senilis,—the dim grayish-white arches or ellipse seen near the borders of the cornea in so many old persons. Its nature, as a true fatty degeneration, consisting in the accumulation of minute oil-drops in the proper tissue of the cornea, was discovered and is fully described by Mr. Canton.* By his and others'† investigations, it has also acquired a larger interest, in being found the frequent concomitant and sign of more widely extended degenerations that are not within sight during life. Thus, it is commonly associated with fatty or calcareous degeneration of the ophthalmic artery; with fatty degeneration of the muscles of the eyeball; and, especially in old persons, with fatty degeneration of the heart and many other organs. In short, the arcus senilis seems to be, on the whole, the best indication that has been yet found of proneness to an extensive or general fatty degeneration of the tissues. It is not, indeed, an infallible sign thereof; for there are cases in which it exists with clear evidences of vigor in the nutrition of the rest of the body; and there are others in which its early occurrence is due to defective nutrition consequent on purely local causes, such as inflammatory affections of the choroid, or other parts of the eye: but, allowing for these exceptions, it appears to be the surest, as well as the most visible, sign and measure of those primary degenerations which it has been the chief object of the last two lectures to describe.‡

* Observations on the arcus senilis, in the Lancet, 1850 and 1851.

† Especially Drs. Quain, Williams, and Virchow (Archiv., B. iv., p. 288).

‡ The degenerations of organs not described in the lectures may be studied by the following references:—

Arteries, Testicles, Lungs, and Liver: Gulliver, in Med.-Chir. Trans., xxvi., p. 86.

Liver: Bowman, in Lancet, 1841-2, vol. i., p. 560.

Kidney: Johnson, in Med.-Chir. Trans., xxix., p. i.; with Appendix in xxx., p. 182; Simon, in Med.-Chir. Trans., xxx., p. 141; Virchow, in his Archiv., B. iv., p. 264, et seq.; and Gairdner, Pathology of the Kidney, Edinb. 1848.

Colorless blood-cells, various Epithelial cells, Cartilage-corpuscles, Nerve-cells: Virchow, in his Archiv., i., p. 144.

Lungs: Rainey, in Med.-Chir. Trans., vol. xxxi., p. 297.

Placenta: Barnes, in Med.-Chir. Trans., xxxiv., p. 183.

Placenta, Decidua, and other tissues of the Uterus, as well as the Muscular: Kilian, as quoted at p. 131.

Cartilage. Redfern, "Anormal Nutrition in the Articular Cartilages," 1850; and Virchow, in his Archiv., B. iv., p. 289.

LECTURE VII.

GENERAL CONSIDERATIONS ON THE REPAIR AND REPRODUCTION OF INJURED AND LOST PARTS.

AMONG the general considerations that may be suggested by the preceding lectures, none, perhaps, is more worthy of earnest thought, than that of the capacity of adaptation to the variety of their circumstances, which is displayed by the several parts of the body. Each part may be said to be conformed, in its first construction, to a certain standard of measure, weight, and power, by which standard it is adjusted to the other parts of the whole organism. The first perfection of the economy is in the justness with which its several parts are thus balanced in their powers; and the mutual adaptation thus established is continued, in ordinary life, by the nutrition of each part being regulated according to a law of direct proportion to the quantity of work that each discharges. But when the external conditions of life vary, and require, for the maintenance of health, varying amounts of function to be discharged by one or more parts; and, still more, when disease disturbs the functional relations of any part to the rest; then each part displays a capacity of adaptation to the new conditions in which it is placed: each can assume a less or greater size and weight; each can acquire a less or more powerful tissue; each can thus rise above, or descend below, its standard of power.

This capacity of adaptation is shown in a yet more remarkable manner in the recovery of parts from the effects of injuries and diseases. It is surely only because it is so familiar, that we think lightly, if at all, of the fact that living bodies are capable of repairing the effects of injury, and that in this capacity they prove themselves adapted for events of which it is not certain whether they will ever occur to them or not. The exact fitness of every part of a living body for its present office, not as an independent agent, but as one whose work must be done in due proportion with many others concurring in operation with it, is a very marvelous thing: but it seems much more so, that in the embryo, each of these parts was made fit for offices and relations that were then

Numerous calcareous degenerations: Dusseau, Het Beenweefsel en Verbeeningen, Amsterdam, 1850.

Pigmental degenerations: Virchow, in his Archiv., B. i.

The chief general histories of degenerations are by Rokitansky, Pathol. Anat.; C. J. B. Williams, Principles of Medicine; and Virchow, in the places cited above, and in his Archiv., B. iv., p. 394.

A remarkable series of instances of fatty degeneration of voluntary muscles has been lately communicated to the Medico-Chirurgical Society by Dr. Meryon, and will be published, I believe, in the 35th volume of the Transactions.

The degenerations of products of disease will be described in future lectures.

future; and yet more marvelous than all it seems, that each of them should still have capacity for action in events that are not only future, but uncertain; that are indeed possible, yet are in only so low a degree probable, that if ever they happen they will be called accidents.

Let us have always in mind this adaptation of the living body to future probabilities, while we consider the physiology of repair. If it be fairly weighed, every part of the process of repair will be an argument of divine design; and such an argument as cannot be impugned by the suspicion that the events among which each living thing is cast have determined its adaptation to them: for all the adaptations here noted prove capacities for things future, and only not improbable.

And let us also keep in view how the reparative processes may illustrate the laws of ordinary nutrition; and especially observe that they furnish evidence of the nature of the formative force exercised in the complete organism. I mentioned in a former lecture (p. 52) that, in many instances of repair and reproduction, the formation of the new replacing structures cannot be ascribed to an assimilative force, or to the development of tissue-germs derived from the injured or lost parts. The completeness of repair after injury, and the extent to which it is sometimes accomplished, become thus most striking evidences of the principle that the formative force, and those that co-operate with it, are, in the completed organism, the same and continuous with those which actuated the formation of the original tissues, in the development of the germ and embryo. There is in every considerable process of repair a remaking of a part: and the new materials assume the specific form and composition of the part that they replace, through the operation of no other, or otherwise directed, force, than that through which that part was first made. For, in all grave injuries and diseases, the parts that might serve as models for the repairing materials to be assimilated to, or as tissue-germs to develop new structures, are lost or spoiled; yet the effects of such injury and disease are recovered from, and the right specific form and composition are regained. In all such cases, the reproduced parts are formed, not according to any present model, but according to the appropriate specific form; and often with a more strikingly evident design towards that form as an end or purpose, than we can discern in the natural construction of the body.

Moreover, it will be observed in the instances of repair of injury, even more plainly than in the maintenance of the body in the successive ordinary stages of its life, that the law of formation is at each period of life the same: that every part is formed after the same method as was observed in the corresponding part of the parent at the same period of life. Thus, when, in an adult animal, a part is reproduced after injury or removal, it is made in conformity, not with that condition which was proper to it when it was first formed, or in its infantile life, but with that which is proper according to the time .of life in which it is reproduced;

proper, because like that which the similar part had, at the same time of life, in members of former generations. In the reproduction of the foot or the tail of the lizard, they grow, as it were, at once into the full dimensions proper to the part, according to the age of the individual. Spallanzani expressly mentions this:—that when a leg is cut from a full-grown salamander, the new leg and foot are developed, as far as form and structure are concerned, just as those of the larva were; but as to size, they from the beginning grow and are developed to the proper dimensions of the adult. The power, therefore, by which this reproduction is accomplished, would seem to be, not the mere revival of one which, after perfecting the body, had lapsed into a dormant state, but the self-same power which, before the removal of the limb, was occupied in its maintenance by the continual mutation of its particles, and is now engaged, with more energy, in the reconstruction of the whole.

The ability to repair the damages sustained by injury, and to reproduce lost parts, appears to belong, in some measure, to all bodies that have definite form and construction. It is not an exclusive property of living

Fig. 10.

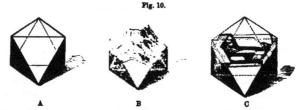

A   B   C

beings; for even crystals will repair themselves when, after pieces have been broken from them, they are placed in the same conditions in which they were first formed.

The diagram represents a series of casts made from a crystal with which I imitated the experiments of Jordan.* A large piece was broken off an octohedral crystal of alum (A). Before the fracture it was perfect in its form, except at one small pit on its surface, where it had what (writing of animal physiology) might be called a congenital defect. Thus broken (B) it was placed again in the solution in which it had been formed, and after a few days its injury was so far repaired as it appears in the figure C. The whole crystal had increased, but the increase on its broken surface was proportionally so much greater than on any other, that the perfect octohedral form was nearly regained. The little congenital defect, also, was completely healed. In a few days more the whole crystal would have been as if it had suffered no injury.

I know not what amount of mutual illustration, if any, the repair of crystals and of living bodies may afford; but, in any case, we may trace

* Müller's Archiv, 1842, p. 46.

here something like an universal property of bodies that are naturally and orderly constructed: all, in favorable circumstances, can repair at least some of the damages to which they are liable from the violence of external forces.

But, to speak only of the repair and reproduction that occur in the several orders of the animal kingdom: among these they exist in singularly different degrees, and in such as can be only partially included in rules or general expressions. The general statement sometimes made, that the reparative power in each species bears an inverse ratio to its position in the scale of animal life, is certainly not proved; and many instances are contrary to it: such as the great reparative power possessed by the Triton and other lizards, and the apparently complete absence of it in the perfect insects. Rather, the general rule which we may expect to find true, and for which there is already much evidence, may be that the reparative power bears an inverse proportion to the amount of power consumed in the development and growth of the individual, and in its maintenance in the perfect state.

Our ideas of the consumption of power in the organization of matter, are, perhaps unavoidably, very vague: yet are there facts enough to prove that the power which can be exercised in a germ is limited, so that the capacity of assuming the specific organic form cannot be communicated to an indefinite quantity of matter; and there are also enough to justify the expression, that the power, thus limited, is in some measure consumed, 1st, in the development of every new structure, and, 2dly, in a less measure, in the growth and maintenance of those already formed.

Thus, first, it appears constantly true, that the reparative power is greater in all parts of the young than in those of the older individuals of all species. Even when we compare individuals that have all attained their highest development and growth, this rule seems to be true. We know it from general observations of the results of similar injuries and diseases in persons of different ages: numerous as the exceptions may be, the general rule seems true. And it is yet more evidently proved in the case of some lower animals. Spallanzani mentions it in regard to the reproduction of the tail of the tadpole. The quickness with which the work of reproduction is both begun and perfected was always, in his experiments, in an inverse ratio to the age. He says the same for the reproduction of the legs of salamanders, and it is only in the young, among frogs and toads, that any reproduction of the limbs will take place. So, too, in experiments on the repair of fractures, the union of tendons and the like, in the mammalia, one may see abundant evidence that the vigor and celerity of the process are in an inverse proportion to the animal's age. There is, indeed, some reason to believe, that in the very early period of embryonic life, a true reproduction of parts of limbs may take place even in the human species. Not to speak of the possibility that supernumerary members may be formed in consequence of accidental fission of the budding limbs of the embryo, there are cases in which fingers are found on the stumps of arms in such circumstances as justify the belief, that after a limb had been accidentally amputated in the uterus, these had been produced on its remaining portion.*

All these facts agree well with the belief that the formative power is gradually diminished in the acts of organizing matter for the mainte- nance of the body; and the difference between the completeness of repair in children and that in adults appears so much greater than the difference in adults of different ages, that it is probable the formative power is more diminished by growth than by mere maintenance.

But, secondly, it seems that the capacity for the repair or reproduc- tion of injured parts is much more diminished by development, than by growth or maintenance of the body; *i. e.*, much more by those transfor- mations of parts by which they become fitted for higher offices, than by the multiplication or maintenance of those that are already perfect in their kind and function. In other words, to improve a part requires more, and more perfect, formative power, than to increase it does.

This, as a general principle, is exemplified in many instances. In the greater part of congenital malformations we find arrest of development, but no hinderance of growth; as a heart, in which a septum fails to be developed, yet grows to its full bulk. If tadpoles be excluded from due light and heat, their development will be much retarded, but their growth will be less checked: in other words, the conditions of nutrition which are enough for growth are not sufficient for development. When a part is, without disease, unduly supplied with blood, it may grow be- yond its normal size, but it is never developed beyond its normal struc- ture: that which is sufficient for increase of growth, is not enough for an advance in development. Again, in the miscalled cultivation and improvement of flowers, growth is increased, but development is hin- dered; and an excess of colored leaves is formed, instead of the due number of male and female organs. In an old ulcer or a sinus, cells may be continually reproduced, maintaining or even increasing the granulations, yet they will not develop themselves in cellular tissue and cuticle for the healing of the part. And so, lastly, even when repair and reproduction have gone far towards their ultimate achievement, that which takes a longer time, and oftener fails, is the improvement, the perfecting, of the new material, by its final development. This is observed in all cases of reproduced limbs, and even in ordinary scars.

These facts (and there are many others like them) seem to justify the expression that, not only more favorable conditions, but also a larger amount of organizing force, are expended in development than in growth, or maintenance; and that the reparative power bears an in- verse ratio to the amount of force already expended in these processes.

* See a paper by Dr. Simpson, in the London and Edinburgh Monthly Journal, Janu- ary, 1848.

If it be so, we might expect that in each species, in its perfect state, the reparative power might be measured by the degree of likeness between the embryonic and the perfect form, structure, and composition.

There are many apparent exceptions to such a rule, especially in the Asteriæ, which, though constructed through manifold metamorphoses, have great capacity of restoring detached rays; yet it is consistent with such a rule that the highest amount of reparative power exists in those lowest polypes in which the materials of the germ-mass are least transformed, but are multiplied, and, as it were, grouped into the shape of their bodies. In the Hydra viridis, and Hydra fusca, it seems literally true that any minute portion derived from the germ-mass, may, after being separated from the perfect body, reproduce the perfect form. This is the general truth of the numerous experiments performed on Hydræ by Trembley, Roesel, and others. They have been so often quoted, that I need not do more than mention the greatest instances of reproductive power that they showed.

Trembley cut an Hydra into four pieces: each became a perfect Hydra; and, while they were growing, he cut each of these four into two or three. These fractions of the quarters being on their way to become perfect, he again divided these, and thus he went on, till from the one Hydra he obtained fifty. All these became perfect; he kept many of them for more than two years, and they multiplied by their natural gemmation just as much as others that had never been divided. Again, he cut similar polypes longitudinally, and in an hour or less each half had rolled itself, and seamed up its cut edges, so as to be a perfect Hydra. He split them into four; he quartered them; he cut them into as many pieces as he could; and nearly every piece became a perfect Hydra. He slit one into seven pieces, leaving them all connected by the tail, and the Hydra became seven-headed, and he saw all the heads eating at the same time. He cut off the seven heads, and, hydra-like, they sprang forth again. And even the fabulist dared not invent such a prodigy as the naturalist now saw. The heads of the Lernæan Hydra perished after excision: the heads of this Hydra grew for themselves bodies, and multiplied with as much vigor as their parent trunk.

Now, these instances may suffice to show not only the great capacity of reproduction in the lowest polypes, but, also, that in them the process of reproduction after injury confounds itself with that of their natural generation by gemmation, or, as it probably more rarely happens, by spontaneous fission. We cannot discern a distinction between them; and there are facts which seem to prove the identity of the power which operates in both. Thus, in both alike, the formative power is limited according to the specific characters of the Hydra: immense as the power of increase is which may be brought into action by the mutilations of the Hydra, yet that power cannot be made to produce an Hydra of much more than ordinary size, or to raise one above its ordinary specific characters. And, again, the identity of the power is shown in this, that the natural act of gemmation retards that of reproduction after injury. Trembley particularly observes, that when an Hydra, from which the head and tentacula had been cut off, gemmated, the reproduction of the tentacula was retarded soon after the gemmule appeared.

Many other species manifest this coincidence of the power of propagating by gemmation of fission, and of producing large portions of the body, and even of reconstructing, from fragments, the whole body. Among them, as chief examples, are the Actiniæ, which after bisection, form two perfect individuals; and the Holothuriæ, which, as Sir J. G. Dalyell has observed, when hurt or handled, will eject all their viscera, leaving their body a mere empty sac, and yet in three or four months will have all their viscera regenerated. And to these may be added, from among the Anellata, the young Nereids, and those species of Nais, on which Bonnet, Spallanzani, and others, made their experiments; experiments of which the climax seemed to be achieved when a Nais was cut by M. Lyonnet into thirty or forty separate pieces, and there were produced from those fragments as many perfect individuals.

Among the instances of greatest capacity of repair, some observed by Sir J. G. Dalyell* seem to illustrate, in a remarkable manner, the general laws of the reparative processes in even the higher animals; and especially the gradual improvement of the repairing part, by which, at length, the effects of injury may be quite annulled.

In the Hydra Tuba, the species of which he traced that marvelous development into Medusæ, he found that when cut in halves, each half may regain the perfect form; but this perfect form is regained only very slowly, and, as it were, by a gradual improvement of parts that are at first ill-formed. The sketch, copied from his plate, shows the succession

Fig. 11.

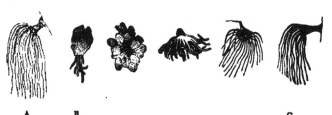

A   B   C

of forms marking these stages of improvement in the stump, or attached part of an Hydra Tuba (A), from which the distal half with the tentacula was cut off.

Through these forms, commencing at B, into which the attached half

* Rare and Remarkable Animals of Scotland, vol. i.

of A was first changed, the perfect state of a Hydra was at length reached; as at C. The fact may possibly be explained (as he suggests) by the mutilation having disturbed the progress of the Hydra in its development of young Medusæ; for the experiment was made in March, nearly at the time when the series of changes should have commenced. But if I may venture not to accept the suggestion of so admirable an observer, I should suspect rather that this is an instance of gradual recovery of perfection, such as we see more generally in the repair of injuries and diseases in the higher animals.

He has noticed something of the same kind, and more definite in the Tubularia indivisa; one of his experiments on which is here illustrated.

A fine specimen was cut near its root, and after the natural fall of its head, the summit of its stem was cloven. An imperfect head was first produced, at right angles to the stem, from one portion of the cleft (A); after its fall, another and more nearly perfect one was regenerated, and, as it grew, improved yet more (B). A third appeared, and then a fourth was yet more nearly perfect, though the stem was thick, and the tentacula imperfect. The cleft was almost healed; and now a fifth head was formed, quite perfect (C); and after it, as perfectly, a sixth and a seventh head. All these were produced in fifteen months.

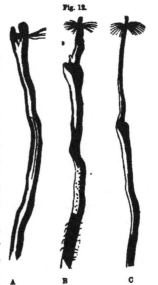

Fig. 12.

The lower half of this specimen had been cut off four months after the separation of the stem. Its upper end bore, first, an abortive head; then, secondly, one which advanced further in development; a third, much better; and then, in succession, other four, which were all well formed.

A B C

The upper portion of this lower half of the stem now showing signs of decay, a portion was cut from its lowest part, and further manifested the reproductive power of the stem; for three heads were produced from the upper end of the piece cut off, and four from the lower end of the upper piece which had seemed to be decaying. In 550 days this specimen had grown twenty-two heads.

Now, I cannot but think that we have, in these instances of gradual recovery from the effects of injury, a type of that gradual return to the perfect form and composition which is noticed in the higher animals. Our theory of the process of nutrition leads us to believe that, in the con-

8

stant mutation of particles in nutrition, those elements of the blood, or of any structure, that have been altered by disease, in due time degenerate or die, and are cast off or absorbed; and that those which next succeed to them partake, through the assimilative force, of the same morbid character; but that, every time of renewal, the new particles approach a step nearer to the perfect state. Thus, as it were, each generation of new particles is more nearly perfect, till all the effects of the injury or the disease are quite obliterated. Surely, in the gradual recovery of perfection by these polypes, we have an apt illustration of the theory; one which almost proves its justice.

The power of reconstructing a whole and perfect body, by the development of a fragment, is probably limited to the species that can propagate by spontaneous fission or gemmation, or that increase their size, as some of the Anellata do, by the successive addition of rings that are developed after the manner of gemmules from those that precede them. Where this power is not possessed, there, whatever be the position of the species in the animal scale, the reparative power appears to be limited to the reproduction of the lost members; such as legs, claws, a part of the body, the head, an eye, the tail, and the like. Within this limit, the rule seems again to hold good, that the amount of reparative power is in an inverse ratio to that of the development, or change of structure and mode of life, through which the animal has passed in its attainment of perfection, or on its way thitherward.

Here, however, even more than in the former cases, we need not perhaps more experiments, but experiments on a larger number of species. It appears generally true, that the species whose development to the perfect state is comparatively simple and direct, have great reparative powers; while many, at least of those in which the development is with such great changes of shape, structure, and mode of life, as may be called metamorphosis, retain in their perfect state scarcely any power for the repair of losses. Yet we want more instances of this; and especially, it were to be wished that we had the results of experiments upon the lowest animals that pass through such metamorphoses; e. g. on the Hydra tuba, not only in its Hydra state, but in all the changes that succeed, till it attains its complete medusal form.

In the absence of such evidence as experiments of this kind might furnish, the best examples of the rule are furnished by the experiments of Mr. Newport. They show that among the insects, the reparative power, in the complete state, is limited to the orders in which that state is attained by a comparatively simple and direct course of development; as the Myriapoda and Phasmidæ, and some of the Orthoptera. These can reproduce their antennæ, and their legs, after removal or mutilation; but their power of reproduction diminishes as their development increases. Even in the Myriapoda, whose highest development scarcely carries their external form beyond that of the larvæ of the more perfect insects, such reparative power apparently ceases, when, after the last casting of their integuments, their development is completed.

In the higher hexapod insects, such reproduction has been seen in only the larval state; none of them, in its perfect state, can reproduce an antenna, or any other member. The Myriapoda, then, are, in their reparative power, equal to the larvæ of the higher insects, and nearly all the power for formation which these manifest, appears to be exhausted in the two later metamorphoses.

The case is the stronger, as illustrating the expenditure of power in metamorphoses, when the higher insects are compared with the Arachnida; for in these, which attain their perfect state through more direct development, the reparative power remains equal to the reproduction of limbs and antennæ. A yet stronger contrast is presented between the higher insects and the several species of salamander, in which so profuse a reproduction of the limbs has been observed; for though they be so much higher in the scale of animal life, yet the amount of change in external form and habits of life, through which they pass, in their development from the embryo to the perfect state, appears less than that accomplished in the metamorphoses of insects.

Many instances, besides those which I have cited, appear to support this rule, that the reparative power, in each perfect species, whether it be higher or lower in the scale, is in an inverse proportion to the amount of change through which it has passed in its development from the embryonic to the perfect state. And the deduction we may make from them is, that the powers for development from the embryo are identical with those exercised for the restoration from injuries: in other words, that the powers are the same by which perfection is first achieved, and by which, when lost, it is recovered.

This is, again, generally confirmed in the instances of the Vertebrata; but of the repair in these or at least in the highest of them, I shall have to speak so exclusively in the future lectures, that I will now only say that, in man and other mammalia, a true reproduction after loss or injury seems limited to three classes of parts:—

1. To those which are formed entirely by nutritive repetition; such as the blood and epithelia.

2. To those which are of lowest organization, and (which seems of more importance) of lowest chemical character; as the gelatinous tissues, the cellular and tendinous, and the bones.

3. To those which are inserted in other tissues, not as essential to their structure, but as accessories, as connecting or incorporating them with the other structures of vegetative or animal life; such as nerve-fibres and blood-vessels.

With these exceptions, injuries or losses in the human body are capable of no more than repair, in its most limited sense; i. e., in the place of what is lost, some lowly organized tissue is formed, which fills up the breach, and suffices for the maintenance of a less perfect life.

I may seem in this, as in some earlier lectures, to have been discussing doctrines that can hardly be applicable to our daily practice, and with illustrations drawn from objects in which surgeons may have but little interest. Let me, then, if only in apology, refer to some of the considerations which are suggested by studies such as these. Let me, first, express my belief that, if we are ever to escape from the obscurities and uncertainties of our art, it must be through the study of those highest laws of our science, which are expressed in the simplest terms in the lives of the lowest orders of creation. It was in the search after the mysteries—that is, after the unknown highest laws—of generation, that the first glance was gained of the largest truth in physiology; the truth of the development of ova through partition and multiplication of the embryo-cells. So may the study of the repair of injuries sustained by the lowest polypes lead us to the clearer knowledge of that law, in reliance upon which alone we dare to practise our profession; the law that lost perfection may be recovered by the operation of the powers by which it was once achieved. Already, in the facts that I have quoted from Sir Graham Dalyell, we seem to have the foreshadowing of those through which the discovery may be made.

Then, let us not overlook those admirable provisions, which we may find in the lives of all that breathe, against injuries that, but for these provisions, would too often bring them to their end before their appointed time, or leave them mutilated to finish a painful and imperfect life. We are not likely to undervalue, or to lose sight of, the design of all such provisions for our own welfare. But we may better appreciate these, if we regard them as only of the same kind as those more abundantly supplied to creatures whom we are apt to think insignificant; indeed, so abundantly, that, as if with a consciousness of the facility of repair, self-mutilation is commonly resorted to for the preservation of life. When the Ophiuræ, or any of the brittle Star-fishes, break themselves to fragments, and disappoint the grasp of the anxious naturalist, they probably only repeat what they are instinctively taught to do, that they may elude the jaws of their more ravenous enemies. But death would be much better than such mutilation, if their rays could not be reproduced almost as easily as they can be rejected. The experimentalist, too, who cuts off one or the other end of any of the Anellata, perhaps only puts them to a necessity to which they are liable from the attacks of their carnivorous neighbors. Almost defenceless, and so easily mutilated, their condition, were it not for their faculty of reproduction, might be more deplorable than that of any other creature; and even their existence as species might have been endangered long ago. It would almost seem as if the species that have least means of escape or defence from mutilation were those on which the most ample power of repair has been bestowed; an admirable instance, if it be only generally true, of the beneficence that has provided for the welfare of even the least (as we call them) of the living world, with as much care as if they were the sole objects of the Divine regard.

Lastly, if I may venture on so high a theme, let me suggest that the instances of recovery from disease and injury seem to be only examples of a law yet larger than that within the terms of which they may be comprised; a law wider than the grasp of science; the law that expresses our Creator's will for the recovery of all lost perfection.   To this train of thought we are guided by the remembrance that the healing of the body, was ever chosen as the fittest emblem of His work, whose true mission was to raise man's fallen spirit and repair the injuries it had sustained; and that once, the healing power was exerted in a manner purposely so confined as to advance, like that which we can trace, by progressive stages to the complete cure.   For there was one, upon whom, when the light of Heaven first fell, so imperfect with his vision, that he saw, confusedly, "men, as trees walking;" and then, by a second touch of the Divine Hand, was "restored, and saw every man clearly."   Thus guided by the brighter light of revelation, it may be our privilege, while we study the science of our healing art, to gain, by the illustrations of analogy, a clearer insight into the Oneness of the plan by which things spiritual and corporeal are directed.   Even now, we may trace some analogy between the acts of the body and those of man's intellectual and moral nature.   As in the development of the germ, so in the history of the human spirit, we may discern a striving after perfection; after a perfection, not viewed in any present model (for the human model was marred almost as soon as it was formed), but manifested to the enlightened Reason in the "Express Image" of the "Father of Spirits."   And so, whenever, through human frailty, amid the violences of the world, and the remaining "infection of our nature," the spirit loses aught of the perfection to which it was once admitted, still its implanted Power is ever urgent to repair the loss.   The same power, derived and still renewed from the same Parent, working by the same appointed means, and to the same end, restores the fallen spirit to nearly the same perfection that it had before.   Then, not unscarred, yet living—"fractus sed invictus"—the Spirit still feels its capacity for a higher life, and presses to its immortal destiny.   In that destiny the analogy ends.   We may watch the body developing into all its marvelous perfection and exact fitness for the purpose of its existence in the world; but, this purpose accomplished, it passes its meredian, and then we trace it through the gradual decays of life and death.   But, for the human Spirit, that has passed the ordeal of this world, there is no such end.   Emerging from its imprisonment in the body, it soars to the element of its higher life: there, in perpetual youth, its powers expand, as the vision of the Infinite unfolds before it; there, in the very presence of its Model, its Parent, and the Spring of all its Power, it is "like Him, for it sees Him as He is."

LECTURE VIII.

THE MATERIALS FOR THE REPAIR OF INJURIES.

In the present lecture I propose to give a general account of the materials employed for the repair of some of the injuries inflicted on the human body.

I hope I do not err in thinking that the most advantageous mode of treating this subject will be to confine myself to that class of injuries which may be called visible breaches of continuity; such as wounds and fractures. For, in regard to the recovery from diseases, our knowledge of the effects of any disease seems, as yet, too imperfect for us to trace the stages by which the morbid state reverts to that which is healthy. We may be sure it is in conformity with the same general laws as those of recovery from injury, and almost sure that it is by the gradual improvement of the particles that in succession replace those altered by disease. But the whole details of the process have yet to be discovered.

Even within the narrower field of the repair of breaches of continuity, I must yet assign to myself a closer limit. A future lecture will be devoted to the healing of fractures; in this, therefore, I shall speak almost exclusively of the healing of divided soft parts; and I shall take, as the chief and typical examples, the repairs of wounds made in operations. References to the healing of other injuries, may, however, be made by the way, and for collateral illustration.

Modern surgery has shown how right Mr. Hunter was, when, in the very begging of his discussion concerning the healing of injuries, he points out, as a fundamental principle, the difference between those two forms of injuries of which one is subcutaneous, the other open to the air. He says: "The injuries done to sound parts I shall divide into two sorts, according to the effects of the accident. The first kind consists of those in which the injured parts do not communicate externally, as concussions of the whole body, or of particular parts, strains, bruises, and simple fractures, which form a large division. The second consists of those which have an external communication, comprehending wounds of all kinds and compound fractures."* And then, he says, "The injuries of the first division, in which the parts do not communicate externally, seldom inflame; while those of the second commonly both inflame and suppurate."

In these sentences Mr. Hunter has embodied the principle on which is founded the whole practice of subcutaneous surgery; a principle of which, indeed, it seems hardly possible to exaggerate the importance.

* Works, vol. iii. p. 240.

For, of the two injuries inflicted in a wound, the mechanical disturbance of the parts, and the exposure to the air of those that were covered, the exposure, if continued, is the worse. Both are apt to excite inflammation; but the exposure excites it most certainly, and in the worse form; i. e., in the form which most delays the process of repair, and which is most apt to endanger life. Abundant instances of this are shown in the difference between a simple and a compound fracture, though the former may have been produced by the greater violence; or, between a simple fracture, even with much violence, extending into a joint, and an open wound, never so gently made into one. Or, for parallel instances, one may cite the rarity of suppurations after even extensive ecchymoses, and their general occurrence when wounds are left open.

I had frequent occasion to observe these differences, in a series of experiments made for the illustration of the healing of divided muscles and tendons. Some of these were divided through open wounds, and some by subcutaneous section; and the recital of a single experiment may afford a fair example of the difference of results that often ensued. In the same rabbit, the tibialis anticus and extensor longus digitorum were divided on the right side with a section through the skin; on the left, with a subcutaneous section, through a small opening. Twelve days afterwards the rabbit was killed. The wound on the left side was well repaired, and with comparatively little trace of inflammation: the gap on the right was closed in with a scab, and an imperfect scar, but under these was a large collection of pus, and no trace of a reparative process. The contrast is the stronger, because in all these cases there is, unavoidably, more mechanical violence inflicted in the gradual subcutaneous division than in the simple open wound. And, it must be added, that a speedy closure of the external wound made in an open section may bring the case into more favorable conditions than those of a subcutaneous wound made with more violence. This, also, I saw in some of the experiments: a clumsy subcutaneous division of one Achilles tendon excited great inflammation about it; while the open section of the other tendon in the same rabbit was quickly and well repaired, if the external wound had been speedily united, and had sufficiently soon converted the open into a subcutaneous injury.

Still, what Mr. Hunter said is true, especially in wounds in our own bodies: subcutaneous wounds seldom inflame; open wounds generally both inflame and suppurate. It will be a principal object of this lecture to show something like an anatomical reason for this difference, in the fact that the materials produced for the repair of open wounds are not usually the same, or, at least, do not develop themselves in the same manner, as those for the repair of closed or subcutaneous ones. The physiological and nearer reason is probably to be discovered in the influence of oxygen abnormally admitted to the tissues, and producing in them such effects as are more nearly traced in the phenomena of inflammation, and will be described in future lectures.

Before speaking of the materials for repair, I must briefly state that the healing of open wounds may be accomplished by five different modes: namely, 1. By immediate union; 2. By primary adhesion; 3. By granulation; 4. By secondary adhesion, or the union of granulations; 5. By healing under a scab. The repair of subcutaneous wounds may be effected by immediate union, but is generally accomplished by connection, or the formation of bonds of union between the divided and retracted parts. Very rarely it is effected by means of granulations without suppuration.

Of these modes, which I hope to describe hereafter in detail, it is the peculiarity of the first, or process of immediate union, that it is accomplished by the mere reunion or re-joining of the divided parts, without the production or interposition of any new material. In all the others, new material is produced and organized. This process of immediate union corresponds with what Mr. Hunter called "union by the first intention." It is not the same as that which, in modern surgery, is called union by the first intention; for that is the same as Mr. Hunter named "union by adhesion," or "by the adhesive inflammation," and is effected, as he described it, by the organization of lymph interposed between two closely approximated wounded surfaces. Mr. Hunter maintained that union by the first intention is effected by means of the fibrine of the blood extravasated between the surfaces of the injured part, which fibrine, there coagulating, adheres to both the surfaces, becomes organized, and forms a vascular bond of union between them.* Doubtless, Mr. Hunter was, in this, in error; but, as the blood extravasated in wounds is not without influence on their repair, I will endeavor to state the several modes in which it may, when thus extravasated, be finally disposed of.

There are ample evidences for believing that masses of effused, or stagnant and coagulated, blood may be organized; i. e., may assume the characters of a tissue, and may coalesce with the adjacent parts and become vascular. These evidences include cases of blood effused in serous sacs, especially in the arachnoid; of clots in veins organizing into fibrous cords, or, after less organization, degenerating into phlebolithes; clots organizing into tumors in the heart and arteries; and the clots so organized above ligatures on arteries as to form part of the fibrous cord by which the obliterated artery is replaced. These last cases afford most conclusive evidence, because they have been very carefully investigated in a series of experiments and microscopic observations, by Dr. Zwicky.†

In 1848, I had the opportunity of examining a specimen which, more fully than any other I had seen, confirmed Zwicky's account of the mode in which blood-clots become organized. It supplied, too, some facts which appear important to the present subject. It was obtained from an

* Works, vol. iii., 253.
† Die Metamorphose des Thrombus. Zurich, 1845.

insane person, by my friend, Mr. Holmes Coote. A thin layer of pale blood-colored and ruddy membrane lined the whole internal surface of the cerebral dura mater, and adhered closely to it. Its color, the existence of patches of blood-clot imbedded in it, and all its other characters, satisfactorily proved that it had been a thin clot of blood,—an example of such as are effused in apoplexy of the cerebral membranes, and are

Fig. 13.

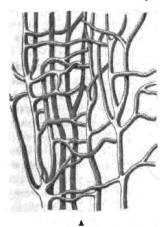 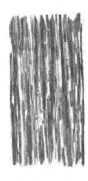

A   B

fully described by Mr. Prescott Hewett.* Numerous small vessels could be seen passing from the dura mater into this clot-membrane; and with the microscope, while they were still full of blood, I made the sketch which is here engraved (Fig. 13, A). The arrangement of the blood-vessels bears a close resemblance, but, perhaps, more in its irregularity than in any positive characters or plan, to that which exists in false membrane formed of organized lymph: but the vessels were, I think, generally larger.

Such were the blood-vessels of this organized clot. Its minute structure, as represented above (B), showed characters which are of peculiar interest, because of their resemblance to those observed in the material that is commonly formed in the repair of subcutaneous injuries. In the substance of what else appeared like a filamentous clot of fibrine, sprinkled over with minute molecules, the addition of acetic acid brought into view corpuscles like nuclei, or cytoblasts, very elongated, attenuated, and, in some instances, like short strips of flat fibre. Of course, such corpuscles are not to be found in any ordinary clot of fibrine; they exactly resemble such as may be found in certain examples of rudimental cellular tissue, and, among these, in the material for the repair of subcuta-

* Med.-Chir. Trans. vol. xxviii.

neous injuries. In short, the minute structure of this clot now organized was an example of what I shall have often to refer to under the name of "nucleated blastema."*

With such evidence as this of the organization of a thin layer of blood-clot, and of the development of its fibrine being apparently identical with that of the material commonly formed for the repair of subcutaneous injuries, I was surprised to find that extravasated blood can, commonly, have no share at all in the reparative process.

One of the best proofs of this is, that scarcely the smallest portion of blood is effused in the cases in which the largest quantity of reparative material is produced in the shortest time, and in which the healing process is most perfectly accomplished. In twenty cases in which I divided the Achilles tendon in rabbits, I only once found, in the subsequent examinations, a clot of extravasated blood in the track of the wound. In this case, I believe, the posterior tibial artery was wounded : for in all others, and in similar divisions of muscles, unless a large arterial trunk were cut, the only effusion of blood was in little blotches, not in separate clots, but effused or infiltrated in the cellular tissue near the wound. In some cases there was blood-stained infiltration of the inflammatory products, but in none were there such clots as could be organized into bonds of union. In short, parts thus divided scarcely bleed : what blood does flow escapes easily through the outer wound, as the surrounding tissues collapse into the space left by the contracting parts ; or, what remains is infiltrated into the tissues, and forms no separate clot.

It is the same with fractures. In a large proportion of these, one finds no clots lying between the fragments where they are united, and only very small spottings of blood, like ecchymoses, in or beneath the periosteum. The abundant extravasations that commonly exist in the subcutaneous tissue are generally confined to it : they are not continued down to the periosteum or bone.

In all these cases, then, we have sufficient proof that extravasated blood is not necessary for union by the first intention, or for any other mode of repair, in the simple fact that where the repair is best, and the material for it most ample, no blood is so extravasated as to form a clot that could be organized.

But, though this may be the usual case, the question still remains— When blood is effused and coagulated between wounded surfaces, how are the clots disposed of ? For, often, though not generally, such clots are found in wounds, or between the ends of a broken bone, or a divided tendon when an artery by its side is cut ; and in most operation-wounds, one sees blood left on them, or flowing on their surfaces, after they are done up. How, then, is this blood disposed of ?

* The description here given has been fully confirmed by the examination of a similar membranous clot, the vessels of which were beautifully injected by Mr. Gray (Pathol. Trans.) ; and more recently by that of one injected by Mr. Coote.

If effused in large quantity, so as to form a voluminous clot, and especially if so effused in a wound which is not perfectly excluded from the air, or if effused in even a subcutaneous injury in a person whose health is not good, it is most likely to excite inflammation; and the swelling of the wounded parts, or their commencing suppuration, will push it out of the wound. Thus we often see blood ejected.

But, in more favorable circumstances, the blood may be absorbed; and this may happen whether it have formed separate clots, or, more readily, when it is infiltrated in the tissues. What I have seen, however, in the experiments to which I have already referred, leads me to dissent from the account commonly given of the absorption of blood thus effused. The expressions generally used imply that the first thing towards the repair of such a wound is the absorption of the extravasated blood; and that then, in its place, the lymph or reparative material is produced. But this can hardly be the case; for the absorption of blood is a very slow process, and commonly requires as much time as would suffice for the complete healing of a wound, or even of a fracture. Not to mention the very slow absorption of the extravasations of blood in apoplexy, or in serious sacs, I have found the blood effused in the subcutaneous tissue and the muscles, after a simple fracture, scarcely changed at the end of five weeks; that in a tied artery was as little changed after seven weeks: and even in common leech-bites we may sometimes find the blood-corpuscles, in little ecchymoses, unchanged a month after their extravasation; yet in much less time than this it is commonly implied that all the blood extravasated in an injury is cleared quite away, that lymph may occupy its place. My impression is, that this opinion is founded on imperfect observations. Blood is supposed to be effused in all subcutaneous injuries; and where it is not found, it is supposed to have been absorbed; the truth rather being, that, where no blood appears, none ever was.

The true method of the absorption of blood left in a wound seems to be, that it is enclosed within the reparative material, and absorbed by the vessels of that material as its organization proceeds. The best instance in support of this that I have seen was in the case of a rabbit's Achilles tendon, divided subcutaneously six days before death. The reparative process had proceeded favorably, and as strong a band of union as is usual at that period was formed of the new reparative material deposited between the retracted ends. On slitting open this band, I found within it a clot of blood, such as must have come from a large vessel; and this clot was completely enclosed within the new material; not closely adherent to it, nor changed as if towards organization; but rather, decolorized, mottled, and so altered as clots are in apoplexy before absorption.

I believe that this case only showed in a very marked manner what usually happens with blood thus effused and not ejected; for it is quite common, after the division of tendons, to find a new reparative material, if not containing distinct clots, yet blotched with the blood that was infiltrated in the tissue in which the reparative material is deposited : and even when the repair of a fracture was nearly perfect, I have still found traces of blood-corpuscles enclosed in the reparative material, and degenerating, as if in preparation for absorption.

Ejection and absorption are, doubtless, the usual means by which blood effused in injuries is disposed of; yet I feel nearly sure it may in some instances become organized, and form part of the reparative material. The cases of manifest organization of blood already referred to leave no doubt of the possibility of this happening : its occurrences can no longer be set aside as a thing quite improbable. The only question is, whether blood effused in injuries has been seen organized. Now I think no one familiar with Hunter's works will lightly esteem any statement of his as to a matter of observation. He may have been sometimes deceived in thinking that he saw blood becoming organized in subcutaneous injuries (for subcutaneous granulations are sometimes very like partially decolorized clots); yet I believe he was often right : for sometimes one finds clots of blood about the fractured ends of bones which have every appearance of being in process of organization. They do not look mottled, or rusty, or brownish, as extravasated blood does when it is degenerating, preparative to its absorption; but they are uniformly decolorized to a pinkish-yellow hue. They have more of appearance of filamentous structure than recent clots have; and they are not grumous or friable, like old and degenerating ones, but have a peculiar toughness, compactness, and elasticity, like firm gelatine. When clots are found in this condition, I believe it is a sign that they were organizing : for this is the condition into which, commonly, the clot in a tied artery passes in its way to be fully organized ; and (which is very characteristic) you may find clots in the track of wounded parts thus changing, as if towards organization, while those about them, and out of the way of the reparative process, are degenerating.

On the whole, then, I believe we may thus generally conclude concerning the part that blood, when it is extravasated, takes in the repair of injuries :—

1. It is neither necessary nor advantageous to any mode of healing.

2. A large clot, at all exposed to the air, irritates and is ejected.

3. In more favorable conditions the effused blood becomes enclosed in the accumulating reparative material; and while this is organizing, the blood is absorbed; and,

Lastly, it is probable that the blood may be organized and form part of the reparative material; but even in this case it probably retards the healing of the injury.

I proceed now to the consideration of the new material which is produced for the repair of injuries that are not healed by the immediate union. It is that to which the general name of lymph, or coagulable lymph, is given.

Our notions concerning the properties of this substance, when once formed for the repair of injuries, are derived almost entirely from examinations of the lymph formed in acute inflammations, with which it is supposed to be identical. This identity is far from being proved, but their similarity is in many particulars evident, and especially in that both manifest, by their spontaneous coagulation, that they contain fibrine. The coagulum which is spontaneously formed in reparative material is, in microscopic characters, like that of fibrine: chemically, too, they appear alike: and the organization of the fibrine of the blood in the complete clot, as well as all the other circumstances which lead to the opinion that fibrine is the principal material for organization into tissues, justifies the belief that the lymph exuded for the purposes of repair has fibrine for its principal constituent. However, when we speak of fibrine as the chief reparative material, we must not have in mind the pure organic compound that minute chemistry might obtain, but rather that which exists in the natural, and seemingly rough, state,—as fibrine, with some fatty matter, and some incidental saline constituents; for all these are found in all the specimens of coagulable lymph that have been examined; and doubtless they are essential, as the so-called "incidental" principles always are, to the due construction of the substance to be organized.

Regarding its vital properties, the essential character of the coagulable lymph is its tendency to develop itself; a tendency which it has of its own properties. It thus displays itself as a plasma or blastema; a fluid to be classed with those others that manifest the capacity to assume organic structure; such as the lymph and chyle that develop themselves to blood, and the semen, which, at first fluid, gradually develops itself into more and more complex structures.

The natural tendency of coagulable lymph is to develop itself into the fibrous, or the common fibro-cellular or connective, tissue—the lowest form of vascular tissue, and the structure which, in nearly all cases in man, constitutes the bond by which disunited parts are again joined. This is commonly formed, whatever be the tissue upon which the lymph is placed, whether containing cellular tissue in its natural structure or not. This, therefore, we may regard as the common or general tendency of lymph; but in certain cases the development of lymph passes beyond this form, or deviates from it into another direction, in adaptation to the special necessity of the part to be repaired. Thus, for the repair of bone, the lymph may proceed a certain distance towards the development of fibrous tissue, as if for a common healing; but this fibrous tissue may next ossify; or, not forming fibrous tissue at all, the lymph may proceed at once to the formation of a nearly perfect cartilage, and this may ossify. In general, moreover, the character of the connective tissue that is formed in repair is adapted to that of the parts that it unites. The bond for the union of a tendon is much tougher than a common scar in the skin; the scar in skin is tougher and less pliant than that in mucous membrane, and so on.

But, passing by, for the present, the instances of special development of the reparative material, in adaptation to special purposes or injuries, let me speak of its development into fibrous, fibro-cellular, or connective tissue. I have said that, in its first production, the reparative material is like the lymph of inflamed serous membranes; at least, no characteristic difference is yet known between these, which we might call respectively, inflammatory and reparative lymph. Neither are there yet any observations to show a difference in the primary characters of the materials effused for the repair of injuries of different parts, or in different circumstances; and yet such a difference, in even the original properties of the reparative lymph, is indicated by the fact, that, in different circumstances, it may proceed to the same end—the formation of fibrous tissue—by two different ways of development. The lymph or new material, which is produced for the repair of open wounds, generally develops itself into fibro-cellular tissue through nucleated cells; that formed for the healing of subcutaneous wounds as generally develops itself into the same tissue through the medium of nucleated blastema.

Now, both these are repetitions of natural modes of development of the same forms of tissue. And it must not appear an objection that there should be two modes of development to the same perfect structure; for this is usual, and has been observed in nearly all the tissues. In the development of the blood-corpuscles, a first set are formed from part of the embryo-cells that form the germinal area, of the whole body of the embryo; and a second set are formed, I believe, exclusively from the corpuscles of lymph and chyle. So it is with the cartilage, the muscular, and other tissues that are formed in the earliest periods of embryo-life. At first they are developed from some of the embryo-cells; yet in later life no such cells are seen among them, but others appropriate to them, and of different form. So also in the bones, which at first are developed through cartilage, but in their subsequent growth are increased by ossification of fibrous tissue; and in the repair of which we shall find even more numerous modifications of these different developments.

The development of the fibro-cellular or connective substance through nucleated cells may be observed in the material of granulations, or in that of inflammatory adhesions (whether in a serous sac or in a wound healing by primary adhesion), in inflammatory indurations, and in the naturally developed fibro-cellular tissue of many parts. The process is, with slight and apparently not essential modifications, the same in all; and is, I believe, almost exactly described by Schwann.

The cells first formed in granulations are spherical, palely or **darkly** nebulous, from about 1-1800th to 1-2500th of an inch in diameter. They contain a few shining, dark-bordered granules, and lie imbedded in a variable quantity of clear pellucid substance, by which they are held together, and which it is hard to see, unless acetic acid be added. When

Fig. 14.*

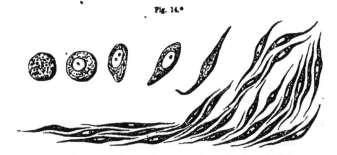

water is added, it penetrates the cells, and as they swell up their walls appear more distinct, and their contents are diffused. Some cells thus become much larger and clearer, and show in their interior numerous vibrating molecules: others display fewer molecules, but a distinct, round, dark-bordered nucleus, which appears attached to the inside of the cell-wall. Such a nucleus is rarely seen in granulation-cells, unless they are distended with water: acetic acid, acting more quickly than water, brings the nucleus more evidently and constantly into view, and often makes it appear divided into two or three portions.†

In the development of cellular or connective tissue from these cells, whether in the natural structures or in those that are formed in disease or after injury, the first apparent change is in the nucleus. It becomes more distinct; then oval (even before the cell does), and at the same time clearer, brighter, like a vesicle tensely filled with pellucid substance. One or two nucleoli now appear distinctly in it, and soon it attenuates itself; but this it does later, or in a less degree, than the cell: for a common appearance is that of elongated cells bellied out at the middle by the nucleus.

While these changes are ensuing in the nucleus, each cell also is developing its structure; first becoming minutely, yet more distinctly, granular and dotted; then having its cell-wall thinned, or even losing it.

* Development of granulation cells; the elongated cells in the group below are sketched as less magnified than those above.

† The granulation-cells are very like the white or lymph-corpuscles of the blood: but the likeness implies nothing more than the general fact that many structures which, in their perfect state, are widely different in form as well as in office, have, as to form, the same rudimental elements. The fact, of which there are many other instances, seems the more remarkable, if we contrast it with that already mentioned,—that the same perfect structure may have more than one original or rudimental form, and more than one method of development.

It elongates at one or both ends, and thus are produced a variety of lanceolate, caudate, or spindle-shaped cells, which gradually elongate and attenuate themselves towards the filamentous form. As they thus change, they also group themselves; so that, commonly, one may find the swollen part of each, at which the nucleus lies, engaged between the thinner parts of the two or more adjacent to it. Thus, the filaments into which the cells are developed are clustered or fasciculated: each cell forming, I think, usually, only one filament, and long filaments being sometimes formed by the attachment of the ends of two or more, each developed from a single cell.

The final disposal of the nuclei of these cells is not clear. In the development of the cellular tissue formed in inflammation or granulating wounds, they seem to waste and be absorbed. Certainly such nucleus-fibres as Henle supposed to be formed from them are not found in recent · scars, though common in those of old standing.

In some granulations, but, I think, only in such as are formed on bones, one may often find large compound cells, or masses or laminæ of blastema, of oval form, and as much as 1-250th of an inch in diameter, containing eight, ten, or more nuclei. They are like certain natural constituents of the medulla of bone (as described by Kölliker* and Robin†); and like the bodies which are found constituting the chief part of fibro-plastic tumors. Sometimes, also, even in the deeper parts of granulations, cells are found expanded, flattened, scale-like, and nucleated, as if approximating to the formation of epidermal cells.

Such, briefly, is the process for the development of fibro-cellular tissue through nucleated cells as observed in granulations. Some modifications of it may be noticed in certain cases, especially in regard to the proportion that the cells bear to the substance in which they lie. In some forms of granulations, as in some natural parts of the embryo, this substance is abundant; and I presume that by its development or fibrillation it takes part in the formation of filaments. But none of the modifications affect the essential characters of the process.

The development of fibro-cellular or fibrous tissue through nucleated blastema is, as I have already said, best observed, among the processes of repair, in the organization of the material by which, in most cases, the bonds of connection after subcutaneous wounds are formed. It is the same process which Henle‡ regards as the only mode of development of the fibro-cellular and fibrous tissues.

Of the union of divided tendons I hope to speak more fully in a future lecture. For the present purpose, and in illustration of the development

* Mikrosk. Anatomie, Fig. 113, 121.

† Bull. de la Société de Biologie, 1849, p. 150.

‡ Allgemeine Anatomie. A similar process is described by Reichert, Zwicky, and Gerlach.

of fibro-cellular or fibrous tissue from nucleated blastema, it may be enough to state that, when the first exudation of the products of the inflammation, excited by the violence of the wound, is completed, a quantity of finely molecular or dimly-shaded substance, like homogeneous or dotted fibrine, begins to appear in the space in which the bond of union is to be formed. This substance is infiltrated in the tissue that collapses into the space between the retracted ends of the tendon. At first there is no appearance of nuclei or cytoblasts in it: it seems to be merely a blastema of fibrine; but, as it acquires firmess and distinctness, the nucle appears in it. These seem to form out of collecting clusters of granules; they presently appear as oval bodies, with dark hard outlines, soon becoming elongated; they have clear contents, without nuclei: they are irregularly scattered, but so firmly imbedded in the blastema that, in general, they cannot be dislodged. They may be seen in very fine fragments without reagents; but, commonly, the application of acetic acid is necessary to make them distinct, by making the intermediate substance transparent, while the nuclei themselves appear to acquire darker edges and shrivel a little. The nuclei undergo comparatively little change, while the blastema in which they are embedded is acquiring, more and more distinctly, the filamentous appearance, and then the filamentous structure. Only, they appear to elongate, and to attenuate themselves, and to grow more irregular in their outlines, as if by shriveling, or by slight branching.

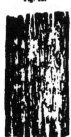

Fig. 15.

The blastema may become at length perfect fibro-cellular or fibrous tissue; a tissue not to be distinguished from that found in normal conditions. I have not been able to find, as Henle describes, that the nuclei are developed into fibres. In the process of repair by tissue thus developed, as well as by that which is formed through cells, my impression is that the nuclei finally shrivel; gradually contracting into little crooked or branched lines, and at length disappearing: for, as I have already said, well-formed nucleus-fibres, or such elastic yellow fibres as might be developed from them, do not generally occur in cicatrices of recent formation, or in the large bonds of union by which divided tendons are healed.

I have been thus minute in the account of these two modes of development of fibro-cellular tissue, prevailing alike in the natural structures and in the materials of repair, because the knowledge of them may enable us to settle some questions respecting all the modes of healing, and because it seems to point out the essential anatomical difference in the healing of open and of subcutaneous wounds, with disconnection of divided parts.

9

The general truth appears to be (as already stated), that the material for repair for subcutaneous wounds of soft parts is developed through the formation of nucleated blastema; while that for repair by primary adhesion, and by granulation, is developed through nucleated cells. Now, since both these methods of development are, as I have already said, imitations of natural methods, we might suppose that they are, therefore, both alike natural or healthy processes; alike sure to pass to their purposed end, safe from disease or degeneration. But, if we consider also the morbid conditions in which these two methods of development occur, we may find that the development through cells is characteristic of a less perfect process of healing than that accomplished with the nucleated blastema that appear to originate in a fibrinous exudation. For, in describing the products of inflammation, I shall have to show, that in general, the inflammatory exudations which occur in plethoric sthenic conditions of the system, or in local diseases in persons otherwise sound, have the aspect of fibrinous substance, like the materials which are produced in subcutaneous injuries, and are developed through nucleated blastema; while, on the other hand, the inflammatory exudations in debilitated persons, and in ascenthic blood-diseases, assume a corpuscular structure, like that of granulations upon open wounds.

Let me, however, in conclusion, state that, although I have described the two modes of development of fibro-cellular or fibrous tissue for the healing of wounds as if they were always as separate as they are distinct, yet they may co-exist, and probably often do so. In the repair of many wounds, the two materials, namely, that which is to be developed through nucleated cells, and that whose progress is to be through nucleated blastema, may be mixed. Thus, in subcutaneous wounds and injuries, the first consequence of the mechanical violence is the exudation of a common inflammatory product, which makes the cellular tissue oedematous, and usually organizes itself into nucleated cells. Thus you find the space between the retracted parts of divided tendons for about two days. But then, the more proper and purer material of repair is produced; and this, increasing in an inverse proportion to the degree of inflammation, soon overwhelms the former product of inflammation, and is developed into the nucleated blastema. Still, for many days, traces of the inflammatory product may be discerned mingled with the blastema, confusing its appearance, but, I believe, finally organizing with it into the bond of union. So, in divided muscles, and in simple fractures, the inflammatory exudation, produced in consequence of the first violence, appears to mingle and develop itself with the more proper material of repair; but they bear an inverse proportion to one another, and the more manifest the signs of the inflammation, the less is the quantity of the proper reparative material, and the slower, in the end, the process of repair.

On the other hand, I think that in the ordinary healing of open wounds, which are soon brought together by sutures, or other appropriate means, there may be less than the commonly observed formation of nucleated cells, and some of the reparative material may be developed through the nucleated blastema. Or, when the different materials are not mingled at the same spot, yet, in a single wound, different parts may be healed by the organization of one or other material, according to the degree of inflammation that is in each part present.

LECTURE IX.

THE PROCESSES OF REPAIR OF WOUNDS.

I PROCEED now to the description of the several modes of healing of wounds, and shall at present speak of only such wounds as are externally open. Among the modes which I enumerated, the first was that which, as I stated in the preceding lecture, is effected by immediate union. It corresponds with what Mr. Hunter called union by the first intention; but, since that term has been applied more recently to another mode of healing, I have adopted the term "immediate union" from Dr. Macartney, who, so far as I know, was the first to observe clearly that the healing of wounds may be effected "without any intervening substance, such as blood or lymph."* He says—"The circumstances under which immediate union is effected, are the cases of incised wounds that admit of being with safety and propriety, closely and immediately bound up. The blood, if any be shed on the surfaces of the wound, is thus pressed out, and the divided blood-vessels and nerves are brought into perfect contact, and union may take place in a few hours; and as no intermediate substance exists in a wound so healed, no mark or cicatrix is left behind.

" We have familiar examples of this mode of healing in slight cuts received on the fingers, which, after being bound up, if no inflammation be induced, perfectly heal without the individual having any unpleasant sensation in the part after the moment of the infliction of the wound. A case has been lately communicated to me, of a considerable cut of the hand having been cured by this mode of direct union, without any sensation of pain, in the short space of four or five hours."

It is singular that Dr. Macartney should speak of the process of immediate union occurring in so few and very trivial instances as these; for it seems certain that many even very large wounds are usually, in favorable circumstances, thus healed. The characteristics of this mode are,

* Treatise on Inflammation, p. 49.

that the divided parts, being placed in exact contact, simply conjoin or reunite: no blood or new material is placed between them for a connecting bond, and no sign or product of inflammation is present. All these characters meet in such cases as the favorable union of flaps of skin, which have been reflected from the subjacent parts, and are then replaced or transferred to some other adjacent wounded surface.

The instances in which I have best observed it have been after wounds reflecting portions of the scalp, and after operations for the removal of the mammary gland. In these operations, as you know, the usual proceeding is to remove some of the skin, including the nipple, and to uncover the rest of the surface of the gland by reflecting from it an upper and lower flap of skin. Then, the gland being removed, these flaps, which are often of considerable extent, are laid down upon the parts on which the base of the gland rested, chiefly upon the fascia over the great pectoral muscle.

One of the first specimens I examined well illustrated the healing that may now ensue. It was taken from a woman thirty-three years old, whose breast and several axillary glands were removed for cancer. Her general health seemed good, and all went on well after the operation. The flaps, which were of course very large, had been carefully laid down, strapped with isinglass plaster, and well tended. They appeared to unite in the ordinary way, and there remained only a narrow space between their retracted edges, in which space granulations arose from the pectoral muscle. Three weeks after the operation these were making good progress towards cicatrization; but erysipelas and phlebitis ensued, and the patient died in four or five days.

I cut off the edges of the wound with the subjacent parts, expecting to find the evidences of union by organized lymph, or, possibly, blood. But neither existed; and the state of parts cannot be better described than by saying that scarcely the least indication remained of either the place where the flap of skin was laid on the fascia, or the means by which they were united. It was not possible to distinguish the relation which these parts held to each other from that which naturally exists between subcutaneous fat and the fascia beneath it. There was no unnatural adhesion; but, as the specimen, which is in the Museum of St. Bartholomew's, will still show, the subcutaneous fat which did lie over the mammary gland was now connected with the fascia over the pectoral muscle, just as (for example) the corresponding fat below the clavicle is naturally connected to the portion of the same fascia that lies there. The parts were altered in their relations, but not in their structure. I could find small points of induration where, I suspect, ligatures had been tied, or where, possibly, some slight inflammation had been otherwise excited; and one small abscess existed under the lower flap. But with most careful microscopic examination, I could discover no lymph or exudation-corpuscles, and only small quantities of what looked like the debris of such oil-particles or corpuscles of blood as might have been between the cut surfaces when the flaps were laid down. In short, we cannot otherwise or more minutely discribe this healing than by the term "immediate union:" it is immediate, at once in respect of the absence of any intermediate substance placed between the wounded surfaces, and in respect of the speed with which it is accomplished.

Opportunities of examining wounds thus healed being rare, I made three experiments on rabbits (with my friend Mr. Savory), and found the description I have just given quite confirmed. A portion of skin, which my extended fingers would just cover, was raised from the back of a rabbit, replaced, and fastened down with a few sutures. Three days afterwards the rabbit was killed. The edges of the wound were slightly retracted, and the space between them was covered with scab : for about half an inch under the edge of the replaced flap of skin, the tissue was inflamed and infiltrated with exudation-matter ; but beyond this no trace of the injury or of its healing could be seen. The parts appeared as they had appeared before the operation. Even the microscope could detect only a slight infiltration of inflammatory matter, which one might certainly ascribe to the wound being open at its edges, and to some hairs having by accident been enclosed under the flap when it was replaced.

Of course, it is only from such examinations as these after death, that we can speak certainly of the absence of inflammation and of all intermediate uniting substances ; yet confirmatory evidence may yet be obtained from the examination of any such wound during life,—I mean in any such case as that of a flap of skin raised up, then laid down on the subjacent wounded surface, and there uniting favorably ; or in any case of that kind of plastic operation in which a flap is raised, and then made to slide to some further position. In such cases, with favorable progress, no sign of inflammation is observed; though, if the skin were in even a small degree inflamed, it could scarcely fail to be manifested by the ordinary appearances of redness and heat. If the flap be pressed, no fluid oozes beneath its edges (I speak, of course, of only such cases as are making favorable progress); and after one or two days, according to the extent of the wound, the flap will move on the subjacent parts, not with the looseness of a part separate from them, nor with the stiffness of one adherent through inflammation, but with the easy and pliant sliding which is peculiar to the natural connection of the skin with the subjacent fascia.

Such is the nature of "immediate union :" the best imaginable process of healing. Two conditions appear essential to it : first, exactness of the coaptation of the wounded surfaces; and secondly, the absence of all inflammatory process.

To obtain the former, the simple replacement of the raised pieces of skin may sometimes be sufficient. But there is a class of cases to which this mode of healing is peculiarly applicable, and in which more than this may be required: I refer to the removal of large subcutaneous tumors,—fatty tumors and the like,—where, after the operation, large cavities are left, and commonly left to granulate. In these cases I believe that modern surgery does not often enough employ the older method of carefully and softly padding the parts, and of so bandaging them that the exposed surfaces may be held in contact for the one, two, or three days necessary for immediate union. Many surgeons, I know, commonly employ these means, but by many they are avoided, through fear of exciting inflammation by over-heating the parts, or hindering the discharge of secreted fluids. Doubtless, no single rule of management would be safe; but I think, with regard to this fear of exciting inflammation, it need not be entertained, if the means I have alluded to be employed only during the first two or three days after the infliction of the wound. For one may generally observe that, for at least two or three days after such an injury as an amputation, the raising of a flap of skin in a removal of the breast, or the like, scarcely any reparative process appears in the parts that are kept from contact; no granulations are formed, no pus secreted, only a little serous-looking fluid oozes from them. Now, during this calm, which would certainly not be disturbed by the parts being softly padded and kept in perfect rest, the immediate union may be accomplished. If, through any untoward circumstance, it be not in this period completed, its occurrence is, I believe, impossible, and then the means more appropriate for other methods of healing may be employed.

The attainment of the other necessary condition, the absence of inflammation, is quite consistent with these means for insuring perfect and continued contact of the wounded surfaces. How the condition is to be fulfilled I need not say: the means are some of those that are commonly laid down for preventing inflammation from being, as it is said, more than is necessary for the union by the first intention; and the best of them are temperance, rest, and uniform temperature. The necessity of observing them will appear the greater, if it is remembered that what is wanted for immediate union is, not a certain undefined slight degree of inflammation, but the complete absence of inflammation; for the probability of the occurrence of immediate union may be reckoned as being in an inverse ratio to the probability of inflammation occurring in the time necessary for its accomplishment.

The second mode of repair that I enumerated, is that by *primary adhesion*.

This is the process which Mr. Hunter named union by adhesion, or union by the adhesive inflammation. My reasons for preferring the term "primary adhesion" will presently appear. He says: "Where the former bond of union" (*i. e.*, the union by blood or by the first intention), "is lost in a part, to produce a new one a second operation takes place, namely, inflammation."* Observe how carefully Mr. Hunter distinguishes the case in which inflammation ensues, from that in which none is necessary: and presently after—"If the divided parts are allowed to remain till the mouths of the divided vessels are entirely shut, inflammation will inevitably follow, and will furnish the same materials for union which are contained in extravasated blood, by throwing out the coagulated lymph; so that union may still take place, though some time later after the division of the parts. This inflammation I have called the adhesive." On this sentence, Mr. Palmer, expressing the opinion entertained by all the pathologists of ten or twelve years ago, says—"It is now generally considered that union by the first intention and adhesive inflammation are essentially the same processes, modified by the degree of inflammation. Union by the first intention is uniformly attended with some degree of pain and swelling, together with increased heat and vascularity, which, taken conjointly, constitute the definition of inflammation." And again: "According to the modern views, the modes of union above detailed" [i. e., the modes of union included by Mr. Hunter under the union by the first intention], "are always accompanied by adhesive inflammation. . . . . . The parts are united, not by the extravasated blood becoming vascular, but by the effusion and organization of coagulable lymph."

After what I have said respecting the process of immediate union, it may appear that Mr. Hunter was more nearly right than his successors. It would be an instructive piece of the history of surgery, to show, exactly, how his truth, being mixed with error, came therefore, to be thrown away, and to make room for an error which had less truth mixed with it. The stages of transition in opinion seem to have been, that, first, sufficient reason was found for disbelieving Hunter's statement, that blood forms the bond of union by the first intention; then, as it was assumed that there must always be some intermediate bond, this, it seemed, could be none but coagulable lymph. Now, coagulable lymph being known only as the product of inflammation, it followed that inflammation must be necessary for the healing of every wound; and then there ceased to be any distinction between the union by the first intention and the union by adhesion; both alike seemed to be the result of lymph, the product of inflammation, being exuded between the wounded surfaces, and united to them both.

Typical examples of union by primary adhesion may be watched in the cut edges of skin that are brought near together. When the cut surfaces are not in exact contact, the wound is exposed, and lymph is formed, and fills up the space; or, when they are in contact, the sutures, or other means employed to keep them so, excite inflammation enough for the production of some lymph between them. The lymph is simply laid on the cut surfaces; and scarcely any is infiltrated in the tissues. Organizing itself, and becoming vascular, it connects the two edges or

* Works, vol. iii. p. 253.

surfaces, and, finally, forms between them a thin layer of cellular tissue, on the thin surface of which, if it be exposed, a very delicate layer of cuticle is developed. The smooth shining surface of this cuticle gives the peculiar character of the scar, and one that scarcely changes, except in the alteration of apparent color when the new material becomes less vascular.

The lymph effused in the healing by primary adhesion always, so far as I know, develops itself through nucleated cells, and, doubtless, the whole process is very similar to that of the adhesion of inflamed serous membranes.

It may be very quickly accomplished. A boy died eighty hours after receiving a lacerated wound of the abdomen ; and, for forty-eight hours, of these eighty, he was so manifestly dying, that I think no reparative process could have been going on. A portion of the edges of the wound was united with lymph, which presented well-marked cells, like those of granulations, and contained looped blood-vessels full of blood.

But it may be accomplished more quickly than in this case. In a rabbit that I operated on as for hare-lip, I found, after forty-eight hours, the edges of the wounds partially, but firmly, united by lymph, many of the cells of which were already elongated, in such development as I have already described. Or, even more quickly than in this instance :—if a small abscess be opened, and the edges of the opening are not gaping or inverted, they may be found united, except at the middle, within twenty-four hours. I have seen them so united, with a distinct layer of soft, pinkish, new substance, in a wound made seventeen hours previously.

There are no cases in which the process of primary adhesion can be better observed than after operations for hare-lip. The inner portions of the wounds made in them may be healed by the immediate union, when the surfaces have been in exact coaptation ; but the edges of the skin and mucous membrane seem always united by the adhesive inflammation, for a scar is always visible—a scar formed by the lymph organized into cellular tissue and epithelium, and one which, as well as any, shows how little of assimilative force can be exercised by adjacent tissues ; for, narrow as it may be, it does not become quite like the adjacent skin, nor, like it, bear perfect epidermis and hair.

The history of union by primary adhesion cannot be conveniently completed till an account has been given of the healing by granulation and by secondary adhesion. Of these I will next speak: now I will only say of this union by primary adhesion, that it is less desirable than the immediate union, because, 1st, it is, probably, not generally so speedy; 2dly, it is not so close, and a scar is always formed by the organization of the new matter ; and, 3dly, the formation of lymph or exudation-cells is a process so indefinitely separated from that of the formation of pus-cells, that union by primary adhesion is much more likely to pass into suppuration than any process is in which no lymph is formed.

In describing the modes of healing by *granulation* and by *secondary adhesion*, I shall venture again to take my account from certain typical examples: such as cases in which, after amputation of a limb, the surfaces of the wound are not united by either of the means already described, but, as the expression is, are "left to granulate;" or such cases as the removal of a breast, and subsequent suppuration of the flaps and the exposed fascia; or such as wounds into inflamed parts, when the edges gape wide asunder, and the spaces left between them are filled up with granulations. These may serve as examples of a process which, although in all cases it may preserve certain general features of similarity, is yet in detail almost infinitely diversified, and often so inexplicably, that any more than a general account of it might fill volumes.*

Granulations will generally arise on all wounded surfaces that are left open to the air and are not allowed to dry. They will do so whether this exposure be continued from the first infliction of the wound, or commence after the edges, which have been brought together, have been again forced asunder by the swelling of the deeper-seated parts, or by hemorrhage, or secretion of fluid, between them. Exposure of a wound to the air is not prevented by any ordinary dressings: the air that is enclosed beneath them, or that can penetrate them, appears to be quite enough to determine all the difference of the events that follow open and subcutaneous injuries.

The simplest case for illustration is that of an open gaping incised wound, which, from the time of its infliction, is only covered, as in ordinary practice, with water-dressing, or some soft and moist substance. Blood gradually ceasing to flow from the surface of such a wound, one may see still some blood-tinged serous-looking fluid oozing from it. Slowly, as this becomes paler, some of it collects, like a whitish film or glazing, on the surface; and this, if it be examined with the microscope, will be found to contain an abundance of the white corpuscles of the blood, imbedded apparently in a fibrinous film. The collection of these corpuscles on the surface of the wound, especially on wounded muscles and fasciæ, appears to depend only on their peculiar adhesiveness. One sees them adhering much more firmly than ever the red corpuscles do to the walls of the minute blood-vessels, and to the glass on which they are examined; and so on cut surfaces, while the other constituents of the blood flow away, the white corpuscles, and, probably, also, some of the fibrine quickly coagulating, adhere.†

.* Some of the most important modifications of the process occur in gun-shot wounds. These are admirably described by Mr. Guthrie in the Lancet, Feb. 14, 1852.

† Reinhardt, by whom, I think, the fact was first clearly noticed (Traube's Beitrage H. ii. p. 188), supposes the white corpuscles may exude separately from the vessels. Perhaps the truth is, that their peculiar adhesiveness makes them flow less readily from the blood-vessels, when the bleeding is about to stop; so that at last, when the vessels finally close and empty themselves, a large proportion of these corpuscles may issue from them and adhere to the cut surface over which they slowly roll.

I am not aware of any facts that would prove what share the white corpuscles thus collected may take in the healing of a wound. They do not hinder it; for it is by many believed to be favorable to union by primary adhesion, to leave cut surfaces exposed, till they appear glazed over with the whitish film, and then to put them into contact. It is probable that corpuscles are organized when the surfaces that they cover are brought together: but I know of no facts bearing on the point, and it is one which I think experiments on animals could hardly be made to illustrate.

If a wound be left open, the glazing remains on such parts as it may have formed on, especially on the exposed muscles. No evident change ensues in it, except that it appears to increase slowly, and makes the surface of the wound look as if covered with a thin grayish or yellowish-white layer of buffy coat. This increase of glazing is the prelude of the formation of granulations; but while it is going on, and, often, for some days later, there is, in and about the wound, an appearance of complete inaction; a calm, in which scarcely anything appears except a slight oozing of serous fluid from the wound. Such a calm continues from one day to eight, ten, or more, according to the nature and extent of the wounded part, and the general condition of the body. In a cut or sawn hard bone, about ten days will generally elapse before any change is manifest; in cancellous bone the change ensues a few days more speedily: on the under surface of a large flap of skin, with subcutaneous fat, three days may thus pass without change; on the cut or excoriated surface of the more vascular part of the skin, two days or three.

These periods of repose after severe injury are of equal interest in physiology and in sugery; but in the former it is chiefly the interest of mystery. Observations on injuries of the frog's web* make it probable that the blood is stagnant in the vessels for some little distance from the wound during several days after the injury: but why it is so, and what are the changes ensuing in and about it, preparatory to its again moving on, we cannot quite tell. The interest to the surgeon watching this period of repose is more practical. The calm may be the brooding-time for either good or evil; whilst it lasts, the mode of union of the wound will, in many cases, be determined: the healing may be perfected, or a slow uncertain process of repair may be but just begun; and the mutual influence, which the injury and the patient's constitution are to exercise on one another, appears to be manifested very often at or near the end of this period. Moreover, in open wounds, the time at which, on each tissue, granulations are produced, is determined by this calm; for they begin to be distinctly formed at its end. Thus, on a stump, after a circular amputation, one may find the margin of the skin and the surface of the

* See especially those detailed by Mr. Travers in his Essay on Inflammation and the Healing Process: and those by Mr. Wharton Jones, On the State of the Blood and Blood-vessels in Inflammation.

muscles well covered with granulations, while the surface of the fat reflected with the skin is barren of them, and the sawn walls of the bone are dry and bare. But from the sawn end of the medullary tube there may already protrude a florid, mushroom-shaped mass of granulations, overhanging the adjacent walls : as if parts in which nutrition is habitually carried on under restraint, within hard and rigid boundary-walls, were peculiarly apt to produce abundant organizable material as soon as they are released.* Generally, also, the granulations springing from these different tissues observe the same order in their rate of development as in their first appearance. Those that first take the lead, keep it, or for a time increase it.

But suppose the period of calm after the violence of the injury to be well over-past—how does the right process of repair set in? Apparently, first of all, by the supply of blood to the injured part being increased.

The experiments on the webs of frogs, to which I have already referred, have shown that, immediately after the infliction of an injury, the blood in the adjacent parts remains for some days quite stagnant ; and we may believe the same occurs, but for a shorter time, in our own case. During this stagnation, materials may ooze from the vessels, enough to form the glazing of the wounded surfaces of certain parts; but before granulations can be formed, the flow of blood must again begin, and its supply must be increased by enlargement, and perhaps by multiplication, of the vessels in the injured part. We cannot often see this increase so well in soft parts as in bone exposed after injury. If, in this condition, compact bone be watched, there may be seen, two or three days before the springing up of granulations, rosy points or minute blotches, which gradually deepen in their hue, and become larger. From these, presently, granulations will arise. The same process may be well seen when a portion of the skull has been exposed, as by suppuration under the pericranium. In such a case, which I watched carefully, nearly one-third of the upper part of the skull was bared, and it became dry and yellowish, and looked quite lifeless ; but after some days a few rosy points appeared on its surface, and these multiplied and enlarged, and from each of them granulations grew up, till the whole surface of the skull was covered. I watched them nearly every day, and it seemed evident, at least to the naked eye, that, in all cases, an increased supply of blood preceded the production of the new material from which granulations were to be formed.

Doubtless just the same happens in soft parts as in bone; so that it may be stated, generally, that the first visible change that ensues after the period of calm—the period of incubation, as it is called—is an in-

---

* One may sometimes observe a similar fact in the growth of granulations out of the very centre of the cut end of a divided tendon, while its margins are unchanged. The abundant growth of substance like brain covered with granulations, in cases of hernia cerebri, is of the same kind.

creased supply of blood to the parts in which repair is to ensue. This, probably, corresponds exactly with the increased afflux of blood which ensues in inflammation; and Mr. Travers's and other observations on the healing of the frog's web, make it nearly sure that this increased afflux is attended with slower movement of the blood, or at first even with stagnation of the blood in the minute vessels nearest to·the cut edges or surface.

Of the force by which this increased afflux of blood is determined, I believe that as yet no sufficient explanation can be rendered; but the fact serves to show that the ordinary process of granulation is, in its commencement, morbid. It is beneficial, indeed, in its end or purpose, but is morbid in its method, being comparable with the process of inflammation more than with any of those that are natural to the body. The process of granulating displays, I think, two points of resemblance to inflammation, and of dissimilarity from natural processes: namely, 1st, that the increased quantity of blood in the part producing granulations, moves more slowly than in health; while in the naturally increased supply its movement is not retarded; and 2dly, that the increased supply of blood precedes the increased production of material. For, in the discharge of natural functions, the increased supply of blood to a part appears always to be a secondary event, the consequence of some increase in the formation of the part. As, in the embryo, many parts form themselves before blood appears, and the growth of these and other parts always a little precedes the proportionate supply of blood to them; so always, subsequently, the increase or diminution of growth, or any other organic act, appears to precede, by some small interval, the proportioned change in the supply of blood. But with unnatural and morbid processes it appears to be usually different; in these, with inflammation for their type and chief example, the increased afflux of blood precedes the increased production of material to be organized, and the decrease of blood precedes the decrease of organic processes.

That which next follows, after the increased afflux of blood, is the effusion of the material that is to be organized into granulations. This is added to, or, perhaps, displaces, the glazing that already exists upon some surfaces; and where none such exists, as on fat or bone, the new material is accumulated on the bare surface of the wound. No account of the process of effusion, so far as it is visible to the naked eye, can be better than Mr. Hunter's (iii. 491). "I have often been able," he says, "to trace the growth and vascularity of this new substance. I have seen upon a sore a white substance, exactly similar, in every visible respect, to coagulating lymph. I have not attempted to wipe it off, and the next day of dressing I have found this very substance vascular; for by wiping or touching it with a probe, it has bled freely. I have observed the same appearance on the surface of a bone that was laid bare. I once scraped off

some of the external surface of a bone of the foot, to see if the surface
would granulate. I remarked, the following day, that the surface of the
bone was covered with a whitish substance, having a tinge of blue; when
I passed my probe into it, I did not feel the bone bare, but only its resistance. I conceived this substance to be coagulating lymph thrown out
from inflammation, and that it would be forced off when suppuration
came on; but, on the succeeding day, I found it vascular, and appearing
like healthy granulations."

To this account, little can be added more than the microscope has
shown. In the minute structure of granulations, or, at least, of such
growths of new substance as present all the characters that we imply by
that term—the bright ruddy texture, the uniformly granulated free surface, the succulency and abundant supply of blood—in these we may
discern two varieties, corresponding with the varieties of lymph that I
have already spoken of. In subcutaneous injuries or diseases, granulations sometimes form which develop themselves into cellular tissue,
through nucleated blastema. So I found in a case of simple fracture in
which the ends of the bone remained long disunited; they were enclosed
in a cavity formed by condensation of the surrounding tissues, but containing no pus, and were covered with a distinct layer of florid granulations. It was just such a case as that which Mr. Hunter had in view,
and preserved,* as an instance of the formation of granulations without
suppuration, in the repair of subcutaneous fractures and other injuries.

But in by far the greater proportion of cases, granulations are only
formed in exposed injuries: and in these, they consist of cells that may
develop themselves into fibro-cellular tissue: and of such as these I will
now exclusively speak.

Cells upon cells, such as I have already described (p. 183), are heaped
up together in a layer from half a line to two lines, or, rarely, more in
thickness, without apparent order, and connected by very little intermediate substance (Figs. 14 and 19). Singly, they are colorless; but in
clusters they are ruddy, even independent of the blood-vessels. In granulations that are making healthy progress—in such as, after three or four
days' growth, are florid, moist, level, scarcely raised above the surrounding tissues, uniformly granular, or like a surface of minute papillæ—one
can conveniently trace the cells in various stages, according to the position they occupy. The deeper-seated ones are always most advanced,
and often much elongated, or nearly filamentous; while the superficial
ones are still in a rudimental state, or, near the edges of the granulating
surface, are acquiring the character of epithelial cells.

The cellular tissue thus constructed by the development of the granulation cells finally assumes all the characters of the natural examples of
that tissue. Thus it is found in the thin layer of substance of which
scars that are formed in the place of granulating wounds, are composed.

* College Museum, No. 16.

After some time, elastic tissue is mingled with the fibro-cellular ; but this, as I have already said, appears to be effected by a later process. I found, in one case, no elastic tissue in scars that had existed, the one twelve months, the other eighteen months ; but in scars several years old I have always found it.

The cuticle, also, that forms on granulations, gradually approximates more nearly to the perfect characters, and, like the fibro-cellular tissue that it covers, presents the interesting fact of adaptation to the purposes of the part on which it is placed. Thus, in granulating wounds or ulcers on the sole of the foot, one may often see that, from the first, the new cuticle is more opaque and thicker than it is on other parts, on which the natural cuticle, in adaptation to the protection required from it, is naturally thinner : and let it be observed that this peculiar formation of the new cuticle is in adaptation to conditions not yet entered upon. It justly excited the admiration of Albinus,* when he saw in the foetus, even long before birth, the cuticle of the heel and palm thicker than those of other parts ; adapted and designed to that greater friction and pressure to which, in future time, they would be exposed. It is the same when, in adult life, new cuticle is to be formed on the same parts. While it is forming, all pressure and all friction are kept away, yet it is constructed in adaptation to its future exposure to them. Surely such a provision is, beyond all refutation, an evidence of design ; and surely in this fact we may discern another instance of the identity in nature and in method of the powers that are put in operation in the acts of first construction and of repair.

But before I end this lecture, let me add, that although one may so clearly trace in the development of granulation-cells, and in the end which they achieve by the formation of fibro-cellular tissue and cuticle, an imitation of the natural processes and purpose of the corresponding developments in the embryo, yet is there a remarkable contrast between them, in regard to the degrees in which they are severally liable to defect or error. We can scarcely find examples of the arrests or errors of development of mere structure in the embryo ; but such events are quite common in the formation of granulations, as well as of all other new products. All the varieties in the aspect of granulating wounds and sores, which the practised eye can recognize as signs of deflection from the right way to healing, are so many instances of different diseases of the granulation-substance ; diseases not yet enough investigated, though of much interest in the study of both the healing process and the organization of new products in inflammation.

A comparatively few observations enable one to trace morbid conditions of these new structures, closely answering to those long known in the older and more perfect tissues. Thus, one may find simply arrested development of granulations; as in the indolent healing of wounds and

* Annotationes Academicæ.

ulcers, whether from locally or generally defective conditions. Herein even years may pass, and the cells will not develop themselves beyond one or other of their lower forms. There is probably a continual mutation of particles among such cells, as in common nutrition; or they may increase, as in growth; but no development ensues, and the wound or the ulcer remains unhealed.

In other cases, the cells not only do not develop themselves, but they degenerate, becoming more granular, losing the well-marked characters of their nucleus, and acquiring all the structures of the pus-cell; thus are they found in the walls of fistulæ and sinuses. Or, worse than this, the granulation-cells may lose all structure, and degenerate into a mere layer of debris and molecular substance. Thus they may be found on the surface of a wound for a day or so before death or exhaustion, or in erysipelas, or fever; and in this state they are commonly ejected when a granulating wound ulcerates or sloughs.

With more active disease, granulations become turgid with blood, or œdematous: such are the spongy masses that protrude beyond the openings leading to diseased bone. Or, they inflame; and abundant large inflammatory granule-cells are found among their proper structures. Or, they suppurate internally, and purulent infiltration pervades their whole mass.

All these are among the many hinderances to healing: these are the dangers to which the healing by granulations is obnoxious; it is the proneness to these things that makes it even slower and more insecure than, in its proper course, it might be. And these are all instances of a class of changes which it is most important to study for exactness in morbid anatomy,—I mean the diseases of the products of disease.

LECTURE X.

THE PROCESSES OF REPAIR OF WOUNDS.

WITH the structural development of the granulation-cells into fibro-cellular tissue and cuticle, as described in the last lecture, there coincides a chemical change which seems to be the contrary of development; for the granulation-substance being converted from albuminous into horny and gelatinous principles, becomes, in chemical composition, less remote than it was from the constitution of inorganic matter. At its first effusion, the reparative material has the characters of a fibrinous principle; afterwards, when in the form of granulations and of young fibro-cellular tissue, its reactions are so far altered that it presents the characters of pyine, a somewhat indefinite principle, yet an albuminous one; finally, in its perfect development, the new-formed fibro-cellular tissue is gelatinous, and the epithelium appears to be like other specimens of horny matter.

These changes are in conformity with what appears to be a general rule; namely, that structures which are engaged in energetic development, self-multiplying, the seat of active vital changes, are generally of the highest organic composition; while the structures that are already perfect, and engaged in the discharge of functions such as are attended with infrequent changes of their particles, are as generally of lower composition. The much higher chemical development (if I may so call it) of the blood, than of the greater part of the tissues that are formed from it, is a general instance of this: in it albumen and fibrine predominate, and there is no gelatine: in the tissues gelatine is abundant, and fatty matter; and both these, through their affinities to the saccharine and oily principles, approach the characters of the lower vegetable and inorganic compounds.

The granulation-substance is a good instance in point: while lowly developed, but in an active vegetative life, it is albuminous; when perfect in its development, its perfected structures are gelatinous or horny. In this state its particles have probably a longer existence: they exchange a brief life of eminence for longevity in a lower station.

I have spoken hitherto of the development of only those structures which form the proper material of granulations, and of the scars that remain after the healing of wounds. But, commensurately with these, blood-vessels, and, perhaps, also, nerves, are formed. Of these, therefore, I will now speak.

In the last lecture I referred to the changes that ensue in the circulation of a wounded part. It first, it appears that the blood stagnates in the vessels immediately adjacent to the wound. This is evident in the wounds made in frogs' webs, and is most probable in the case of wounds in our own tissues; for else we could hardly understand the total absence of bleeding from a surface on which, as in every large wound, myriads of small vessels must be cut, and lie exposed. But after a time, of various duration in the different tissues, the movement of the blood is renewed, though not to its former velocity; the vessels of the wounded parts enlarge, and they all appear more vascular. Then the material of granulations, already in part effused, accumulates, and very soon blood and blood-vessels appear in this material.

By what process are these new vessels formed? Mr. Hunter's opinion was (and it is still held by many), that both the blood and its vessels form in the granulation-substance, as they do in the germinal area of the chick; and that, subsequently, they enter into communications with the vessels and blood of the part from which the granulations spring.

This is certainly not proved; although the development of the new vessels is according to a method equally natural.

In embryos, we may discern three several modes according to which blood-vessels are formed,—a good example of the manifold ways by which, in development, the same end may be reached.* In the first and earliest method, they are constructed around the blood corpuscles, which, being gradually developed from some of the embryo-cells, are laid out in the plan of the earliest and simplest circulation of the blood.

In this case, the vessels appear to be formed of the cells, or of the plasma which lies around the forming blood-cells, and gradually assumes the condition of a membrane, and is then developed into the more complex structures of the blood-vessels and the heart.

After this earliest period of embryo-life, it is probable that blood is never formed except within the vessels already constructed. It would seem as if none but the original embryo or germ-cells could be directly transformed into blood-corpuscles; all those that are later made derive their materials through a process of gradual elaboration in lymph or blood-vessels, to which process no resemblance can be discerned in the substance of granulations.

To increase the extent and number of vessels that must be added in adaptation to the enlargement and increasing complexity of the embryo, two methods are observed. In one, primary cells, in the interspaces of vessels already existing, enlarge and elongate, and send out branches in two or more directions. These branches are hollow: and while some of them are directed into anastomosis with each other, others extend towards, and open with dilatations into the vessels already formed and carrying blood. Then, these fine branches of each cell becoming larger, while the main cavity of the cell, from which they issued, attenuates itself, they are altogether transformed into a network of tubes of nearly uniform calibre, through which the blood, entering by the openings of communication with the older vessels, makes its way. Thus the wide network formed in the primordial circulation is subdivided into smaller meshes, and each part receives a more abundant supply of blood.

The other of these secondary modes of formation of new blood-vessels, is, I believe, the only mode in which blood-vessels are ever formed for granulations, or for superficial deposits of lymph, adhesions, and the like. The sketch is made from what may be seen in the growing parts of the tadpole's tail, and it accords with what Spallanzani observed of the extension of vessels into the substance of the tail when being reproduced after excision. Mr. Travers[†] and Mr. Quekett watched the same

* They are described in Kirke's Physiology, p. 661; and in the Supplement to the Translation of Muller's Physiology, p. 101. See also Garlach; Gewebelehre, p. 200.

[†] On Inflammation, and the Healing Process. See, also, on a similar formation, Virchow, in the Wurzburg Verhandlungen, B. i., p. 301.

process in the new material formed for the filling up of holes made in
the frog's web; and the same is indicated in the specimens illustrating
the repair of similar wounds which are in the College, from the Museum
of the late Dr. Todd, of Brighton.   There is, I think, no sufficient reason
to suppose that any other method prevails for the supply of blood-vessels
to any granulations, or similar new productions.   For, though the process in granulations or in lymph cannot be exactly watched during life,
yet every appearance after death is consistent with the belief that it is
the same as has been traced in the cases I have cited, and I have never
seen any indications of either of the other methods of development having
occurred.

The method may be termed that by *outgrowth* from the vessels
already formed.   Suppose a line or arch of capillary vessels passing

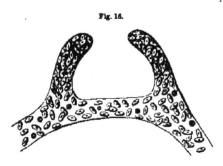

Fig. 16.

below the edge or surface
of a part to which new material has been superadded.
(Fig. 16.)   The vessel will
first present a dilatation at
one point, and coincidently,
or shortly after, at another,
as if its wall yielded a little
near the edge or surface.
The slight pouches thus
formed, gradually extend, as
blind canals or diverticula,

from the original vessel, still directing their course towards the edge
or surface of the new material, and crowded with blood-corpuscles, which
are pushed into them from the main stream.   Still extending, they converge; they meet; the partition-wall, that is at first formed by the meet-
ing of their closed ends, clears away, and a perfect arched tube is
formed, through which the blood, diverging from the main or former
stream and then rejoining it, may be continuously propelled.

In this way, then, are the simplest blood-vessels of granulations and
the like outgrowths formed.   The plan on which they are arranged is
made more complex by the similar outgrowths of branches from adjacent
arches, and their mutual anastomoses; but, to all appearance, the whole
process is one of outgrowth and development from vessels already formed.
And I beg of you to consider the wonder of such a process; how, in a
day, a hundred or more of such loops of fine membranous tube, less than
1-1000th of an inch in diameter, can be upraised; not by any mere
force of pressure, though with all the regularity of the simplest mechanism, but each by a living growth and development, as orderly and exact
as that which we might trace in the part most essential to the continuance
of life.   Observe, that no force so simple as even that of mere extension
or assimilation can determine such a result as this: for, to achieve the

construction of such an arch, it must spring with due adjustment from two determined points, and then its flanks must be commensurately raised, and these, as with mutual attraction, must approach and meet exactly in the crown. Nothing could accomplish such a result but forces determining the concurrent development of the two outgrowing vessels. We admire the intellect of the engineer, who, after years of laborious thought, with all the appliances of weight and measure and appropriate material, can begin at points wide apart, and force through the solid masses of the earth one tunnel, and can wall it in secure from external violence, and strong to bear some ponderous traffic; and yet he does but grossly and imperfectly imitate the Divine work of living mechanism that is hourly accomplished in the bodies of the least conspicuous objects of creation—nay, even in the healing of our casual wounds and sores.

The wonder of the process is, perhaps, in some degree enhanced by the events that will follow what may seem to be an accident. When the new vessel has begun to project, it sometimes bursts; and the diagram shows what then will happen. I have to thank Mr. Quekett for the sketch, which he made while assisting Mr. Travers in the examinations already cited. The blood-corpuscles that issue

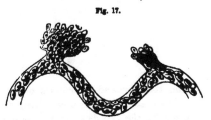

Fig. 17.

from the ruptured pouch or diverticulum collect in an uncertain mass within the tissue, like a mere ecchymosis; but, before long, they manifest a definite direction, and the cluster bends towards the line in which the new vessel might have formed, and thus opens into the other portion of the arch, or into some adjacent vessel. For this mode of formation from vessels, the name of *channeling* seems more appropriate than that of outgrowth; for it appears certain that the blood-corpuscles here make their way in the parenchyma of the tissue, unconfined by membranous walls. That they do so in a definite and purposive manner, though their first issue from the vessel has appeared so accidental, may be due to the fact that in the more regular development by outgrowth, the cells of the parenchyma concur with the extension of the new vessels, by clearing away from them as they approach; so that, even before the outgrowth, the way for it, or for its contents (should they happen to escape), is, in some measure, determined.

The occurrence of such a process of channeling as is here indicated, loses all improbability, when we remember that in many insects and mollusca the blood habitually flows, in a considerable and important part of its course, through lacunæ, spaces, or channels without proper walls, such as are here supposed to exist only for a time.

The general plan of arrangement of the blood-vessels in granula-

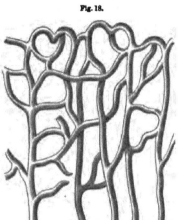

Fig. 18.

tions, represented in the adjoining sketch, agrees with this account of their development by outgrowth. Some of Sir A. Cooper's prepara-tions in the Museum of the Col-lege* show how the new vessels extend from the parts on which the granulations lie, in lines directed vertically towards their surface, not often dividing, but communi-cating on their way by frequent transverse or irregular branches. Of these branches, some, probably, represent the loops or arches suc-cessively formed in the deepening layer of granulation-cells, while others must be formed by offshoots from the sides and other parts of the several arches. Near the surface of the granulations, at a very little distance below the outermost layer of the cells, the vessels communicate much more frequently, and form their loops or terminal arches—arches of junction between the outgoing and the returning streams of blood.

On the same plan are formed the vessels of the walls of abscesses lined with granulations; but here (at least in the specimens I have been able to examine) the vertical vessels are not so long, and the whole num-ber of vessels is generally greater. I believe the vessels of granulating ulcers are always similarly arranged; so they are represented by Mr. Liston† in a common ulcer; so, also, Sir A. Cooper‡ described them in granulations from an ulcerated scirrhous cancer; and I have found the same general plan in the warty ulceration of soot-cancer on the scrotum. The structure of the new vessels formed in granulations also agrees with the described mode of development. In the earliest period of their appearance they present no indication of being formed by fusion, or any transformation, of the granulation-cells, but consist of thin membrane, in which, if it be not quite simple, nuclei or cytoblasts are imbedded. These nuclei pass through stages of development, by narrowing and elongation, similar to that which I have described in the nucleated blas-tema; and thus they become like the pieces of flat fibre that one sees on the walls of the original vessels of the same size. Like them, also, they are arranged, some longitudinally, and some transversely to the axis of the vessels; and it is often noticeable, that the development of the tissues

* Nos. 19, 20, 556.
† Medico-Chirurgical Transactions, vol. xxiii. p. 85.
‡ Catalogue of the Pathological Museum of the College, vol. i. p. 111.

of the blood-vessels makes more progress than that of the granulation-cells which they subserve.

Respecting the purpose of the supply of blood thus sent to granulations, one traces, in the development of vessels, a series of facts exactly answering to those in ordinary embryonic development. Organization makes some progress before ever blood comes to the very substance of the growing part; for the form of cells may be assumed before the granulations become vascular. But, for their continuous active growth and development, fresh material from blood, and that brought close to them, is essential. For this, the blood-vessels are formed; and their size and number appear always proportionate to the volume and rapidity of life of the granulations. No instance would show the relation of blood to an actively growing or developing part better than it is shown in one of the vascular loops of a granulation, imbedded, as this sketch shows it, among the crowd of living cells, and maintaining their continual mutations. Nor is it in any case plainer than in that of granulations, that the supply of blood in a part is proportionate to the activity of its changes, and not to its mere structural development. The vascular loops lie imbedded among the simplest primary cells, or, when granulations degenerate, among structures of yet lower organization; and as the structures are developed, and fibro-cellular tissue formed, so the blood-vessels become

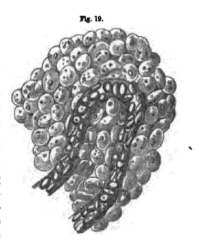

Fig. 19.

less numerous, and the whole of the new material assumes the paleness and low vascularity of a common scar. But, though the quantity of blood-vessels is determined by the state of the substance they supply, the development of their tissue has no such relation. It is often complete while the granulation-cells are rudimental, and remains long unchanged when they are degenerate. The fact may be regarded as evidence of the formation of the new blood-vessels by outgrowth from the older ones; for it is not probable that well-developed blood-vessels and ill-developed granulation-cells should be formed out of the same materials at the same time.

Of the development of Nerves in granulations I know nothing; I have never been able to see any in either granulations or cicatrices. The exquisite pain sometimes produced by touching granulation would indicate the presence of nerves: but it would be more satisfactory to see them; for the force of contact, or the change that it produces, may be propagated through the layer of granulations, and stimulate the nerves beneath them, as contact with the exterior of a tooth excites the nerve-filaments in its pulp. The sensibility that granulations seem to have may, therefore, be reatly that of the tissues from which they spring.

Lymphatics do not exist in granulations. Professor Schroeder van der Kolk has demonstrated them in false membranes by mercurial injections:* but in a letter he tells me that they cannot, either by these or by any other means, be traced in either scars or granulations; and, he adds, "they cannot be demonstrated in the skin, even in the healthy state, except in the scrotum."

The subject of suppuration should perhaps be considered now; but I had rather defer it till I have spoken briefly of the two remaining modes of healing open wounds; those, namely, by *secondary adhesion*, and by *scabbing*.

The healing by secondary adhesion, or union of granulations, has been long and often observed; yet it has been only casually described, and having never been distinguished by a specific name, has not received that attention to which its importance in practice seems to entitle it. It occurs wherever surfaces of granulations, formed in the manner just described, well-developed, but not yet covered with cuticle, are brought into contact, and so retained at rest. As often as this happens, the cells of which the surfaces are composed adhere together; vessels passing through them form mutual communications; and the surfaces, before separate, are connected; out of the two layers of granulations, one is formed, which pursues the normal development into fibro-cellular tissue.

In all its principal characters, therefore, the process of secondary adhesion is like that adhesion for which, to mark at once their likeness and their differences, I have suggested the term of primary. In the primary adhesion, the layer of lymph, placed between the wounded and bare surfaces, is probably formed equally and coincidently from both; and, being developed in the same manner as the granulations, of which I have spoken, it probably receives vessels from both surfaces, and so becomes the medium through which the vessels communicate and combine the severed parts. In the process of secondary adhesion, the superficial cells on the surfaces of two layers of granulations are placed together, and receiving vessels from both combine them into one.

Mr. Hunter observed this process, and says of it— "Granulations have the disposition to unite with one another when sound or healthy; the great intention of which is to produce the union of parts, somewhat similar to that by the first intention, although possibly not by the same means." And "I have seen two granulations on the head—viz.: one from the dura-mater after trepanning, and the other from the scalp—

* Lespinasse, De Vasis Novis Pseudo-membranarum, figs. iii., iv.

unite over the bare bone which was between them so strongly, in twenty-four hours, that they required some force to separate them, and when separated they bled."*

In illustration of this process he put up a preparation† which in his MS. Catalogue he described as "granulations under the skin in an abscess in the leg, which were opposed by others on the muscles, and which were to unite. Those under the skin only are saved, and folded towards each other, to show the opposition of two granulating surfaces."

There are several circumstances in which the healing by secondary adhesion should be attempted. For example: after an ordinary amputation of the thigh, no immediate union, and no primary adhesion, took place, and the whole interior of the stump was granulating. Had it been, as the expression is, "left to granulate," or "to fill up with granulations," the healing process would have occupied at least a month or five weeks more, and would have greatly exhausted the patient, already weakened by disease. But Mr. Stanley ordered the stump to be so bandaged that the opposite surfaces of granulations might be brought into close contact: they united, and in a week the healing of the stump was nearly perfected.

In all such cases, and I need not say that they are very frequent, the healing by secondary adhesion may be attempted without danger, and often with manifest advantage.

Again: Mr. Hunter operated for hare-lip, and no primary adhesion of the cut surfaces ensued. He let them both granulate, then brought the granulations together, as in the common operation, and they united, and healed soundly.

Or, again: Mr. Skey, not long since, operated for fissure of the soft palate. The edges of the wounds sloughed and retracted, and the case seemed nearly hopeless; but he kept in the sutures, and granulations sprang up from the edges of the cleft, after the separation of the sloughs: they met in the mid-space of the cleft, and coalesced, and formed a perfect scar.

Doubtless, cases like these are of no rare occurrence; but I am induced to mention them, as illustrations of a process of which the importance and utility are not generally considered, and which is rarely applied in practice.

In applying it, certain conditions are essential to success; especially that—1st, the granulations should be healthy, not inflamed, or profusely suppurating, or degenerated, as those in sinuses commonly are; 2dly, the contact between them should be gentle, but maintained; and perhaps they should be as much as possible of equal development and age.

The healing of wounds by scabbing may be regarded, as Mr. Hunter‡

* Works, vol. iii., p. 493.   † Pathological Museum of the College, No. 27.
‡ Works, vol. iii., 262.

says, as the natural one, for it requires no art. It is the method by
which one sees nearly all open wounds healed in animals; for in them,
even in the warm-blooded, it is difficult to excite free suppuration from
the surfaces of wounds; they quickly become coated with a scab, formed
of the fluids that ooze from them and entangle dust and other foreign
bodies; and under such a scab the scar is securely formed.

In general, the scabbing process is effected by some substance which
is effused on the surface of the wound, dries there, and forms a hard and
nearly impermeable layer. The edges of this substance adhere over
those of the wound, so as to form for it a sort of air-tight covering,
under which it heals without suppuration, and with the formation of a
scar, which is more nearly like the natural parts than any scars formed
in wounds that remain exposed to the air, and which does not, like them,
contract, so as to produce deformity of the parts about it.

The scab may be formed of either dried blood, dried lymph, and
serum, or dried purulent fluid. Instances of the healing of wounds under
dried blood are not rare. It is especially apt to occur in the cases of
wounds in which a large flat surface is exposed, as after the removal of
the breast with much integument. The most remarkable case of this
kind is recorded by Mr. Wardrop.* The largest wounded surface he
ever saw, remaining after the removal of a diseased breast, almost
entirely healed under a crust of blood, which remained on for more than
thirty days.† But the most common examples of healing under blood-
scabs are in small wounds, such as are made in bleeding, or more rarely
in some compound fractures. The excellent, though nearly obsolete,
practice of laying on such wounds a pad of lint soaked in the blood, was
a good imitation of the most natural process of their repair.

If a blood-scab be not formed over a wound, or if such an one have
been detached after being formed, then at once a scab may be derived
from the serum and lymph that ooze from the surface of the wound.
Thus it is commonly with wounds in animals that are left to themselves,
and in many small wide-open wounds in our own case. Thus, also, I
imagine, the best healing of superficial burns and scalds is effected, when
the exposed surface is covered with cotton-wool or other substance, which,
as the oozing fluids become entangled with it, may help them to form a
scab.

At a yet later period, the pus produced from exposed granulating
wounds may concrete on them, and they will heal under it excluded from
the air. Such a process may also ensue in the healing of ulcers, and
has been successfully imitated in Mr. Stafford's plan of filling deep ulcers
with wax.‡ In any case, the healing process is probably just the same

* In his Lectures on Surgery, in the Lancet for 1832-3, vol. ii.

† Mr. Henry Lee tells me that a similar case has occurred in his practice. An excellent
instance of healing under blood-scabs is also related by Dr. Macartney (Treatise on Inflammation, p. 208).

‡ On the Treatment of the Deep and Excavated Ulcer. 1829.

as that under scabs of blood or serum; but I believe it has not yet been exactly determined what are the changes that ensue in the surface beneath the scab. So far as one can discern with the naked eye, the wounded surface forms only a thin layer of cuticle on itself; no granulations, no new fibro-cellular tissue, appears to be formed; the raw surface merely skins over, and it seems to do so uniformly, not by the progressive formation of cuticle from the circumference towards the centre, as is usual in open wounds.

The healing of a wound by scabbing has always been thought a desirable process; and when one sees how quickly, by means of this process, wounds in animals are healed, and with how little general disturbance, one may well wish that it could be systematically adopted. But to this there seems some hinderance. Many surgeons have felt, as Mr. Hunter did, that the scabbing process should be permitted much oftener than it is, in the cases of both wounds and ulcers; but none have been able to lay down sufficient rules for the choice of the cases in which to permit it. Probably, the reason of this is that, at the best, in the human subject, the healing by scabbing is an uncertain process. When the scab is once formed, and the wound covered in, it is necessary that no morbid exudation should take place. Whenever, therefore, inflammation ensues in a wound or sore covered with a scab, the exuded fluid, collecting under the scab, produces pain, compresses the wounded surface, or forces off the scab, with discomfort to the patient and retardation of the healing. I suspect that the many instances of disappointment from this cause have led to the general neglect of the process of scabbing in the treatment of wounds. The observance of perfect rest, and of the other means for warding off inflammation, will, however, make it a valuable auxiliary in the treatment of wounds, especially of large superficial ones: in the treatment of small wounds, collodion appears sufficient to accomplish all that scabbing would do; and in deep wounds, fluid is too apt to collect under the scab.

Such are the several methods of healing observed after wounds of soft parts;* and in connection with them, two subjects remain to be considered, namely, the process of suppuration, and that of the perfecting of scars.

Respecting the process of suppuration, it cannot be necessary that I should give a minute account of pus, or of its general or chemical characters: I will rather endeavor to show its relations to the healing pro-

---

* I have not been able to recognize what Dr. Macartney named the *modelling process*, as a method of healing distinct from that which ensues in the most favorable instances of healing by granulations. I have, therefore, not enumerated it among the modes of healing; yet it may occur in some conditions that I have not met with: I would not, with only my present experience, impute confusion to so good and independent an observer as Dr. Macartney.

cess, by illustrating the points of resemblance and of difference between it and the materials of which granulations are formed.

Let me remind you that the formation of granulations is not necessarily attended with the production of pus.. I have already referred to this fact in speaking of the formation of subcutaneous granulations, such as are sometimes seen on the end of bones that do not unite, in the ordinary way, after simple fractures. Mr. Hunter also expressly describes these cases; and the same kind of granulations without suppuration may be sometimes seen springing from the ulcerated articular surfaces of bones, in cases of diseased joint without any external opening.

However, when granulations are formed on an open wound, there is always suppuration; i.e., an opaque, creamy, yellowish-white or greenish-white fluid, pus, or matter, is produced on the surface of the granulations. If the surface be allowed to dry, the pus may form a scab: if it be kept moist, fresh quantities of pus are produced, till the surface of the granulations is covered with the new cuticle. Granulations that are skinned over no longer suppurate.

The essential constituents of pus are cells, and the liquid (*liquor puris*) in which they are suspended. In pus produced during healthy granulation, no other material than these may be found. But, often, minute clear particles, not more than $\frac{1}{15000}$ of an inch in diameter, are mingled with the pus-cells, to which they seem to have some relation as rudiments. And when the process deviates from health, we find not only variations in the pus-cells, but multiform mixtures of withered cells, molecular and fatty matter, free or escaped and shrivelled nuclei, blood-corpuscles, fragments of granular substance like shreds of fibrine, and other materials. All these indicate defects or diseases of pus, corresponding with those of the granulations, to which I have already referred.

Pus-cells, in their ordinary state, are represented in the adjoining sketch.

Fig. 20.

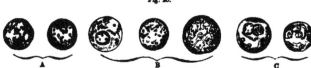

A　　　　　　　　B　　　　　　　　C

As shown at A, they are spherical, or spheroidal, or even discoid, bodies, the differences in shape depending apparently on the destiny of the fluid suspending them. In the same proportion as it becomes less dense, they tend to assume the more perfectly spherical shape. They have an uniform nebulous or grumous aspect; distinct granules, more or less numerous, are commonly seen in them; and they appear more darkly nebulous and more granular in the same proportion as the fluid becomes more dense. Their usual diameter is from $\frac{1}{1700}$ to $\frac{1}{3000}$ of an inch. Sometimes a distinct, circular, dark-edged nucleus may be seen

in the paler corpuscles; and, more rarely, two or even three particles
like a divided nucleus.

When, as in the corpuscles B, water is added to pus, it usually penetrates the cells, expanding them, raising up a distinct fine cell-wall, and
separating or diffusing their contents. Sometimes the contents are uniformly dispersed through the distended cell, which thus becomes more
lightly nebulous, or appears filled with a nearly clear substance in which
minute particles vibrate with molecular movement, while in or near the
centre a dark-edged well defined nucleus may appear. Sometimes, while
the cell-wall is upraised, the whole contents of the cells subside into a
single ill-defined darkly nebulous mass, which remains attached to part
of the cell-wall, looking like a nucleus, but differing from a true nucleus
in the characters just assigned, as well as in the absence of the two or
three shining particles like nucleoli. Lastly, a few pus-corpuscles appear
unchanged by the action of water: they seem to be merely masses of
soft colorless substance having the shape and appearance, but not the
structure, of cells.

When dilute acetic acid is added to pus (as in Fig. C), it produces the
same effects as water, but more quickly, and with a more constant
appearance of two, three, or four small bodies like nuclei. These bodies
are remarkable, though far from characteristic, features of pus-cells.
They are darkly edged, usually flattened, clear, and grouped, as if
formed by the division of a single nucleus; and commonly each of them
appears darkly shaded at its centre. When the acetic acid has been too
little diluted, these bodies alone may be at first seen; for the cell-wall
and the rest of its contents may be rendered so transparent as to be
scarcely visible.

Such are the pus-cells found in healthy suppurating wounds. The
liquor puris contains albumen, a compound called pyin, regarded by some
as identical with that which Muller described as tritoxide of protein,
abundant fatty matter, and inorganic substances similar to those dissolved in the liquor sanguinis.

Pus not distinguishable from that of granulating wounds is formed in
many other conditions; as in inflamed serous and mucous cavities, and
in abscesses. In these relations it will be considered in the lectures on
Inflammation. But the histories of all cases of the formation of pus
concur, with that of suppurating wounds, to the conclusion that pus may
be regarded as a rudimental substance ill-developed or degenerated; as
a substance essentially similar to the materials of granulations, or of the
lymph of inflammatory exudation, but which fails of being developed
like them, or, after having been developed like them to a certain stage,
degenerates.

To illustrate this relation between the pus and the granulations of
healing wounds, I may state that the last figure was copied from sketches
that I made, at the same time, of some granulation-cells from the walls

of a sinus, and some pus-cells from a healthily granulating wound. I chose those sources purposely, that I might be able to compare ill-developed granulation-cells with well-constructed pus-cells; and a comparison of them showed that, whether as seen without addition, or as changed by the action of water and acetic acid, they were not to be distinguished from one another. Had I not seen the vessels in the tissue that the granulation-cells formed, I might, in the first examination, have almost thought I was deceived in thinking they were not pus-cells. The six varieties of the appearances of the cells which are represented might have been taken from either source; so might some other varieties: but these may suffice to show the apparent identity of structure between well-formed pus-cells and ill-developed or degenerate granulation-cells, such as are found in the walls of sinuses and the like half-morbid structures. I do not mean to say, generally, that granulation-cells and pus-cells cannot be distinguished; for between well-formed granulation-cells, such as are found in healing wounds, and any particles that are usually found in pus, certain distinctions are almost always manifest. The pus-cells are darker, more and more darkly, granular, more various in size, and more various, not in shape, but in apparent structure, more often containing numerous particles, like fatty molecules, more rarely showing a nucleus when neither water nor acetic acid is added, and much more commonly showing a tripartite or ill-formed nucleus under the action of the acid. None, however, of these characters is indicative of essential difference; and between even the widest extremes there are all possible gradations, till distinction is impossible; so that when you place, as I have often done, ill-developed or degenerate granulation-cells on one side of the microscope-field, and pus-cells on the other, there is not a form of corpuscle on the one which is not repeated on the other.

From this, one cannot but conclude that the cells of pus from wounds are ill-developed or degenerate granulation-cells. Some of them may be degenerate, i. e., they may have been, as granulation-cells, attached for a time to the surface of the granulation-layer, and having lived their time, may, in ordinary course, have been detached and shed, as epithelial cells are from healthy surfaces. They may be thus detached after more or less degeneration, and hence may result some of the modifications that they present. But some pus-cells, I imagine (at least in the healing of wounds), may be ill-developed; that is, imperfectly formed of material which exudes from the surface of the granulations, and which, being exposed to the air, or being too remote from the supply of blood, cannot attain its due development, and, in an imperfectly developed state, is soon cast off. It cannot but be that organizable matter is constantly oozing from such a surface as that of granulations; but the conditions into which it enters on that surface are such as are very likely to hinder any but the lowest or some imperfect organization.

The many characters of imperfection or of degeneracy that pus-cells show, accord with this view: such as the general imperfection of their nuclei; the frequent abundance of fatty-looking granules in them; the large quantity of fatty matter that analysis detects in pus; and the limitation of the cells to certain forms, beyond which they are never found developed, though none of these forms is more highly organized than that of the youngest or most rudimental granulation-cell.

A further confirmation of the opinion that pus-cells are ill-developed or degenerate granulation-cells, is furnished in the cases, to which I shall hereafter refer, in which pus-cells are produced after, or together with, inflammatory lymph-cells; as in abscesses, inflamed membranes, and the like. Now such lymph-cells are not distinguishable in apparent structure from granulation-cells, and, like these, they may show every gradation of form to that of the pus-cell.*

But it is not only in the cells that we may trace this appearance of the degeneracy or incomplete development of pus. It is equally shown in the fluid part, or *liquor puris*, which, unlike the intercellular substance of granulations and inflammatory lymph, is incapable of organization, even when, by evaporation or partial absorption, it assumes the solid form. The liquor puris answers to the solid and organizable blastema of granulations; and as undue liquidity is among the most decided marks of ill-formed pus, so the abundance of the blastema, in proportion to the cells, is one of the best signs that granulations are capable of quick development.

These considerations may suggest, in some cases, the imperfection of the liquor puris; and an observation, which any one may easily make, seems to indicate that it may, in other cases, be the product of the degeneration and liquefaction of the solid blastema, as the pus-cells are, in the same cases, of the granulation or inflammatory lymph-cells imbedded in it. If the formation of abscesses be watched, one may see, on one day, a large solid and inflamed swelling, firm and almost unyielding, giving no indication of containing any collection of fluid; but, next day, one may detect in the same swelling the signs of suppuration; the border may feel as firm as before, but all the centre and the surface may be occupied with an ounce or more of matter. And observe, this change from the solid to the liquid state may have ensued without any increase of the swelling. Such an increase must have occurred had the pus been secreted in a fluid state into the centre of the solid mass: and the changes cannot, I think, be explained except on the admission, that the inflammatory product, which was effused and infiltrated through the

* Valentin, Gerber, and many others, have held nearly the same view as this of the character of pus-cells; but I think they have not sufficiently, if at all, dwelt on the probability that some pus-cells are ill-developed, others degenerate from a previously higher development. The many varieties of form, and the many differences of the conditions in which they occur, may be thus explained. I think, too, that the characters of degeneracy, or imperfect development, in the liquor puris, have been too much overlooked.

tissue in a solid form, has been liquefied: its cells degenerating into pus-cells, its blastema into liquor puris.*

Can we assign any use or purpose to the process of suppuration? In the case of abscesses and acute inflammations we may discern no more of purpose than in any other disease. But, in the case of granulating wounds, the use commonly assigned to pus, that it serves as a protection to the granulations, is probably ascribed to it with reason. It does this even in the fluid state; but the devices of surgical treatment, having regard to present comfort, rarely let us see how much better it protects a wounded surface when, as in animals, it is allowed to dry into a scab.

Let us now consider the case of a wound completely healed, and the scar that occupies its place.

It is hard to describe in general terms the characters of scars, varying as they do in accordance with the peculiar positions, and forms, and modes of healing of wounds. But two things may be constantly ob-served in them: namely, their contraction, and the gradual perfecting of their tissues.

A process of contraction is always associated with the development of granulations. Mr. Hunter has minutely described it, and preserved several specimens to illustrate it: among which are two stumps,† in which its occurrence is proved by the small size of the scars in compari-son with that of the granulating surfaces which existed before them. This healing of stumps, especially after circular amputations, will always show the contraction of the granulations, even before the cicatrix is formed; for one sees the healthy skin drawn in and puckered over the end of the stump, before any cuticle is formed on the granulations, except perhaps on the very margin. And many injuries, but especially burns, show the contraction of the scar continuing long after the appa-rent healing is completed.

To what may we ascribe this contraction of both the granulations and the scars? It has been regarded as the result of some vital power of contraction; and possibly it may be so in some measure. Yet, on the whole, it seems rather to be the necessary mechanical effect of the changes of form and construction that the parts undergo. The same change ensues in the organization of inflammatory products: as, e. g., in false membranes, indurations, thickenings of parts, and the like con-sequences of the exudation and organization of lymph.

Now, in all these cases, the form of the cell, while developing itself into a filament, is so changed that it will occupy less space. The whole

* Such a liquefaction is not that assumed in the older doctrines, which held that pus was partly formed of the dissolved materials of the original tissues. The original tissues doubtless remain, unless partially absorbed: yet there appears to be thus much of lique-faction in the formation of an abscess, that part of the inflammatory product, first formed as a soft solid, degenerates and becomes fluid.

† Nos. 28 and 29 in the Museum of the College.

mass of the developing cells becomes more closely packed, and the tissue that they form becomes much drier; with this, also, there is much diminution of vascularity. Thus, there results a considerable decrease of bulk in the new tissue as it developes itself; and this decrease, beginning with the development of the granulation-cells, continues in the scar, and, I think, sufficiently accounts for the contraction of both, without referring to any vital power.

The force with which the contraction is accomplished is often enormous. One sees its result in the horrible deformities that follow the healing of severe burns. Deep scarred and seamed depressions, even of the bones, may be produced by the contraction of granulations and scars over them. The whole process shows the error of such expressions as "filling up with granulations," commonly applied to deep healing wounds, as if granulations increased in thickness till they attained the level of the upper margins of deep hollows. The truth is, that, even in the deepest open wounds, the granulation-layer is, as usual, from one to three lines thick; and that, when such a wound grows shallower in healing, it is not by the rising of the granulations, but by the lowering of its margins. The granulations and the scars of deep open wounds remain alike thin and depressed.

The improvement and perfecting of the tissue of the scar is, again, a very slow process. It is often thought remarkable that nerves and some of the higher tissues should require so long time for their repair; but scarcely less is necessary for the perfecting of a common scar. The principal changes by which it is accomplished include the removal of all the rudimental textures, the formation of elastic tissue, the improvement of the fibrous or fibro-cellular tissue, and of the new cuticle, till they are almost exactly like those of natural formation; and the gradual loosening of the scar, so that it may move easily on the adjacent parts.

All these changes are very slowly accomplished. One sees their effects, it may be, only after the many years in which, as it is said, the scars of childhood gradually wear out; i.e., in which the new-formed tissues gradually acquires the exact similitude of the old ones. Thus, the remains of the rudimental cellular tissue, imperfectly developed, may be found in apparently healthy scars of ten months' duration. After second operations, in which the scar of some former wound was removed, I have still found imperfectly developed granulation-cells in the tissue of the scar. Elastic tissue, also, I think, is not commonly formed in the first construction of a scar, but appears in it sometimes as much as twelve months after its first formation, and then gives it the common structure of the mixed fibro-cellular and elastic tissues which exist in the cutis.

But, an occurrence which may appear more singular than this slow perfecting of the tissues, is, in all good scars, as they are called, that gradual loosening of the tissue which at first unites the scar to all the adjacent parts. Thus, in such a wound as is made for tying a deep artery, or in lithotomy, at first the new tissue, the tissue of the scar, extends down to the bottom of the wound, equally dense in all parts, and fastening the skin to the parts at the very deepest portion of the wound. But after a time this clears up. The tissue of the scar in the skin becomes more compact and more elastic; but that beneath it becomes looser and more like natural cellular tissue ; and the morbid adhesions of one part to another are freed. So, after injuries or diseases followed by scars about joints, the stiffness depending on the adhesion of the scar to the deeper tissues gradually decreases: and, so, in like manner, the scars of burns often become gradually and of themselves more pliant, and the parts which they held become more freely movable, though some- times scarcely seeming to change for a year after the first healing of the injury.

Now, in all this gradual return of tissues to the healthy state, we may trace, I think, a visible illustration of the recovery from the minute changes of disease. In all there is a gradual approach of the new par- ticles that are successively produced, to a nearer conformity with the specific character of the parts they should replace, till repair becomes almost reproduction. And how, let me ask, can all this be reconciled with any theory of assimilation ? How can assimilation alter the charac- ters of a scar ? how make one part of it assume one character, and another part a character quite different, till, at length, that which looked homo- geneous, as a mass of new formed tissue, acquires, in separate parts, the characters of the several tissues in whose place it lies, and whose office it is destined, though still defectively, to discharge ?

LECTURE XI.

THE REPAIR OF FRACTURES.

THE necessity, which I have felt in the preceding lectures, of describing the healing process as it is observed in a few typical examples, is in- creased, when I come to the consideration of the repair of fractures. A volume would not suffice for all that should be said of it; for there are no examples of the reparative process which present so many features of interest as this does, whether we consider its practical importance, or the wide field which it offers alike for the science and for the art of surgery, or the abundant illustrations of the general principles of recovery from injury which are present in every stage of the process, or the perfect evidences of design which it displays, of design that seems unlimited in the variety and point with which it is adapted to all the possible diversities of accident. To consider the repair of fractures completely, in any of these views, would be far beyond my purpose, and farther beyond my ability. I shall therefore limit myself almost entirely to an account of the repair of the simple fractures of long bones. What is true of this will be so nearly true of the repairs of other fractures, that a few words may suffice in reference to the chief modifications of the process in them. Moreover, I shall in general describe only what occurs in the adult human subject.

The injury inflicted in the fracture of a long bone is rarely limited to the bone. The two or more fragments, driven in opposite directions, penetrate the adjacent tissues, wounding and bruising them, and giving rise to bleeding of various amount. Provided all these injuries are subcutaneous, and the air has no access to the damaged parts, their repair is perfectly, though slowly, effected. It is not unfrequent, in recent fractures, to find portions of muscle or other soft parts completely crushed by the bones, or even, in minute fragments, enclosed in the reparative material or the inflammatory exudations; and yet, when similar fractures are examined a year or more after their occurrence, the tissues round the bone appear quite normal in their structure, however disturbed they may be in their relations.

The periosteum is rarely much damaged in fractures of long bones. It is seldom stripped off the broken ends. Commonly, it is cleanly rent across at the same level as the bone is broken, and maintains its close union, having only its fibres somewhat frayed or pulled from their natural direction. Sometimes, indeed, it remains entire, even in extensive fractures; and in this case, thickening, it contributes to the security of the repair of the injury.

The extravasation of blood about fractures is not only uncertain in amount, but unequal in the several tissues. Its abundance in the subcutaneous tissue is often so remarkable, as to be among the useful signs for diagnosis, in cases of doubtful fracture near joints; but in the deeper soft tissues less blood is shed; and, commonly, in the periosteum, near the broken ends of the bone, only a few spots of blood are seen. I have already spoken (p. 123) of the manner in which the extravasated blood is disposed of; and since it rarely appears to take part in the reparative process, I shall make no further mention of it.

Some days elapse, after a fracture, before any clear marks of a reparative process can be found. An early consequence of the injury appears to be the exudation of a small quantity of inflammatory lymph; so that the cellular tissue in and near the seat of injury appears more succulent than is natural, being infiltrated with a serous-looking fluid, in which are cells like those of granulations of lymph.

In bad cases, this exudation may increase, and add to the swelling that is often seen to augment in the second or some later day; but, in

11

better instances of repair, and when the parts, even though much injured, are kept at rest, I think the inflammatory exudation usually ceases after the second or third day, and that, then, some days pass before the proper reparative material is produced.* The state of the injured parts during this period of calm, or of incubation, is probably like that observed in wounds of soft parts (page 138). Its duration is uncertain, but I think, in the adult, is rarely less than one week or more than two.

In this long period of inaction we find the first contrast between the repairs of fractures in man, and in the animals that have been used for experimental inquiry into the process, as dogs, rabbits, pigeons, and others. In any of these, an abundant reparative material will be produced, and organized into cartilage or bone, in a time little longer than elapses before the first commencement of the process in a man.† We cannot, therefore, from the rapidity of repair in any lower animals, form any just calculation of its rate of progress in ourselves.

The proper reparative process, commencing after this period of rest, may usually be divided into two chief parts; namely, the process of uniting the fragments, and that of shaping or modeling them and their combining substance. The uniting and the modeling parts of the process are so different in nature and in time, that they may well be considered separately. They are comparable with the forming and the subsequent perfecting of the scars of wounded soft parts; and in the union of fractures, even more evidently than in any other instance of repair, we may note how safety is first provided for, then symmetry; how the welfare of the individual is first secured, and then the conformity of the repaired part to the typical or specific form: for the modeling scarcely begins before the uniting is completed.

The union of fractures is commonly effected by the organization of new material connecting the fragments. Sometimes, indeed, immediate union occurs. When portions of bone are placed and held in exact apposition, they may be united without any new material being formed for their connection; a continuity of tissues and of blood-vessels being restored, as in the cases of healing by immediate union of soft parts. But this is rare, and has not yet been sufficiently studied.

The material deposited for the more usual method of repair of simple fractures,—the callus, as it is called, when it has become firm or hard,—is, I think, in the first instance, not visibly different from the material formed for the repair of other subcutaneous injuries. Its peculiarity is shown in the direction and end of its development; and, in this respect, the repair of fractures supplies an extreme case of the variety of ways through which the same end of development may be attained.

* More concerning this inflammatory exudation will be related in the account of the repair of tendons in the next lecture.

† See Nos. 418, 419, 420, in the Museum of the College; and Series iii., Nos. 69, 70, 71, &c., in that of St. Bartholomew's.

In its first production, the reparative material is a structureless, or dimly-shaded, or granular substance, like fibrine; or, perhaps at a later period, it is ruddy, elastic, moderately firm and succulent, like firm granulation-substance. Of the manner in which it is placed, in the space and in the tissues around or between the fragments to be connected, I will speak presently. At first, it has none of the firmness belonging to the "callus:" this, however, it soon attains, as it makes progress towards being transformed into bone. Its ossification, as I have said, may be accomplished through several transitional forms of tissue, which might be distinguished as so many varieties of callus, if the term be worth retaining. It may become, before ossifying, either fibrous or cartilaginous, or may assume a structure intermediate between these; and, in either of these cases, ossification may ensue when the previous tissue is yet in a rudimental state, or may be delayed till the complete fibrous or cartilaginous structure is first achieved.

I cannot tell the conditions which will determine, in each case, the route of development towards bone that the reparative material will take; nor in what measure the differences that may be observed are to be ascribed to the seat or nature of the injury, or to the condition of the patient. All these things have yet to be determined; and I believe that years of patient and well-directed investigation will be requisite for them. I can do little more than point out the modes in which the ossification may be accomplished.

And, first, it may be accomplished through perfect fibrous tissue. Thus I found it in a case of fracture of the lower part of the femur after six weeks, and in a fracture of the radius after about nine weeks; thus, too, I think, whatever new bone is formed after fractures of the skull is developed; and thus one may find, in the neighborhood of fractures and other injuries of bone, ossifications of interosseous fibrous membranes, and of the tissue of the periosteum, or just external to it.[*]

But, secondly, the new bone may be formed by ossification of the fibrous tissue in a rudimental state. And this rudimental state may be that either of nucleated cells or nucleated blastema. Through nucleated cells, as the embryo-forms of fibrous tissue, bone is formed when granulations or inflammatory exudations ossify. The process may be often seen in the union of compound fractures, or of simple ones when much inflammation has been excited. But, best of all, though here only for illustration of what may occur in fractures, the ossification of nucleated cells, in granulations may be observed, when bone is formed in the mushroom-shaped mass of granulations that is protruded through the medullary canal of a bone sawn across in an amputation.[†] In all these cases there

---

[*] The thin plate of bone which closes in the exposed medullary canal of the end of a fractured long bone, where one fragment overlaps another, will usually, I think, present a good example of ossification of fibrous tissue.

[†] College Museum, Nos. 552, 553.

appears to be a direct transformation into bone, without the intervention of either cartilage or perfect fibrous tissue.

The ossification of nucleated blastema, such as I have described as a rudimental form of fibrous tissue, may also be seen in simple fractures; and my impression is, that it is an ordinary mode of ossification in simple fractures of adult long bones that unite well and quickly. In such a case, in a fracture of the tibia of five weeks' date, I found, in long-continued examinations, that the bone is formed without any intermediate state of cartilage; a finely and very closely granular osseous deposit taking place in the blastema, and gradually accumulating so as to form the delicate yet dense lamellæ of fine cancellous tissue. The nuclei of the blastema appeared to be enclosed in the new-forming bone, and I thought I could trace that they became the bone-corpuscles; but I could not be sure of this.

Thus, the new material produced for the repair of fractures may be ossified through an intermediate fibrous stage. In other instances it may pass through a cartilaginous stage. In animals, perfect cartilage, with its characteristic homogeneous intercellular substance, its cells, and all the characters of pure fœtal cartilage, may be produced. Through the ossification of such cartilage, Miescher[*] and Voetch,[†] and others, describe the repair of fractures as accomplished in dogs, pigeons, and other animals. I have not yet found the very same process in the human subject; but I should think it would occur in favorable instances of simple fracture in children. In youths and adults, I have found only varieties of fibrous cartilage; and these have presented numerous gradations from the fibrous towards the perfect cartilaginous structure. In different specimens, or sometimes even in different parts of the same, the reparative material has displayed, in one, fibrous tissue with a few imbedded corpuscles like the large nearly round nuclei of cartilage cells; in another, a less appearance of fibrous structure, with more abundant nucleated cells, having all the characters of true cartilage-cells; and in a third, a yet more nearly perfect cartilage.[‡]

Through any of these structures the reparative new bone may be formed. It may be formed, first, where the reparative material is in contact with the old bone, and thence extending, it may seem as if it grew from the old bone; or it may be formed in the new material, in detached centres of ossification, from which it may extend through the

[*] De Inflammatione Ossium, 1836.
[†] Die Heilung der Knochenbruche, 1847.
[‡] I do not describe the minute methods of ossification occurring in the callus, or reparative material; for my opportunities of studying it in man have been too few for me to conclude from: and, although I have seen nothing opposed to the belief that the normal methods of ossification are imitated, yet the process seems capable of so many modifications that I think it would not be safe to adapt, unconditionally, to the case of the reparative material in man, such conclusions as are drawn from the normal ossification of his skeleton, or from the ossification of the reparative material in lower animals.

intervening tissues, and connect itself with the old bone. (See figs. 21 and 23.)

The new bone, through whatever mode it is formed, appears to acquire quickly its proper microscopic characters. Its corpuscles or lacunæ, being first of simple round or oval shape, and then becoming jagged at their edges, subsequently acquire their canals, which appear to be gradually hollowed out in the preformed bone, as minute channels communicating with one or more of the lacunœ. The laminated canals for blood-vessels are later formed. At first, all the new bone forms a minutely cancellous structure, which is light, spongy, soft, and succulent, with a reddish juice rather than marrow, and is altogether like fœtal bones in their first construction. But this gradually assimilates itself to the structure of the bones that it repairs; its outer portions assuming a compact laminated structure, and its inner or central portions acquiring wider cancellous spaces, and a more perfect medulla. It acquires, also, a defined periosteum, at first firm, thin, and distinctly lamellar, and gradually assuming toughness and compactness. But, in regard to many of these latter changes in the bonds of union of fractures, there are so many varieties in adaptation to the peculiarities of the cases, that no general account of them can be rendered.

A subject of chief interest in the repair of fractures is the position of the reparative material, and in relation to this we find a greater difference than any yet mentioned between the processes traced respectively in man and in the animals submitted to experiments.

There are two principal methods according to which the reparative material or callus may be placed. In one, the broken ends or smaller fragments of the bone are completely enclosed in the new material; they are ensheathed and held together by it, as two portions of a rod might be by a ferrule or ring equally fastened around them both. In such a case, illustrated by fig. 21, the new material, surrounding the fracture, has been usually called "provisional callus," or "external callus:" but the term "ensheathing callus" will, I think, be more explanatory. In the other method (as in figs. 22 and 23), the new material is placed only between those parts of the broken bone whose surfaces are opposed; between these it is inlaid, filling the space that else would exist between them, or the angle at which one fragment overhangs another, and uniting them by being fixed to both. Reparative material thus placed may be called "intermediate callus." In either method (as in figs. 21 and 22), there is usually some reparative material deposited in and near the broken medullary tissue; and this may be still named "interior callus."

The method of repair with an ensheathing or provisional callus is rarely observed in man, but appears to be frequent in fractures of the long bones in animals.* From these it has been admirably described by Dupuytren

* Even in animals it is not constant. To obtain what would be called good specimens of provisional callus, the injuries must be inflicted upon young animals, and among these I

and others. The chief features of the process are as follows (omitting dates, which have not been ascertained in man, and cannot well be calculated for him):—

In the simplest case, when the fragments (represented in this dog's tibia; fig. 21) lie nearly in apposition, and nearly correspond,

Fig. 21.

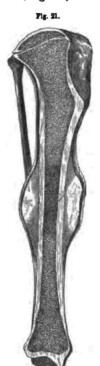

the reparative material accumulates at once around and within them, and in any interspaces that may be left between them, that is, the unsheathing callus, forms most quickly and in greater abundance, and lies chiefly or solely between the wall of the bone and the periosteum, which is thus lifted up from the wall, the bloodvessels that passed from it into the bone now passing to their destinations through the callus. The distance from the broken ends to which the callus extends up each fragment is uncertain: in the long bones of dogs, and the ribs of men, it is usually about half an inch. The thickness of the callus is greatest at a little distance from the plane of the fracture: exactly in that place, it is usually less thick than either above and below; so that, even when it is ossified, it is often marked with a slight annular constriction.

The interior callus fills up the spaces in the cancellous tissue, extending in the medullary canal of each fragment to a distance somewhat short of that to which the ensheathing callus reaches. At the end of each fragment there is usually an abrupt contrast between the firm reparative material that forms this interior callus, and a softer substance, like that of granulations, which remains between the fragments even till the callus without and within is quite ossified. As the section drawn in fig. 21 shows, the reparative material is abundant and

cannot but suspect that particular instances have been selected for description; those in which less callus was formed having been put aside as imperfect instances of repair, though, in truth, they may have displayed the more natural process. Such good specimens are in the Museum of the College, Nos. 418 to 426; and in that of St. Bartholomew's, Ser. iii., 69, 70, 71, 81, 82, 92, 96, 106. Fig. 21 is drawn from No. 96. It is very desirable to obtain examinations of fractured long bones recently united in young children; for it is probable that in these the process would be very like that described from the experiments on animals. No opportunity for such an examination has yet occurred to me.

well developed both around and within the fragments: but between them, i. e., in the plane of the fracture, it is sparingly formed and soft, so that the fragments, if the ensheathing callus were removed, would be no longer held together; they are, in fact, combined long before they are united.

The ossification of the ensheathing callus is accomplished chiefly or solely by outgrowth of bone from the fragments on which it is placed. Here, also, the same method of progress is observed, in that the formation of new bone extends gradually towards that part of the callus which exactly corresponds with the plane of the fracture. This part of the callus is last ossified; but, at length, its ossification being complete, the fragments are combined by and within a sheath or ferrule of new bone. The interior callus, ossifying at about the same time, consolidates the cancellous tissue of the fragments, and, at a later period, unites them. The walls remain still longer disunited. The ossified callus is, indeed, sufficient to render the bone fit for its office, but it retains the nearly cancellous tissue of new bone, and it is still only provisional: for when the walls of the fragments are themselves united, and their continuity is restored, all, or a part, of the external callus is removed, and the cancellous tissue loses its solidity by the removal of the internal callus.

Such is the process of repair with an ensheathing callus. It is, as I have said, usual in animals; but in man I have never seen its occurrence as a natural process in any bones but the ribs. In these it may be traced as perfectly as I have described it from the instances of repaired fractures of long bones in the rabbit and dog. Sometimes, indeed, a similar process occurs in other human bones: I have seen it in the clavicle and humerus;[*] but in both these cases the more proper mode of repair had been disturbed by constant movement of the parts, and in the humerus the process had manifest signs of exaggeration and disease.

The normal mode of repair in the fractures of human bones is that which is accomplished by "intermediate callus." The principal features of difference between it and that just described are, (1) that the reparative material or callus is placed chiefly or only between the fragments, not around them; (2) that, when ossified, it is not a provisional, but a permanent bond of union for them; (3) that the part of it which is external to the wall of the bone is not exclusively, or even as if with preference, placed between the bone and periosteum, but, rather, in the tissue of the periosteum, or indifferently either in it, beneath it, or external to it.

When the fragments are placed in close apposition and correspondence, they may, I believe, be joined by immediate union; but if this do not

[*] Museum of St. Bartholomew's, Ser. iii., 92, 65, and 66. The clavicle was broken twelve weeks before death; but the fracture was not detected, and the fragments were allowed to move unrestrained. The humerus was taken from a man who died some weeks after the fracture, and whose arm had, for several days after th͏ . . . h͏ . . the s͏ . of severe spasms. See Mr. Stanley's " Illustrations of . . . .

happen, a thin layer of reparative material is deposited between them; it does not, in any direction, exceed the extent of the fracture; neither does it, in more than a trivial degree, occupy the medullary canal; but, being inlaid between the fragments, and there ossifying, it restores their continuity. The process may be compared with that of union by primary adhesion.

When, as more commonly happens, the fragments, though closely apposed, do not exactly correspond, but, at certain parts, project more or less one beyond the other, the reparative material is, as in the former case, inlaid between them, and, to a slight extent, in the medullary canal: but it is, also, in larger quantity, placed in the angles at which the fragments overhang one another. Its position is, in these cases, well shown in the specimens drawn in the 22d and 23d figures. In the fractured radius* (fig. 22) the carpal portion, laterally displaced, projects beyond the

Fig. 22.   Fig. 23.

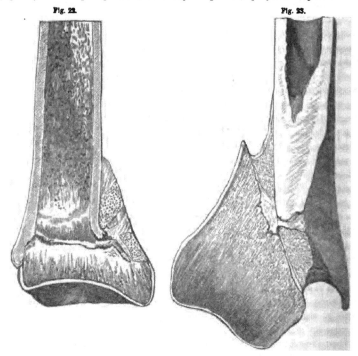

radial margin of the upper and impacted portion; and the angle between them is exactly filled, without being surpassed, by a wedge-shaped mass of reparative material. So, but less perfectly, is the angle on the other side. In the fractured femur† (fig. 23), with great displacement of the

* Museum of St. Bartholomew's, Ser. iii., No. 94.
† The same Museum, Ser. iii., No. 103.

fragments, the same rule is observed; the interspace between the fragments, and parts of the angles at which the one projects beyond the other, are filled with partially ossified reparative material. In neither case is there an ensheathing callus; in neither is any reparative material placed on that aspect of the one fragment which is turned from the other.

Lastly, when the fragments neither correspond nor are apposed, when one completely projects beyond or overlaps another, and when, it may be, a wide interval exists between them, still the reparative material is only placed between them. It just fills the interval; it does not even cover the ends of the fragments, or fill any part of the medullary canal: much less does it enclose both ends of the mutually averted surfaces, as the provisional callus would in a similar fracture in a dog or a rabbit; it passes, bridge-like, from one fragment to the other, and thus, when ossified, combines them. Thus it appears in the fractured femur, part of which is repr.sented in fig. 24.*

The three instances which I have cited, of different relative positions of the fragments, may suffice as examples of classes in which nearly all simple fractures of long bones might be described. But, whether the displacement were like either of these, or of any other kind, I have seen no examples (other than the exceptions already mentioned) in which the reparative material has been placed according to a different method.† It is always an intermediate bond of union; it is inlaid between the fragments; and when formed in largest quantity, is only enough to smooth the chief irregularities, and to fill up the interspaces and angles between them. And, regarding the particular position which it may in each case occupy, I do not know that it can be more exactly described, than by saying, that it is deposited where it is most wanted for the strengthening of the bone; so that, wherever would be the weak part, if unhealed, there is the new material placed, in quantity as well as in position just adapted to the exigencies of the case, and restoring, as much as may be, the original condition and capacities of the bone.

If, now, it be inquired why this difference should exist in the corresponding processes in man and other animals, I believe it must be ascribed principally to two causes, namely, the quietude in which fractures in our

* Museum of St. Bartholomew's Hospital, Ser. iii. No. 98.

† I exhibited at this lecture all the specimens of fractures examined within six months or the injury that are contained in the Museums of the College and St. Bartholomew's; and they all, with the exceptions already mentioned, exemplified this account of the repair by intermediate callus, and of the absence of provisional or ensheathing callus. They included a radius, four weeks after the fracture; another, four or five weeks; a tibia, five weeks; a femur, six weeks; another of the same date; a third, about eight or nine weeks: a radius, of somewhat later date; a tibia, eight weeks; a fibula, eleven weeks; a tibia, twelve weeks; a tibia, sixteen weeks after the injury; and many others of various but unknown dates, all in process of apparently natural repair. Since the lecture was given, the description has been confirmed by many examinations by myself and others. It is similarly approved by specimens in which the union has been long completed; but less satisfactorily, because it might be said that we cannot tell how much callus may have been removed.

bones are maintained, and the naturally greater tendency to the production of new bone which animals always manifest. Even independently of surgery, in the case of fractures of the lower extremity, the human mode of progression almost compels a patient to take rest: and in fractures of the upper extremity, the circumstances of human life and society permit him to do so far more than other animals can. The whole process is, therefore, more quietly conducted; and, as we may say, there is comparatively little need of the strength which the formation of provisional callus would give a broken limb.

The exceptions to the rule, of difference in the repair of human bones and those of animals, confirm it as thus explained; for they are found in the ribs, which are certainly never kept at rest during all the time necessary for repair after fracture, and in bones of which, from various causes, the repose of the fragments has been disturbed, or which have been the seats of disease, with inflammatory deposit, during or subsequent to the reparative process.

The comparative restlessness of animals is, however, I think, not alone sufficient to account for all the difference in the processes. The remainder may be ascribed to their greater tendency, in all circumstances, to the formation of new bone. Not in fractures alone, but in necrosis this is shown. It is very rarely that such quantities of new bone are formed in even children, as are commonly produced after necrosis of the shafts of bones in dogs or other animals; nor is there in the human subject any such filling up of the cavities from which superficial sequestra have been separated, as the experiments of Mr. Hunter showed, after such exfoliations from the metatarsal bones of asses.*

It remains, now, that I should describe the later part of the repair of fractures—that which consists in the shaping or modeling of the fragments and of their bond of union.

Omitting the removal of the provisional callus, where such an one has been formed, this modeling is best observed when there has been much displacement of the fragments. In these cases, the chief things to be accomplished are, 1st, the removal of sharp projecting points and edges from the fragments; 2dly, the closing or covering of the exposed ends of the medullary tissue; 3dly, the forming a compact external wall, and cancellous interior, for the reparative new bone; and lastly, the making these continuous with the walls and cancellous tissue of the fragments.

The first of these is effected by the absorption of the offending points and angles; and an observation sent to me by Mr. Delagarde tells much

* Museum of the College, Nos. 641 to 653.
The denial of the formation of an ensheathing callus in the repair of fractures is sometimes met by the statement that such a callus can be often felt during life. The deception is produced either by thickening and induration of the softer parts around the fracture; or by the two overlapping ends of the fragments being grasped at once; or, much more rarely, by new bone accumulated about the fragments in consequence of inflammation.

of the process: "A patient in the Exeter Hospital had a bad commi-
nuted fracture of the leg, and a long spike of the tibia, including part
of its spine, could not be reduced to its exact level, but continued sensibly
elevated, though in its due direction. At the end of five weeks (union
having taken place) the end of the spike began to soften; at six, it was
quite soft and flexible; at the conclusion of the seventh week it was
blunt and shrunken. Six months later, the cartilaginous tip had disappeared, and the spike was rounded off."

Fig. 24.

I have since, in a similar case, seen
the same process repeated. Both
cases seem to show that the absorption
of the bone is accomplished, as Mr.
Hunter described it in cases of necrosis,
by removing first the earthy matter,
and then the softened remains of animal substance.

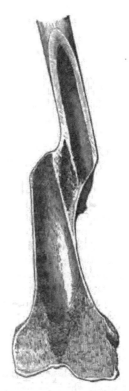

The closing or covering-in of the
parts of the broken medullary tube,
which are exposed in fractures with
much displacement, is slowly accomplished by the formation of a thin layer
of compact bone, like that which covers
the cancellous tissue at the articular
ends of bones. It is well shown in the
original of the 24th figure.* In a
fracture of the femur, after six weeks,
I have seen the exposed medullary tube
covered-in with a thin fibrous membrane, tense like a drum-head, new-
formed, and continuous with the periosteum. The permanent closure appears
to be effected by the ossification of such
a membrane; and the new bone becomes smoothly continuous with the
rounded and thinned broken margins
of the walls of the old bone. So are
the ends of stumps covered-in; and
neither in these nor in fractures have I seen new bone extending into the
medullary canal, as if formed by the ossification of an internal callus.

The same sketch shows the nearly completed formation of distinct
walls and medullary tissue in the bridge of new bone connecting the
two fragments of the femur. At an earlier period we may be sure that
all this new bone was soft and cancellous; it has now acquired the tex-

* From the Museum of St. Bartholomew's, Ser. iii. No. 98.

tures proper to the bone which it repairs, and, as if to complete its conformity with the structures among which it was thus, by accident, introduced, the process was begun by which the new and the old compact and medullary tissues would become respectively continuous. Already those parts of the walls of the shaft that intervene like partitions, separating the new from the old medullary tissue, are thin, uneven on their surfaces, and in their interior half-cancellous. At some later time they would, probably, have been reduced to mere cancellous tissue, and the repair of the fracture would have been completed. crookedly, indeed, but with unbroken continuity of tissue.

. To adapt the forgoing account to the case of compound fractures, it is, I believe, only necessary (so far at least as the normal process of repair is concerned) to say that the reparative material is more mingled with products of inflammation ; that that part of it which is formed within reach of the air, or in a suppurating cavity, is developed to bone through the medium of granulations, like those formed in open wounds of soft parts ; and that the whole process of repair is, generally, slower, less secure, and more disturbed by morbid growths of bone, and other effects of what has been named " ossific inflammation."

The data, at present collected, concerning the times in which the several parts of the reparative process are usually completed after fractures of adult human bones, are not sufficient for more than a general and approximate estimate. They may be thus generally reckoned. To the second or third day after the injury, inflammatory exudation in and about the parts ; thence to the eighth or tenth, seeming inaction, with subsidence of inflammation ; thence to about the twentieth, production of the reparative material, and its gradual development to its fibrous or cartilaginous condition ; thenceforward its gradual ossification, a part of the process which is, however, most variable in both its time of commencement and its rate of progress, and which is, probably, rarely completed before the ninth or tenth week, although the limb may have long previously recovered its fitness for support or other use. From this time the rate of change is so uncertain, that it is impossible to assign the average time within which the perfection of the repair is, if ever, accomplished.

The consequences of failure in the process of repair may be illustrated by what I have described as its normal course. In a large part of the cases of ununited fracture the fragments are connected by fibrous or fibro-cartilaginous tissue, inlaid between them. Such is the defective union of most cases of fracture of the neck of the femur within the capsule, and of the olecranon and the patella when their fragments are not held close ; and such a defect may occur in any long bone. It is an example of arrested development of the reparative material; and may be, in this respect, compared with the condition of granulations whose cells persist in their rudimental form. Every other part of the process may be complete; but this part fails, and the fragments are combined by a yielding, pliant, and almost useless bond.

In other cases, the failure seems to occur earlier. No reparative material is formed, and the fragments remain quite disunited. This may be the result of accidental hinderances of the normal reparative process: but it sometimes appears like a simple defect of formative power; a defect which, I believe, cannot be explained, and which seems the more remarkable when we observe the many changes which may, at a later time, be effected, as if to diminish the evil of the want of union. Thus, commonly, the ends of bones thus disunited become covered with a thin layer of fibrous tissue, polished as if with a covering of epithelium, and as smooth as an articular surface: similar smooth linings form in the cavities that enclose them; the tissues immediately around them become condensed and fibrous; and thus, at length, the ends of the fragments are brought to the imitation of a joint, in which they may move without mutual injury. Or else, in the place of such a false joint, the end of each fragment has a kind of bursal sac formed on it, protecting the adjacent parts from injury in its movements. But, much as may be thus accomplished, new bone is not spontaneously produced. As the result of disease, it may be formed; and in this case it is often formed uselessly, and without evident design, in heaps or nodules about the ends of the fragments; yet it is of such disease that surgery may often make happy use when it can excite inflammation of the fragments, and so hold them close that the new bone may grow between or around them, and fasten itself to both.*

* It will diminish the defects of the foregoing description of the repair of fractures, which I have drawn almost entirely from my own observations, if I subjoin a list of the works especially or chiefly devoted to this subject, in which the reader may find the best help to a larger knowledge of the subject.

Dupuytren: Exposé de la Doctrine de M. Dupuytren sur le Cal, par Sanson. In Journ. Univ. des Sciences Médicales, t. xx.

Breschet: Recherches ... sur la Formation du Cal; Thèse. Paris, 1819.

Howship: On the Union of Fractured Bones. Med.-Chir. Trans., vol. ix.

Miescher: De Inflammatione Ossium eorumque Anatome. Berlin, 1836.

Flourens: Sur le Développement des Os et des Dents. Paris, 1842.

Lebert: Sur la Formation du Cal. In his Physiologie Pathologique, t. ii. Paris, 1845.

Voetsch: Die Heilung der Knochenbrüche. Heidelberg, 1847.

Stanley: Illustrations of the Effects of Disease and Injury of the Bones, p. 27. 1849.

Malgaigne: Traité des Fractures et des Luxations, t. i. Paris, 1847.

Dusseau: Onderzoek van het Beenweefsel en Verbeeningen in sachte Deelen. Amsterdam, 1850.

LECTURE XII.

HEALING OF INJURIES IN VARIOUS TISSUES.

THIS last lecture on the process of repair I propose to devote to the consideration of the modes of healing of several different tissues; modes which, although they be all consistent with what has been said of the general rules and methods of the healing process, yet present each some peculiarity that seems worthy of observation.

And first (though it matters little which I begin with), of the healing of wounds and other injuries of cartilage.

There are, I believe, no instances in which a lost portion of cartilage has been restored, or a wounded portion repaired, with new and well-formed permanent cartilage, in the human subject. When a fracture extends into a joint, one may observe that the articular cartilage remains for a long time unchanged, or else has its broken edges a little softened and rounded off. In one case, I saw no other change than this in six weeks; but at a later period the gap is filled with a tough fibrous tissue, or, rather, the gap becomes somewhat wider and shallower, and the space thus formed is so filled up.

The excellent researches of Dr. Redfern* have ascertained the method of this process in incised wounds of the articular cartilages of dogs. As showing the slowness of the repair, he found in one instance, in which he made three incisions into the cartilage of a patella, and two into that of the trochlear surface of the femur, that no union had taken place in twenty-nine weeks. No unusual cause for the want of union had been apparent, yet a reparative process had but just commenced. In another case, twenty-five weeks and four days after similar incisions, he found them completely and firmly united by fibrous tissue formed out of the substance of the adjacent healthy cartilage. The cut surfaces of the cartilage were very uneven, and were hollowed into small pits, produced by the half-destroyed cartilage-cells, the former contents of which were now lying on the surface. No evident change had taken place in the texture of the cartilage at a little distance from the cut surfaces, except that here and there the intercellular substance presented a fibrous appearance. The substance uniting the cut surfaces consisted of a hyaline, granular, and indistinctly striated mass, in which were numbers of rounded oblong, elongating, or irregularly-shaped corpuscles. A nucleated fibrous membrane, formed by the conversion of the superficial layers of the cartilage bordering the wounds, was continuous with their uniting medium. "The essential parts of the process [of union of such incised wounds]

* Anormal Nutrition in Articular Cartilages: Edinburgh, 1850. And, On the Healing of Wounds in Articular Cartilages: in the Monthly Journal of Medical Science, Sept., 1851.

appear to be," Dr. Redfern concludes, "the softening of the intercellular substance of the cartilage, the release of the nuclei of its cells, the formation of white fibrous tissue from the softened intercellular substance, and of nuclear fibres by the elongation of the free nuclei."

Such a process has peculiar interest as occurring in a tissue which has no blood-vessels, and in which, therefore, the reparative material is furnished by transformation of its own substance, not by exudation from the blood. In the same view the results of inflammation of articular cartilage will have to be particularly noticed.

In membraniform cartilages that have perichondrium, the healing process is, probably, in some measure, modified; a reparative material being furnished, at least in part, from the perichondrial vessels. The cartilaginous tissue was less changed than in Dr. Redfern's cases, in an example of wounded thyroid cartilage that I examined. A man, long before death, cut his throat, and the wound passed about half an inch into the angle of his thyroid cartilage. In the very narrow gap thus made, a gap not more than half a line in width, there was only a layer of tough fibrous tissue; and with the microscope I could detect no appearance of a renewed growth of cartilage. The edges of the cartilage, to which the fibrous tissue was attached, were as abrupt, as clean, and as straight, as those would be of a section of cartilage just made with a very sharp instrument. The cut cartilage was unchanged, though the union between it and the new-formed fibrous tissue was as close and as firm as that of the several parts of a continuous tissue. The perichondrium on both sides was equally firmly attached to the fibrous bond.

In some instances (but I suppose in none but those of cartilages which have a natural tendency to be ossified in advancing years) the fractures of cartilage may be united by bone. This commonly happens in the costal cartilages; and it has been noticed in fractures of the thyroid cartilage. The union of a fracture of the cartilaginous portion of a rib is usually effected, as that of one in the osseous portion is, by an enclosing ring of bone, like a provisional external callus; and the ossification extends to the parts of the cartilage immediately adjacent to the fracture.*

HEALING OF TENDONS.—I have already often referred to the phenomena that follow the division of tendons by subcutaneous and by open wounds; but the practical interest of the subject will justify my giving a connected account of the process, as I observed it in a series of numerous experiments performed, with the help of Mr. Savory, on rabbits from three to six months old. Such experiments are, I know, open, in some measure, to the same objection as I showed in the last lecture to those on fractures in the lower animals; but the few instances in which exami-

* Museum of the College, No. 377; and of St. Bartholomew's, Ser. iii., Nos. 48, 73. Numerous examples of the partial repair of larger injuries of articular and other cartilages will be found in Hildebrandt's Anatomie, B. i. p. 306.

nations have been made of human tendons, divided by subcutaneous section, have shown that the processes in man and in animals are not materially different. The chief differences are, we may believe, that, as in the repair of bones, the production of reparative material is more abundant, and its organization more speedy, in animals than in man.

I have already, in the second lecture, stated generally the differences in the several consequences of open and subcutaneous wounds. In the case of divided Achilles tendons, the disadvantages of open wounds, i. e. of wounds extending through the integuments over and on each side of the tendon, as well as through it, were as follows:—1. There were always more·inflammation in the neighborhood of the wound, and more copious infiltration of the parts, than in a subcutaneous division of the tendon in the same rabbit; 2. Suppuration frequently occurred, either between the retracted ends of the divided tendon, or beneath its distal end; 3. The skin was more apt to become adherent to the tendon, and so to limit and hinder its sliding movements, when the healing was completed; 4. The retracted ends of the tendon were more often displaced, so that their axes did not exactly correspond with each other, or with that of the reparative bond of union. Such mishaps were often observed in the open wounds, but were rare after the subcutaneous operations. In the cases of open wounds, they were avoided as often as the wound through the integuments healed quickly; and, whenever this happened, the case proceeded like one in which the subcutaneous division had been made. It was evident that the exposure of the wounded parts to the air

Fig. 25.

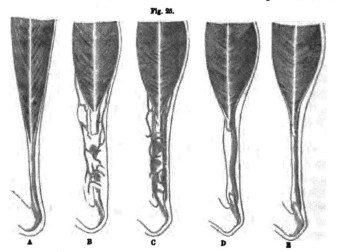

A   B   C   D   E

did little harm, if it was continued for only a few hours; a fact that may be usefully remembered when operations must be performed on tendons which it is not convenient to divide unseen.

These same cases of speedy healing of the opening in the integuments served to show, that it is unimportant for the healing of divided Achilles tendons, whether the cellular sheath or covering of the tendon be divided or not. In all the cases of open division in these experiments, it was completely cut through; yet, when the external wound healed quickly, the union of the divided tendon was as speedy and as complete as in any case of subcutaneous division in which it might be supposed that the sheath of the tendon was not injured.

I will describe now the course of events after subcutaneous division of the Achilles tendon; stating only what was generally observed, and illustrating it, as far as may be, with the annexed diagram (fig. 25), in which, as in longitudinal sections, A may represent the natural condition of the tendon and its muscles, and the succeeding figures the effects of its division and the successive stages of its repair.*

At the instant of the division, the ends of the tendon separate to the distance of nearly an inch, the upper portion of the tendon being drawn up the leg by the action of the gastrocnemius and soleus muscles (B). The retraction is comparatively much greater than is usual in operations on the human Achilles tendon; for where these are done, the muscles are seldom capable of strong or extensive contraction. It is in all cases to be remembered that the separation is effected entirely by the withdrawal of the upper portion of the tendon; the lower, being not connected with muscle, remains with its end opposite the wound. To this we may ascribe the general fact that the reparative process is more active, and the inflammatory process less so, at the upper than at the lower portion of the tendon: for the latter lies in the very centre of the chief inflammatory action; while the former is removed far from it, being drawn away, at once from the seat of the injury, and from even the slightest exposure to the air.

I have already said that very little blood is effused in the subcutaneous operations. Commonly, only a few blotches of extravasation appear in and near the space from which the upper part of the tendon is retracted (B). The first apparent consequence of the division of the tendon is the effusion of a fluid or semi-fluid substance, which, like the product of common inflammation, quickly organizes itself into the well-known forms of lymph or exudation-cells. These, speedily becoming more distinctly nucleated and elongated, undergo the changes which I mentioned in describing the development of cells in granulations. The exuded lymph makes the tissues at and near the wound succulent and yellow, like parts infiltrated in anasarca. The blood-vessels near the

---

* The account here given agrees in all essential respects with that by Lebert, in his Abhandlungen . . . . der prakt. Chirurgie, p. 403. Neither do the accounts materially differ, except in being less minute, which are given by Von Ammon (De Physiologia Tenotomiæ), Duval (Bull. de. l'Acad. Royale de Médecine, 1837), and Duparc (Nederlandsch Lancet, 1837).

12

divided tendon enlarge, as in an inflamed part, and appear filled with blood (B, C). The exudation, together with the enlargement of the vessels, swells the parts, so that the skin is scarcely at all depressed between the separated ends of the tendon. But in well-made subcutaneous sections, this inflammatory product is of small amount, and takes, I believe, little or no share in the healing of the injury ; for the exudation ceases after the first twenty-four hours, and I think that its cells are not developed beyond the state in which they appear spindle-shaped. I have never seen indications of their forming filaments of cellular or fibrous tissue.

In rabbits, forty-eight hours usually elapse before there are distinct signs of the production of the proper reparative material. This is deposited in the fibro-cellular tissue that lies between and close round the separated ends of the tendon, as well as in the interspaces of the tendinous fasciculi of those ends. It thus swells up the space between the separated ends, and makes the ends themselves larger, and somewhat ruddy, soft, and succulent. Some portion, at least, of it being deposited where the inflammatory effusion was, one finds their constituents mingled ; but I believe that, while the proper reparative material develops itself, the product of the inflammation is either arrested in its development, or even degenerates ; its cells shriveling and gradually wasting.

I need not now describe the mode of development of the reparative material provided for divided tendons: for I have taken it as a typical example of the development of lymph into nucleated blastema, and thence into fibrous tissue (p. 129). To the naked eye it appears after three days as a soft, moist, and grayish substance, with a slight ruddy tinge, accidentally more or less blotched with blood, extending from one end of the tendon to the other, having no well-marked boundary, and merging gradually into the surrounding parts (C). In its gradual progress, the reparative material becomes commensurately firmer, tougher, and grayer, the ruddiness successively disappearing from the circumference to the axis : it becomes, also, more defined from the surroundings parts, and, after four or five days, forms a distinct cord-like vascular bond of connection between the ends of the tendon, extending through all the space from which they have been retracted, and for a short distance ensheathing them both (D, E).

As the bond of connection thus acquires toughness and definition, so the tissue around it loses its infiltrated and vascular appearance : the blood-vessels regain their normal size, the inflammatory effusion clears up, and the integuments become looser and slide more easily. In every experiment, one finds cause for admiration at the manner in which a single well-designed and cord like bond of union is thus gradually formed, where at first there had been a uniform and seemingly purposeless infiltration of the whole space left by the retraction of the tendon.

With the increase of toughness, the new substance acquires a more decidedly filamentous appearance and structure. After the fourth day, the microscope detects nuclei in the previously homogeneous fibrine-like reparative material; and after the seventh or eighth day there appear well-marked filaments, like those of the less perfect forms of fibrous tissue. Gradually perfecting itself, but with a rate of progress which becomes gradually less,* the new tissue may become at last, in all appearance identical with that of the original tendon. So it has happened in the valuable specimens presented to the Museum of the College by Mr. Tamplin.† They are the Achilles tendon and the tendons of the anterior and posterior tibial muscles of a child nine months old, in whom, when it was five months old, all these tendons were divided for the cure of congenital varus. The child had perfect use of its feet after the operation, and, when it died, no trace of the division of any of the tendons could be discerned even with microscopic aid.

In the instances of divided human tendons, less retraction, I have already said, takes place than in those of lower animals. The connecting bond is therefore comparatively shorter; and it is yet more shortened when, like a scar, it contracts as it becomes firmer. It is impossible, therefore, to say what length of new material was, in this case, formed into exact imitation of the old tendon. But, however little it may have been, such perfect repair as these specimens show is exceedingly rare. More commonly the differences between the original tendon and the new substance remain well-marked. The latter does not acquire the uniform arrangement of fibres, or the peculiar glistening thence accruing to the normal tendons: it is harder and less pliant, though not tougher; its fibres appear irregularly interwoven and entangled, dull-white, like those of a common scar. And these differences, though as time passes they become gradually less, are always seen when a longitudinal section is made from behind, through both the ends of the tendon and the new substance that ensheaths and connects them. In such a section (as in fig. 25, E), one sees each of the retracted ends of the divided tendon preserving nearly all its peculiar whiteness, only somewhat rounded or misshapen, swollen, and imbedded in the end of the new substance, which is always grayer, or less glistening, and looks less compact and regular. In the retracted ends of the tendon, one may discern the new substance mingled with the old and interposed between its fasciculi, with which one may believe it is connected by the finest dove-tailing.‡

The strength, both of the new substance itself, and of its connection

---

* One may remark this as a general fact, that when once the reparative process has commenced, much more appears to be done in it in the first few days than in any equal subsequent period of time. It may be another instance justifying the general expression, that production is easier than development or improvement, and that the earlier or lower developments require less organizing force than the higher or later.

† Nos. 358, 359, 360.

‡ The appearances are shown in specimens in the College Meseum, Nos. 348 to 354; and in those from the experiments on rabbits in the Museum of St. Bartholomew's.

by intermingling with the original substance, is worthy of remark. To test it, I removed from a rabbit an Achilles-tendon, which had been divided six days previously, and of which the retracted ends were connected by a bond of the size and texture usual at that period of the reparative process. I suspended from the half-section of this bond gradually increased weights. At length it bore a weight of ten pounds, but presently gave way with it: yet we may suppose the whole thickness of the bond would have borne twenty pounds. In another experiment, I tried the strength of a bond of connection which had been ten days forming: this, after bearing suspended weights of twenty, thirty, forty, and fifty pounds, was torn with fifty-six pounds. But surely the strength it showed was very wonderful, when we remember that it was not more than two lines in its chief diameter; and that it was wholly formed and organized in ten days, in the leg of a rabbit scarcely more than a pound in weight. With its tenacity it had acquired much of the inextensibility of the natural tendon. It was indeed stretched by the heavy weights suspended from it, yet so slightly that I think no exertion of which the rabbit was capable would have sufficed to extend it in any appreciable degree.

THE HEALING OF MUSCLES, subcutaneously divided, presents many things exactly similar to those just described as observed in the healing of tendons similarly divided, and the structure of the connecting reparative bond is of the same kind; new muscular fibres, I believe, are never formed. But, in the experiments I made on the triceps extensor brachii, and the tibialis anticus of rabbits, there are always observed a peculiar inversion, subsidence, or *tucking-in* of the muscular fibres at the divided parts; so that nearly all the fasciculi directed their cut ends towards the subjacent bone or fascia. Thus it sometimes appeared to happen that, though the retracted portions of the muscle were imperfectly united, yet the action of the muscle was not lost; for one or both its ends, acquiring new attachments to the subjacent parts, could still act, though with diminished range, upon the joint over which its fibres passed.

In general, it appeared that the reparative material was less quickly produced than after the division of tendons; but this might be because of the greater violence inflicted in the operation, more than because of the structure of the divided parts. The usual method and end of the development of the reparative material were the same as after division of the tendons; and at length, but always, I think, more slowly than with them, the ends of the retracted portions became inclosed in a tough fibrous bond of union.

After the formation of this bond, the healing of divided muscles is improved, both by the clearing up of the surrounding tissues infiltrated with inflammatory products, and by the contraction of the new bond, which thus draws together the retracted portion of the muscle, so that they very nearly coalesce. Thus, in a man who had cut his throat long before his death, and had divided the left sterno-hyoid, omo-hyoid, and sterno-thyroid muscles, I found that the ends of these muscles, though they must at first have retracted considerably, had all been drawn to attachments on the cricoid cartilage, over which their several portions nearly united.

THE HEALING OF INJURED ARTERIES AND VEINS is commonly a more complicated process than those already described, on account of the changes that ensue in the blood that is stagnant within, or shed around, the injured vessel.*

Small wounds of either arteries or veins may heal by immediate union, or primary adhesion, as those of any other tissue may, and the blood shed into the adjacent tissues may be absorbed as from a common ecchymosis. An artery divided in only part of its circumference, although it may be for a time contracted, yet does not remain so; neither is it commonly, in such a case, obstructed by clot within its canal. Hence, after such wounds, the pulse in the distal or lower part of the artery is often unaffected. After the first outrush of blood, some that remains extravasated among the tissues usually clots, and covers the wound in the artery; but the closure is often ineffectual, or only for a time, and fresh bleedings ensue, either increasing the accumulation of extravasated blood, or pushing out the clots already formed. In this way, with repeated hemorrhages at uncertain intervals, the wound in an artery is often kept open, and at the end of two or three weeks may show no trace of healing, but, rather, appear widened and with softened averted edges. In such a case, it is possible that the wound in an artery may still heal by granulations, either rising from its edges or coalescing over it from adjacent parts; but the event is too unlikely to justify the waiting for its occurrence, if there be opportunity for surgical interference.

In the case of an artery divided quite across, three chief things are to be considered; namely, the natural immediate arrest of the bleeding, the closure of the two orifices, and the disposal of the blood that may become stagnant at and near the ends of the divided vessel.

The bleeding is arrested, mainly by the contraction of the muscular coat of the artery. Stimulated by the injury and by exposure to the air, and relieved from much of the pressure of the blood, whose onward course is less resisted, the muscular tissue of the divided artery contracts and closes, or, at least, diminishes, the canal. In some instances the contraction is narrowly funnel-shaped, and the end of the artery may be open, while, at a little distance within, its canal is closed or much

---

* Nearly all that follows relates to the healing of wounds of arteries. The process in veins appears to be essentially the same, but more quickly accomplished. See Stilling : " Die naturlichen Processe bei der Heilung durchschlungener Blutgefasse :" Eisenach, 1834, p. 147 and 289.

narrower. In some, the exterior layers of the muscular fibres seem to contract rather more than the interior, and the end of the artery appears prominent or pouting. Many, perhaps trivial, differences of this kind may be noticed in different arteries cut across in amputations.

The retraction of the divided artery within its sheath, or among the adjacent tissues, assists to stay the bleeding, by giving opportunity for the blood to become diffused, as it flows over the tissues that collapse over the end of the artery before it closes. But the degree to which this retraction can take place is very uncertain. It depends chiefly on the laxity or the closeness of the attachment of the artery to the surrounding tissues, and on the extent to which they with it are divided, and with it are capable of retraction. In amputations, one sees many differences in these respects. Arteries divided close to ligamentous parts and the origins of the muscles appear much retracted, because the tissues about them are scarcely at all drawn back; so it is in amputations just below the knee: but those that are divided where there is much cellular tissue, or where muscles are far from their origins, as in the middle or lower part of the forearm, appear less retracted, because these surrounding parts are retracted as much or more than they. In like manner, arteries from which branches are given off just above the place of division retract less than others, the branches holding them in place.

Equally various is the degree to which the bleeding from a wounded artery is arrested by the blood collecting around it, and in front of its orifice. It depends mainly on the degree of retraction of the artery, and on the facility with which the blood can escape through the external wound. It is assisted, in case of large hemorrhage, by the weakening of the action of the heart, and, perhaps, by the readier coagulation of the blood which ensues in syncope.

The efficacy of these means for the arrest of bleeding from all but the principal arterial trunks, is evident enough immediately after the amputation of a limb. However many arteries may need ligatures, they are probably not more than a tenth of those that were just now traversed by quick streams of blood. The rest are already closed by their own muscular action, needing no assistance, from a diminished action of the heart, or the effusion of blood around them.

I know no observations showing the method of healing and permanent closure of the small arteries that thus spontaneously cease to bleed. All the accurate inquiries that I am aware of relate to the closure of the torn umbilical arteries, which have hardly a parallel in other vessels, or else to the more complicated cases of large arteries on which ligatures have been tied, or which have been closed by some artificial means, such as the "Durchschlingung" of Stilling; a defect much to be regretted, since the ligature, or any similar means, introduces such a disturbance into the process of repair, as makes it a morbid process, however advantageous its end may be. Indeed, when a divided artery is tied, the injury to be repaired is not that of the wound, but that of the ligature; an injury in which a bruised wound dividing the middle and internal coats of the artery, a bruise with continued compression of its external coat, and the continued presence of a foreign body, are superadded to the injuries which preceded the application of the ligature.

For simplicity's sake, let us consider the repair of such an injury in only that part of an artery which is above the ligature, i. e., nearer to the heart. The changes in the part beyond the ligature are, according to Stilling, the same, but more quickly accomplished.

Now, in this repair, three parts are chiefly concerned; namely (1), the injured walls of the vessel at and immediately adjoining the ligature; (2), the part of the vessel between the ligature and the first branch above it, through which the blood can flow off; and (3) the blood which, within the same part of the vessel, i. e., between the ligature and the first branch nearer to the heart, lies nearly stagnant. The healing of the artery may indeed be accomplished without the help of this blood, but certain changes in it commonly concur with the rest of the process.

(1.) The injured walls of the vessel, and the tissue immediately around them, inflame, and exudation of lymph takes place in them, especially at and just above the divided part of the coats constricted and held in contact by the ligature. Thus, as by primary adhesion, or by an adhesive inflammation, the wound made by the ligature in the middle and internal coats is united; and, through the same process, this union is strengthened by the adhesion of these coats to the outer coat, and of the outer coat to the sheath or other immediately adjacent tissues. There is a general adhesion of these parts to one another; they appear thickened, infiltrated, and morbidly adherent; beneficial as the result is, it is the result of disease. Through the same disease, the portion of the outer coat of the artery included within the ligature ulcerates, permitting the removal of the ligature, and a more natural process of organization of the inflammatory products among which it lay, and which its presence had tended to increase.

(2.) When any part of an artery, through any cause, ceases to be traversed by blood, its walls tend to contract and close its canal. The application of a ligature brings into this condition all that part of the tied artery which lies between it and some branch or branches higher up, through which the stream of blood may be carried off. The walls of this part therefore slowly contract, gradually reducing the size of its canal, and, in some instances probably, closing it. There is not in this, as in the last described part of the process, any disease: the contraction is only the same as that of the ductus arteriosus, the umbilical arteries, and other vessels, from which, in normal life, the streams of blood are diverted; and the closure may, as in them, according to Rokitansky,* be assisted by deposit from the blood thickening with an opaque white layer the in-

* Pathologische Anatomie, B. ii, p. 623.

ternal coat. The time occupied by this contraction, and its extent in length along the artery, are too various to be stated generally. When it is permanent, the coats of the artery, at its completion, waste, lose their peculiar structures, and are slowly transformed into fibrous tissue, such as that which composes the solid cord of the ductus arteriosus.

(3.) Respecting these two consequences of the application of ligatures, little difference of opinion can exist ; and it may be repeated, that either of these may suffice for the safe closure of the artery. Thus, on the one hand, we sometimes see an artery pervious to the very end of a stump, but there safely closed as the seat of the ligature ; and, on the other, the naturally torn umbilical arteries of animals, and, I suspect, the arteries which in common wounds are divided, and spontaneously cease to bleed, are closed and obliterated without inflammation. However, much more commonly, the blood contained in and near the end of the tied artery becoming stagnant, concurs with both the processes just described, to the closure of the canal.

Concerning this third constituent of the process, more questions have been raised. I shall describe it from the admirable observations of Stilling[*] and Zwicky.[†] They were made in large series of experiments on the arteries of animals : those of Stilling refer chiefly to the changes visible to the naked eye, those of Zwicky to the more minute.

When an artery is tied, the blood, as already said, becomes nearly stagnant in the canal; from the ligature upwards to the first principal branch. In an uncertain time, varying from one to eighteen hours, a part of this blood coagulates ; and the clot commonly assumes a more or less conical form. The base of this " conical clot," "internal obturator," "plug," or "thrombus," rests in and fills the end of the artery, at the wound made by the ligature ; its apex usually lies nearly opposite the first branch above, in the axis of the artery : it is surrounded by fluid, but still nearly stagnant, blood, which, except at its base, intervenes between it and the internal surface of the artery. At its base, and higher up if it fills the artery, the clot is dark and soft, like a common blood-clot : its upper part and apex are denser, harder, and whitish, like coagulated fibrine ; and layers of white substance are often gradually superadded to its middle and apex, and increase its adhesion to the walls of the vessel.

In course of time, the clot becomes marked with paler spots, and then porous, spungy, and cavernous, as if it were being gradually channeled from its surface towards its central parts. In this state, injection impelled into the artery will enter and distribute itself in the clot, making it appear vascular, or like a cavernous tissue.[‡] While thus changing,

* Die natürl. Processe bei der Heilung durchschlungener Blutgefässe. Eisenach, 1834.
† Die Metamorphose des Thrombus. Zurich, 1845.
‡ It was such an injection probably, that half deceived Hunter into the belief that he had found the beginning formation of new blood-vessels in the clot (Works, vol. iii. p. 119 ; and

also, it becomes gradually more decolorized, passing through ruddy, rosy, and yellowish tints, till it is nearly colorless. As it loses color, it gains firmness, and its base and the greater part of its length become more firmly adherent to the inner surface of the artery, directly or through the medium of the lymph deposited in it. In this increasing firmness, the clot, moreover, is acquiring a more definitely fibrous texture; and, as the same change is gradually ensuing in the inflammatory products deposited near the ligature, the clot and they unite more firmly than before. The walls of the artery, also, gradually closing in on the clot, unite with it; and, finally, as they also lose their peculiar texture and become fibrous, the clot and they, together, form the solid fibrous cord by which the tied portion of the artery is replaced; a cord which commonly extends, as did the clot, from the seat of the ligature to the first principal branch above it.

The minuter changes in the clot, associated with those visible to the naked eye, are, chiefly, that it acquires a fibrous or fibro-cellular texture, and becomes vascular. I have already said (p. 120), that Zwicky has traced the development of the fibrine of the clot into fibrous tissue through the formation of nucleated blastema; and, probably, I need not add to the descriptions of this process already drawn from other though similar instances of it (pages 128 and 178). The development, or, at least, the later part of it, is accomplished much more slowly than in the reparative material of tendons in rabbits; needing more than ten weeks in the clots formed in dogs, and more than two years in those in men. The retardation may depend in some measure on the presence of the blood-corpuscles in the clot; for these, though they seem not to affect, or take part in, the development of the fibrine, yet probably, as they suffer degeneration preparatory to removal, may retard it.*

The blood-vessels usually enter the organizing clot, in dogs, in the fourth week, when already it has acquired a nucleated and imperfectly fibrous tissue, and firmness in the place of the spongy texture from which it had derived a spurious appearance of vascularity. They pass into it, apparently, from the vessels formed in the lymph exuded within the artery, in and just above the situation of the ligature; hence they enter its lower part, and gradually extend towards its apex.

Such is the important process for the healing of tied arteries. In applying the description drawn from experiments on animals to the cases of human arteries, the same allowance must be made as in the repairs of fractures and of divided tendons. The process is less speedy, less simple, less straightforward (if I may so speak), more prone to deviate

the Museum of the College, No. 11); and this led Stilling into one of the few errors in his essay, inducing him to believe that the clot thus became vascular independently of the vessels of the surrounding parts.

* The changes ensuing in the blood-corpuscles are described by Zwicky; but I omit them, since they take no evident part in the reparative process, and are, as yet, not clearly ascertained.

and to fail, through excess of that disease, by a measured amount of which the security of the artery is achieved.*

THE HEALING OF DIVIDED NERVES may be accomplished in two methods, which may be named, respectively, primary and secondary union, and may, probably, be compared with the processes of primary adhesion (p. 135), and of connection by intermediate new-formed bonds (p. 177).

I know no instances in which nerves healed in the first method have been examined, but the nature of the process may be explained by the history of a case in which it occurred :—

A boy, eleven years old, was admitted into Saint Bartholomew's Hospital, under Mr. Stanley, with a wound across the wrist. This wound, which had been just previously made with a circular saw, extended from one margin to the other of the forearm, about an inch above the wrist-joint. It went through all the flexor tendons of the fingers and thumb, dividing the radial artery and nerve, the median nerve and artery, and extending for a short distance into the radius itself. The ulnar nerve and artery were not injured; the condition of the interosseous artery was uncertain, but the interosseous ligament was exposed at the bottom of the wound. Half an inch of the upper portion of the divided median nerve lay exposed in the wound, and was distinctly observed and touched by Mr. Stanley, myself, and others. All sensation in the parts supplied from the radial and median nerves below the wound was completely lost directly, and for some days after the injury.

The radial artery was tied, and the edges of the wounded integuments put together. No particular pains were taken to hold the ends of the divided median nerve in contact, but the arm was kept at rest with the wrist bent.

After ten days or a fortnight the boy began to observe signs of returning sensation in the parts supplied by the median nerve, and these increasing, I found, a month after the wound, that the nerve had nearly recovered its conducting power. When he was blindfolded, he could distinctly discern the contact of the point of a pencil with his second finger, and the radial side of his third finger; he was less sure when his thumb or his forefinger was touched, for, though generally right, he sometimes thought one of these was touched when the contact was with the other; and there were a few and distant small portions of the skin supplied by the median nerve from which he still derived no sensation at all.

Now all this proves that the ends of the divided median nerve had coalesced by immediate union, or by primary adhesion with an exceedingly small amount of new substance formed between them. In the

* Rokitansky (B. ii., p. 616) may be referred to concerning some events in the process which are not yet clearly ascertained : such as the amount to which, in some cases, the clot may be absorbed, and the share taken by deposit from the blood producing opaque-white thickening of the inner coat of the artery.

ordinary secondary healing of divided human nerves, twelve months generally elapse before, if ever, any restoration of the function is observed; in this case, the nerve could conduct in a fortnight, and perhaps much less, after the wound. The imperfection of its recovery is just what one might expect in such a mode of union. One might anticipate that some of the fibres in one of its portions would fail to be united to any in the other portion: and the parts supplied by these filaments would necessarily remain insensible. So, again, one might expect that some of the fibres in one portion would unite with some in the other, with which they were not before continuous, and which supplied parts alien from those to which themselves were destined: in all such dislocations of filaments there would be confused or transferred sensations. But, among all the fibres, some would again combine in the same continuity in which they had naturally existed; and in these cases the function would be at once fully restored.*

While this case was under observation, Mr. Gatty sent me, with the permission of Mr. Heygate, in whose practice the case occurred, the following particulars of a similar instance of repair.

A lad, near Market Harborough, thirteen years old, had his hand nearly cut off at the wrist-joint by the knife of a chaff-cutting machine. The knife passed through the joint, separating a small portion of the ends of the radius and of the ulna, and leaving the hand attached to the forearm by only a portion of integument about an inch wide, connected with which were the ulna vessels and nerve, and the flexor carpi ulnaris muscle—all uninjured. The radial artery and some small branches being tied, the hand and arm were brought into apposition, and after removing a small portion of extensor tendon that protruded, were retained firmly with adhesive plaster and a splint of pasteboard. The wound went on very well, and was left undisturbed for a week. The warmth of the hand returned; in ten or twelve days after the injury there was slight sensation in the fingers, but in the thumb none was discernible till more than a fortnight had elapsed. Finally, the sensation of the hand and fingers, and most of their movements, were perfectly restored.

In this case, again, it seems impossible to explain the speedy restoration of the conducting power of the nerve, except on the supposition that its divided fibres had immediately reunited. We have no evidence that new nerve-fibres could in so short a time be formed; all the cases of

* I saw this boy again nearly a year after the injury. He had almost perfect sensation in all the distribution of the median nerve, except in the last phalanges of the thumb and forefinger. These had not decreased or changed in texture; but they were very liable to become cold, and he came to the hospital because large blisters had formed on them. He had been warming his hands at an open fire, and the heat, which was not uncomfortable to the rest of the hands, had blistered these parts, as boiling water would have blistered healthy ones. He had almost completely recovered the movement of his fingers.

less favorable healing show that they require a year or more for their formation.

I need hardly add the practical rule we may draw from these cases. It is, briefly, that we may, with good hope of great advantage, always endeavor to bring into contact, and immediately unite, the ends of divided nerves; and that we need not in all such cases anticipate a long-continued suspension of the sensation and other function of the part the nerves supplied.

The secondary healing of divided nerves presents many features similar to that of divided tendons. A bond of new substance is formed, which connects the ends of the retracted portions of the nerve, and in which, though at first it is like common reparative material, new nerve-fibres form, and connect themselves with the fibres in the portions above and below. I need not dwell on the formation or development of this connecting bond: the subject is amply treated in several works on physiology;* and it is thoroughly illustrated, so far as the appearances to the naked eye are concerned, by the valuable series of preparations given to the Museum of the College by Mr. Swan.† But the observations of Dr. Waller‡ have added some remarkable facts to those hitherto ascertained. Watching the process that follows the division of the glosso-pharyngeal nerve in frogs, he has found that after a nerve is divided, the old fibres, in the distal portion, never recover their functions. They degenerate, and new fibres are gradually formed in the whole length of the nerve, from the place of division to the peripheral distribution. These new fibres connect themselves with those in the connecting bond of repair, and through these with the old fibres in the proximal portion of the nerve. They are, and permanently remain, like the nerve-fibres of the embryo: they lie between the shriveled older fibres; and are not formed unless union have first taken place between the divided parts of the nerve.

The repair of nervous centres has been comparatively little studied. The experiments of M. Brown-Sequard§ have proved that, after complete division of the mid-dorsal part of the spinal cord of pigeons, and after division of more than half of that of guinea-pigs, the sensibility and movements of the hinder part of the body may be almost completely restored in about twelve months; and that the substance by which the injury of the cord is healed contains, with fibro-cellular tissue, abundant

* See especially Müller's Physiology, by Baly, i. 457; Valentin's Physiologie, i. 702; Hildebrandt's Anatomie, i. p. 291.

† Nos. 2169 to 2175. All these specimens, and the appearances of the formation of new nerve-fibres which they display, are described and illustrated by Mr. Swan, in his "Treatise on the Diseases and Injuries of Nerves." In Nos. 2165 to 2168 in the College Museum, Mr. Hunter has shown the formation of the bulb at the ends of divided nerves, and the extension of nerve-fibres into it.

‡ London Journal of Medicine, July, 1852.

§ Comptes Rendus de la Soc. de Biologie, t. i. p. 17; t ii. p. 3; t. iii. p. 77.

well-formed nerve-fibres connected with those of the cord above and below, and sparing nerve-cells.

Schrader's experiments of dividing and removing small portions of the cervical ganglia, and the ganglion of the vagus, of rabbits, found union by fibrous bonds, but no regeneration of ganglion-cells after eleven weeks.[*] Valentin's similar experiments had scarcely a more positive result.[†]

After wounds and losses of substance of the brain, a large quantity of new material may be formed to fill up the gap;[‡] but observations are wanting to show how much this may contain of proper cerebral substance. I have found nerve-fibres in it after thirty-three years (see p. 66); but in the same specimen there was no appearance of gray matter.

The last tissue to the healing of which I shall particularly refer, is the skin. I need not indeed describe the whole process, because nearly all that was said of the healing processes generally was chiefly illustrated by instances of wounds involving the skin. Yet it may be useful to indicate the skin as, on the whole, the part which, being most exposed to injury, is capable of the best repair ; that which heals most commonly by the immediate union, most quickly by primary adhesion ; that which produces the most rapidly and securely organizing granulations. The healing of skin is further favored by its extensibility and loose connection with adjacent parts; so that, when large surfaces are to be healed, the contracting granulations can draw over their borders the loose skin around. Moreover, the new-formed skin imitates the old skin very well, if we consider the complexity of its structure. I am not aware that the smooth muscular fibres, or any of the glandular structures of the skin, are formed in its scars; but its fibro-cellular and elastic tissues, its papillæ and epidermis, are all well-formed in them. It is commonly said that the smoothness of a scar is due to the absence of papillæ, but I believe it depends only on the tightness of the new-formed skin, and its want of such wrinkled and furrowed lines as naturally exists. If a thin section be made of the border of a healing wound, so as to include the

new-formed layer of epidermic, the granulations now skinned over will be found, as in the annexed diagram (fig. 26, A), presenting the papillary form. They consist still of nucleated cells, but the shape of papillæ is acquired, or, rather, is retained ; for the likeness of a granulating surface to a finely papillary one is evident, and may be regarded as an example of the general tendency of new-formed struc-

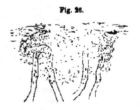

Fig. 26.

* Experimenta circa Regenerationem in Gangliis nerveis. Göttingen, 1850.
† Physiologe, i. 703.
‡ See especially Arnemann: Versuche über das Gehirn und Rückenmark. Göttingen, 1787.

tures, even in disease, to assume a plan of construction similar to that of
the adjacent parts. The likeness ex-

Fig. 27.

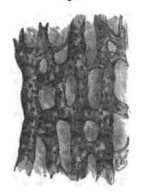

tends to the arrangement of the
blood-vessels; and the papillary structure is not lost in the later development
of the scar. If the epidermis of a
scar be separated, its under surface
will present a series of depressions
corresponding with the elevations of
the papillæ on which it was adapted.
The adjoining sketch represents the
under surface of epidermis so reflected
from a scar on the arm of a negro:
and may illustrate not only the plan of
the papillæ, of which it was like a
mould, but, by its color, the complete
reproduction of a rete nigrum.*

In concluding the lectures on Repair, and before beginning those on
Inflammation, let me briefly state the relations of the one process to
the other.

It is not because we have any well-defined idea of inflammation that
it is desirable to refer to it, as if it were a standard with which we
might compare other organic processes; but such a reference seems
necessary, because some idea of inflammation mingles itself with nearly
everything that is considered in surgical pathology. Nowhere is this
more manifest than in what has been written in surgical works upon the
methods of repair; concerning which a general impression seems still to
be, that a process of inflammation forms part of the organic acts by
which even the smallest instance of repair is accomplished.

Now the process we have traced appears to warrant these general
conclusions :—

1. In the healing of a wound by immediate union, inflammation forms
no necessary part of the process; rather, that its presence always hinders, and may completely prevent it. The healing by immediate union
should be a simple rejoining of the several parts, without the production of any new material; and in the same proportion as, in any case,
inflammatory matter is effused, either in or between the wounded parts,

* For the further study of the healing process, especially in the tissues and organs not
mentioned in this lecture, I must refer the reader either to special treatises on the pathology
of those parts, or to the chief works on General Anatomy, especially in relation to all but
microscopic observations, to that of Hildebrandt, edited by E. H. Weber; and to the chapters on Reproduction in Müller's Physiology, by Baly, vol. i. p. 440, and in Valentin's
Physiologie, i. 700. The power of repair in the cornea is illustrated especially by Dr.
Bigger, in the Dublin Journal of Med. Science, 1837; and by Donders, in the Onder-
zoekingen. . . . der Utrechtsche Hoogeschool, D. i. p. 31.—The repair of fractured
teeth by bone is described by Mr. Tomes in his "Dental Surgery." The Museum of the
College has the best specimens illustrating repair, that I am acquainted with.

in that proportion does the healing deviate from the true and best process of immediate union.

2. For subcutaneous wounds and injuries, as in divided tendons, simple fractures, and the like, nearly the same may be said. Inflammation is excited by the local injury, but its products form no necessary part of the material of repair; rather, the more abundant they are, the more acute the inflammation is, and the longer it continues, the less speedy and the less perfect is the process of repair. For here the necessary or best reparative material is a substance which is produced without the signs of co-existent inflammation, and of which the development is different from that of the inflammatory products that are mingled with it. And this, which is most evident in the case of the healing of subcutaneous injuries by bonds of connection, is probably equally true in the case of subcutaneous granulations.

3. In the healing of a wound by primary adhesion, or by open granulations, we, usually, have evidence of a process of inflammation, in the first instance, in the presence of its ordinary signs, in a degree generally proportioned to the severity and extent of the injury.

4. Still, in these cases, the signs of an inflammatory process are often absent; and even when they exist, the process appears necessary for no more than the production of the organizable matter, and, in the case of granulations, for the production of only the first portions of it. The right formation of the cells, and, yet more evidently, their higher organization into cellular and other tissues, ensue only while the signs of inflammation are absent. They are manifestly hindered or prevented when signs of inflammation are present, or when its existence may be suspected in consequence of the presence of some irritation, as a foreign body, dead bone, or the like. The continuance of suppuration, also, during the process of healing, is no proof of the continuance of inflammation, if the account that I have given of pus be true.

In these two modes of healing, therefore, we may conclude that inflammation is sometimes absent, and is, in any case, only partially, and at one period, requisite; and that, in regard to its requisite degree, the least amount with which an exudation of lymph is possible, is that which is most favorable to repair.

5. For the process of healing by scabbing, the absence of inflammation appears to be essential: indeed, the liability of our own tissues to the inflammatory process, and to the continued exudation that it produces, appears to be that which prevents their injuries from being healed as easily and surely, by the scabbing process, as nearly all open wounds are in animals.

Lastly, in certain cases, the artificial production of an inflammatory process is necessary for repairs for which the natural processes are insufficient or insecure. Among these, are the cases of fractures remaining disunited, and of arteries and veins needing ligatures.

Such may be regarded as the relations of the reparative process to that of inflammation, as it is commonly understood; but, I repeat, such a comparison can be made only for the sake of deference to the general state of opinion in matters of surgical pathology. In truth, we know less of inflammation than of the reparative process.

LECTURE XIII.

PHENOMENA OF INFLAMMATION.

It is no more than the truth which Mr. Travers has well expressed in his work on the "Physiology of Inflammation and the Healing Process" —"that a knowledge of the phenomena of inflammation, the laws by which it is governed in its course, and the relations which its several processes bear to each other, is the keystone to medical and surgical science."

I shall not attempt to define inflammation in any set terms; for as yet we are not, I think, in a position to do this. Just definitions cannot be made in any science till some of its broad and very sure principles have been established. Such principles we cannot boast to have yet attained in the study of pathology; and the attempts at precise definitions that have been made hitherto, seem to have led to confusion, or to false and narrow views of truth. Besides, to define inflammation is the less necessary, because, practically, we all know sufficiently well what the term implies: we know the signs of the presence of the disease in all its chief forms; and, when we watch these signs in any external part. we see them so often followed by peculiar changes in the part, that we are justified in recognizing the changes as effects of inflammation, and in believing that wherever we find them, the similar or corresponding signs of inflammation have preceded them.

But the very difficulty of exactly defining the process of inflammation may be our guide to the most hopeful method of investigating it. When we see such gradual transitions from the normal process of nutrition to the disease of inflammation, that we cannot draw a definition-line between them, we may be sure that the main laws of physiology are the laws alike of the disease and of the healthy process; that the same forces are engaged in both; and that, though interfered with by the conditions of the disease, they are not supplanted or annulled.

Now, such transitions from the normal processes to that of inflammation are not rare. We may trace them, for example, in the gradual passage from the active exercise of the brain, or of the retina, to its "irritation" when overworked, and thence to its complete inflammation and impairment of structure, after long exposure to what had been a natural stimulus, or to what, in a less degree, might be so. Or, on the introduction of medicines, such as certain diuretics, into the blood, we may trace gradations from the normal increase of the functions of the kidneys, under what is regarded as no morbid stimulus, to their intensest inflammations. Or, again, in the application of an abnormal stimulus, such as that of a heat greater than the natural temperature of the body, where shall we mark the line at which inflammation begins to supervene on health? We may, indeed, say that stagnation of blood, or effusion of liquor sanguinis, or some exudation, or some degenerative change in the elements of the affected tissue, shall be the condition *sine quâ non* of inflammation; we may call whatever falls short of these, "active congestion," "irritation," or by any other name; but, in reality, such distinctions are often impossible, and sometimes untrue, and in study, the terms are convenient for the sake of brevity rather than of clearness.

Evading, then, the question of the precise definition of inflammation, I shall endeavor, first, to describe the state of an inflamed part, giving to the description such a plan and direction as may best help the chief design—first, of contrasting the inflammatory with the normal method of nutrition ; and, secondly, of showing that the immediate causes, and the chief constituents, of the inflammatory state are to be found in alterations of those things which are necessary conditions of the healthy nutrition of a part. It will be easy to connect with such a description the explanations, so far as they can be given, of the constituent signs or phenomena of inflammation,—the redness, swelling, heat and pain, and the disturbed function of the part.

The conditions of the healthy maintenance of any part by nutrition, are, as illustrated in former lectures (p. 26)—1st, a regular and not far distant supply of blood; 2d, a right state and composition of that blood; 3d (at least in most cases), a certain influence of the nervous force; and 4th, a natural state of the part in which nutrition is to be effected. All these are usually altered in inflammation.

I. The supply of blood to an inflamed part is altered, both by the changes of the blood-vessels, especially by their enlargement, and by the mode in which the blood moves through them.

The enlargement of the blood-vessels is, I suppose, a constant event in the inflammation of a part; for, although in certain parts, as the cornea, the vitreous humor, and the articular cartilages, some of the signs or effects of inflammation may be found where there are naturally no blood-vessels, yet I doubt whether these ever occur without enlargement of the vessels of the adjacent parts, and especially of those vessels from which the diseased structure derives its natural supply of nutritive material, and which may therefore be regarded as its blood-vessels, not less than those of the part in which they lie. Thus, in inflammation of the cornea, the vessels

13

of the sclerotica and conjunctiva are enlarged, and in ulceration of articular cartilages those of the surrounding synovial membrane or subjacent
bone.

The enlargement usually affects alike the arteries, the capillaries, and
the veins, of the inflamed part; and usually extends to some distance
beyond the chief seat or focus of the
inflammation. To it we may ascribe
the most constant visible sign of inflammation, the redness, as well as much of
the swelling. Its amount is various; it
may be hardly perceptible, or it may
increase the vessels to two or three
times their natural diameter. Extreme
enlargement is admirably shown in
Hunter's specimen* of the two ears of
a rabbit, of which one was inflamed by
thawing it after it had been frozen.
"The rabbit was killed when the ear
was in the height of inflammation,
and, the head being injected, the two
ears were removed and dried." A
comparison of the ears, or of the drawings from them (fig. 28), shows all the
arteries of the inflamed ear three or four
times larger than those of the healthy
one, and many arteries that in the
healthy state are not visible, are, in the inflamed state, brought clearly
into view by being filled with blood.

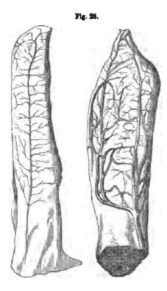
Fig. 28.

I have repeatedly seen similar enlargements of both arteries, and veins,
and capillaries, in the stimulated wings and ears of bats. The like phenomena occur in the webs of frogs, and other cold-blooded animals; but
in these, I think, the amount of enlargement is generally less.†

The redness of an inflamed part always appears more than is proportionate to the enlargement of its blood-vessels; chiefly, because the red
corpuscles are much more closely crowded than they naturally are in the
blood-vessels. The vessels of an inflamed part are not only dilated, but
appear crammed with the red corpuscles, which often lie or move as if no
fluid intervened between them: their quantity is increased in far greater
proportion than that of the liquid part of the blood.

This peculiarity is even more manifest in the frog than in the bat; for

* Museum of the College, No. 71. See, also, Hunter's Works, vol. iii., p. 323, and
pl. xx.

† Emmert, who is among the few that have measured it, says it is equal to one-half or
one-third of the normal diameter of the vessels. Lebert says one-sixth to one-third (Gazette Médicale, Mai 15, 1852).

in the former, the crowding of corpuscles may occur in vessels that appear to have undergone no change of size on the application of the stimulus.*

Another, but a minor, cause of the increased redness of the inflamed part, is sometimes to be observed in the oozing of the coloring matter of the blood-corpuscles, both into all the interspaces between them, and through the walls of the small vessel into the adjacent tissue. During life this may be noticed, especially when the blood is stagnant in the vessels, and it may give them a hazy, ruddy outline; but it is generally much more considerable after death, when we may ascribe to it no small portion of the redness that an inflamed part may still present.

In the state of inflammation no new blood-vessels are formed. Many more may come into view than were at first seen in the part; but these are only such as were invisible till the flood of blood-corpuscles filled and distended them. So it was in the rabbit's ears; in the healthy ear no trace can be seen, with the naked eye, of any vessels corresponding with one of the largest, or with many of those of inferior size, in the inflamed ear. So it is, too, in microscopic examinations. Within half an hour after stimulating a bat's wing, many vessels may come into view which could not be seen before by the same lens, and with which none can be seen corresponding in the other wing, though doubtless such vessels exist there of smaller size.

It is only when the inflammation has subsided, and the lymph exuded from the blood-vessels begins to be more highly organized, that new vessels are formed, and pass into the lymph, as if for the maintenance of its increase or development.† So long as the inflammation lasts, the intensest redness in parts naturally colorless,—even such as we see in acute inflammation of the conjunctiva, or yet more remarkably in those of periosteum,‡ or in congestion of the stomach,—is due to the enlargement of the natural blood-vessels to their admitting crowded red corpuscles, and in a much less degree, and, perhaps, in only certain cases, to the diffusion of the coloring matter of the blood.

With the enlargement of the blood-vessels a change of shape is commonly associated. Being usually elongated as well as dilated, they are thrown into curves and made more or less wavy or tortuous. Thus we may see the larger vessels in an inflamed conjunctiva, and, more plainly,

* I do not more particularly refer to what is described as the encroachment of the red blood-corpuscles on the lymph-space, or the layer of fluid that lies in apparent rest adhering to the walls of the vessels. The too pointed description of this layer has led to exaggerated notions concerning it. Its existence is certain, but it is too thin for any blood-corpuscle to lie at rest in; and when white corpuscles remain by the walls of the vessel, it is evident that they do so more because of their own adhesiveness than because a small portion of the fluid about them is at rest.

† Mr. Hunter held this opinion; but more lately the contrary one has been commonly held. See his Works, vol. iii. p. 322.

‡ As illustrated in Mr. Stanley's plates; plate vii. fig. 1, which represents a specimen in the Museum of St. Bartholomew's, Series i. No. 195. The whole inner surface of the inflamed periosteum of a tibia is bright scarlet.

the subperitoneal arteries in cases of peritonitis; so, too, they are represented in the inflamed rabbit's ear.

A more remarkable change of shape of the small vessels of inflamed parts is that in which they become aneurismal or varicose. The first observations of this state were published, I believe, by Kölliker and Hasse, in an account of a case of inflammatory red softening of the brain, in which many of what, at first sight, appeared to be points of extravasated blood, proved to be dilatations of capillary vessels filled with blood. After this they found the same changes, but in a much less degree, in some cases of inflammation artificially excited in the brains of rabbits and pigeons.* Many, as well as myself, have since made similar observations, most of which, however, seem to show, that the peculiar dilatation has its seat in the small arteries and veins, as well as in the capillaries of the inflamed part.

Among the various forms of partial dilatation, some are like gradual fusiform dilatations of the whole circumference of the vessel; some like

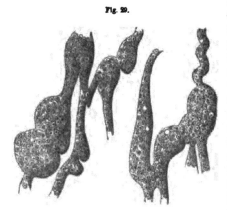

Fig. 29.

shorter and nearly spherical dilatations of it; some like round, or oval, or elongated pouches, dilated from one side of the wall: in short, all the varieties of form which we have long recognised in the aneurisms and aneurismal dilatations of the great arteries may be found in miniature in the small vessels of such inflamed parts. Some of these forms are represented in fig. 29, from the small vessels of an inflamed pericardium.

Frequently, however, as this state of the small vessels has been observed in inflamed parts (and I believe some measure of it may be found in the inflammations of most membranes),† yet, I think, we may not assume it to have a necessary or important connection with the other phenomena of inflammation. It is often observed, as Virchow‡ especially has shown, in other, besides inflammatory, diseases; and in all alike, may be referred to a gradual deterioration of the structure of the vessels, weakening them, and rendering them unable to resist the

---

* Zeitschr. für wissensch. Zoologie, B. i. p. 262. Mr. Kiernan had observed the same changes some years previously. See Dr. Williams's Principles of Medicine, 2d edit. p. 387.

† Leibert says it is a constant occurrence in experimental inflammations of the subcutaneous tissue of frogs. Gazette Médicale, Mai. 22, 1852.

‡ In his Archiv, B. iii. p. 432.

uniformly increased pressure of the blood. Perhaps, in some cases, as Mr. Quekett has suggested to me, the punch-like dilatations may represent a disturbed effort for the production of new blood-vessels by dilatation, or outgrowth of the walls of those already extant.

Such is the ordinary state of the blood-vessels of an inflamed part; all dilated and elongated, tensely filled with blood, of which the red corpuscles are in excess, often wavy and tortuous, and sometimes variously aneurismal.

But the supply of blood to an inflamed part is affected by its mode of movement, as well as by the size of the blood-vessels: this, therefore, I must now describe.

. Nearly all the observations hitherto recorded, on the morbid changes in the movement of the blood, have been made with the webs of frogs; and it has been objected that it is not safe to apply conclusions drawn from them to the case of warm-blooded animals. I have therefore employed the wings of bats, in which (when one has acquired some art in quieting them with chloroform or gentle management) nearly all the phenomena of the circulation, as affected by the application of stimuli, may be watched as deliberately as in the frog, and in some respects even more clearly.

I think we may believe that what may be seen in the wings of bats occurs, in the like circumstances, in all warm-blooded animals. It is true that, like the other hybernants, the bats, while they are in their winter-sleep, resemble the cold-blooded animals, in that their temperature is conformed to that of the external air, and scarcely exceeds it. It is true, also, that when they are ill nourished, their temperature, even in their active state, is comparatively low, ranging from 65° to 80° F., in an atmosphere of 60°; and that generally they are liable to much greater diversities of temperature than our own bodies are.* And the

---

* For instance, I found the temperature of a strong and active Noctule-Bat (*Vespertilio Noctula*) thus various in two days:—

April 29th, at noon, after he had been nearly two hours under the influence of chloroform, and on awaking had been struggling very actively, his temperature was 99° F. At 9 P. M., having sometimes been quiet, hanging by his hind feet, and looking sickly, his temperature was only 70°. When disturbed he became very fierce and active, shrieking and biting the bars of his cage; and at 9h. 40m. his temperature was 92°. Soon after this he became quiet again, and at 10h. 30m. his temperature was 80°. The temperature of the atmosphere during these examinations had gradually increased from 61° to 67°.—April 30th, at 8 A. M., he was feeble, but not torpid: the temperature of the room during the night had been between 40° and 45°, and was now 57°; the temperature of the bat was only 59°. At 11 A. M., after struggling violently for half an hour, it rose to 69°. After being long under chloroform, and nearly dying, he remained all the afternoon only one or two degrees warmer than the atmosphere. But at night, at 12h. 15m., he recovered and became active; and, while the atmosphere was at 65°, he was at 85°. At 12h. 40m., after being made very fierce, he was at 88°; and at 1h. 30m. remained at 85°. Next morning he was again scarcely warmer than the atmosphere. The temperature was always taken with a small thermometer applied to the surface of the abdomen.

remarkable condition, discovered by Mr. Wharton Jones,* that those veins in the wing that have valves contract with regular rhythm for the acceleration of the venous stream, may affect in some measure the morbid as well as the normal movement of the blood. Still, since in the development of their nervous system, and the commensurate development of their heart and respiratory organs, and in the close reciprocal relations in which these act, the bats resemble the other warm-blooded vertebrata, we may, I think, fairly assume a close resemblance also in their processes and conditions of nutrition.

The simplest effects upon the blood-vessels are produced by a slight mechanical stimulus. If, as one is watching the movement of blood in a companion artery and vein, the point of a fine needle be drawn across them three or four times, without apparently injuring them or the membrane over them, they will both presently gradually contract and close. Then, after holding themselves in the contracted state for a few minutes, they will begin again to open, and, gradually dilating, will acquire a larger size than they had before the stimulus was applied.†

Simple as this observation is, it involves some cardinal facts in our pathology. It illustrates, first, the contractile power of both arteries and veins; it shows that this is possessed by the smallest, just as it is by the larger, vessels of both kinds; and, by the manner of their contraction, which follows at some interval after the application of the stimulus, and is slowly accomplished, it shows that their power of contraction is like that of parts with smooth or organic muscular fibres.

But, again, the experiment shows the vessels reopening and becoming wider than they were before; either yielding more to the pressure of the blood which previously they resisted with more strength, or else dilating, as of their own force, with that which Mr. Hunter called active dilatation, and compared with the act of dilatation of the os uteri. In whichever way the dilatation is effected, whether it be active or passive, the vessels will not at once contract again under the same stimulus as before affected them. The needle may be now drawn across them much oftener and more forcibly, but no contraction ensues, or only a trivial one, which is quickly succeeded by dilatation. Yet with a stronger sti-

* Philos. Trans. 1852, Part I.

† Some doubt must exist as to the contraction of the veins here described; for Mr. Wharton Jones has not been able to convince himself of it. He considers, also, that in the frog's web the veins are capable of but slight variation in diameter through the operation of contractile power; and this accords with E. H. Weber's observations (Müller's Archiv, 1847). Lebert, on the other hand, expressly says that he has observed the same various states of contraction in the veins as in the arteries of the frog's web. In most other points relative to the condition of the blood-vessels, and the movement of the blood in them, my observations accord with those which Mr. Wharton Jones had completed, but not published, when his lectures were delivered. The reader may, however, find in his admirable essay (Guy's Hospital Reports, 1850) many minute details which I had not learned, and many illustrations of singular beauty and accuracy. I cannot doubt that his later researches with the bat's wing will much improve the description I have given.

mulus, such as that of great heat, they will again contract and close. And such a contraction excited by a cautery may last more than a day, before the vessels again open and permit the flow of the blood through them.

Moreover, we may observe in this experiment the adapted movement of the blood. As the vessels are contracting the blood flows in them more slowly, or begins to oscillate : nay, sometimes, I think, even before the vessels begin visibly to contract, one may observe that the blood moves more slowly in them, as if this were an earlier effect of the stimulus : nor have I ever seen (what has been commonly described) the acceleration of the flow of blood in the contracting vessels. Such an acceleration, however, is manifest, as the vessels reopen ; and as they dilate, so, apparently in ·the same proportion, does the flow of blood through them become more free, till, at length, it is manifest that they are traversed by both fuller and more rapid streams than passed through them before the stimulus was applied. How long this state may last depends on many circumstances hard to estimate : but at length it ceases, and the vessels, and the circulation through them, assume again their average or normal state.

Such are the effects of the mechanical stimulus of blood-vessels.

The effects of other stimuli applied to wings of bats correspond in kind, but differ in degree and extent. If a drop of acetic acid, of tincture of capsicum, of turpentine, or of ethereal solution of cantharides, be placed on a portion of the wing, or washed over it, one sees a quickly ensuing dilatation of the blood-vessels, and a rapid flow of blood through them all. I am not sure that the dilatation is preceded by contraction. Certainly the contraction is very slight, if it occur at all ; but the dilatation is usually much more extensive. When the stimulus has been applied to only one small spot upon the wing, the whole of the blood-vessels in the corresponding metacarpal space, and even those of the adjacent spaces, may enlarge. One might imagine that the dilatation of vessels was due to an increased action of the heart, if it were not that (as I think) it is always greater at the very point to which the stimulus was applied than in any other part of the same wing, and is never at all imitated in the corresponding parts of the opposite wing.

The state which is thus induced by stimuli is what is commonly understood by the expressions "active congestion," or "determination of blood," in a part. It consists, briefly, in general enlargement of the blood-vessels of the part, with an increased velocity of the blood in them. It is, probably, just such a state as this that is felt by suckling women in what they term the "flow of milk." It seems to be an increased flow of blood in the mammary gland just before a quicker secretion of the milk. Less normally, it is such a state as this that we observe in the skin after the application of mustard, or sharp friction, or a heat from 20° to 50° above its own, or, in the most striking instance, when a drop of strongest nitric acid is placed on the skin, and, in a few seconds, all the surrounding area seems to flush, and feels burning hot. Such, too, we may suppose to be the state of the vessels of the conjunctiva, when stimulated by dust that is soon dislodged; and such the condition of many internal organs, when we might doubt whether they are inflamed, or are only very actively discharging their natural functions. Herein, indeed, in what I have described, is one of the pieces of neutral ground between health and disease: a step in one direction may effect the return to health; in another, the transit to what all might admit to be the disease of inflammation.

Now this transit appears to be made when the circulation, which was rapid, begins to grow slower, without any diminution, but it may be with an increase, of the size of the vessels. This change one may see in the bat's wing. After the application of such stimuli as I have already mentioned, the movement of the blood may become gradually slower, till, in some vessels, it is completely stagnant. The stagnation commences, according to Mr. Wharton Jones, in the capillaries: and first in those which are least in the direct course from the artery to the vein [in the stimulated frog's web]: thence it extends to the veins and to the arteries.

A corresponding state of retardation of blood, leading to partial stagnation of it, may be well seen after such an injury as that of a fine red-hot needle driven into or through the membrane of the wing.

The first effect of such an injury (in addition to the charring and searing of the membrane, the obliteration of its blood-vessels, and the puckering of the portion of it adjacent to the burn) is to produce contraction of the immediately adjacent arteries and veins. They may remain closed, or, as I have already described, after being long closed, may open again, and become wider than they were before. This dilatation follows more certainly, and perhaps without any previous contraction, in the arteries and veins at a little distance from the burn. In these, there speedily ensues such a state of "determination of blood" as I have already described: in arteries and veins alike the stream is full and rapid; and the greater accumulation, as well as the closer crowding, of the red corpuscles, makes the vessels appear very deep-colored. The contrast of two diagrams, showing the natural and the stimulated conditions in a single segment of the vascular plan of the wing, illustrates this difference sufficiently well* (Figs. 30, 31). The vessels of the one, nearly twice as large as those of the other, darker, and more turgid with blood; and, in the one, numerous capillaries which are not visible in the other. But diagrams cannot show the changes in the mode of movement. Close by the burn, the blood which has been flowing rapidly begins to move more slowly, or with an uncertain stream; stopping, or

* The plan of vessels drawn is copied from Mr. Wharton Jones's plate. Philos. Trans. 1852, Part I.

sometimes ebbing, and then again flowing on, but, on the whole, becoming gradually slower.   Thus it may, at length, become completely stagnant;

Fig. 30.

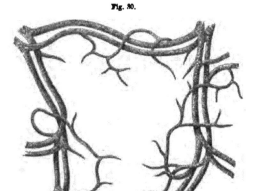

and then, in the vessels in which it is at rest, it seems to diffuse and change its color, so that its crowded corpuscles give the vessel a brilliant carmine appearance, by which, just as well as by the stillness of

Fig. 31.

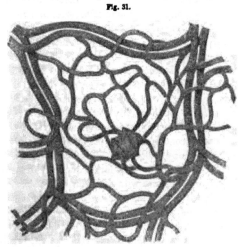

the blood, they may always be distinguished.   As one surveys an area surrounding this part, one sees streams the more rapid and more distant they are from the focus of the inflammation.   And often, when there is stagnation in a considerable artery, one may see the blood above or behind it pulsating with every action of the heart, driven up to the seat of stagnation, and thence carried off by the collateral branches; while, in the corresponding vein, it may oscillate less regularly, delaying till an accumulated force propels it forward, and, as it were, flushes the channel.* In the area still more distant, one sees the full and rapid and more numerous streams of "determination" or "active congestion," which extend over a space altogether uncertain.

Such is the general condition of the circulation in and around a part that is inflamed. In a few words, there is, in the focus of severe inflammation, more or less of *stagnation* of blood; in and close around it, there is *congestion*,—i. e., fulness and slow movement of blood; more distantly around there is *determination*,—i. e., fulness and rapid movement of blood. The varieties in lesser points that may be presented cannot be described. These must be seen; and, indeed, the whole sight should be viewed, by every one who would have in his mind's eye a distinct image of what, in practice, he must often too obscurely contemplate.

The phenomena that I have described as seen in a bat's wing correspond very closely with those observed in a frog's web. Only I think the stagnation of blood is neither so constant nor so extensive in the bat: it is seen in portions of single vessels, rather than in districts of vessels; often in corresponding portions of arteries and veins, as they lie side by side. The stagnation usually extends into such branches as may be given from the vessels that are its principal seats; and three or four such seats of stagnation may appear placed irregularly about the burn, or other focus of the inflammation; but I have never seen a general stagnation of blood in all the vessels of even a severely stimulated part. My impression is, that, in strong and active warm-blooded animals, stagnation of blood would be found in only the most severely inflamed parts; in others, I think, retardation alone would exist.†

To sum up now what concerns the supply of blood in an inflamed part. We seem to have sufficient evidence that, in general, in the focus of the inflammation, blood is present in very large quantity, distending all the vessels, gorging them especially with red corpuscles, but often moving through them slowly, or even being in some of them quite stagnant; that all around this focus, the vessels are as full, or nearly as full, as they are in it, but the blood moves in them with a quicker stream, or may pulsate in the arteries, and oscillate in the veins; that, yet further from the focus, the blood moves rapidly through full but less turgid vessels. And this rapidity and fulness are not to be ascribed, I think, merely to the blood, which should have gone through the inflamed part, being driven through collateral channels, but are such a state as is commonly

* What I thus described was, no doubt, the result of the rythmical contraction of the veins, which Mr. Wharton Jones has since discovered.

† M. Lebert expresses the same belief: Gazette Médicale, Mai 22, 1852.

understood as an "active congestion," or "determination of blood" in the part.

I have already said, that we may believe that what is seen in the bat represents fairly the state of inflamed parts in all warm-blooded animals. I am quite conscious that the most one can see with the microscope, in these experimental inflammations, is but a faint picture of such inflammations as we have to consider in practice; that it is very trivial in both its appearance and its results. Still, it is a picture of a disease of the same kind; and a miniature, even faintly drawn, may be a true likeness. Besides, all that can be observed of the complete process of inflammation in man is consistent with what we can see in these lower and lesser creatures. The bright redness of an inflamed part testifies to the fullness of its blood-vessels, and the crowding of the corpuscles; the occasional duskiness or lividity of the focus is characteristic of stagnation; the throbbing of the part, and about it, and the full hard pulse in the ministrant arteries, are sure signs of obstruction to the passage of blood; the gush of blood on cutting into the tissues near an inflamed part, or in bleeding from one of their veins, tells of the determination of the blood in these, and of the tension in which all the containing blood-vessels are held.

It is particularly to be observed, that the stagnant or retarded blood is not apt to coagulate. I have found it fluid after at least three days' complete stagnation, and so I believe it would remain till it is cleared away, unless the part sloughs. In the latter case it would coagulate, as it does in carbuncles and the like, which hardly bleed when we cut them through, but so long as the blood is fluid, though stagnant, it may be driven from the vessels with full force, as soon as an easy exit for it is made by cutting into the inflamed part, or opening one of its large veins. I need only here refer to Mr. Lawrence's well-known and instructive experiment. In a patient with an inflamed hand he made similar openings into veins in both arms. From the vein on the diseased side three times more blood flowed than from the vein in the healthy arm, in the same time. This increased flow represented at once the greater determination of blood about the focus of the inflammation, and the greater tension in which the walls of the blood-vessels, and, indeed, all the tissues of the inflamed and swollen part, were held.

Now, to what can we ascribe these changes in the movement of the blood?

It has been commonly said that, as the vessels contract, therefore the movement of blood becomes more rapid in them, as when a river entering a narrow course moves through it with a faster stream; and that then, as the vessels widen, so the stream becomes, in the same proportion, slower. But this is far from true. The stream becomes slower as the artery or vein becomes narrower by contraction; and then, as the tube again dilates, the stream grows faster; and then, without any appreciable change of size, it may become slower again, till complete stagnation ensues in at least some part of the blood-vessel.* I think I can be quite sure that the velocity of the stream, in any vessel of an inflamed part, is not wholly determined either by diminution or enlargement of the channel, or by the stagnation or congestion of blood in the vessels beyond. That much of the change in rate of movement depends on these conditions cannot be doubted; and it may seem unnecessary to question their sufficiency for the explanation of that change, after Mr. Wharton Jones's observations. But I think other forces must still be considered, whose disturbance may contribute to the result. Whether we name it vital affinity, or by any other terms, or (which may, as yet, be better) leave it unnamed, I cannot but believe there is some mutual relation between the blood and its vessels, or the parts around them, which, being natural, permits the most easy transit of the blood, but, being disturbed, increases the hinderances to its passage. Such hinderances appear to be produced by the addition of salts of baryta, or of potash, to the blood; and by an excess of carbonic acid in the blood that should traverse the minute pulmonary vessels. The presence of an excess of urea in the blood probably produces the like effect: and some of the facts connected with other than traumatic inflammations appear quite inexplicable without such an hypothesis as this. At any rate, the belief that the more or less rapidity of movement of blood through small vessels may depend on other than evident mechanical relations, cannot appear absurd to any one who has seen the movements of fluid in the Chara or Vallisneria, or any such plants, in which a circulation is maintained without any visible source of mechanical power.

II. I mentioned, as the second condition necessary to the healthy nutrition of a part, a right state and composition of the blood. In former lectures (p. 26, et seq.) I pointed out that, by this state, we must understand not merely such purity of the blood that chemistry cannot detect a wrong constituent in it, or a wrong quantity of any of the normal ones, but that natural constitution of the blood by which it is exactly adapted to every tissue that it has to nourish; with an adaptation so exact that· chemistry often cannot approach to the determination of whether it is maintained or lost.

That this adaptation is disturbed, in many cases of inflammation, is proved by the instances to which I shall have to refer, in which they plainly have their origin in morbid conditions of the blood. But I fear that the nature of this disturbance cannot yet be chemically expressed, and that the facts, which chemistry has discerned, in the condition of the blood in inflammations, cannot yet be safely applied in explanation

* As Mr. Wharton Jones has shown, the retarded stream exists only when the vessel is generally contracted, and the accelerated stream when it is generally dilated: when a single vessel presents successive enlargements and diminutions of calibre, the rate of the stream in it diminishes in the former and increases in the latter.

of the local process. For, first, we observe the phenomena of inflammation where we cannot suppose the whole blood disordered; as after the application of a minute local stimulus, such as a foreign body on the conjunctiva : secondly, the changes observed in the blood during inflammations are not peculiar to that state, but are found more or less marked in pregnancy, and in other conditions in which no inflammatory process exists: and, thirdly, among the changes observed in inflammatory blood, the principal one, namely, the supposed increase of fibrine, is ambiguous ; it may be at once an increase of fibrine and of the white corpuscles of the blood. These two constituents of the blood, the fibrine and the white or rudimental corpuscles, cannot be well separated by any process yet invented ; and in all the estimates of fibrine, whether in health or in disease, the weight of the white corpuscles is included. Now in many inflammations these corpuscles are increased ; and in such cases we have no means of clearly ascertaining how much of an apparent increase of fibrine is really such, and how much is due to the corpuscles entangled in the fibrine. Till this can be settled, I think we may not deduce any of the local phenomena of inflammation from the increase of fibrine in the blood; neither, more assuredly, can we trace, as some do, the fever and other general signs of inflammation to the abstraction of fibrine and albumen by the exudation from the blood.

The other principal changes of the blood in inflammation—the diminution of its red corpuscles and increase of water—are even less adapted to explain any of the phenomena of the local process. Whatever may be their strength or value as facts, they are as yet isolated facts, such as we cannot weave into the pathology of the disease.

I fear, too, that the structural condition of the blood will not, more than the chemical, help us to explain the phenomena of inflammation. Some of our most worthily distinguished pathologists have ascribed much to the existence of large numbers of the white blood-corpuscles, and their accumulation in the vessels of the inflamed part ; indeed, they have taken this for the foundation of nearly their whole doctrine of inflammation, ascribing to it both the stagnation of the blood and the changes it is presumed to undergo; such as the increase of the fibrine, and many others. But the facts on which they have rested are unsound: their observations have been made on frogs, and do not admit of application to our own case, or, perhaps, to that of any warm-blooded animal.

In many frogs, especially in those that are young, or sickly, or ill-fed, the white corpuscles are abundant in the blood. They are rudimental blood-cells, such as may have been formed in the lymph or chyle; and in these cases they are probably either increasing quickly in adaptation to quick growth, or else relatively increasing because, through disease or defective nutriment, although their production is not hindered, yet their development into the perfect red blood-cells cannot take place. In either case, their peculiar adhesiveness making them apt to stick to the walls of the blood-vessels, they may accumulate in a part in which the vessels are injured or the circulation is slow, and thus they may sometimes augment the hinderances to the free movement of the blood. But I believe nothing of the kind happens in older or more healthy frogs, or in any ordinary inflammation in the warm-blooded animals. I have drawn blood from the vessels in the inflamed bat's wing, in which it was quite stagnant, and have found not more than one white corpuscle to 5000 red ones. I have often examined the human blood in the vessels of inflamed parts after death, and have found no more white corpuscles in them than in those of other parts. In blood drawn from inflamed parts during life, I have found only the same proportion of white corpuscles as in blood from the healthy parts of the same person. I therefore cannot but accord with the opinion, often expressed by Mr. Wharton Jones and Dr. Hughes Bennett, that an especial abundance of white corpuscles, in the vessels of an inflamed part, is neither a constant nor even a frequent occurrence; and I believe that, when such corpuscles are numerous in an inflamed part, it is only when they are abundant in the whole mass of the blood.* Now, as already stated, they are thus abundant in some cases of inflammation; especially, I think, in those occurring in people that are in weak health, and in the tuberculous; but, even in these cases, I have never seen an instance in which they were present in sufficient quantity to add materially to the obstruction of the blood in the inflamed part, nor one in which any influence of theirs could be suspected to alter peculiarly the constitution of the blood therein.

Mr. Wharton Jones was the first to describe accurately a remarkable condition presented by the red blood-cells in inflammation. When healthy blood is received on a glass plate and immediately examined, the corpuscles lie diffused in the liquor sanguinis, but in about half a minute run together into piles or rouleaux, which arrange themselves in a small-meshed network, as in the following figure (A). But, if a drop of blood from a patient with acute rheumatism or inflammation be similarly examined, the piles of corpuscles are found to be instantly formed, and they cluster into masses, in a network with wide meshes, as in the same figure (B). In such an arrangement they give the thin clot outspread on the glass the peculiar mottled pink and white appearance, which Mr. Hunter observed as one of the characters of inflammatory blood. The same condition is observed in the blood of pregnant women, and appears natural in that of horses; and in all these cases it may be regarded as the chief cause of the formation of the buffy coat, inasmuch as the clustered blood-cells, sinking rapidly, generally subside to some distance below the surface of the liquid part of the blood, before the coagulation of the fibrine is begun.

* Dr. Hughes Bennett's researches on Leucocythæmia have shown that even the extremest abundance of white corpuscles in the blood has no tendency either to produce or to aggravate inflammations.

Some have supposed that a similar adhesion of the blood-cells may occur in the vessels of an inflamed part, and produce, or materially

Fig. 32.

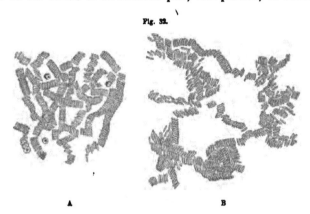

A   B

affect, the inflammatory process. I have seen nothing of the kind in either the inflamed bat's wing, or in the vessels of inflamed organs examined after death. When the blood is not stagnant, the corpuscles are indeed closely crowded, but they are not clustered, nor do they appear adherent: neither does such clustering appear even in stagnant blood; the change here appears to be a diffusion of the coloring matter, so that the outlines of individual blood-cells cannot be seen, and all the contents of the vessel present a uniform bright carmine tint.

But although we can see so little of the changes that may ensue in blood thus stagnant or much retarded, yet we may be nearly sure that the blood in an inflamed part does undergo important changes, when we remember what general effects, what constitutional disturbance, may ensue in the train of an inflammation of purely local origin. Changes probably ensue in the blood similar to some of those that we shall have to trace in the lymph effused from it into the parts around the vessels; particles of fibrine may coagulate in it, and corpuscles like those of lymph may be formed and degenerate within it; and these, when the stagnation is not constant, or is incomplete, or is passed away, may be carried into the general circulation, infecting the whole blood, exciting general disturbance, as in traumatic fever, or producing various and wide-extended suppurations, as in the purulent diathesis following local injury. All these, and many other concomitants of inflammation, may be reasonably ascribed, at least in part, to the changes that the blood undergoes in the inflamed tissue; but I must repeat that nothing that either the microscope or chemistry has yet discerned will suffice to explain these changes: they belong rather to the theory than to the facts of inflammation.

III. The third enumerated condition for the healthy nutrition of a part is a certain influence of the nervous force. The change that this undergoes in an inflamed part is, therefore, next to be considered; or, rather, the evidence that it is changed is to be cited; for, as we have no exact knowledge of the manner in which the nervous force operates in ordinary nutrition, so neither can we tell how its operation is affected in inflammation, though we may be sure that it is not normal.

The expression that the nerves of an inflamed part are in an "excited" state, is suggested by the existence of pain; by a slight stimulus being acutely felt; by the natural heat, or a slight increase of the heat, being felt as a burning; and by the part being, even independent of any known stimulus, the seat or source of subjective pains and heat. But the very frequent cases in which pain exists, and abides long, without any other sign of inflammation, and the cases in which the pain bears no kind of proportion to those other signs, or to the effects of inflammation,—these may suggest that, besides this "excited" state of the nervous force which is felt as pain in the inflamed part, there may be some other state by which the nervous force is more intimately connected with the inflammatory process; a state of disturbance which may indeed be felt as pain, but which more properly affects the influence of the nervous force in the process of nutrition.

We obtain some evidence of the existence of such a state in the fact that, without relation to pain, it is communicable from the nerves of inflamed parts to those of other parts; in which parts, then, a kind of sympathetic inflammation may be generated. This transference or communication of the disturbance of nervous force is, indeed, evident enough in relation to that state which is felt as pain; for pain is not limited to the inflamed part but is diffused around it, and is, in sympathy, often felt where no other sign of inflammation exists. But besides, and sometimes, I repeat, independent of this condition which is felt as pain, the inflammatory condition, if I may so name it, of the nervous force, may be similarly communicated or transferred. The simplest may be the most proving instances. Whoever has worked much with microscopes may have been conscious of some amount of inflammation of the conjunctiva, in consequence of over-work. Now the stimulus exciting this inflammation has been directly applied to the retina alone; and I have often had a slightly inflamed left conjunctiva, after long working with the right eye, while the left eye has been all the time closed. I know not how such an inflammation of the conjunctiva can be explained, except on the supposition that the excited state of the optic nerve is transferred or communicated to the filaments of the nerves of the conjunctiva, generating in them such a state as interferes with its nutrition. It is true that, in these simpler cases, the retina is not itself evidently inflamed; but after yet severer stimulus it commonly is so, and the conjunctiva shares in the evil effects of the communicated stimulus: effects which we cannot ascribe to any alteration in the blood, or the size of the blood-vessels.

I may mention another case; the occurrence of inflammation of the testicle in cases of severe irritation of the uretha. The most unexceptionable cases of the kind are those in which the irritation is produced by a calculus impacted in a healthy uretha. I have a specimen,* in which extensive deposits of lymph and pus are seen in the testicle of a man, in whose uretha a portion of calculus was impacted after lithotrity. Here is such an inflammation as we cannot refer to diseases of the blood, and attended by such changes as we cannot explain by any enlargement or paralysis of the blood-vessels: nor do I know how it can be at all explained, except by the disturbance of the exercise of the nervous force in the testicle, which disturbance was excited by transference from the morbidly affected nerves of the primary seat of irritation in the uretha.

In like manner, I believe that the extension or transference of inflammation, after or with pain, may be ascribed, at least in part, to the coincident transference of the disturbed plasturgic force of the nervous system. In paroxysms of neuralgia, we see sometimes a transient inflammatory redness or œdema of the part; so, when a more abiding pain has been excited, by sympathy with some inflamed part, there may presently supervene the more palpable effects of inflammation.

I feel that in discussing such a point as this, one passes from the ground of demonstrable facts; but there is, I hope, less fault in this than in the belief that the very little we can see of a morbid process can guide us to its whole pathology. When we look at an inflamed part, we should not think that, if we could see its blood-vessels and test its blood, we should detect all that is in error there: rather, we should think that all the forces are at fault which should be concurring to the due maintenance of that part; and while we are ignorant of the nature of some of these forces, it is better that their places in our minds should be occupied by reasonable hypotheses, than that they should be left blank, or be overspread with the tinge of one exaggerated theory, such as those are which ascribe all inflammation to a change in some one of the conditions of nutrition.

IV. The last condition necessary to healthy nutrition in a part is the natural or healthy state of the part itself.

The manner in which this is changed in the inflammatory state cannot be well considered till an account has been given of the exudation that takes place from the blood-vessels, and of some other changes in the very process of nutrition. Let it, for the present, suffice to say (1), that a disturbance in the condition of a part may be the cause, independently of blood-vessels or nerves, of an inflammation in it, as in wounds and other injuries of non-vascular and other parts; and (2), that when an inflammation is thus, or in any other way, established, the proper

* Museum of St. Bartholomew's Hospital, Ser. xxviii. No. 55.

14

elements of the effected part continually suffer change. Such changes
are due, first, to the degenerations which, as in other cases of hindered
nutrition, the elemental structures spontaneously undergo : and, secondly,
to the penetration of the inflammatory product into them and the interstices between them. Each of these sources of change may, in different
cases, predominate : in certain cases, it is probable that one alone of them
may be effective; and either or both of them may affect either the elemental structures that are already perfected, or, probably in a greater
degree, the materials that are in progress of development.

All these things will be subjects of future lectures, but before proceeding to them, let me add a few words, to prevent misunderstanding.

I have spoken so separately of the changes in the several conditions of
nutrition, that I may have seemed to imply that inflammation may consist
in the disturbance sometimes of one, sometimes of another, of these states.
It is true that inflammation may have its beginning in any one of these
conditions,—as in an alteration of the blood in rheumatism, in an alteration of the nervous force in irritation of the retina, in an alteration of
the proper elements of the tissue in inflammation of the cornea; but,
probably, it is never fully established without involving in error all the
conditions of nutrition; and both the manner in which they may be
thus all involved, and their subsequent changes, should be studied as
concurrent events, rather than as a series of events, of which each stands
in the relation of a consequence to one or more of those that preceded it.
Nowhere more than here is the mischief evident, of trying to discern in
the economy of organic beings a single chain or series of events, among
which each may appear as the consequence of its immediate predecessor:
most fallacious is the supposition that, starting from a turgescence and
stagnation of blood in the vessels of a part, we may explain the pain, the
swelling, the heat, and all the other early and consecutive phenomena of
inflammation. The only secure mode of apprehending the truth in this,
as in every other part of the economy of living beings, is by studying
what we can observe as concurrent, yet often independent, phenomena,
or as events that follow in a constant, but not necessarily a consequent,
order.

LECTURE XIV.

PRODUCTS OF INFLAMMATION.

THE state described in the last lecture may, without further change,
cease and pass by, and leave the part, apparently, just as it was before.
And there are two chief modes in which this may happen; namely, by
resolution or the simple cessation of the inflammation, and by metastasis,

in which, while the inflammation disappears from one part, it appears in another. So far as the inflamed part itself is concerned, I believe the changes are in both these cases the same, and consist in a more or less speedy return to the normal method of circulation, and the normal apparent condition of the blood and of the nerves; the tissue itself presenting no change of structure.

I do not know that any description of the process of recovery, from the inflammatory state, would tell more than is implied by calling it a gradual return to the natural state, a gradual retracing of the steps by which the natural actions had been departed from. As it has been watched in the frog's web, and in the bat's wing, the vessels, that were filled with quick-flowing blood, became narrower, the streams in them also becoming slower, and less gorged with red blood-corpuscles, till the natural state is restored. The pulsating or slower streams are equalized with those about them, and, gradually making their way into the stagnant columns, drive them on or disperse them. In the frog, clusters of blood-corpuscles have been seen to become detached, by a stream breaking off portions of the stagnant blood, and then to float into the current, where, gradually, they disperse. So, too, in the tadpole, after injury, I have seen fragments of fibrine, washed from the blood in the vessels of the injured part, floating in some distant vessels. Dr. Kirkes's observations leave no doubt that similar changes may occur in the warm-blooded animals, and may be the source of great evil, by carrying the materials of diseased or degenerate blood from a diseased organ to one that was previously healthy (p. 103).

It may be difficult to explain this discovery in the case of complicated inflammations. When a slight mechanical stimulus has been applied, and the vessels, after contracting, have dilated, we may see some signs of weakened muscular power, in the fact that the same stimulus will not make them contract again; and then their gradual recovery may be the consequence of their regaining their weakened and exhausted power, just as a wearied muscle does when left at rest. This must always be one element in the recovery of the natural state by a part that has been inflamed; indeed, it is probably that part of recovery which is most slowly achieved. Still, it is, probably, only one element in the process of recovery. In an inflammation in which all the conditions of nutrition are at fault, each must recover its normal state; but of the manner in which they severally do so we have no knowledge. The order in which they are restored is scarcely less uncertain: probably it is not constant, but may depend, in great measure, on the order in which they were involved in error. But we have no clear facts in this matter; only we may observe that, in many cases, if we correct the error of one of the conditions of nutrition, the rest will be more apt to correct themselves. Thus, of the remedies for inflammation, few can act upon more than one of the conditions on which it depends; yet they may be remedies for the whole disease; for, as it were, by abstracting one of its elements, they destroy the consistence and mutual tenure of the rest.

The cessation of the disease may be regarded as the most perfect cure of which inflammation admits. It is in many cases an unalloyed advantage; but in some it is not so, though the local change may be the same; for materials accumulated in the stagnant blood of the inflamed part, or absorbed from its morbidly altered tissues, may, when the inflammation subsides, pass into the general current of the blood, and infect its whole mass, or disturb the nutrition of an organ more important than that which they have left. Such are the events in the metastasis of gout, and the premature subsidence of cutaneous eruptions.

We have now considered how, in the inflammatory state, the conditions of nutrition are affected : and, in a future lecture, I hope to show how a change in any one of these conditions may appear as the cause of inflammation, by being the first in the series of changes in which, in the complete morbid process, they are all involved.

The next subject may be the changes in the nutritive process itself; those which are commonly observed as the effects of inflammation, when the process does not subside in the manner just described. They are chiefly manifest (1) in a change of the material that is separated from the blood into or upon the affected tissue; and (2) in changes of the tissue itself. These changes usually coincide : and it may be generally said, that in all inflammations, at least of vascular parts, there is at once an increased exudation of fluid from the blood-vessels, and a deterioration of the structures of the affected part. Either of these events may, in certain cases, predominate over the other; in some instances, one alone of them may be observed; but they so generally concur, that a natural division of the inflammatory changes of the nutritive process may be into those that are *productive* and those that are *destructive*.

Adopting, then, such a division, as of the effects of inflammation, the description of the productive changes will include the histories of the several effusions or exudations from the blood-vessels into the inflamed part, their developments, degenerations, and other changes. In the account of the destructive effects may be comprised that of the various defects of nutrition, the degeneration, absorption, ulceration, and death, to which the proper elements of the inflamed part, and, with them, the products of the inflammation, are liable.

I proceed, then, to these histories; and first of the *products of inflammation* or *inflammatory exudations*.

The materials that may be effused from the blood-vessels of inflamed parts are chiefly these: serum; blood; lymph, or inflammatory exudation especially so-called; and mucus. The last two may be regarded as primary forms, from which, by development, or degeneration, many others may be derived.

I. *The effusion of serum*, except as the result of the lowest degrees of inflammation, or as a diluent of other products, is probably a rare event. That which is usually regarded as a serous effusion in inflammation, is, in many cases, a fluid that contains fibrine, and resembles the *liquor sanguinis* rather than mere serum. It is this kind of effusion on which Vogel[*] has fully written, under the designation of "Hydrops fibrinosus." A good example of it may be seen in the fluid contained in blisters, raised by the action of cantharides or heat applied to healthy persons. And another form of liquid effusion differs from serum, in that, though it does not coagulate, it contains a material capable of organization into cells: such is the fluid that fills the early vesicles of herpes, eczema, and some other cutaneous diseases.

The fluid that contains fibrine, and is most generally described as a serous effusion, may have the ordinary aspect of serum; more rarely it is colorless or opalescent, like the liquid part of the blood which one sees collecting for the formation of a buffy coat. The fibrine that it contains may remain in solution, or without coagulation, for an indefinite time within the body, but will coagulate readily when withdrawn. For example, the so-called serous effusion, which is abundant in the integuments near the seat of an acute inflammation in deeper parts, and which flows out like a thin yellowish serum after death, will soon form a soft jelly-like clot, that is made succulent with the serum soaked in it. The fibrine appears tough, opaque-white, and stringy, when the fluid is expressed from it, and shows all the recognized characters of the fibrine of the blood. Thus, to mention but one case which was remarkable for the delay of the coagulation. A man received a compound fracture of the leg, and it was followed by phlegmonous inflammation and abscesses up the limb. As soon as the inflammation had subsided enough, the limb was amputated; and, three days afterwards, in examining it, a quantity of serous-looking fluid oozed from the cut through the integument. I collected some of this, and, after four hours, it formed a perfect fibrinous clot; yet the fibrine in this case had remained among the tissues without coagulating, for three days after the death of the limb, and for many more days during the life of the patient.

Such, too, are the effusions like serum in blisters raised on the skin by heat or cantharides; such the serous effusions of peritonitis, as in hernia, and of many cases of pleurisy and pericarditis. All these fluids, though they may retain their fluidity for weeks or months within the body, during life, may yet coagulate when they are removed from the body. With these, too, may be reckoned, but as the most nearly serous of the class, the fluid of common hydrocele; for I have seen a small coagulum form in such fluid spontaneously; and the presence of fibrine may always be proved by the formation of a clot, when a small piece of blood-clot, or of some organized tissue, is introduced into the fluid.

[*] Pathologische Anatomie, p. 23.

One can rarely tell why the coagulation of the fibrine in these cases should be delayed : there are, here, the same difficulties as are in all the exceptions from the general rules of the coagulation of the blood. But, it may be observed, the delay of the coagulation is a propitious event in all these cases; for, so long as the effusion is liquid, absorption may ensue on the subsidence of the inflammation ; but absorption is more unlikely and tardy when the fibrine has coagulated. Thus, large quantities of fluid, which we may be sure contained fibrine, may disappear by absorption from the seats of acute rheumatism or gout, or from the pleura or peritoneum, or from the subcutaneous tissues, and leave only inconsiderable adhesion, or thickening of the affected part. But, on the other hand, when, in the same class of cases, the fibrine coagulates, it may be organized, and the usual consequent phenomena of inflammation will ensue. Thus it is in the cases of what has been called solid œdema, where, in the neighborhood of acute inflammation, an effusion long abides with all the characters of ordinary serous œdema ; but, at length, the tissues are found indurated and adhering, the œdema having consisted in the effusion of serum with fibrine, which has coagulated and become organized in the seats of its effusion. Thus, too, it is that the damage done by rheumatism in a part is, on the whole, in direct proportion to the length of time it has subsisted there, and the opportunity given by time for the coagulation of the fibrine.

From what I have said, it will appear that nearly all of what are called serous effusions in inflammation are effusions of fluid containing either fibrine, or a material that will organize itself into cells. But it may be said that we often find, after death, effusions which contain nothing but the constituents of serum, though produced in an inflammatory process. If, however, we examine these cases more closely, they will appear consistent with the others : some of the fluids will coagulate if kept for several hours, or if mixed with other serous fluids, or if fragments of fibrine be placed in them; in others we find flakes of molecular matter, indicating that fibrine had been already coagulated, or that corpuscles had been formed, but that subsequently they were disintegrated, or even partially dissolved ; and in some we may believe that similar materials were decomposed in the last periods of life, or after death.

On the whole, it seems sure that an effusion of serum alone is a rare effect of inflammation, and that generally it is characteristic of only the lowest degrees of the disease. Among the instances of it are, probably, the cases of the chronic forms of hydrops articuli, some forms of hydrocephalus, and some cases of inflammatory œdema of the mucous membrane, as in the œdema of the glottis, and chemosis of the conjunctiva.

In the nearly constant fact of the presence of organizable materials in the products of inflammation, we have one evidence of the likeness between inflammation and the normal process of nutrition, and of its difference from the merely mechanical obstructions or stagnations of the blood. In these, the material effused from the blood is usually the merely serous part: the fluids of anasarca and ascites will not coagulate; they present neither fibrine nor corpuscles, except in the cases of extremest obstruction, when, as in cases of ascites from advanced disease of the heart, one may find flakes of fibrine floating in the abdomen, or masses of it soaked and swollen up with serum.*

II. The second of the so-called inflammatory effusions is Blood.

Among the effusions of blood that occur in connection with the inflammatory process, many, as Rokitansky has explained, are examples of hemorrhage from rupture of the vessels of lymph recently become vascular. The new vessels, or their rudiments, are peculiarly delicate; and being apt to rend, like the vessels of new granulations, with a very slight force, especially when they are made turgid or dilated by an attack of inflammation of the lymph, they will commonly be sources of considerable bleeding. So, for example, it probably sometimes happens when, as the expression is, a hydrocele is converted into an hematocele; some lymph becoming vascular, and being submitted to even slight violence, its vessels break, and blood is poured into the sac. So, too, probably, it is with many or all the cases of what are called hemorrhagic pericarditis. But of these, which may be called *secondary hemorrhages*, I will speak hereafter.

Primary effusions of blood, *i. e.*, effusions of blood poured from the ruptured vessel of the inflamed part, and mingled with the lymph or other inflammatory product, appear to be rare in some forms or localities of inflammation, but are almost constant in others. Thus, *e. g.*, in pneumonia, extravasated blood-corpuscles give the sputa their characteristic rusty tinge. In the inflammatory red softening of the brain, blood is also commonly effused; and the condition of the vessels, which I described in the last lecture (p. 196), may well account for their rupture. There are also other cases of these effusions of blood in inflammation; but I believe these imply no more than accidents of the disease.

We must not confound with hemorrhages the cases in which the inflammatory products are merely blood-stained, *i. e.*, have acquired a more or less deep tinge of blood, through the oozing of some dissolved coloring matter of the blood. The natural color of inflammatory exuda-

---

* It has been supposed that, in mechanical dropsies, the effusion of serum takes place through the walls of the small veins, and that in inflammations an equally mechanical effusion of liquor sanguinis takes place through the walls of the capillaries and small arteries: and this supposition is assumed for an explanation of the difference between a dropsical and an inflammatory effusion. But I think that in a merely mechanical obstruction of the blood, as by diseases of the heart or compression of veins, the pressure of the blood cannot but be increased alike in the veins, capillaries, and arteries, and that, in correspondence with this uniformly diffused pressure, the increased effusion wall take place at once through all these vessels, in direct proportion to the permeability of their walls.

tions is grayish or yellowish-white, and, even, when they have become
vascular, their opacity in the recent state prevents their having any uniform tint of redness visible to the naked eye.   When inflammatory products present the tinge of redness, it is either because of hemorrhage
into them, or because they have imbibed the dissolved coloring-matter of
the blood : and when this imbibition happens during life, or soon after
death, it is important, as implying a cachectic, ill-maintained condition
of the blood, in which condition the coloring-matter of the corpuscles
becomes unnaturally soluble.   Thus blood-stained effusions are among
the evil signs of the products of inflammation during typhus, and other
low eruptive fevers, in syphilis, and in scurvy.

III. Serous effusions, then, appear to be rare as the results of inflammation ; and effusions of blood are but accidents in its course.   The characteristic primary product of the inflammatory process is the liquid
which the elder writers named "lymph," "coagulating or coagulable
lymph," and which more lately has been called "exudation," or "inflammatory exudation."*   It is, probably always, at its first exudation, a
pellucid liquid, which passes through the blood-vessels, especially the
capillaries,† of the inflamed part ; and its most characteristic general
properties are, that it is capable of spontaneously organizing itself, even
while its external circumstances remain apparently the same, and that,
thus organized, it may proceed by development to the construction of
tissues like the natural structures of the body.
    The form assumed by inflammatory lymph in its primary organization
is not always the same.   There are, rather, two chief forms of organization, which, though they are often seen mixed in the same material, are
yet so distinct as to warrant the speaking of two varieties of inflammatory lymph, by the names of *fibrinous* and *corpuscular*.‡
    To the fibrinous variety belong, as typical examples, all the instances
in which inflammatory lymph, effused as a liquid, coagulates into the
solid form, and yields, when the fluid is pressed from the solid part, either
an opaque-whitish, elastic substance, having the general properties of the

    * It is to be regretted that we have no distinctive appellation for this substance.   To call
it "lymph" is objectionable, while, already, the same word is employed for the fluid in the
lymphatic vessels, with which it is probably not identical, though they are in many respects
similar.   And the term "exudation" is yet more objectionable, since it has to be employed
as well for the act of separation from the blood, as for the material separated ; or, even if
it be limited, as the Germanized "Exsudat" is, to what has oozed from the blood, still, it is
equally applicable to all the liquid products of inflammation, and not more to any one of
them than to the serum of a dropsy, or the material separated for normal nutrition.   On
the whole, in accordance with the generally good rule of retaining an old term till a better
new one is proposed, the words "inflammatory lymph" appear least improper.
    † Or, perhaps, only from them : see a remarkable case by Mr. Bowman ; Lectures on the
Eye, p. 44.
    ‡ Corresponding varieties are distinguished or implied by Vogel, p. 30, Dr. Andrew Clark
(Medical Gazette, vol. xlii. p. 286), and others.

fibrine of the clot of blood, or the softer, and, as it is supposed, the less perfect or less developed, fibrine of the chyle or the absorbed lymph.

Such examples of nearly pure fibrinous inflammatory lymph are found, in the cases already referred to, among what have been supposed to be effusions of mere serum. Such are many instances of effusions produced by blisters and other local irritations of the skin in healthy men: such, too, are most of the effusions in acute inflammations of serous membranes, especially in those of traumatic origin, and in those that occur in vigorous men. If, in any of these cases, the lymph be examined after coagulation, or, possibly, deposit in the solid form, it may be hard to distinguish it from the fibrine of the clot of blood. The layers of fibrinous lymph thus formed may be known to the naked eye, when on serous membranes, by their peculiar elasticity and toughness, their compact and often laminated structure, their grayish or yellowish-white and semi-transparent aspect, and their close adhesion to the membrane, even before they have become vascular.

In the corpuscular variety of inflammatory lymph, no coagulation, in the ordinary sense of the word, takes place; but corpuscles form and float free in the liquid part. Typical examples of this variety are found in the early-formed contents of the vesicles of herpes, eczema, and vaccinia; in the fluid of blisters raised in cachectic patients; in some instances of pneumonia; and in some forms of inflammation of serous membrane.

The lymph or exudation-corpuscles or cells, found in such lymph as this, present numerous varieties in their several developments and degenerations; but, in their first appearance, resemble very nearly the primordial condition of the corpuscles of chyle and absorbed lymph, the white corpuscles of the blood, and those of granulations.*

The first discernible organic form in the lymph of herpes, for example, is that of a mass of soft, colorless, or grayish-white substance, about $\frac{1}{1000}$th of an inch in diameter, round or oval, pellucid, but appearing, as if through irregularities of its surface, dimly nebulous or wrinkled. It does not look granular, nor is it formed by an aggregation of granules; nor, in its earliest state, can any cell-wall be clearly demonstrated, or any nucleus, on adding water. But, in a few hours, as the development of this cell-germ proceeds, a pellucid membrane appears to form as a cell-wall over its whole surface; and now, when water is added, it penetrates this membrane, raising up part of it like a clear vesicle, while upon the other part the mass retreats, or subsides, and appears more nebulous

---

* I have already (p. 184) referred to this fact of a single primordial form existing in the rudiments of many structures, which in later periods of their existence are widely different. It is a repetition of a fact in the first development of beings. In the early embryo, the most various ultimate forms are developed from a nearly uniform mass of primordial embryo or germ-cells. And so it is in later life; many of both the normal and the morbid structures start from one primordial form, and, thence proceeding, diverge more and more widely in attaining their several perfect shapes.

or grumous than before. In yet another state, which appears to be a later stage of development, the action of water not only raises up a cell-wall, but breaks up and disperses the outer part of the contents of the cell, and exposes in the interior a nucleus, which is commonly round, clearly defined, pellucid, and attached to the cell-wall.

From the various developments of these cells are derived, in the products of inflammation, all the several forms of corpuscles that are described as plastic cells, fibro-cells, caudate or fibro-plastic cells, and some forms of filaments. These correspond with the development of granulation-cells already described (p. 127). On the other hand, from their various degenerations descend those known as pus-corpuscles, granule-cells, granule-masses, inflammatory globules, and much of the molecular and debris-like matter that makes inflammatory effusions turbid.

The examples of inflammatory lymph which I have quoted are such as may be considered typical of the two varieties : the first, in which, spontaneously coagulating, it presents fibrine, either alone or mingled with very few corpuscles; and the second, in which corpuscles are found alone, or with only a few flakes of fibrine. But, in a large number of examples of inflammatory lymph, the fibrine and the corpuscles occur together, mixed in various proportions, the one or the other preponderating. Such instances of mixed lymph are found in the fluid of blisters in all persons not in full health ; in all but the freshest inflammations of serous membranes ; in most of the inflammatory deposits in cellular tissue, and in most of the viscera; and in the false membranes of croup and other similar inflammations of mucous membranes.

Now, in general, and in the first instance, the proportions of fibrine and of corpuscles that are present in the lymph of an inflammation, will determine the probability of its being organized, or of its degenerating. The larger the proportion of fibrine in any specimen of inflammatory lymph (provided it be healthy fibrine), the greater is the probability of its being organized into tissue ; such as that of adhesions, indurations, and the like. On the other hand, supposing the other conditions for development or degeneration to be the same, the larger the proportion of corpuscles in lymph, the greater is the probability of suppuration or some other degenerative process, and the more tardy is any process of development into tissue. In other words, the preponderance of fibrine in the lymph is generally characteristic of the " adhesive inflammation;" the preponderance of corpuscles, or their sole existence, in the liquid, is a general feature of the " suppurative inflammation."*

* In this view, the fibrinous and the corpuscular varieties of lymph nearly correspond with those which Dr. Williams, in his Principles of Medicine, and others, have named plastic and aplastic; but they do not completely do so. In different instances of both varieties, very diverse degrees of plastic property may be found ; and the occurrence of development or degeneration depends on many things besides the primary characters of lymph. They more nearly correspond with what Rokitansky (Pathologische Anatomie, i. 96) has distinguished as fibrinous and croupous; the varieties which he names croupous

The knowledge of this fact may help us to learn the several conditions on which, in the first instance, depend these two forms of inflammation, the contrast between which has lost none of its importance since the time of Hunter. I will therefore at once enter on this question :—what are the conditions that determine the production of one or the other variety of lymph ; the fibrinous, which, apt for development, is as the symbol of the adhesive inflammation, or the corpuscular, which, prone to degenerate, may be that of the suppurative inflammation ?

The conditions which are chiefly powerful in determining the character and tendency of inflammatory lymph, are three; namely—
1. The state of the blood ;
2. The seat of the inflammation ;
3. The degree of the inflammation.

First, in regard to the influence of the state of the blood in determining the characters of an inflammatory product, Rokitansky has happily expressed it by saying that "the product of the inflammation exists, at least in part, in its germ preformed in the whole blood." Some, indeed, have supposed that lymph is only the liquor sanguinis exuded in excess through the walls of the blood-vessels; but of this opinion we cannot be sure; and many facts, such as the occurrence of inflammatory lymph which does not spontaneously coagulate, e. g., in herpes, will not agree with it. Still, it is not difficult to show that a certain character is commonly impressed by the state of the blood on the inflammatory product from it.

I will not refer here to the cases of inoculable diseases, in which some of the morbid material that was in the blood may be incorporated with the product of a local inflammation, though in these the correspondence of the blood and the inflammatory product is manifest enough; but I will refer to cases that may show a more general correspondence between the two, a correspondence such that, according to the state of the blood, so is the lymph more fibrinous or corpuscular; more characteristic of the adhesive, or of the suppurative inflammation.

Some of the best evidence for this is supplied by Rokitansky, in the first volume of his Pathological Anatomy ; a work that I cannot again

α, β, and γ, representing the several grades of lymph in which the corpuscles gradually predominate more and more over the fibrine, and assume more of the characters of the pus-cell. I would have used his terms, but that, in this country, we have been in the habit of considering croupous exudations to be peculiarly fibrinous.

I described the healing of subcutaneous wounds as usually accomplished by a fibrinous material, and that of open wounds by cells developing into fibres (p. 125). These materials exactly correspond in appearance and modes of development with the fibrinous and corpuscular varieties of inflammatory lymph. And what was then said of the liability of the cells formed in the repair of open wounds to be arrested in their development, or to degenerate into pus-cells and lower forms, and of the consequent insecurity of this mode of repair as compared with the subcutaneous, is confirmed by the corresponding history of the two varieties of lymph.

mention without a tribute of respect and admiration for its author, since in it, more than in any other of his writings, he has proved himself the first among all pathologists, in knowledge at once profound, minute, and accurate, in power of comprehending the vastest catalogue of single facts, and in clear discernment of their relations to one another, and to the great principles on which he founds his systems.   In this work, he has shown clearly, that the characters of inflammatory deposits, in different diatheses, correspond very generally and closely with those of the coagula found in the heart and pulmonary vessels; and that, in general, the characters of inflammatory lymph, formed during life, are imitated by those of clots found in the body after death, when the fibrine of the blood may coagulate very slowly, and in contact with organic substances.

Other evidence may be obtained by examining the products of similar inflammations excited in several persons, in whom the state of the blood may be considered dissimilar.   And here, the evidence may be more pointed than in the former case; for, if it should appear that the same tissue, inflamed by the same stimulus, will, in different persons, yield different forms of lymph, we shall have come near to certainty that the character of the blood is that which chiefly determines the character of an inflammation.

To test this matter, I examined carefully the materials exuded in blisters, raised by cantharides-plasters, applied to the skin in thirty patients in St. Bartholomew's Hospital.   Doubtless, among the results thus obtained, there might be some diversities depending on the time and severity of the stimulus applied; still, it seemed a fair test of the question in view, and the general result proved it to be so.   For, although the differences in the general aspects of these materials were slight, yet there were great differences in the microscopic characters; and these differences so far corresponded with the nature of the disease, or of the patient's general health, that, at last, I could generally guess accurately, from an examination of the fluid in the blister, what was the general character of the disease with which the patient suffered.   Thus, in cases of purely local disease, in patients otherwise sound, the lymph thus obtained formed an almost unmixed coagulum, in which, when the fluid was pressed out, the fibrine was firm, elastic, and apparently filamentous. In cases at the opposite end of the scale, such as those of advanced phthisis, a minimum of fibrine was concealed by the crowds of corpuscles imbedded in it.   Between these were numerous intermediate conditions which it is not necessary now to particularize.   It may suffice to say that, after some practice, one might form a fair opinion of the degree in which a patient was cachectic, and of the degree in which an inflammation in him would tend to the adhesive or the suppurative character, by these exudations.   The highest health is marked by an exudation containing the most perfect and unmixed fibrine; the lowest, by the formation of the most abundant corpuscles, and their nearest approach, even in their early state, to the characters of pus-cells. The degrees of deviation from general health are marked, either by increasing abundance of the corpuscles, their gradual predominance over the fibrine, and their gradual approach to the characters of pus-cells: or, else, by the gradual deterioration of fibrine, in which, from being tough, elastic, clear, uniform, and of filamentous appearance or filamentous structure, it becomes less and less filamentous, softer, more paste-like, turbid, nebulous, dotted, and mingled with minute oil-molecules.

I would not make too much of these observations. They are not enough to prove more than the rough truth, that the products of similar inflammations, excited in the same tissue, and by the same stimulus, may be in different persons very different, varying especially in accordance with the several conditions of the blood. Yet, simple as the observations are, they may illustrate what often seems so mysterious; namely, the different issues of severe injuries inflicted on different persons. To what, more than to the previous or some acquired condition of the blood, can we ascribe, in general, the various consequences that follow the same operations on different patients? The local stimulus, and the conditions by which the inflammatory product finds itself surrounded, may be in all alike; but, as in the simpler case of the blister, the final events of the inflammation are according to the blood.

I cannot doubt that a yet closer correspondence between the blood, and the products of inflammation derived from it, would be found in a series of more complete observations; in such, for instance, that the characters of the blood drawn during life, or, much better, of the clots taken from the heart after death, might, in a large number of patients, be compared with those of inflammatory exudations produced, as in the cases I have referred to, by the same stimulus applied to the same tissue.

In the few cases in which I have been able to make such examinations, this view has been established; and it is confirmed by the parallelism between the varieties of lymph that may be found in blisters, and the varieties of the fibrinous coagula in the heart described by Rokitansky.* The varieties of solidified fibrine which he classes as fibrines 1, 2, 3, 4, are very nearly parallel with what I have enumerated as the stages from the best fibrinous to the corpuscular lymph; and, as I have already implied, he regards these clots found in the heart and vessels as representing the different "fibrinous crases" or diatheses of the blood.

I mentioned, as the second condition determining the character of inflammatory lymph, the seat or tissue which the inflammation occupies.

I need hardly remind you that, since the time of Bichat, there has been a general impression that each tissue has its proper mode and pro-

* Pathologische Anatomie, B. i., p. 142.

duct of inflammation. The doctrines of Bichat on this point were, indeed, only the same as Mr. Hunter held more conditionally, and, therefore, more truly; but they gained undisputed sway, among the principles of that pathology which rested on general anatomy as its foundation.

The facts on which it is held that, in general, each part or tissue is prone to the production of one certain form of inflammatory exudation, are such as these: that, *e. g.* in the apparently spontaneous inflammations of the skin, lymph with corpuscles alone is produced, as in herpes, eczema, erysipelas; that in serous membranes, the lymph is commonly fibrinous, and has a great tendency to be organized, and form adhesions; that in mucous membranes there is as great a tendency to suppuration; that in the lungs, both fibrine and corpuscles are abundant in the lymph, and the corpuscles have a remarkable tendency to degenerate into either pus-cells or granule-cells; that in the brain and spinal cord the tendency is to the production of a preponderance of corpuscles, that quickly degenerate into granule-cells; while in the cellular tissue, both fibrine and corpuscles appear, on the whole, equally apt to degenerate into pus, or to be developed into filamentous tissue.

Now these are, doubtless, facts; but the rules that it is sought to establish from them are not without numerous exceptions. The instances I have lately quoted show that, in one tissue at least, the skin, the products of inflammation will vary according to the condition of the blood, although the inflammation be always similarly excited by the same stimulus. So, too (as Mr. Hunter remarks*), if it were the tissue alone that determines the character of an inflammation, we ought to have many forms of inflammation in the same stump after amputation: whereas, all is consistent; or the differences among the tissues are only differences of degree; they all adhere, or all granulate and suppurate, or all alike inflame and slough.

It is therefore not unconditionally true that each tissue has its proper mode and product of inflammation. It has been too much overlooked that a morbid condition of the blood, or perhaps of the nervous force, may determine, at once, the seat of a local inflammation, and the form or kind of inflammatory product. Thus, *e. g.* the variolous condition of the blood may be said to determine, at once, an inflammation of the skin, and the suppurative form of inflammation; for, in variola, whatever and wherever inflammations arise, they have a suppurative tendency. So, in rheumatism, whether it be seated in muscles, ligaments, or synovial membranes, in serous membranes, or in fibrous tissues, there appears the same tendency to serous and fibrinous effusions, which are slow to coagulate or organize, and even less prone to suppuration. The same might be said of the local inflammations that are characteristic of typhus and of

* Works, vol. iii., p. 313.

gout, and, I believe, of all those diseases in which a morbid condition of the blood manifests itself in some special local error of nutrition. And all these cases are illustrative of the general truth, that each morbid condition of the blood is prone both to produce an inflammation in a certain part, and to give to that inflammation a certain form or character.

Cases, however, remain, that prove some influence of the tissue in determining the product of its inflammation; in determining, I mean, the primary form, as well as the later development, of the product: and the true influence of the tissue in this respect is best shown in some of the cases in which the inflammation, excited, apparently, by the same means, has happened coincidentally in two or more very different parts in the same person. Thus we may find, e. g. that, in pleuro-pneumonia, the lymph on the pleura is commonly more fibrinous than that within the substance of the lung; and adhesions may be forming in the one, while the other is suppurating. In cases of coincident pneumonia and pericarditis, the lymph in the lung may appear nearly all corpuscular, and all the corpuscles may show a tendency to degenerate into granule-cells, while the lymph on the pericardium may have a preponderance of fibrine, and what corpuscles it has may tend to degenerate into pus-cells. So too, one may find, in the substance of an inflamed synovial membrane abundant lymph-cells, while all the exudation on its surface may appea. purulent.

I have said that the fluid of the sac in cases of strangulated hernia coagulates on withdrawal from the body: it may be regarded as a mixture of serum and fibrinous lymph from the inflamed serous membrane. But, in a case in which I was able to examine a pellucid fluid contained in large quantity in the cavity of the strangulated intestine, and which appeared to be the nearly pure product of inflammation of the mucous membrane, there was no fibrine; the fluid was albuminous, and contained abundant lymph-cells.

Other instances of this might be mentioned. These, however, may seem enough to establish the influence of the second condition that I mentioned; namely, the seat of an inflammation, as determining the character of its products.

The third condition on which the character of the lymph chiefly depends is, the degree of the inflammation producing it.

The influence of a tissue, in determining the character of the lymph formed in its inflammations, may be in some measure explained, by believing that the primary product of inflammation is, often, a mixture of lymph, and of the secretion, or other product, of the inflamed part, more or less altered by the circumstances of the inflammation.

When it is seen that in inflammations of bone the lymph usually ossifies; in those of ligament, is converted into a tough ligamentous tissue; and that, in general, lymph is organized into a tissue more or less corresponding with that from whose vessels it was derived; it is usually concluded that this happens under what is called the assimilative influence of the tissues adjacent to the organized lymph. But we may better explain the facts, by believing that the material formed in the inflammation of each part partakes, from the first, in the properties of the natural products of that part; in properties which, we know, often determine the mode of formation independently of any assimilative force (p. 52).

We have some evidence of this in the products of inflammation of secreting organs, the only structures of which we can well examine the natural products in their primary condition. In a moderate amount of inflammation of a secreting gland, the discharge is usually a mixture of the proper secretion in a more or less morbid state, and of the inflammatory product. Thus we find morbid urine mixed with fibrine, or albumen, or pus. In cases of inflamed mucous membranes, the product is often a substance with characters intermediate between those of the proper mucous secretion and those of lymph. Or again, in serous membranes, we may perceive a relation between their natural secretion and the usual products of their inflammation.

Now, these considerations are equally illustrative of the influence of the third among the conditions enumerated as determining the character and tendency of inflammatory products; namely, the degree or severity of the disease. For, as a general rule, the less the degree of inflammation is, the more is the product like that naturally formed in or by the part, till we descend to the border at which inflammation merges into an exaggerated normal process of secretion; as in hydrops articuli, hydrocele, coryza, &c.

These, it may be said, are only instances of secretions. But the instances of the so-called inflammatory hypertrophies may be regarded as parallel with those just referred to; for the analogies between secretion and nutrition are so numerous, the parallel between them is so close, that what can be shown of one may be very confidently assumed of the other. We may therefore believe, that in the inflammation of any part, the product will, from the first, have a measure of the particular properties of the material employed in the normal nutrition of the part: that, as in the inflammation of a secreting organ, some of the secretion may be mingled with the product of the inflammation, so in that of any other part, some of the natural plasma, i. e. some of the natural material that would be effused for the healthy nutrition of the part, may be mingled with the lymph. The measure of likeness to the natural structure acquired by the inflammatory product in its development, will thus bear an inverse proportion to the severity of the inflammation; because the more the conditions of nutrition deviate from what is normal, the more will the material effused from the vessels deviate from the normal type. In severest cases of inflammation we may believe that unmixed lymph is produced, the conditions of the due nutrition of the part being wholly changed; but when the inflammation is not altogether dominant, its product will be not wholly contrary to the natural one, and will, from the first, tend to manifest in its development some characters correspondent with those of the natural formations in the part. Thence, onwards, this correspondence will increase as the new tissue is itself nourished: as scars improve, so do false membranes and the like become more and more similar to natural tissues.

To sum up, then, what may be concluded respecting the conditions that, in the first instance, may determine the adhesive or suppurative characters of an inflammatory exudation: they are, 1st. The state of the blood—its diathesis or crasis—the power of which is evident in that the same material may be exuded in many inflamed parts in the same person; in that this material may exhibit peculiar characters correspondent with those of the blood itself; and in that, in different persons, an inflammation excited in the same tissue, and by the same stimulus, will produce different forms of lymph, corresponding with the differences of the blood. 2d. The seat of inflammation, and the tissue or organ affected; of which the influence is shown by cases in which, with the same condition of blood, different forms of lymph are produced in different parts or organs. 3d. The severity, and acute or chronic character, of the inflammatory process, according to which the product deviates more or less from the character of the natural secretion or blastematous effusion in the part.

The primitive character or tendency of any case of inflammation might be represented as the resultant of three forces issuing from these conditions.

The last product of inflammation of which I have to speak, is *Mucus*.

Peculiar difficulties, owing to imperfect investigations of what normal mucus really is, beset this portion of our subject.

Normal mucus, so far as it has been examined, is a peculiar, viscid, ropy, pellucid substance, which, of its own composition, has no corpuscles or organized particles. Such mucus is to be found in the nasal cavities of sheep and most large mammalia, and in the gall-bladder when its duct has been totally obstructed. In these parts, mucus may be found without corpuscles; and probably there are other examples of such pure and unmixed mucus.

With all these, however, accidental mixtures commonly occur, of epithelial particles from the mucous membrane, and of corpuscles from the imbedded mucous follicles. And these particles vary according to the seat of the membrane, the fluid with which the mucus may be mixed, as gastric acid, intestinal alkali, &c., the time the mucus may lie before discharge, and other such conditions.

The first effect of a stimulation, within the normal limits, is to increase

15

the secretion of the proper mucus, making it also more liquid; to increase the quantity of the epithelium cast off with the liquid; and, often, to induce the premature desquamation of the epithelium, so that particles of it imperfectly formed may be found in the mucus. Many of these immature epithelial particles have been named mucus-corpuscles or mucus-cells.

In an established inflammation of a mucous membrane, there appear, mixed with mucus, and with imperfect or degenerate epithelium, materials which closely resemble, if they are not identical with, the lymph-products of inflammation in other parts. I am, indeed, disposed to think that we should not draw a strong contrast between the inflammatory products of mucous membranes and those of serous membranes, and other parts, except in relation to the material, with which, in the several cases, they are mixed. For, in certain inflammations of mucous membranes, we find fibrinous exudations; as in Hunter's experiment of injecting strong irritants into the vagina of asses;[*] they are found also, but less pure, in croup and bronchial polypus;[†] and I have seen them in the renal pelvis, ureters, and bladder in a case of calculus. In other cases, we find, either without fibrine, or mixed with minute soft flakes of it, corpuscles, which are, also, commonly called mucus-corpuscles, but which appear to differ from those in the lymph already described, only because of the peculiarly viscid fluid in which they lie. All appear to be, alike, lymph-corpuscles: but in the one case they lie in a serous, in the other, in a mucous fluid, in which they appear clearer, more glistening, more perfectly pellucid, less plump, and are less acted on by water.

From these inflammatory products in mucus may be derived, by various degenerations of the fibrine, the flaky and molecular materials which commonly make morbid mucus look turbid and opaque; and by corresponding degenerations of the corpuscles (i. e. of the lymph-corpuscles, not of any normal cells or nuclei), the more frequent pus-cells, which make the transition to the complete pus formed on mucous membranes in active inflammation.

Such degenerations are more frequent in the products of inflamed mucous surfaces than are any forms of development. Development of fibrine, I suppose, never happens here; but in the corpuscles some indications of it may be found, especially when the inflammation is very slight, as in the end of a bronchitis. In this case, among the corpuscles, many may be found enlarged, having distinct cell-walls, and clear, well-defined nuclei and nucleoli.

But among these there are usually many that present a peculiar pigmental degeneration. In the gray, smoke-colored mucus, commonly expectorated at the close of bronchitis, the peculiar color, though commonly ascribed to the mixture of inhaled carbon, is due to the

* Works, vol. iii. p. 341. Museum of the College, Nos. 83, 84.
† See Henle, in his Zeitschrift, t. ii. p. 178.

abundance of cells containing more or less numerous black pigment-granules. Particles of carbon or soot may by chance be present, but

Fig. 33.

they only trivially contribute to the color: it depends on the number of these pigment-cells, to which it is easy to trace the transitions from the lymph or mucus-corpuscles. The chief stages of transition are seen in that the cells enlarge to a diameter of about $\frac{1}{1400}$th of an inch, become clearer, and acquire one or two clear oval nuclei; but, at the same time, minute black granules, almost like those of melanotic cells, accumulate in them; and these, increasing in number and clustering, may at length fill the whole cell, while the nucleus disappears. Subsequently, the cell-wall may burst or dissolve, and the black granules be set free.

It can hardly be supposed that the black granules are in any way derived from inhaled carbon, although it seems that this kind of mucus is most abundant in those who are exposed to atmospheres laden with coal-smoke; for the color is completely destroyed by immersing the mucus in nitric acid or solution of chlorine. The occurrence of such pigment-cells being, I believe, peculiar to the mucus of the air-passages, may be connected with the general tendency of inflammatory products to imitate the properties of the natural products of the inflamed part; for they closely resemble the black pigment-cells from which the lungs and bronchial glands derive their black spots and streaks and other marks. And it may be added, that their peculiar abundance in the slightest forms of bronchitis, compared with their absence in acute cases, affords another example, that the likeness of the morbid to the natural product is inversely proportionate to the severity of the inflammation.

LECTURE XV.

DEVELOPMENTS OF LYMPH.

In the last lecture I considered part of the contrast between the processes of nutrition in the normal and in the inflammatory state, endeavoring to illustrate the nature of the materials exuded from the blood-vessels of inflamed parts. The contrast in this particular cannot,

indeed, be accurately drawn: for we have, as yet, no certain knowledge
of either the properties or the quantity of the material separated from
the blood, for the ordinary nutrition of each part; we have no normal
standard wherewith to compare, in this respect, the processes of disease.
It is evident that the exudation in an inflamed part is superabundant;
but its error in quality can be proved only by its diversity in various
cases, and by the differences which it commonly presents in the rate and
method of its development or degeneration. It is one of those processes
in the exuded lymph, and of the contrast between them and the normal
maintenance of a part, that I propose next to speak.

The biography of the lymph-product comprises much of the most
important part of the pathology of inflammation: and if it were required
to point out what, since Hunter's time, has contributed most to the progress of general pathology, one could scarcely hesitate to name the full
appreciation of the fact, that inflammatory lymph, and other primary
products of disease, have an independent life, and are, of their own
nature, capable of appropriate development, degeneration, and disease.
We may regard this as one of the best achievements of the observations
which Schleiden and Schwann began to generalize; for, till it was clearly
apprehended, the idea of a part being organizable meant scarcely more
than it admitted of being organized by the forces of the parts around it;
that it could be built up by the arteries, and modeled by the absorbents,
as a material plastic, yet passive, in the hands of workmen. Hence was
derived the erroneous direction of inquiries, which sought for blood-
vessels as the essential characters of organic life in part; and for their
varieties of size, and number, and arrangment, as the measure of the
ability and method of development.

Now, more truly, we may study the lymph, as having a life only so
dependent on the blood and vessels as are all the tissues of the body—
dependent on them as conditions of life, but not as sole arbiters of the
method of direction of the vital transformations. And I venture to
think, that the chief aim of our observations, in this part of the pathology
of inflammation, should be to learn, now, the exact relation in which the
several products of inflammation stand to certain primary forms, as developments or degenerations from them. The catalogue of various corpuscles is already swollen to an extent that is confusing to those who
are familiar with them, and repulsive to those who would begin to study
them. It would be an easy task to increase it, and it might have a seeming of accuracy to do so; but what we want, is such a history of the
imflammatory lymph, that we may arrange the components of this catalogue as indicating so many progressive stages of development, degeneration, or disease, in the primary products of inflammation. An attempt
to construct such a history is the more advisable, for the sake of the
illustration which it may afford to the history of normal structures.
There are, as I have already said, no normal instances in which we can

see the materials that are effused for the nutrition of parts; but we may assume something concerning them and their progressive changes from the analogy of the materials that are more abundantly produced in inflammations.

I propose, then, to devote the present lecture to some general, and only a very general, account of the development of lymph. But let me first state the sense in which the term development is here to be employed.

I have said (p. 19 and 77) that, in the generally accepted meaning of development, we have adopted an arbitrary standard of comparison, in the assumption that the nearest approach to organic perfection is in the human body, at the age of manhood. The assumption may be right on the whole; and a less arbitrary definition of development would, proba- bly, be less useful; yet it may be observed, that in what we take for the period and standard of perfection, many parts that were once highly organised and active have passed away, as the thymus gland; and some are, in certain respects, rather degenerated than developed, as the renal capsules and the bones. Development, in its highest sense, should imply not merely that a part becomes more fit for membership under the most perfect economy, but, also, that such fitness is acquired with greater complexity of chemical composition, or with greater evidence of formative or other organic power, or with greater difference from the structure or composition of lower beings. With none of these characters of develop- ment does such a process as that of ossification agree; and, therefore, as I have said before, when we call it the development of bone from carti- lage, it should be with the understanding that the term is applicable only because bone is the proper material of the skeleton of the adult human body.

This distinction is important in the pathology of inflammation. In all true or complete development we may believe there is a larger ex- penditure of vital force than in any other organic act: for all such de- velopment, too, the external conditions need to be the most complete, and the least interfered with; such development is the highest achieve- ment of the formative force, the highest instance of what might be understood as "increased action" in a part.

To speak, therefore, of the development of inflammatory products, when already the normal development of the body is completed, may seem to imply the exercise of unusual vital force; the renewal, as it were, of the pristine embryonic vigor; and the existence of conditions more favorable for nutrition than even those of health are. But we may be led to judge differently, if it should appear that most or all of the so-called developments of inflammatory products are instances in which the tissues, though they are formed into the likeness of such as exist in the perfect human frame, yet acquire characters of lower organization than those they had in their earliest state. It will appear that they are such; and that however much the inflammatory products may become, by their changes, better suited for the general purposes of the economy, they are, in relation to their own condition, rather degenerated than developed. The changes that they undergo are, therefore, not always declaratory of a large expenditure of a vital force; they are not such as the term "sthenic," or "increased action," applied to the inflammatory process, would suggest; not such as to imply that it is an exaggeration of any normal method of nutrition.

With this understanding, however, the changes I shall presently describe may be called developments of inflammatory lymph or exudation; they are developments in the sense of being approximations to the likeness of the natural tissues of the adult human body.

In the last lecture I spoke, generally, of the conditions upon which depends the production of such inflammatory lymph as may be most apt for development. They are all such as favor the production of a lymph rich in fibrine, and that fibrine clear, homogeneous, elastic, tough, and filamentous. But even such lymph as this may altogether fail to be developed, or may be arrested in any stage of its development, and turned into the downward course of degeneration, unless favorable external conditions are present with it. For the development of lymph, of whatever form, nearly all those conditions are requisite which are necessary for the normal development of the proper constituents of the body. It needs, in general, the due supply of healthy and appropriate blood, the normal influence of the nervous force, and, for the highest and latest forms of development, the normal condition of the proper elements of the affected part.

Now, the existence of these conditions for the development of lymph implies a cessation of the inflammatory process, and a recovery from whatever originated or maintained the inflammation. So long as inflammation lasts, no high development of the exudation already formed will take place; rather, fresh lymph will be continually exuded, hindering the due process of development, and hindering it the more, because, as the general health suffers through the continuance of the disease, so the lymph freshly formed will be less and less prone to organization. We may see this illustrated in bad cases of pleurisy. The layers of lymph next to the pleura are always more prone to organization than the later-formed layers that lie next the cavity; while within the cavity all the lymph may retain its fluid form, or may have degenerated into pus. So, more openly, we may see an illustration of the ill effects of abiding inflammation, in the healing of wounds by granulation. An inflammation, ensuing or continuing in the wound, hinders all development of granulation-cells, even though it may be too slight to hinder their formation, and may be favorable to the production of the ichor and pus-cells. We may truly say, that the conditions most favorable to the abundant production of lymph are among the most unfavorable to its development, *i. e.* to its complete and higher organization.

Even when the inflammation has ceased, and fresh lymph is not formed, still, development is often prevented or retarded for want of some necessary condition. The blood-vessels, long dilated, may remain in a state of congestion, distended as if paralyzed, and filled with slowly moving blood. In such a state of "passive congestion," so apt to follow more acute attacks, development will not happen in even well-disposed lymph. We have parallel facts in the tardy development of granulations on the legs, in the healing of ulcers; and how much this depends on the defective movement of the blood is well illustrated by a specimen* appropriate to an observation of Mr. Hunter's. It shows three ulcers of the integuments of a leg; they were all granulating, and all healing; but their progress in healing was inversely proportionate to the hinderances of the blood. The lowest of the three, that most distant from the heart, and of which the vessels were subject to the pressure of the highest column of blood, was least advanced in healing; while the uppermost of the three was most advanced, and was nearly cicatrized.

But let us suppose all the conditions for development provided; what will now determine the direction or result of the process? Into what tissues will the lymph be formed? Two chief things will determine this: first, the general natural tendency of organizable lymph, produced in inflammation, is to form filamentous, *i. e.* fibro-cellular or fibrous tissue; and, secondly, all lymph has some tendency to assume, sooner or later, the characters of the tissue in or near which it is seated, or in place of which it is formed.

The natural tendency of lymph to the construction of fibro-cellular or connective tissue, such as composes false membranes or adhesions, and many permanent thickenings and indurations of parts, is shown by the production of this tissue under all varieties of circumstances, and in nearly all parts; even in parts which, naturally, contain little or none. Thus, it is found in the brain, and in glands, as in the testicle; within joints, even where adhesions only pass from one articular cartilage to another; in the adhesions and thickenings of the most diverse serous membranes; in the thickenings of the most diverse mucous ones. And with all these, we have the corresponding facts in the healing of wounds. All granulations, springing from what surface they may, tend, at least in the first instance, to the formation of filamentous tissue, such as we see uniting all parts in a stump; and a large proportion of subcutaneous injuries are repaired by similar tissue, whatever parts may have been divided. And, sometimes, we may find incomplete instances of this development where the lymph is not even in continuity with any tissue, but floats free; as in ascites, or in effusions into joints.

* Museum of the College, No. 26.

But besides this general tendency, we may recognize in inflammatory lymph a disposition to assume characters belonging to the part in which it was produced; so that, for instance, that about fibrous and ligament-ous parts will be developed into peculiarly tough fibrous tissue; that about bone will become osseous; that in the neighborhood of epithelium will form for itself an epithelial covering; and so on. I referred to this fact in the last lecture, and suggested that this tendency of the developed lymph, to conform to the characters of the parts around it, is probably due to the original and inherent quality of the lymph; that the material formed in the inflammation of each part partakes, from the first, in the properties of the natural products of that part, and partakes of them in an inverse proportion to the severity of the inflammation; because, the more the normal conditions of nutrition are deviated from, the more will the material produced be unlike the normal product. Besides, when the conditions are restored to the normal type, the organized product of in-flammation will constantly approximate more and more to the characters of the parts among which it is placed, or with which it has acquired membership. As scars improve, i. e. gain, gradually, more of the cha-racters of skin, so do false membranes, and the like structures, formed by the organization of inflammatory lymph, acquire, by their own nutri-tion and development, more nearly the characters of the parts with which they are connected. Thus false membranes in the serous cavities acquire a covering of epithelium exactly like that which covers the original serous membrane, and their tissue becomes perfectly fibro-cellular; ad-hesions of the iris may become black, apparently from the production of pigment-cells like those of the uvea; thus, too, in adhesions of the pleura, even when they are long and membranous, pigment may be formed as in the pulmonary pleura itself; and thus many other inflammatory products are gradually perfected, till we may come to doubt whether they be of normal or of morbid origin, so complete is the return from the aberrant action.

I will endeavor, now, to describe more particularly the transitions to the several tissues that may be formed from inflammatory lymph. I need not, indeed, describe the minute changes of development; for, as the fibrinous and corpuscular varieties of lymph resemble very nearly the two forms of reparative material, so (as far as they are yet studied), their respective methods of development are equally similar. On these points, therefore, I may refer to former lectures (p. 126, 128, 141, 163, &c.); and, if it seem strange that disease should thus so closely imitate health, let it be repeated, that this process of development of the lymph is not disease. The lymph is, indeed, produced in inflammation, but it is de-veloped in health, when all the natural conditions of nutrition are re-stored.

The instances are very numerous in which the inflammatory lymph, following its natural tendency, becomes fibro-cellular, or fibrous, tissue. The general forms which, in these instances, it assumes (1) are adhesions, where the new-formed tissue is between free surfaces, and unites them; (2) thickenings, where the formation is in the substance of membranes; (3) indurations, with or without contractions, where it is in the substance of organs; (4) opacities of certain parts that were transparent.

The best examples of the formation of fibro-cellular tissue from inflammatory lymph are in the adhesions, or false membranes, found after inflammation of serous or synovial membranes. In the former, especially, the lymph is apt, in such favorable conditions as I have specified, to be thus developed. In an acute peritonitis, or pleuritis, for instance, it is usually, in the first instance, deposited in layers of uncertain thickness on the opposed surfaces of the membrane. The condition of these layers is variable. The lymph is sometimes grayish, half-translucent, compact, and laminated, consisting chiefly of fibrinous material, and peculiarly apt for development: in other cases, it is yellowish, opaque, soft, succulent, or almost creamy, having a great preponderance of corpuscles, and being less fit for development: and between these forms are many connecting varieties of appearance.

In the first instance, the connection of the lymph with the surface of the serous membrane is, usually, such that it may be cleanly stripped off. Its free surface presents great varieties; it may be flocculent, or villous, reticular, perforated, or nearly smooth. Commonly, at first, the surfaces of the two layers (the visceral and parietal layers as they may be called, after the portions of the serous membrane on which they are severally placed) are separated by serous fluid exuded, in various quantity, with the lymph. But they may be, in parts, continuous, or connected by bands or columns; and, usually, when the inflammation ceases, and such a state of circulation is restored as is favorable to the organization of the lymph, the same state is equally adapted to the absorption of the superabundant fluid. In this case, the opposed surfaces of the two layers of lymph are gradually brought into contact with one another, and with portions of lymph which had floated in the fluid: and now, as the organization proceeds, they are all united; they become continuous, and form "adhesions" between the opposite surfaces of the serous membrane, whether these be the surfaces of adjacent organs, as the abdominal viscera, or of any organ and of the cavity enclosing it, as in the case of the testicle and tunica vaginalis.

The method, and the chief part of the plan, of the organization of lymph in these cases, are, I believe, similar to those described in the healing of wounds by primary or by secondary adhesion; and the general results are the same. Various as are the forms and other conditions of adhesions and false membranes (depending as they do on the relative positions and mobilities of the parts that they connect), yet their structure, when complete, is, I believe, uniform. They consist of well organized fibro-cellular or connective tissue, with which (perhaps only at a late period) elastic tissue may be mingled : they possess abundant blood-vessels, the chief of which are parallel to the direction of their filaments; and their free surfaces are covered with an epithelium like that of the membranes which they connect.

Fibro-cellular tissue is formed in adhesions of synovial membranes as well as of serous membranes; and, probably, in the same manner. In both cases, moreover, it is very usual for lymph to be exuded in and just beneath the membrane, as well as on its surface; and this infiltrated or interstitial lymph, becoming organised, produces thickening and opacity of the membrane. The coincident organization of the lymph, in both positions, is well shown in the frequent instances of white spots in the cardiac pericardium, with adhesions between the pericardial surfaces.— Such white spots, when completely formed, consist of new fibro-cellular tissue, exactly like that of the adhesions. It is by similar interstitial exudation of lymph, and by its development into fibro-cellular tissue, that the frequent adhesions take place between parts which, though connected, should slide freely upon one another: such as adjacent tendons, &c.— From this is derived a large share of the stiffness that remains about injured joints; the parts that should slide pliantly over them are fixed by the new-formed interstitial fibro-cellular tissue. So, too, are formed various morbid thickenings of parts: as of pieces of integument, capsules of joints, &c. But, in many of these cases, the lymph retains very long its rudimental structures, and is, perhaps, on this account, peculiarly apt to degenerate and permit absorption or the ulcerative process. I know no better example, for microscopic examination of interstitially deposited lymph, than an indurated chancre: but I have never found one in which the lymph-cells had reached a further development than the elongated caudate form.

FIBROUS TISSUE, as the result of the development of lymph, is found when the exudation is interstitial in any fibrous tissue; as in ligaments, capsules of joints, and the like. The best examples of it are in the laminated nodular thickenings of the capsule of the spleen, or the thickening and induration of the periosteum, or the capsule of the hip-joint in chronic rheumatic arthritis. In all these cases, the new material is derived from repeated, but not acute, inflammations; therefore, probably, though excessive, it is not widely different from the normal material for nutrition: and, the conditions for nutrition being little disturbed, it is developed into the exact likeness of the original texture with which it is intermingled and confused.

As the fibro-cellular and fibrous tissues, formed from inflammatory lymph, become more perfectly organized, they are prone to contract: imitating the contraction already described in granulations and scars (p. 159). Hence, in part, the contraction of the wall of the chest after pleurisy, and the various displacements and deformities of organs that have become adherent to adjacent parts: hence, in part also, the contractions of inflamed organs, as of the liver in cirrhosis: hence, too, an addition to the rigidity of joints when the parts around them have been inflamed; and hence, with yet greater mischief, the contractions of the thickened valves and tendinous cords of the heart.

ADIPOSE TISSUE may be formed, if not directly from inflammatory lymph, yet in the fibro-cellular tissue of completely organized adhesions. I think it is not often so formed: but, lately, Dr. Kirkes found a lung of which all the anterior part was covered with well-organized false membrane; and in part of this was a quantity of perfect adipose tissue, more than four ounces in weight.

ELASTIC TISSUE is sometimes abundantly formed in the adhesions developed from inflammatory lymph. I have not seen it except in such as are completely organized: and I think it is, in this case, as in the formation of scars, a late production (see p. 129 and 159). I believe, also, with Virchow,* that its formation depends, in some measure, on the membrane that is inflamed; pleural adhesions being most favorable to it. In these it is often abundant; its principal, but always slender, filaments lying in the same general direction as those of the fibro-cellular tissue.

EPITHELIUM I have already mentioned as covering the surfaces of well-formed adhesions. I know of no observations proving whether the epithelial cells are developed directly from the lymph, or are a later construction from materials derived from the blood of the adhesion's vessels: but it is not rare to find, in inflammation of serous membranes, recent lymph-cells presenting many characters indicative of development towards epithelium; flattened and enlarged, and having circular or oval clear nuclei.

BONE is often formed from inflammatory lymph. It may appear as a late transformation of lymph that has been organized into perfect fibrous tissue; as in the osseous plates that are sometimes found in the false membranes of the pluera, or in the pericardium. In most of these, however, there is not true bone, but an amorphous deposit of earthy matter, which is imbedded in the fibrous tissue, or which (as Rokitansky holds) is the residue of the degenerated and partially absorbed tissue.

The proper condition for the transformation of lymph into bone is that in which the exudation takes place in an inflammation seated in the

---

* Verhandl. der Phys.-Med. Gesellschaft in Würzburg, 1850, p. 142. He describes here a peculiar thorny or dentate structure often presented by the elastic filaments in old adhesions.

bone itself, or, else, in or near the periosteum. Such inflammations have been called "ossific;" and the Museum of the College, like every other, abounds with specimens of their various results.

There is a great lack of minute observations respecting both the characters of the lymph exuded in inflammations of bone or periosteum, and the methods of its ossification. Such as have been made, indicate, as might be expected, a close resemblance to the processes described in the repair of fractures* (p. 162, et seq). The lymph produced in moderate inflammation, and therefore likely to ossify, is, at first, according to Rokitansky, a dark-red exudation, like gelatine, which, being gradually decolorized, becomes white, and at the same time acquiring firmness, becomes like soft flexible cartilage, and then like ruddy succulent bone. But though it be like cartilage, I suspect that cartilage is very rarely, if ever, formed in inflammation of bone; for it seems to be formed in the repair of fractures only when the conditions are more favorable than they are likely to be in any inflammations. Probably the lymph is more or less developed towards the fibrous tissues when it ossifies; and, as in the repair of fractures, so here, we may believe that ossification may be postponed till the fibrous tissue is quite formed, or that it may ensue in the rudimental state of the tissue, whether in a nucleated blastema, or in cells like those of granulations.

It would be hardly possible to explain, without illustrative specimens, all the various appearances of bone new-formed in or after inflammations. It may be produced in the very substance of compact bone, after the softening and expansion of the original tissue which occur in the earlier parts of the inflammatory process, and to which I shall have again to refer. Or, it may be produced in the medullary or cancellous tissue; and here, commonly, it appears as a gradual thickening of the minute cancellous lamellæ and fibres of bone, which, as they increase, gradually exclude the proper structures of the diploe or medulla, and finally coalesce into hard solid bone.

But, by far the most common seat of the formation of new bone, and that in which it is almost always found when it exists in either of the former situations, is on the surface, between bone and periosteum, or even in the periosteum itself. Here it forms the various growths to which the general term Osteophyte has been given. In a series of specimens of common inflammation of bone or periosteum, it is not difficult to trace the changes of construction to the new bone, by which, like that formed in a process of repair, it gradually approximates to conformity with the bone on which it grows.†

* Köstlin, Müller's Archiv, 1845, p. 60; Rokitansky, ii. p. 172 ; Virchow, in his Archiv, p. 135.

† Any large Museum will supply such specimens. Those in the College of Surgeons are minutely described in the Catalogue, vol. ii. p. 83, e. s., and vol. v. p. 43, e. s. : those at St. Bartholomew's may be studied through the Indices, pp. 1 and 57. Even different parts of a single specimen will show much of what is described.

At first, it is, when dried, light and friable, with a close, filamentous, velvety texture, and a smooth surface, gradually rising from that of the surrounding healthy bone. As it increases in thickness it becomes longitudinally grooved, as if lodging blood-vessels passing, through it, from the periosteum to the old bone. Then, as fresh formations of new bone take place, they assume the form of nodules and thick plates, laid over the longitudinal grooves, and leaving large apertures for the passage of blood-vessels. Such plates, like nearly all bone new-formed in disease, present, at first, a porous surface and a finely cancellous lung-like texture. But, gradually, in whatever form, the new bone tends to become harder and heavier : the apertures that made its surface porous gradually diminish till they are obliterated, and thus the new bone, while still cancellous within, acquires a compact external layer, and becomes more firmly united to the bone beneath it. The process of induration continuing, the new bone acquires throughout a hard compact texture: its outer surface, no longer porous, becomes nearly as smooth as that of the old bone; its color also changes to that of the old bone; and, finally, the two unite so closely that the boundary line between them can hardly be discerned.

Such is the gradual assimilation of the inflammatory product to the characters of the normal structure from whose disease it issued: a process peculiarly worth studying in the bones, because in them, more than in any other tissue, the changes can be leisurely examined. Those which I have described occur in common inflammations : such, e. g. as follow injuries, or exist in the neighborhood of necrosis, or ulceration, or foreign bodies. They are generally observed, also, in specific inflammations of bone : but among these it is worth observing how characteristic of different diseases are certain formations of the new bone. The pustules of variola, or the vesicles of herpes, are scarcely more characteristic of those diseases, than are the hard nodules of cancellous bone, clustered about the articular borders of bones that have been the seat of chronic rheumatism ; or the porous, friable, dirty, and readily ulcerating thin layers formed on the shafts in syphilis.*

CARTILAGE, I have said, is probably not formed in inflammatory lymph in the process of its ossification. Neither does it appear to be formed in the more acute inflammations of articular cartilage; but, we must not exclude it from the possible developments of inflammatory products, while we remember the observations of Mr. W. Adams† respecting the enlargements of the ends of bones in chronic rheumatic arthritis. In these, which are marked by such formations of new bone, and such thickenings of fibrous tissue, as we constantly ascribe to inflammations, there is manifest increase of the articular cartilage, and a subsequent ossification both of that which is new-formed, and, more

* As in Nos. 572, 628, and others, in the College Museum.
† Trans. of Pathol. Soc. of London, vol. iii. 1851.

slowly, of that which normally covered the head of the bone. The early conditions of the increase of the cartilage are not traced: but that it depends on inflammation, rather than on true hypertrophy, is probable, both from the concurrent signs and results of inflammation, and from the new cartilage falling short of the perfect characters of the old; for it has a fibrillated intercellular substance, and scattered nuclei, and is prone to ossification.

It remains that I should describe the adjunct structures of organized inflammatory lymph. But this may be briefly done, because the account of the formation of new blood-vessels in granulations and other reparative materials might, I believe, be transferred hither (p. 145). The question is, indeed, often raised, as in the corresponding instance of granulations becoming vascular, whether the blood-vessels are formed entirely of the material of the lymph, and, as it were, by its own power of development, or whether they are outgrowths from adjacent natural or original vessels, which, as the expression is, shoot out into the lymph.

I think it nearly certain, for the following reasons, that the lymph forms neither vessels nor blood, but receives those that are projected into it from the parts on or in which it is placed.

1. The direct observations supposed to prove that blood is formed in lymph are very liable to fallacy, through the facility with which blood may be accidentally mixed with the lymph, in consequence of hemorrhage during life or after death, or in the preparation of the specimens. Where these sources of fallacy have been avoided, I have never seen anything suggestive of a transformation of lymph into blood.

2. The development of blood from tissue-cells is limited, naturally, to the earliest period of embryo-life, as if it needed the greatest amount of force for development; afterwards, blood is not formed except through a long process of elaboration, and with the aid of many organs. Its formation, therefore, in the malconditions of inflammation is very improbable.

3. In no specimen of inflammatory lymph have I seen appearances of transitions from lymph-cells to blood-cells, such as we may see in the lymph of the lymphatics, both before and after it is poured into the blood-vessels.

4. Neither in any lymph have I seen appearances of such stellate cells as the interstitial blood-vessels of the early embryo are formed from; nothing comparable with them has ever come into view.

5. In the formation of vessels for granulations and the walls of chronic abscesses, all is favorable to the belief that they grow up from the blood-vessels of the adjacent parts; and there are no structures to which the lymph bears so close analogy as it does to these, or to which it is so likely to be conformed in the production of its vessels.

On the whole, therefore, although direct observations are wanting, I think we may conclude that all the vessels of inflammatory lymph are formed by outgrowth from adjacent vessels, as in the process of repair, and that through these vessels, not by its own development, it derives its supply of blood.

In the first instance, the blood-vessels of lymph appear to be usually very numerous and thin-walled; therefore easily bursting, or dilated by congestions during life, or in the attempt to inject them after death.

The College collection contains an extremely beautiful specimen of soft recent lymph from the pericardium of a Cheetah, the vessels of which, injected by Mr. Quekett, appear as numerous and close-set as those of some of the more vascular mucous membranes. They present occasional slight and gradual dilatations, especially when they branch or anastomose.

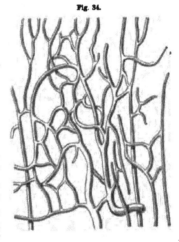

Fig. 34.

But after an uncertain time, as the lymph becomes more highly organized, so its vessels waste and diminish in number; and while it acquires the proper structure of the fibro-cellular tissue, so it descends to the low degree of vascularity of that tissue. The vessels of false membranes, as represented here (fig. 34), from an instance in which they were naturally injected with blood, are usually rather wide apart, long, slender, and cylindriform. In all these particulars they differ from those of more recently vascularized lymph; and their changes are, in these respects, parallel with those of the vessels of granulations during the gradual formation and perfecting of scars.

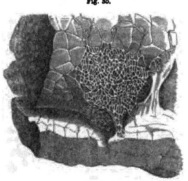

Fig. 35.

Perhaps the most perfect instance of the conformity with the natural tissues of the body to which the developed lymph can attain, is manifested in its acquiring a supply of lymphatic vessels. We owe the knowledge of the lymphatics of false membranes to the masterly skill of Professor Schroeder van der Kolk, whose preparations of them are described and represented by his pupil, Dr. de Les-

pinasse.* In fig. 85, copied from one of his plates, beautiful networks
of lymphatics, with their characteristic beaded forms and abundant
anastomoses, are shown traversing adhesions extending between two
lobes of a lung; while yet closer networks are seated in the thickened
and opaque-white substance of the pleura, or of false membrane covering
it, beneath the adhesions.

It seems to be in only the most perfect state, and when blood-vessels
have long existed, that lymphatics are formed in false membranes. In
recent lymph Schroeder v. d. Kolk has never succeeded in injecting any;
and we can only suppose that they are, like the blood-vessels, produced
by outgrowth from the lymphatics of the membrane with which they are
cohnected.

Virchow† has twice seen nerve-fibres in adhesions. In one case, two
fine nerve-fibres passed through an adhesion of the pleuræ; in the other,
a single fibre extended into, but not through, an adhesion between the
liver and diaphragm.

The time in which these complete developments of lymph may be
accomplished must vary so much, according to the circumstances of the
inflammation, that perhaps no reasonable estimate of it can be made.
The experiments of Villermé and Dupuytren‡ upon dogs assign twenty-
one days as the earliest time in which new vessels are formed; but I am
disposed to agree with Dr. Hodgkin, that a shorter time is sufficient.
On the other hand, I am sure that the supposition of their being formed
in one or two days is incorrect. The principal case in support of this
opinion is that recorded by Sir Everard Home; but the specimens preserved in the College Museum§ show that he was deceived as to the true
nature of the case. He says‖ that he operated for strangulated hernia
in a man, and found in the sac a portion of ileum, which was healthy,
except in that its vessels were turgid with blood. The patient died
twenty-nine hours after the operation; and on examination "several
small portions of exuded coagulable lymph" were found adhering to the
intestine that had been protruded. When the vessels of the intestine
were injected, the injection passed into vessels in all these portions of
supposed lymph, each "having a considerable artery . . . . and a returning vein." Sir Everard Home, therefore, concludes "that the whole

---

* Spec. Anat. Path. de Vasis novis Pseudo-membranarum, 8vo. Daventriæ, 1842, fig.
iii., iv. In another instance he injected lymphatics in an adhesion between the liver and
diaphragm. A similar injection of these in adhesions between an ovarian tumor and the
small intestines is described by Lebert: Traité des Maladies Cancereuses, p. 40.

† Würzburg Verhandlungen, i., 144.

‡ Quoted by Dr. Hodgkin, in his Lectures on the Morbid Anatomy of the Serous Membranes, p. 42.

§ Nos. 81 and 82 in the Pathological Museum.

‖ In his Dissertation on Pus, p. 41. The whole case is given in the College Catalogue,
vol. i., p. 37.

operation of throwing out coagulable lymph, and supplying it with blood-vessels after it had become solid, was effected in less than twenty-four hours."

Now, one of these specimens was figured by Mr. Hunter,[*] "to show a small portion of coagulating lymph . . . . which is supplied with vessels;" but neither here, nor in his manuscript catalogue, does he allude to a probability of the vessels having been formed in twenty-four hours, although, had he believed it, he would scarcely have failed to record it.[†] An examination of the specimens show that the small, shred-like portions of membrane, attached by little pedicles to the intestine, have not the appearance of recently coagulated lymph, but are fully organized, with traces of filaments and fat-cells.   They are also very regularly disposed, at distances of from half an inch to an inch from each other, and are nearly all placed in two rows on each side of the intestine, about half an inch from the attachment of the mesentery, like very minute appendices epiplocæ, such as are occasionally met with on the coats of the small intestine.   Whether they be such appendices or not, it is in the highest degree improbable that they were formed after the operation ; especially since they are too minute and delicate to have prevented the intestine from exhibiting, when exposed in the sac, the natural polished appearance of its surface.

I am not aware of any other case adapted to prove the earliest period at which blood-vessels may be formed in lymph.   Serous surfaces may, indeed, become adherent in twenty-four hours, but this does not imply vascularity of the lymph between them ; it is simply adhesion by the coaptation of the intermediate lymph.

———

LECTURE XVI.

DEGENERATIONS OF LYMPH.

HAVING given, in the last lecture, a general history of the chief developments of the lymph exuded in the inflammatory process, I propose, now, to tell a corresponding history of its degenerations ; and herein to describe what appear to be the transitions, from the ordinary forms of lymph in its primary state, its fibrine and its corpuscles, to those many lower forms enumerated as molecular and granular matter ; as pus-cells, granule-cells, inflammatory globules, and the rest.

* Works, pl. xxi. fig. 2.
† In the Treatise on the Blood (Works, vol. iii. p. 350) he speaks of nine days as a short time for the complete organisation of adhesions.

16

I said that, for the development of lymph produced in inflammation, it is requisite that the inflammation shall have ceased, and the conditions of healthy nutrition be restored. In the failure of this event, if the inflammation continue, or the due conditions of nutrition be in any way suspended, then, instead of development, degeneration will occur, with more or less rapidity, according to the original character of the lymph. And this may happen in any of the stages of formation which I described in the last lecture : it may happen alike to the rudimental fibrine, or to the earliest lymph-cell, or to either, in any part of its progress to complete development.

The following appear to be the chief degenerations of the fibrinous part of lymph, or of the materials derived from its earliest stages of development, whether in the purely fibrinous, or in any of the mixed, forms of lymph :—

1. It may wither : wasting, becoming firmer and drier, passing into a state which Rokitansky has designated *horny*. One sees the best examples of this change of fibrine in the vegetations on the valves of the heart, or in the large arteries, when they become yellow, stiff, elastic, and nearly transparent. The fibrine may, in this state, show no marks of development into tissue, but may have all the simplicity of structure of ordinary fibrine, being only drier and more compact. A nearly similar character is acquired when lymph is deposited over a lung which is extremely compressed in empyema, or in hydrothorax. The tough dry lymph that here forms the grayish layer over all the lung, is not always developed, though it may adhere firmly : it may be withered, wasted, and dried (as the lung itself may be), apparently in consequence of the compression.

2. The fibrine of lymph is subject to a degeneration which we may compare in many respects with fatty degeneration, or, more closely, with the changes by which lymph-corpuscles are transformed into those of pus, with which changes, indeed, this is commonly associated in the mixed forms of lymph. In the solid parts of effusions, that are found in the lower forms of inflamation, or in very unhealthy persons, the fibrine of the lymph is usually not clear and uniform and filamentous, but rather opaque or turbid, nebulous or dotted, presenting just such an appearance as marks the earliest stages of fatty degenerations in the muscular fibrils. In such lymph, also, one sees, not unfrequently, minute, shining, black-edged particles, which we may know to be drops of oil ; while some general alteration in the composition of the fibrine is shown by its not being made transparent with acetic acid. In all such cases as these the fibrine is very soft, and easily broken : it is devoid of all that toughness and elasticity which is the peculiar characteristic of well-formed fibrine ; and by breaking it up, one may see the meaning of what one so often finds in the lowest forms of inflammatory exudation, such as occur in erysipelas and typhus ; namely, films and fragments of molecular and

dotted substance, floating in fluid that is made turbid by them, and by abundant minute molecules and granules and particles of oily matter. These represent the disintegration of fibrine that has degenerated after clotting, or has thus solidified in an imperfect coagulation. Of such changes, also, an excellent instance is presented in the softening and disintegration of clots within the heart, which Mr. Gulliver * first described. These, indeed, or any of the instances of the apparent suppuration within clots in the blood-vessels, might be studied for the illustration of the corresponding changes in inflammatory lymph; especially, in relation to the likeness which, in both cases, the degenerate fibrine bears to the molecular matter in the thinner and more turbid kinds of pus.

We have examples of numerous varieties of this degenerate and disintegrated fibrine exuded in inflammation. It is a principal constituent of most of what has been called "aplastic lymph," in inflammation of the serous membranes. Similar fibrine occurs, mingled with mucus, in the severer inflammations of the mucous membranes. And to the same source we may trace much of that molecular and granular matter which is usually mingled with all the less perfect forms of pus: e. g. with that formed in the suppuration of chronic inflammatory indurations; with the variously changed corpuscles of "scrofulous matter;" or with the granule-cells, and other corpuscles of pneumonia, and the like inflammations.

The general characters of the materials here described, and the coincident changes ensuing in the corpuscles that may be mingled with the fibrine, make it probable that the changes are of the nature of fatty degeneration occurring in the fibrinous lymph. But when, as I have said elsewhere (p. 157), we see how a large mass of inflamed hard substance will become fluid, as it suppurates, and this with scarcely any, if any, increase of bulk, we may believe that another change ensuing in the fibrine is that which I called liquefactive degeneration (p. 78). In such a swelling, we may be nearly sure there is coagulated fibrine, both from the general circumstances of the inflammation, and because neither corpuscles alone, nor fibrine in the liquid state, would give such hardness. The suppuration, therefore, if without increase of bulk, can hardly be explained, except on condition of the fibrine, which had solidified, becoming again liquid. The occasional liquefaction of clots out of the body † makes this more probable; but I am not sure that it can be proved by any more direct facts.

A point of some practical importance it connected with these forms of degeneration of lymph, whether affecting fibrine or corpuscles. When the fibrine has withered and become dry, it is probably put out of the capacity of being further developed, and is rendered passive for further

---

* Medico-Chirurgical Transactions, vol. xxii. p. 136.

† As in cases by Nasse and De la Harpe, quoted by Henle, in his Zeitschrift, B. ii. p. 169. See also Virchow on the same subject, in the same Zeitschrift, B. iv. Henle refers to this same liquefaction the changes that ensue in emitted semen.

harm or good, except by its mechanical effects. But the fatty and liquefactive degenerations may be yet more beneficial, in that they bring the lymph into a state favorable to its absorption, and, therefore, favorable to that which is termed the "resolution" of an inflammation in which lymph has been already formed. I suppose it may be considered as a general truth that the elements of a tissue cannot be absorbed so long as they retain their healthy state. There is no power of any absorbent vessels that can disintegrate or decompose a healthy portion of the body; for absorption, there must, in general, be not only an absorbing power, but also a previous or concurrent change—as it were a consent—in the part to be absorbed; so that it may be reduced (or, rather, may reduce itself) into the minutest particles, or may be dissolved. And this change is probably one of degeneration, not death, in the part; for dead matter is usually rather discharged from the body than absorbed.

Now such degeneration of the fibrine products of inflammation as I have described, brings them into a state most favorable for absorption; indeed, one may see in lymph thus changed many things which, in regard to the fitness for absorption, would make it parallel with chyle.* Of such absorption of fibrine we may find many instances. In rheumatic iritis we may believe the lymph to be fibrinous; but we see its complete absorption taking place; and the observations of Dr. Kirkes on the rarity of adhesions of the pericardium, in comparison with the frequency of pericarditis,† may be in the same manner explained. In rheumatic pericarditis we may be sure fibrine is exuded; and the observed friction-sound has, in some cases, proved its coagulation; yet in these cases, when death occurred months afterwards, scarce a trace of fibrine was found in the pericardium: it had been absorbed, and the degeneration I have been describing was probably the preparation for its absorption.

3. I am not aware of any direct proof of the calcareous degeneration ensuing in the fibrinous part of an inflammatory exudation; but we have the strongest evidence from analogy for believing that this change may be a frequent one. For there are numerous instances of calcifications of fibrine within the vessels: as, e. g. in the ordinary formation of phlebolithes from clots of blood, in the branching and irregular pieces of bone-like substance found in obliterated veins, and in the lumps and grains of substance like mortar imbedded in fibrinous deposits on the heart's valves. We can, therefore, hardly doubt that the fibrine, even before development, may take part in formations of earthy matter in inflammatory products; but the calcareous degeneration seems much more frequent in purulent fluids, and in the later developments of lymph.

4. Lastly, we have examples of the pigmental degenerations of fibrinous lymph in the various shades of gray and black which often pervade

* See also the ingenious contrast of the progress of chyle and the regress of pus drawn by Gerber, in his Allgem. Anatomie, p. 49.

† Medical Gazette, April, 1849.

the lymph formed in peritonitis, and which are produced, not by staining or discoloration of the blood by intestinal gases, but, according to Rokitansky, by the incorporation of free pigment-granules.

Such appear to be the degenerations of the fibrine of inflammatory lymph: such at least are the changes in it which we may refer to defects in its power or conditions of nutrition, because they correspond with changes that may be traced in the gradual degenerations of old age. I need hardly say, that it is chiefly by such correspondence that we can interpret them; for when we find them, it is often beyond our power to tell, by direct observation, whether or in what way, the conditions of nutrition were defective.

The corpuscular constituents of lymph, in any of their stages of development, may retrograde, and present degenerations corresponding and usually concurrent with those which I have just described.

1. Their withering is well seen in some forms of what is called scrofulous matter, such as occurs in chronic and nearly stationary scrofulous enlargements of lymphatic glands. In the dull ochre-yellow-colored and half dry material imbedded in such glands, may be found abundant cells, such as are sketched in fig. 86. They are collapsed, shriveled, wrinkled, glistening, and altogether irregular in size and form. One might suppose them to be the remnants of pus dried up, or the corpuscles of chronic tuberculous matter, if it were not that among them are some with nuclei shriveled like themselves, and some elongated and attenuated, which are evidently such as withered after they had been developed into the form of fibro-cells; into which form it is certain that neither pus-corpuscles nor those of tubercle are ever changed.

Fig. 86.

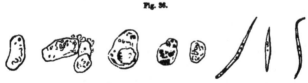

These are the best examples of withered lymph-corpuscles; but they may be also found in the pus of chronic abscesses, especially, of course, in that of such abscesses as ensue by suppuration of lymph-deposits like those just referred to. It may be hard, sometimes, to say whether corpuscles in these cases may not be pus-corpuscles shriveled up, but on the whole, I am inclined to believe that the shriveled corpuscles of the pus of chronic abscesses are asually derived from the lymph, in which, having withered, they had become incapable of further change.

2. The fatty degeneration of lymph-cells is shown in their transition into granule-cells.* We owe the first demonstration of this to the ex-

* The inflammatory globules of Gluge.

cellent observations of Reinhardt,* who has also shown how, by similar degenerations, corresponding forms of granule-cells may be derived from the primary cells of almost all other, both normal and abnormal, structures.†

This method of degeneration appears peculiarly apt to occur in the inflammations of certain organs; as, especially, the lungs, brain, and spinal cord; but it may be found occasionally prevalent in the lymph of nearly all other parts and in the granulations forming the walls of abscesses or of fistulæ. It may occur alike in the early forms of lymph-cells, and after they have already elongated and attenuated themselves, as for the formation of filaments, and after they have degenerated into pus-cells. The changes of transition (as shown in fig. 37), are, briefly, these:—The lymph-cells, which may have at first quite normal characters, such as I have described (p. 217), present a gradual increase of

Fig. 37.

shining, black-edged particles, like minute oil-drops, which accumulate in the cell-cavity, and increase in number, and sometimes in size also, till they nearly fill it. The fatty nature of these particles is proved by their solubility in ether: and their accumulation is attended with a gradual enlargement of the cell, which also assumes a more oval form. Moreover, while the fatty matter accumulates, the rest of the contents of the cell become very clear, so that all the interspaces between the particles are quite transparent; and, coincidently with all these changes, the nucleus, if any had been formed, gradually fades and disappears, and the cell-wall becomes less and less distinct.

I need hardly say, that, in these particulars, the changes of the lymph-cells (which may also occur when they have been already developed into the form of fibro-cells), correspond exactly with those of the fatty degenerations observed in the cells of the liver or kidney, or in the fibres of the heart. There can be hardly a doubt of the nature of this process: and it presents an important parallel with the similar changes described in fibrine. For, we may observe, first, that where this degeneration is apt to occur in lymph, it is least likely to be developed. A proper induration and toughening of the lungs and brain, such as might happen through development of the products of inflammation, is extremely rare;

* Traube's Beiträge, B. ii. 217.

† Observations similar to those of Reinhardt were made independently by Dr. Andrew Clark. (Medical Gazette, vols. xlii. xliii.) See also Dr. Gairdner's description of the formation of granule-cells from epithelium-cells in pneumonia (Contributions to the Pathology of the Kidney, p. 20); and the list of references, p. 105.

it is rarely seen, except in the scars by which the damages of disease are healed. And, besides, this degeneration is a step towards the absorption of the lymph; for commonly we may trace yet later stages of degeneration in these granule-cells. They lose their cell-walls, and become mere masses of granules or fatty particles, held together for a time by some pellucid substance, but at last breaking up, and scattering their components in little clusters, or in separate granules.

Thus, if at no earlier period of their existence, or after no fewer changes, the lymph-corpuscles may pass into a condition as favorable for absorption as is that of the fibrine when similarly degenerate and broken up: and such as this, we may believe, is a part of the process by which is accomplished that "clearing up" of parts indurated and confused in inflammation, and, especially, that of the solidified lung, which is watched with so much interest in pneumonia.

8. Calcareous degenerations of the lymph-cells appear in cases, such as Henle* refers to, in which granule-cells are composed not wholly of fatty matter, but in part also of granules of earthy matter. In this combination they correspond with a common rule; for the fatty and earthy degenerations are usually coincident: they are combined in the advanced stages of the degenerations of arteries, and may be said to have their normal coincidence in ossification.

4. Of the pigmental degeneration of lymph-cells there are, I suppose, examples in the black matter effused in peritonitis: but the best examples are in the cells in bronchial mucus, to which I have already referred (p. 226).

The most frequent degeneration of inflammatory lymph is into pus. It may ensue in nearly all the cases in which lymph is placed in conditions unfavorable to its development; as in the persistence of inflammation, or in exposure to air, or in general defects of vital force. It affects alike the fibrinous and the corpuscular parts of lymph. For although we do not call any liquid "pus," unless it have the characteristic pus-corpuscles, yet the materials of degenerate fibrine are commonly mixed with these; and indeed many of the varieties of the pus formed in inflammations owe their peculiarities to the coincident degenerations of the fibrine.

The facts proving the transformation of inflammatory lymph into pus correspond very nearly with those already cited (p. 155) concerning the similar relations of granulations to pus in the process of repair. But a few may be mentioned here:—

1. The fluid of such vesicles as those of herpes, is, in the first instance, a pure inflammatory lymph, containing corpuscles which might be taken as types of the lymph or exudation-corpuscles, and which may be as easily distinguished from any cells of pus, as the cells of well-formed gra-

* In his Zeitschrift, B. ii.

nulations may be.   If we watch these vesicles, we see their contents not increased,—rather, by evaporation, they are diminished; but the lymph is converted into pus, and pus-cells are now where lymph-cells were. And the change may ensue very quickly: I think I have known it accomplished in twelve hours at the most.

2. In like manner, as I said before (p. 157), when we watch the progress of an abscess, we may find one day a circumscribed, hard, and quite solid mass, and in a few days later the solid mass is fluid, and this with little or no increase of bulk.   Now the solidity and hardness are due to inflammatory lymph; the later fluid is pus; and the change is the conversion of lymph into pus.

3. As in common suppuration of a granulating wound, the granulation-cells appear to be convertible into pus-cells; superficial cells being detached in pus, while deeper ones are being developed into filaments; and as in worse-formed granulations, the cells are often by no characters, except by their forming a solid tissue, distinguishable from pus-cells; so, in an inflamed serous membrane, pus-cells may float in the fluid, such as cannot be distinguished from cells in the vascularized lymph that lines the cavity.   In the fluid exudation, and in that which is solid, the same forms may be found; though, by comparison, we may be able to trace that in the former none of the cells were being developed, and many were proceeding beyond the degeneration to which any had attained in the latter.

3. One may see the same conversion of inflammatory lymph into pus thus illustrated.   An amputation through the thigh was performed when all the parts divided were infiltrated with lymph, effused in connection with acute traumatic inflammation of the knee-joint.   Next day pus flowed freely from the wound.   Now, in amputation through healthy tissues, free suppuration does not appear till after three or four days: the pus here seen must have been formed by the conversion of the inflammatory lymph previously infiltrated in the divided tissues.*   Similar facts may be less strikingly observed in any wound.

From these and the like facts we have an almost exact parallel, in their relations to pus, between the material for repair by granulations and that exuded in the inflammatory process; and between, if they may be so called, the reparative and the inflammatory suppurations.   And in some of the facts we may trace a transition from the one process to the other.   In the formation of an acute abscess, for example, inflammatory lymph is transformed into pus; then the pus, say, is discharged; the signs of inflammation cease; the process of repair is established, and

* These facts, while they prove that the pus-cells are commonly the result of degeneration of lymph-cells, may also serve to show that the question often asked, whether pus-cells are ever an original or primary product of inflammation, cannot be precisely answered. We cannot always discern a preliminary lymph-stage; but neither can we always distinguish lymph-cells from pus-cells, whether in serous fluid or in mucus, nor can we say in how very brief a time the transformation from the one to the other may be accomplished.

reparative granulations line the abscess-cavity in the place of, or formed by, the peripheral layer of the lymph. Now, pus continues to be formed; but this pus is derived, not from inflammatory lymph, but from granulation-substance. So, also, when an inflamed part is cut, the first pus is from lymph: the latter pus, when repair is in progress, is from granulation-substance. In both cases, alike, the pus manifests itself as a rudimental substance ill-developed or degenerated (see p. 156); and the transition from the one condition to the other is an evidence of the impossibility of exactly defining between the inflammatory and the reparative processes, unless we can see their design and end.

Much, therefore, of what was said respecting suppuration in connection with repair, might be repeated here. But, avoiding this, let me only point out the principal methods in which inflammatory suppuration ensues, and the relation of the pus in each to the previous or coincident inflammatory product. In this last respect, the suppuration of disease differs importantly from that of the reparative process, in that the degeneration may take place in any of the different varieties of lymph, and that according to the primary character of the lymph, there may be traced (though as yet too obscurely) different appearances of the pus.[*]

The methods of such suppuration may be named the circumscribed, the diffuse, and the superficial. The first may be exemplified by the formation of an abscess or a pustule; the second by phlegmonous erysipelas, or purulent infiltration of any organ; the third by purulent ophthalmia, or gonorrhœa: and in these and the like instances we may often, at the close of the disease, watch the transition from the suppuration that depends on the inflammatory process, to that which is coincident with repair.

In circumscribed suppuration, which has its most usual seat in the cellular tissue, we can generally observe the previous signs of inflammation, and of an exudation of lymph in a certain area of the tissue. The exudation is interstitial, or by infiltration; and, probably, in most acute abscesses, is of a mixed kind, containing both fibrine, which may solidify, and a liquid material of which corpuscles may form themselves. The proper elements of the tissue are separated or expanded by the lymph thus inserted among them; and the inflamed part derives from it much of its swelling, and much of its hardness while the fibrinous part of the lymph is solid. Generally, such a swelling is at first, comparatively, ill-defined; and if it be near the skin, the visible inflammatory redness very gradually fades out at its borders, where, in the deeper tissue, we may believe, the exudation is gradually less abundant. But, in time, the swelling usually becomes more defined; the inflammation, as it were, concentrates itself, and appears more completely circumscribed. Now the lymph, in such a case, may be absorbed, or may be developed so as to form a long-continuing thickening and induration of the part: but, in

* See especially Rokitansky: Pathol. Anat., B. i., p. 210.

the case I am supposing, it is transformed into pus; its corpuscles
changing their characters in the manner already described (p. 156), and
its previously solidified part becoming liquid. The change almost always
begins at or near the centre of the lymph, where, we may believe, the
conditions of nutrition are most impaired. It may extend from a single
point, or from many which subsequently coalesce. In either case, the
central collection of matter remains surrounded by a border or wall of
indurated tissue, in which the infiltrated lymph is not transformed into
pus, but, rather, tends to be more highly organized. This border or
peripheral layer of lymph now forms the wall, as it is called, of the abscess, and the finger may detect, as the best sign of abscess, a soft or
fluctuating swelling with a firm or hard border. The expressions commonly used are, that the suppurative inflammation has taken place in
the centre of the swelling, and that its effects are bounded by the adhesive inflammation: it might be said, with the same meaning, but perhaps
more clearly, that, of a certain quantity of lymph deposited in the original area of the inflammation, the central portions have degenerated into
pus, and the peripheral have been maintained or more highly developed:
and, probably, we may add in explanation, the difference has depended
on the degrees in which the conditions of nutrition have been interfered
with in the places in which the two portions have been seated. In the
central parts of an inflammatory swelling, the circulation, if not wholly
arrested, must be less free than in the peripheral; the blood, moving
very slowly, or stagnant, must lose more of its fitness for nutrition; the
tissues themselves are more remote from the means of maintenance by
imbibition: in these parts, therefore, degeneration, if not death, ensues;
while, in the peripheral parts, maintenance, or even development, is in
progress.*

Now, in the ordinary course of such an abscess, the purulent matter
is discharged. (I shall speak in the next lecture of the manner in which
this takes place, as well as of the changes that ensue in the tissues among
whose elements the lymph is infiltrated.) On the interior of its wall,
especially if its course have been very acute, we may find a thin, opaque,
yellowish-white layer, easily to be detached, flaky, or grumous. It is
usually formed of lymph-cells or pus-cells imbedded in flakes of soft
fibrinous substance. It has been made to seem more important than it
is, by being called by some a "pyogenic membrane," and by its being
supposed that it is the work of the cells to secrete the pus. But the

* Expressions are sometimes used which imply that the wall of the abscess is formed by
an adhesive inflammation following, and purposely consequent on, the suppurative. This
certainly happens, if ever, very rarely: it only seems to take place when suppuration is
accompanied by extending inflammation. In such a case, that which is to-day the indurated abscess-wall, may, to-morrow, have become pus; and new inflammatory products,
deposited around it during its degeneration, will form then, the boundary of the enlarged
abscess. It may be, indeed, that the lymph deposited at the centre of the inflammatory
process is, naturally, less organizable than that at the periphery; but this is not proved.

existence of such a layer is far from constant in abscesses; it is, often,
a sign of the imperfect organization of the abscess-wall; its materials
are probably oftener detached and mingled with the pus than they are
vascularized; and no such layer is found when free suppuration continues
in an open abscess. A more normal course is observed when the progress of suppuration has been slower. In this case, the wall of the abscess becomes more highly organized after the discharge of the contents;
the circulation being restored to the infiltrated tissues of which the wall
is formed, the lymph is developed, or at least, if I may so speak, more
highly vivified, and its cells, or new ones formed next to the abscess-
cavity, are constructed into granulations, and are supplied with blood-
vessels, like those on the surface of a healing suppurating wound. Such
vessels are represented in this sketch.

Fig. 38.

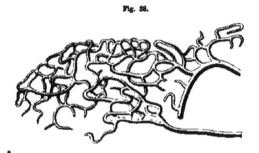

With, or soon after, the evacuation of the purulent matter, the disease
on which the abscess depended may cease; and, if this be so, the later
progress of the case is a process of healing which may, in every essential character, be likened to the healing of a wound by granulation.
There is the same gradual development of the lymph-cells, or, as they
might now be called, the granulation-cells of the walls of the abscess,—
first of the deeper, and then of the more superficial cells. The same
contraction, also, attends this process, and serves to diminish the area of
the cavity, and to bring its walls more nearly into correspondence and
proximity with the external opening, till, coming into contact, the opposite surfaces of granulations may unite, as in healing by secondary adhesion; or till, as the edges of the opening are retracted and depressed,
and the floor of the abscess is raised, they are brought nearly to a level,
and heal as a single granulating surface.

Such an abscess as I have described is often called acute or phlegmonous, in contradistinction from those collections of pus which, being formed
without the observed signs of inflammation, and, generally, slowly, are
named cold or chronic abscesses. Observations are wanting, I believe,
which might show how far the chronic abscesses differ from such as I
have described in their early condition; and, especially, whether there

be first a circumscribed infiltration of lymph, of which part degenerates and the rest is developed. It is probable the phenomena are essentially the same; for instances of all possible gradations between the two forms may be observed; and, in the complete state of the chronic abscess, the structures are not widely different from those of the acute. The abscess-wall is usually firmer, more defined, so that it can often be dissected entire from the adjacent parts, and has its tissue more developed, and more like those of a membranous cyst: the lining is generally less vascular, smoother, and less distinctly granulated; the contents are usually thin and serous, and indicate not only that the material of which they are composed was peculiarly unapt to be organized, but that, even after its transformation into pus, further degenerations ensued in it.

The diffuse suppuration, as I have said, may be exemplified by phlegmonous erysipelas. Here, with well-marked phenomena of inflammation, lymph is exuded through a wide extent of the subcutaneous cellular tissue, and, from first to last, the boundaries of the exudation are ill-defined: the suppuration is, indeed, most certain and complete at the centre, or where the inflammation began; but it may be nearly coextensive with the exudation, and most rarely presents a well-defined boundary wall, as in abscess. The lymph, in its primary character, is mixed; its fibrinous constituent is evident in the coagulation that ensues when it is let out (see p. 213), and, usually, in the abundant molecular matter in the pus. The exudation is even more distinctly interstitial than in an abscess; the tissue is thoroughly infiltrated with it, and is, comparatively, little expanded: and when suppuration has ensued, and we cut into the inflamed parts, the pus often flows out slowly, or even remains entangled in the tissue. The same condition is, often, yet more plain in the purulent infiltrations of such organs as the lung; their tissues are completely soaked with pus. The infiltrated tissues themselves are usually softened, not only by the mixture of the unorganized inflammatory matter, but through their own degeneration; and, very generally, large portions of them perish, and are found as sloughs infiltrated with pus.

In regard to their structural changes, there may appear little difference between this condition and that of acute abscess, except in the contrast of the one being less, the other more circumscribed. But in regard to the materials exuded, they are, probably, in the phlegmonous erysipelas, much less naturally apt for organization than in the abscess. The central suppuration of an abscess, while the lymph around is organizing, implies that the degeneration depends much on the local defect of the conditions of nutrition: the diffuse suppuration seems due, in a larger measure, to original defect of the lymph; and these differences correspond with those of the constitutional states attending the two diseases.

After the discharge of the pus, the healing of the diffuse suppuration is, in all essential respects, similar to that of the abscess; but the methods of discharge are much more diverse. Sometimes, after extensive sloughing of the skin, wide-spread suppurating cavities are exposed, which then granulate and heal like wide-open wounds; sometimes, numerous isolated suppurations ensue, whence the pus is discharged as from so many small ill-defined abscesses, in each of which ordinary healing occurs, while the intermediate parts are indurated by the imperfect organization of the lymph; sometimes, from a comparatively small opening, large sloughs are discharged, and then the boundaries of the subcutaneous cavities which they leave granulate, and healing takes place as by secondary adhesion.

The superficial inflammatory suppuration is such as we observe in gonorrhœa, and in purulent ophthalmia, and generally in the inflammations of mucous membranes. Here, the material exuded is least apt for organization, partly because of the situation in which it is produced, and through its own natural condition; for though exudation takes place, in these cases, within the tissue of the inflamed membrane, as well as on its surface, yet the amount of thickening, or other structural change, that takes place is slight, if we compare it with the changes that, in the same duration and severity of inflammation, would ensue in fibro-cellular tissue, or in serous membranes.

I have already spoken of the changes of mucus in the inflammatory process, and of the mixture of lymph that then occurs. The lymph is chiefly of the kind that forms corpuscles; and there is no instance in which the rapidity of formation of such corpuscles, and of their change into the characters of pus-cells, can be watched. It is, indeed, chiefly, in some of these cases of inflamed mucous membranes, that one may doubt whether it is reasonable to speak of the formation of lymph-cells as preceding that of pus; for, especially in the more acute inflammations, the characters of pus-cells seem to be acquired in the very beginning of organization of the exuded liquid. And this character of the cells is often retained, even after the product of the inflamed membrane has regained, to the naked eye, a more mucous appearance; for here (unless ulceration of the membrane have ensued) the process of recovery from inflammatory suppuration is not through such healing by granulation, as in the former cases, but by a gradual return to the secretion of a more normal material; and in this recovery, the inflammatory exudation becoming gradually less, the corpuscles that are formed, though they may assume the characters of pus-cells, are not sufficient to give a purulent character to the liquid.*

* The question of the diagnosis between mucus and pus should, perhaps, be here referred to. Between normal mucus and pus there can be no confusion (see p. 225). Between the mucus and the pus of an inflamed mucous membrane, the difference corresponds, in some measure, with that between lymph and pus; depending, first, on the proportion in which the inflammatory material is mingled with proper constituents of the mucus, and, secondly, on the degree in which the former tends to assume the purulent characters. In other words, the diagnosis required is not, strictly speaking, so much between mucus and pus, as between the lymph and pus which are, in different cases, mingled with the mucus of inflamed mem-

' ' The superficial suppuration from inflamed mucous membranes is closely related to that from an ulcerated surface. I think, indeed, that an inflamed mucous membrane may yield purulent matter, even though it remain covered with an epithelium. I believe this happens in gonorrhœa and in purulent ophthalmia : the vascular tissues, in these affections, appear still to have epithelium on them, though perhaps it is too thin and immature, and is reduced to a condition analogous to that of the thin and moist glistening epidermis on the inflamed "weeping" leg. But observations are wanting on this point. The transition to the suppuration from an ulcerated surface takes place when the epithelium is wholly removed from a mucous membrane. This constitutes its abrasion or excoriation ; in the next stage, the surface of the membrane itself is cast off, and this is its ulceration or erosion.*

Such are the several chief methods of inflammatory suppuration, and the relations of the pus to other products of the disease. In all the cases, a point of contrast between pus and any form of lymph is to be found in its complete incapacity for organization.

When once formed, the pus-cells, if they are retained within the body, have no course but to degenerate further ; it is characteristic of their being already degenerate, that they can neither increase nor develop themselves. Various corpuscles found in pus, besides those I have already mentioned, may find their interpretation in these degenerations ; for the pus-cells are prone to all the degenerations that I described as occurring in the lymph-cells.

They may wither, as in the scabbing of pustular eruptions, or in long-retained and half-dried strumous abscesses.

Or, they may be broken up, whether before or after passing into the fatty degeneration, which is one of their most common changes, and in which they are transformed into granule-cells. It is this breaking up into minute particles which, probably, precedes the final absorption of pus.

Or, lastly, both the cells and the fluid part of the pus may alike yield fatty and calcareous matter, and this may either remain diffused in fluid, or may dry into a firm mortar-like substance.

It is to such degenerations as these, in various degrees and combinations, and variously modified by circumstances, that we must ascribe the diverse appearances of the contents of chronic abscesses, and of the

branes. And this diagnosis is one which it is easy to make, in many cases, according to such characters of the corpuscles as have been already described ; but, in other cases, it is impossible, if it so chance that the materials are in the transition-stage from lymph to pus.

* The whole of the subjects of this paragraph are clearly and very fully illustrated, in relation to the affections of the mucous membrane of the uterus and vagina, by Drs. Tyler Smith and Hassal, in a paper which will appear in the 35th vol. of the Medico-Chirurgical Transactions, and of which an abstract is in the Lancet and the Medical Times of July 31, 1852.

substances that remain when abscesses close without complete final discharge of their contents. In such abscesses we may find mixtures of pus-cells, granule-cells, and molecular matter, diffused in more or less liquid; or pus-cells, half-dried, shriveled, and showing traces of their divided nuclei; or, all cells may be broken up, and their débris may be found mingled with minute oily particles, which appear in such cases to be always increasing; or, with these may be abundant crystals of cholesterine; or, such crystals may predominate over all other solid contents. In yet other chronic abscesses (though, still, without our being able to tell why the pus should degenerate in these rather than in the foregoing methods), we find molecules of carbonate and phosphate of lime, mixed with fat molecules and crystals, which are diffused in an opaque-white fluid, and look like a deposit from lime-water, or like white oil-paint; and as these contents dry, in the healing of the abscess, so are formed the mortar-like deposits and the hard concretions, such as are found in the substance of lymphatic glands, or other organs that have been the seats of chronic abscesses.

Time and patience would fail in an attempt to describe all the varieties of material that may thus issue from the transformations of pus. What I have enumerated are the principal or typical forms with which, I believe, nearly all others may be classed; though not without consideration of the various substances that may be accidentally mixed with the pus; as blood, débris of tissues, &c.

In conclusion of this part of the subject,—of this biography of inflammatory lymph,—a few words must be added respecting the degenerations and diseases which may occur after it is completely organized. The degenerations to which I have now so often referred, may be observed in full-formed adhesions, or in the corresponding organized tissues in the substance of organs.

Of the wasting of adhesions we often see instances in the pericardium, where films of false membrane are attached to one layer of the membrane, while the opposed portion of the other layer is only thickened and opaque. A more remarkable instance is presented in a case by Bichat, in which a man made twelve or fifteen attempts at suicide, at distant periods, by stabbing his abdomen. In the situations of the more recent wounds, the intestines adhered to the walls of the abdomen; in those of the older wounds, the older adhesions were reduced to narrow bands, or were divided and hung in shreds.

To similar wasting atrophy we may refer the extreme thinning and perforation of false membranes, by which, as Virchow[*] has well described, they became fenestrated like wasted omentum.

Of fatty degeneration I have seen no good examples in adhesions or similar inflammatory products, but of calcareous degeneration, or of such

[*] Würzburg Verhandlungen, B. i., p. 141.

as present a combination of fatty and earthy matter, museums present abundant specimens. Among these are most of the plates of bone-like substances imbedded in adhesions of the pleura, in thickened and opaque portions of the cardiac pericardium, in the tunica vaginalis in old hydroceles, in the thickened and nodulated capsule of the spleen, in the similarly altered mitral and aortic valves. So, too, many of the so-called ossifications of muscles and ligaments are examples of calcareous degeneration of fibrous tissue, formed in consequence of inflammation of these parts, and imbedded, in masses of fibrous-looking bands, within their substance. In some of these cases, indeed, there may be an approximation to the characters of true bone; but in nearly all, the earthy matter is deposited in an amorphous form, and seems to take the place of the former substance, as if, according to Rokitansky, it were a residue of the transformation of the more organized tissue, whose soluble parts have been, after decomposition, absorbed.*

Pigmental degeneration of adhesions may be seen, sometimes, in those of the pleura, in which black spots appear like the pigment-marks of the lungs and bronchial glands.† Adhesions of the iris, also, may become quite black, by the formation of pigment like that of the uvea.

Lastly, it must be counted among the signs of its attainment of complete membership in the economy, that the organized product of inflammation is liable to the same diseases as the parts among which it is placed; that it reacts like them under irritation; is, like them, affected by morbid materials conveyed to it in the blood; and, like them, may be the seat of growth of new and morbid organisms. No more complete proof of correspondence with the rest of the body could be afforded than this fact presents; for it shows that a morbid material in the blood, minute as is the test which it applies, finds in the product of inflammation the same qualities as in the older tissue to which it has peculiar affinity.

The subject, however, of the diseases to which these substances, themselves the products of disease, are liable, has been little studied. I can only enumerate the chief of them.

Lymph, while it is being highly organized, is often the seat of hemorrhage; its delicate new-formed vessels bursting, under some external violence, or some increased interior pressuee, and shedding blood. Such are most of the instances of hemorrhagic pericarditis, and other hemorrhages into inflamed serous sacs.

Even more frequently, the lymph, when organized, becomes itself the seat of fresh inflammation. Thus, in the serous membranes, we may find adhesions, in the substance or interstices of which recent lymph or pus is deposited;‡ or, in other cases, adhesions, or the thickenings and

* Numerous specimens of the calcareous degeneration of adhesions are in the College Museum; e. g., Nos. 103, 1493, 1494, 1516, &c.

† As in No. 96 in the College Museum.

‡ As in No. 1512 in the College Museum. The specimen has some historic interest. It

opacities of parts, become highly vasaular and swollen. It is, indeed, very probable that, in many of the instances of the recurring inflammations that we watch in joints, or bones, or other parts, the seat of the disease is, after the first attack, as much in the organized product of the former disease as in the original tissue.

I suppose, also, that to such inflammations of organized inflammatory products, we may ascribe many of the occasional aggravations of chronic inflammations in organs; the renewed pains and swellings of anchylosed joints, of syphilitic nodes, and the like; which are so apt to occur on exposure to cold, or in any otherwise trivial disturbances of the economy. In such cases we may believe that the former seat of disease becomes more inflamed, and that with it are involved the organized products of its previous inflammations. And in such cases there are, perhaps, none of the effects of inflammation which may not ensue in the newly organized parts: evidently, they may be softened, or thickened and indurated, and made more firmly adherent; or they may be involved in ulceration, or may slough with the older tissues among which they are placed.

Lastly, the products of inflammation may be the seats of the morbid deposits of specific diseases. In their rudimental state they may incorporate the specific virus of inoculable diseases, such as primary syphilis, variola, and the rest; and, when fully organized, they may be the seat of cancer and tubercle.

<hr>

LECTURE XVII.

CHANGES PRODUCED BY INFLAMMATION IN THE TISSUES OF THE AFFECTED PART.

THE account of the results of inflammation, in the tissues of the part in which it has its seat, will include the chief among those destructive processes which, I said in a former lecture (p. 212), may be reckoned as a second division in the inflammatory changes of the nutritive process. For I believe that all the effects of inflammation are injurious, if not destructive, to the proper tissues of the part in which it is seated. All the changes I shall have to describe are characteristic of defect of the normal nutrition in the parts: they are examples either of local death, or of some of the varieties of degeneration, modified and peculiarly accelerated by the circumstances in which they occur. The degenerations are observed, most evidently, in the processes of softening and

is one of those by which, in 1808, attention was first drawn, by Sir David Dundas, to the connection between acute rheumatism and disease of the heart.

17

absorption of inflamed parts. These I shall, first, endeavor to illustrate; and then, after some account of the minute changes that are associated with them, I will describe the process of ulceration; reserving for another lecture the account of the death of parts that may occur in inflammation. Let me, however, at once state, that the changes in the proper tissues of an inflamed part are, generally, of twofold origin. (1.) They are due to the natural degeneration of the tissue. That degeneration, which would be progressive in the healthy state, but which would then be unobserved, being constantly repaired, is still progressive in the inflamed state of the part, and is the more rapid because of the suspension or impairment of the proper conditions of nutrition. (2.) They are due, also, to the penetration of the products of inflammation into the very substance of the affected tissue; not merely into the interstices of its elemental structures, but into those structures themselves. These two methods of change are not essentially connected; but they are generally, in various proportions, coincident and mutually influential; and when concurring it is hardly possible to assign to each its share in the result to which they lead.

One of the most common effects of inflammation in an organ is a more or less speedy *softening* of its substance; and this is due not only to infiltration of it with fluid, but to a proper loss of consistency, a change approaching to liquefaction, or to disintegration, of which, indeed, it is often the first stage. Of such softening, some of the best examples are in the true inflammatory softening of the brain and spinal cord, in which the softened part is usually found to consist of broken-up nervous substance, together with more or less abundant granular products of inflammation. Such softening also may be found in the lungs: the peculiar brittleness and rottenness of texture, which exist with the other characters of hepatization, are evidently due to changes in the proper tissue, more than to incorporation of the products of inflammation. In staphyloma of the cornea, similar softening ensues in connection with the opacity and other changes of appearance. But, perhaps, the most striking instance of softening in inflammation (and it is the more so because the softening probably precedes the other evident signs of inflammation*) is to be found in bones. One may generally notice that an acutely inflamed bone is soft, so that a knife will easily penetrate it. Thus it may be found in the phalanges of the fingers when they partake in deep-seated inflammation, and thus, sometimes, in the neighborhood of diseased joints. The change depends partly on an absorption of the earthy matter of the bone, this constituent being removed more quickly, and in greater proportion, than the animal matter;† but the entire material of the bone is softened.

* See Küss, as quoted by Virchow, in his Archiv, i. p. 121.
† Gendrin, Hist. des Inflammations, i. p. 383.

The softening of bones may permit peculiar subsequent changes, especially their swelling and expansion. Thus in a remarkable case communicated by Mr. Arnott to Mr. Stanley, after excision of the bones of an elbow joint, inflammation ensued in the shaft of the humerus, and after four months the patient died. The end of the humerus was dull-red, and swollen, with expansion or separation of the layers of its walls (fig. 39). And the case showed well the coincidence of absorption and of enlargement by expansion; for though the inflamed humerus was thus enlarged and contained more blood than the healthy one, "yet it was found not to weigh so much by half."

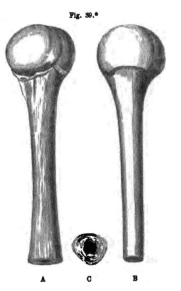

Fig. 39.*

A   C   B

Similar expansions of bone, with all the characters of inflammation, and such as could not have happened without previous softening of the tissues, form part of the many swollen and enlarged bones which are common in all museums.† Doubtless, in many of these cases, the disease has been of very slow progress, and the separation of the several layers of the compact bone, which the specimens display, must be ascribed to their gradually altered form, as they have grown about the enlarging blood-vessels and interlaminar inflammatory deposits. But, in other cases, the expansion has in all probability been more rapid, the softened bone yielding and extending, as the naturally softer tissues do, in an inflammatory swelling.

The characters of a bone thus expanded are easily discerned. Its substance may be irregularly cancellous or porous; but the most striking change is a more or less extensive and wide separation of the concentric laminæ of the walls of the bone, so that, as in the section of the femur (fig. 40), the longitudinal section of the enlarged wall appears composed of two or more layers of compact tissue, with a widely cancellous tissue between them: and these layers may sometimes be traced into continuity with those forming the healthy portion of the wall. Usually, the separated layers are carried outwards, and the bone appears outwardly

---

* A, the inflamed humerus. The swelling of its lower part is shown by contrast with that of the corresponding part of the healthy humerus B. The separation of laminæ is shown in c: all the figures are reduced one-half. From Mr. Stanley's Illustrations, pl. i. figs. 4, 5, 6.

† In the College Museum, Nos. 593 to 600, and 3085 to 3094; and in the Museum of St. Bartholomew's, Series i. Nos. 56, 94, 138, 196, 197, 198, &c.

enlarged; but sometimes the inner layers of the wall are pressed inwards, and encroach upon the medullary tissue. In the first periods of the

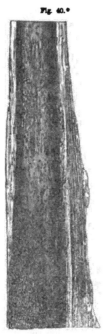

Fig. 40.*

disease, the cancellous tissue between the separated layers of the wall has wide spaces, which are usually filled with a blood-colored medulla: but this tissue, like the often coincident external formations of new bone, appears to have a tendency to become solid and hard; and its fibrils and laminæ may thicken till they coalesce into a compact ivory-like substance, harder than the healthy bone.

Again, for examples of softening in inflammation, I may adduce the softening of ligaments, such as permits that great yielding of them which we almost always see in cases of severely inflamed joints. This is not from mere defective nutrition; for it does not happen in the same form, or time, or measure, in cases of paralysis or paraplegia engendering extreme emaciation. Neither is it from the soaking of the ligaments with the fluid products of the inflammation; for it does not happen in the abundant effusions of the slighter inflammations of the joints; and when ligaments are long macerated in water they yet retain nearly all their inextensibility. It appears to be a peculiar softening, or diminished cohesion, of the proper tissue of the ligaments: the result of a degeneration, combined with infiltration of inflammatory products.

We may see such changes in the ligaments of all joints; in the hip, in the cases of spontaneous dislocation occasionally seen, independent of suppuration or ulceration of the parts belonging to the joint; in the wrist, when the ulna after disease becomes so prominent; in the vertebræ, especially in the ligaments of the atlas and axis. But we see the effects of this softening best in diseased knee-joints and elbow-joints; and in all these cases we may often observe an interesting later change when the inflammation passes by. The ligaments, softened during the inflammation, yield to the weight of the limb, or more rarely, to a muscular force, and the joint is distorted. Then, if the inflammation subsides, and the normal method of nutrition in the joint is restored, the elongated ligaments recover their toughness, or are even indurated by the organization and contraction of the inflammatory products deposited in them.

* From a specimen in the Museum of St. Bartholomew's, Series i. No. 04.

But they do not recover their due position; and thus the joint is stiffened in the distortion to which its ligaments had yielded in the former period of inflammation.   In the crowds of stiff, distorted, and yet not immovably fixed joints, that one sees as the consequences of inflammation, these changes must generally have happened to the ligaments: first softening and yielding; then recovery, with induration, and perhaps some con- traction, due to their atrophy and the organization of the inflammatory deposit.   The cases are aggravated by similar changes in the adjacent parts; for the stiffness of such joints is not due to the ligaments alone; all the subcutaneous tissues are apt to be adherent and indurated.

The ABSORPTION of the affected tissues is another example of the de- structive changes ensuing in the inflammatory process.   Like the degene- rations, which, arobably, always precede it, it is, in many inflammatory conditions, a peculiarly rapid event; and it may affect, at once, the proper elements of a part, its blood-vessels, and the inflammatory products that may have been previously deposited among them.

I shall refer here only to that which has been called *interstitial absorp- tion;* to the removal of parts from within the very substance of the tissues, as distinguished from the removal by the ejection of particles from the surface, of which I shall afterwards speak as occurring in *ulceration.*

Interstitial absorption of inflamed parts is seen very well in inflamed bones.   The head of a bone may be scarcely enlarged, while its anterior is hollowed out by an abscess; what remains of the bone may be indu- rated, as by slight and tardy inflammation, but so much of the bone as was where now the abscess is, must have been inflamed and absorbed. The changes in the instance of abscess in the lower end of the tibia are well shown in fig. 41, page 262.*   Here, too, the evidence of absorption is completed by the similar excavations formed in bones within which cysts and tumors grow; for in these cases no other removal than by absorption seems possible.   •

To similar absorption of inflamed tissue we may refer the wasting that we notice in the heads of bones that have been the seat of chronic rheu- matism.   The best examples of this are in the head and neck of the femur; and the retention of the compact layer of bone, covering in the wasted cancellous tissue of the shortened neck and flattened head, is characte- ristic of interstitial absorption, as distinguished from ulceration, by which the cancellous tissue is commonly exposed.   In these cases of chronic inflammation of the bones, we may notice, also, an appearance of dege- neration that precedes a peculiar mode of absorption or of ulceration. While the articular cartilages are passing through the stages of fibrous degeneration, and are being gradually removed, the subjacent bone is assuming the peculiar hardness which has been termed "eburnation," or "porcellaneous" change.   Now this change is effected by the formation of

* Museum of St. Bartholomew's, Series i. No. 82.

very imperfect bone; of bone that has no well-formed corpuscles; and it resembles the result of mere calcareous degeneration rather than a

Fig. 41.

Fig. 42.

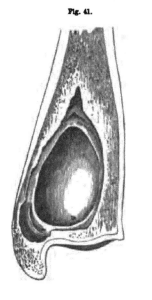
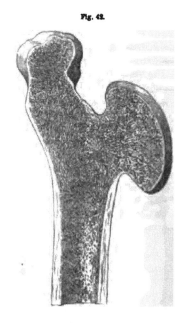

genuine ossifying induration. And its character as a degeneration is further declared in this, that it is prone to destructive perforating ulceration, which often gives a peculiar worm-eaten appearance to the bones thus diseased.*

With these changes in rheumatic bones we may also cite, as instances of absorption during slow inflammation, the changes which Mr. Gulliver† first described as apt to ensue after injuries about the trochanter of the femur (fig. 42). In such cases, without any appearance of ulcerative destruction, the head and neck of the femur may waste by absorption, the neck becoming shortened and the head assuming a peculiar conical form. We might regard these effects as simple atrophy, if it were not that they are like the effects of the more manifest inflammation in the

* A change, which appears to correspond with the eburnation of bone, is described by Mr. Tomes, as occurring in a part of a tooth which lies beneath a carious cavity. In both cases, the induration might suggest that it is calculated to retard the progress of the disease, but we have no evidence that it does this in an effective manner; and in the case of the bones there is every appearance that the destruction is most rapid where there is most induration.

† Edinburgh Med. and Surg. Journal, vol. xlvi. His illustration of a well-marked case is here copied.—The change is illustrated in No. 3312 in the College Museum.

rheumatic cases, and that the existence of inflammation during life is often declared by the abiding pain and other symptoms following the injury.

Again, other examples of the absorption of inflamed parts, or of parts that have been inflamed, are presented in the wasting of glands after inflammation; as in cirrhosis of the liver, in some forms of granular degenerations of the kidney, in the indurated and contracted lung after pneumonia.

No doubt, in these cases, the reduction of the organ depends, in a measure, on the contraction of the diffused inflammatory product, as it organizes; but in many cases the quantity of new tissue is extremely small (it is so in the shriveled granular kidney); and, in all the cases, we may well doubt whether the contraction of organizing lymph would produce such extensive and uniform absorption of the proper substance of an organ, if there were not a previous condition favoring the absorption. The most probable explanation of these cases seems to be, that as, in the early periods of inflammation, the softening and the degeneration of the inflamed tissues coincide with the production of the lymph; so, as the inflammation subsides, and subsequently, the absorption of the degenerated tissues may often coincide with the full organization and contraction of the lymph. And it is altogether most probable that these events are independent though concurrent; and that each occurs as of itself, not as the cause or consequence of the others.

To all these cases must be added the fact of the absorption of the blood-vessels, and other necessary apparatus, of the inflamed tissues. The absorption of the absorbents themselves must coincide with that of the tissues. What a problem is here! These, that have once been the apparatus of maintaining life, that had been adjusted to its energy and fashion, now, as it fails, remove themselves in adaptation to its failure. How can this be? We can only guess that its method is just the reverse of the method of formation; that, as in growth the blood-vessels and lymphatics follow in the course of evolution of the growing parts, opening and extending into each new part as it forms, so, in decrease, they follow, and closing in harmoniously with the general involution, mingle their degenerate materials with those of the tissue, and are absorbed by the nearest remaining streams of blood.

Once more; not only the original elements of the tissues may be absorbed, but, even more rapidly, the new-formed products of inflammation. We have the best example of this, as well as, indeed, of many of the facts which I have been mentioning, in the spontaneous opening of a common abscess; which, though it be so common a thing, I will venture to describe here.

Let us suppose the case of an abscess formed in the subcutaneous tissue; of such an one as I described some pages back, and may illustrate by the following sketch of an imaginary section through its cavity and the superjacent skin (fig. 43). It has had its origin in lymph infiltrated through a certain area of the tissues, and forming therein a hard, circumscribed, inflamed mass.   Of this lymph all the central portion is suppurated, and forms the purulent contents of the abscess; while the peripheral part acquires more abundant blood-vessels, assumes the character of a granulation layer on its surface, and forms the proper wall of the abscess.

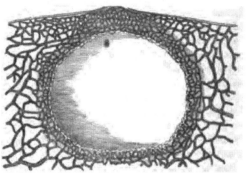

The pus of such an abscess as this will contain probably, besides its proper constituents, some of the disintegrated tissue of the part in which it has its seat.   We cannot, indeed, be quite sure of this; for it may be, that while the lymph is being formed, or being converted into pus, the proper tissue of the infiltrated part is undergoing absorption; and although, in the pus of abscesses thus formed, we often find abundant molecular and granular matter, yet this may be the débris, not of the tissue, but of the cells or fibrine of the inflammatory product.   We cannot, I think, be sure on this matter: but we may be sure that one of these two events occurs: that the circumscribed portion of the tissue, in which such an abscess has its seat, degenerates; and is then either absorbed, or else disintegrated, so as to mingle more or less of its substance with the pus.

The abscess thus formed has a natural tendency to open, unless all the inflammation in which it had its origin subsides.   Inflammation appears to be not only conducive, but essential, to the spontaneous opening of abscesses; for where it is absent, the matter of chronic abscesses will remain, like the contents of any cyst, quiet for weeks, or months, or years; and when in chronic abscesses or in cysts, inflammation ensues through the whole thickness of their coverings, it is usually certain that their opening is near at hand.   This difference between acute and chronic abscesses makes it very doubtful whether the inflammation of the coverings of an abscess can be ascribed to any local influence of the pus.   But to whatever it may be ascribed, we may refer to this inflammation, and to the degenerative changes that accompany it, the comparatively quick absorption of the integuments, and of the infiltrated lymph, over the collection of pus: and thus the fact, however me may account for it, that the integuments are more prone to inflammation, and more actively engaged in it, than the other tissues about an abscess are, may be used to explain the progress of matter towards the surface. Possibly (though this, I think, is much less probable) the tissues and the lymph between an abscess and the surface may, after the degeneration which accompanies the inflammation, be disintegrated, and may mingle their molecules with the purulent contents of the abscess. But, in favor of the belief that they are absorbed, we have the evidence of analogy; for just the same thinning and removal of integuments takes place when they inflame over a chronic abscess with a thick impenetrable cyst, or over an encysted or even a solid tumor. In these cases, absorption alone is possible; and the cases are so similar to the ordinary progress of abscesses, that I think we may assign all the changes of the integuments over these to the same interstitial absorption.

During, or preparatory to their absorption, the integuments over an abscess become softer and more yielding. The change is, most probably, due to such softening as I have described in degenerating inflamed parts. It takes place especially in the portion of the integuments over the middle, or over the most dependent part, of the abscess; and this most softened portion, yielding most to the pressure of the pus, becomes prominent beyond the parts around it, and *points*. Mr. Hunter refers to this as "the relaxing or elongating process." He says: "Besides these two modes of removing whole parts, acting singly or together [that is, besides the interstitial and the progressive absorption], there is an operation totally distinct from either, and this is a relaxing and elongating process carried on between the abscess and the skin, and at those parts only where the matter begins to point. It is possible that this relaxing, elongating, or weakening process, may arise in some degree from the absorption of the interior parts; but there is certainly something more, for the skin that covers an abscess is always looser than a part that gives way from mere mechanical distension, excepting the increase of the abscess is very rapid.

"That parts relax or elongate without mechanical force, but from particular stimuli, is evident in the female parts of generation, before the birth of the fœtus; they become relaxed prior to any pressure. The old women in the country can tell when a hen is going to lay, from the parts becoming loose about the anus."*

While these changes of degeneration, leading to softening and absorption, are ensuing in the cutis and the lymph over such an abscess as I have described, we commonly notice that the cuticle separates, leaving

---

* On the Blood, &c. Works, vol. iii. p. 477. The last fact is, probably, not appropriately cited. The change in the state of parts before the birth is most likely due to relaxation of the abundant muscular fibres that they all contain.

the very point, or most prominent part, of the abscess bare (fig. 43). The cuticle is sometimes raised as a blister; but much more often it cracks and separates, and then, with its broken edges raised, peels off like dead cuticle: and we may believe that it is dead, partaking in the failure of nutrition in which all the parts over the abscess are involved, and being removed as a dead, not as a merely degenerated, part.

At length, after extreme thinning of the integuments, they perish in the centre of the most prominent part. Sometimes the perished part becomes dry and parchment-like, with a kind of dry gangrene; but much more commonly a very small ordinary slough is formed, and the detachment of this gives issue to the purulent matter. The discharge is usually followed by a more or less complete cessation of the inflammation in the integuments, and then the wall of the abscess, having the character of a cavity lined with healthy granulation, heals.

The softening and absorption of inflamed tissues of which I have been speaking, are the chief consequences, or attendants, of minuter molecular changes, to which I must now refer. These changes are derived, as I have already said, from one or both of two sources; namely, the natural degenerations of the inflamed tissues, and their penetration by the inflammatory product.

The rapid softening of an inflamed tissue is, probably, in most cases, dependent on both these conditions; and yet in some cases, and in some measure in all, it may be ascribed to a simple degeneration, such as might be classed with those named liquefactive. Thus, in the case of the integuments over an abscess, we find it associated with infiltration of degenerating lymph-products, and probably in some measure due to their presence; but in the brain and spinal cord, the softenings of inflammation are, in structure, and probably also in nature, very like those of mere atrophy.

Less rapid softening is often connected with a well-marked fatty degeneration of the inflamed tissues. This is especially the case in the muscles, bones, cartilages, cornea, and certain glands, as the liver and kidney.

I found such a degeneration well-marked in the fibres of the heart of a man, who thrust a needle through his left ventricle four days before his death. There were evident signs of pericarditis, and of inflammation of the portion of the heart close by the wound; and both in this portion, and, in a less degree, in all other parts of the heart, I found such a fatty degeneration of the muscular fibres as I could not have distinguished from that which occurs in the corresponding atrophous degeneration.* The same changes may be oftener observed at later

* I spoke with some hesitation about this case when the lecture was given; for I could scarcely believe in the occurrence of such an acute degeneration. The admirable observations of Virchow (Archiv, B. iv. H. i.) leave no doubt that such a change is a general atten-

periods after inflammation of the substance of the heart; and in some
of these cases the interstitial deposits of lymph are organized into fibrous
tissue, while the muscular fibres themselves are degenerate.   The extended observations of Virchow, on the inflammations of muscles,[*] show
that such fatty degeneration of the fibres usually occurs in nearly all but
the most acute cases; in these, softening and disintegration of the muscular fibrills rapidly ensue, and fatty particles appear subsequently, if at
all, in the inflammatory exudation and disintegrated tissue that are mingled within the sarcolemma.   He shows, also, very clearly, how the
changes in the muscular fibres may be associated with the effects of
lymph deposited interstitially among them, as well as within them, and
passing through its ordinary progress of development or degeneration;
and that they may be followed by the complete wasting, or absorption,
of the degenerate tissue, in the place of which the new fibrous tissue
formed by the developed lymph may remain like a scar or a tendinous
spot.

In inflamed bone, also, Virchow has traced fatty degeneration as a
part of the process of softening which precedes its expansion or absorption.   The change is observed not constantly, yet very often, as a fatty
degeneration of the bone-corpuscles, in the interior of which small fatty
molecules appear.   After, or sometimes without, such previous changes
in the corpuscles, he has also traced their enlargement and the gradual
softening, disintegration, and final liquefaction and separation of the
proper bone-substance, immediately surrounding and including each corpuscle.   The changes he has thus traced accord completely with those
described by Goodsir and Redfern in the cartilage; and, as he well
observes, they have peculiar interest in relation to the occurrence of
fatty degeneration, as a part of the inflammatory process, inasmuch as
they are the results of the same process as that by which, normally, the
medullary spaces and areolæ of growing bone are formed, by which, as
the bone grows, the compact cortical tissue is gradually changed into
areolar or spongy tissue, and by which the peculiar "mollities ossium,"
or "osteo-malacia," is produced.

Changes like these in inflamed bone have been found in ulcerating and
articular cartilage; and they are here the more important, as showing
a process essentially similar to the degeneration of inflammation, although
occurring in a tissue that has no blood-vessels, and into which we have
no evidence of the penetration of lymph.   They have been chiefly observed
by Dr. Redfern;[†] but have been confirmed by many.   They consist,
essentially, in the enlargement of the cartilage-cells, with increase of the

dant of inflammation of muscles.   Few things could be more assuring than to find the
opinions I expressed concerning this and other parts of the inflammatory process completely confirmed by him.

[*] In his Essay on Parenchymatous Inflammation, cited above, p. 266.

[†] Anormal Nutrition in Articular Cartilages: Edinburgh, 1850. And "On the Healing
of Wounds in Articular Cartilages," in the Monthly Journal of Medical Science, Sept. 1851.

nuclei, or of peculiar corpuscles contained in them, or with fatty degeneration of their contents, and fading, or similar degeneration of their nuclei. The hyaline intercellular substance at the same time splits up, and softens into a gelatinous and finely molecular and dotted substance, or else is gradually transformed in the less acute cases, into a more or less fibrous tissue. The enlarged cartilage-cells on the surface are released, and may discharge their contents on the surface of the ulcer; and the intercellular substance is gradually disintegrated and similarly discharged, or, whatever part of it remains, is transformed into fibrous tissue, and becomes the scar by which the ulceration is, in a measure, healed.

Lastly, in the cornea, a series of observations on the effects of inflammation, purposely excited in it by various stimuli,* have shown that the changes in it are not due to any free exudation of lymph in it, but to alteration in its proper constituent textures. They consist, chiefly, in swelling and enlargement of its corpuscles, the appearance of minute fatty molecules in them, and the increase and enlargement of their nuclei. The intercellular substance becomes, at the same time, turbid, more opaque, denser, more fibrous, and, sometimes, finely granulated; and in some cases fatty molecules appear in it. The changes thus produced in the cornea are not essentially different from those that follow its idiopathic inflammations; and, as Virchow concludes, they are extremely like those of the arcus senilis.

Now, from all these cases, with which others of similar import might be combined, we may conclude that the degeneration of the proper tissues of inflamed parts, which we recognize in the mass as a softening of their substance, or an aptness to be absorbed, is, very often, essentially like the fatty degeneration which we have studied as a form of atrophy of the same parts; that the changes of structure are, in both, essentially the same; differing in rate of progress, but not in method or result. And the cases of the bones, cartilages, and cornea, are the more to be considered, because the changes described in them cannot be referred, in any considerable measure, if at all, to a process of exudation into the elements of their tissues.

The fatty degeneration and that of softening, as by progressive liquefaction, are, doubtless, the most general forms in which the defective nutrition in an inflamed part is manifested. But something allied to the calcareous degeneration occurs in the ossifications of the laryngeal cartilages when they are involved in inflammation, and of such other cartilages as are prone to an imperfect ossification in old age. These are frequent events; and as Virchow observes, the ossification occurs

---

* They are published briefly in Virchow's essay already cited; and in detail in a dissertation—" Der normale Bau der Cornea und die pathologischen Abweichungen in dimselben," Würzburg, 1851—by Fr. Strube, by whom the observations were made under the superintendence of Virchow.

constantly and often exclusively in the very part of the cartilages which corresponds with the seat of the inflammation. To the same class of cases we may refer the ossifications of parts of the articular cartilages in chronic rheumatic arthritis (p. 237), and the formation of the imperfect dentine or osteo-dentine which ensues in inflammatory affections of the tooth-pulp, or in the pulp of the elephant's tusk round bullets lodged in it. In all these cases, it may be observed, the inflammatory process is attended with such changes as occur almost normally at some later period of life, or in old age ; such changes, then occurring, are reckoned among the natural degenerations, the signs of simply defective formative power: the difference, therefore, between the natural degeneration and that of the inflammatory process seems to be one of time more than of kind; the inflammatory is premature and comparatively rapid, and ensues with the characters of disturbed, rather than of merely defective, nutrition.

Such are some of the evidences of degeneration ensuing in the proper tissues of inflamed parts. The cases I have selected are of the simplest kind; whose results are least confused by the changes that may ensue in lymph penetrating the degenerating tissue. When this happens, it is perhaps impossible, at present, to separate the two series of changes: those, I mean, which are due to the degeneration of the elements of the tissue, and those which are occurring in the lymph within them. The latter are especially described by Virchow, in the muscular fibres, and in the renal cells, in what he calls the parenchymatous form of granular degeneration of the kidney. In the latter he says,* that while, as in the croupous form, fibrinous cylinders of free inflammatory exudation may be found in the straight, and a part of the convoluted tubes, other changes are ensuing in the epithelial cells; and by these chiefly, and sometimes alone, the characteristic altered structure of the kidney is induced. They occur especially in those parts of the tubes which run transversely or obliquely. In the first stage of the disease these cells enlarge, and their molecular nitrogenous contents increase, by the pene-tration of the inflammatory product into them. In the second stage, the increase is such that the cells break up, and the urine-tubes appear filled with a molecular albuminous substance ; or else the fatty transformation ensues in them, and they are filled with finely granular fatty matter, and appear as granule-cells, or granule-masses. In the third stage the fat granules depart, and an emulsive fluid is formed which may be absorbed or discharged with the urine.

Virchow describes similar changes in the hepatic cells: but it may suffice only to refer to these. What has been already described will be enough, I hope, to justify the expressions used at the beginning of the lecture : namely, that the changes (short of death) which ensue in the

* In his essay, referred to at p. 320. Many of his facts were published by one of his pupils, Dr. Niemann, in his dissertation, De inflammatione renum parenchymatosa, Berol. 1848.

proper elements of an inflamed part are twofold: first, those of a degeneration, such as might ensue in simply defective or suspended nutrition; and secondly, those which depend on the penetration of the exuded inflammatory product. Either of these may, perhaps, occur alone, but the first can be rarely, if ever, absent. When they are concurrent, their several effects cannot be clearly separated; and when they both take place rapidly, the degeneration is apt to lose all likeness to such as naturally occur, and to appear as only contributing to the rapid disintegration and liquefaction of both the tissue and the inflammatory product. This appears to be the case in many instances of ulceration; a process which I have deferred to the very end of the history of inflammation, because all the other parts of the disease appear to be engaged in it.

I need hardly say that, ever since Hunter's time, confusion has existed in the use of the terms employed for various kinds or methods of absorption and ulceration. Of all that Hunter wrote, nothing, I think, is so intricate, so difficult to understand, as his chapter on ulcerative inflammation; and much of the obscurity in which he left the subject remains. Some of this depends on the same terms having been used in different senses, and may be avoided if it is agreed to speak of the removal of those particles of inflamed parts, which are not on an open or exposed surface, as the "interstitial absorption" of inflamed parts. Then, the term "ulceration" may be employed to express the removal of the superficial or exposed particles of inflamed parts: or, rather, when the epithelium or epidermis of an inflamed part is alone removed, it may be called "abrasion" or "excoriation;" and when any of the vascular or proper tissue is removed from the surface, it may be called "ulceration." If, in such ulceration, the superficial particles may be supposed to be absorbed, the process of removing them may be termed "ulcerative absorption;" but if, as is more probable, their removal is effected entirely by ejecting them from the surface of the inflamed part, then the term "ulceration" may sufficiently express this ejection, and will stand in stronger contrast to the "interstitial absorption" of the particles that are not so ejected, but are taken into the blood.

I have lately referred to the uncertainty whether, as the cavity of an abscess enlarges or opens, the tissues, and the infiltrated lymph, that are removed from the inner surface of its boundary walls, are absorbed, or are disintegrated and mingled with its fluid contents; in other words, whether they are absorbed or ejected. The same uncertainty exists, in some measure, in the case of ulceration, concerning which, indeed, all that was said (p. 264), respecting the necessity of inflammation to the opening of abscesses, might be here repeated, inasmuch as inflammation seems essential, not only to the formation, but to the extension or enlargement, of an ulcer. The ulcerative process cannot take place in healthy tissue; previous degeneration of the tissue, and that such as occurs in the inflammatory process, is a condition essential to it.

But, when this condition is provided, is the enlargement of an ulcer effected by absorption of its boundaries, or by the ·gradual detachment and casting off of particles from their free surface? Both methods of enlargement may, perhaps, in some cases, ensue; but the probabilities are in favor of the enlargement being, as a general rule, effected by the ejection of particles.

Thus :—1. Parts to be removed from a surface are generally cast off rather than absorbed, as cuticles of all kinds are, and the materials of secretions; so that, by analogy, we might assume that the particles of the surface of a spreading ulcer would also be cast off.

2. The materials of the ulcerating tissue may be sometimes found in the discharge from the ulcer. In most cases, indeed, this is impossible; but perhaps it is so only because, when the tissues, and the lymph deposited in them, are degenerate, and broken up, or decomposed and dissolved, we have no tests by which to recognize them. In the ulceration of cartilage, however, in which inflammatory exudation has no share, the process of ejection of the disintegrated tissue is clearly traced; and we might deem this almost a proof of the same process being observed in other tissues, if it were not that in the cartilage a necessary condition of absorption, the presence of a circulation, is wanting. The same process of ejection, however, is traceable in ulcerating bone, where absorption might occur. It is shown by the observations which I have quoted from Virchow; and Mr. Bransby Cooper has observed that, while in pus from soft parts only traces of phosphate of lime are found, the pus from around diseased bone contains in solution nearly $2\frac{1}{2}$ per cent.[*] A similar, but less complete, observation has been made by Mr. Thomas Taylor,[†] and by v. Bibra;[‡] and we may believe that at least some of the phosphate of lime, in these cases, was derived from the diseased bone.[§]

3. It strengthens this belief to observe, that, in many cases small

---

[*] Medical Gazette, May, 1845.

[†] Stanley: Treatise on Diseases of the Bones, p. 89.

[‡] Chemische Untersuchungen verschiedener Eiterarten, p. 85.

[§] The belief may seem the more reasonable, because of the similar fact of the quick absorption of bone-earths in inflamed but not ulcerating bones. Still, it must be admitted, more evidence is needed than the quantity of bone-earths discharged with the pus is proportionate or equal to the quantity lost by the ulcerating bone. For if what has been said (p. 231) of the conformity of the properties of inflammatory and reparative products with those of the tissues from which they are produced, be true, then will also pus from diseased bone possess more bone-earths than pus from any other tissue, even though the bone be not ulcerating. Granulations upon bone doubtless contain more bone-earths than those on soft parts, and they may ossify: now the relation of pus to granulations is commonly that of degenerating cells to the like cells developing; therefore we might expect that pus from bone, like granulations from bone, will contain a large proportion of bone-earths, independent of what may be derived from the ulceration of the bone.

fragments of bone and other tissues are detached, and cast out with the fluid from the ulcerating part. These, indeed, when they are not fragments of tissue detached by ulceration extending around them, are good examples of the transition that may be traced from ulceration to sloughing or gangrene of parts, between which, if ulceration be always accomplished by ejection, the only essential difference will be one of degree; the ulceration being a death and casting off of invisible particles of a tissue, while gangrene implies the death and casting off of visible portions.

4. And it may be proved of many that we call ulcers, that they begin as sloughs which are cast off, and leave the ulcerated surface beneath. We may often see this, on a large scale, in the instances of what are called sloughing ulcers; but Dr. Baly has proved it for a much wider range of cases, in his observations on dysentery, in which he has traced how even the smallest and most superficial ulcers of the intestine are preceded by the death and detachment of portions of the mucous membrane, with its covering of basement-membrane and epithelium.*

From these considerations, we may hold it as probable that ulceration is, usually, the result of the detachment of dead portions or molecules of an inflamed tissue, and that the substance removed in the process is not absorbed but ejected. There are, indeed, some cases which may make us unwilling to admit, at present, that all ulceration is by ejection; such as those of bone ulcerating under cartilage, or in the rapid extension of inflammation within it, or such as the spreading ulceration of the vertebræ, or of the heads of bones, that is not attended with external discharge of fluid. These may, for the present, interfere with the universality of the rule, but not with its generality.

But, if we may believe that the removal of a tissue by ulceration is generally effected by ejection of its substance, the question may be asked, in what form is it ejected? Dr. Baly's observations enable us to say that, in the first instance, a visible slough is detached, a portion of the tissue dying and being disconnected from the adjacent living tissue. But, after this is done, when an ulcer enlarges, or extends and spreads, is the material of the tissue still removed in visible sloughs or fragments? Certainly it is so sometimes; for we may find little fragments of bone in the discharge from ulcerating bone, especially in strumous ulceration. But in other cases we have no evidence of this kind; we cannot detect even microscopic fragments of tissues in the discharges, and we must suppose that they are removed, in a state of solution or of molecular division, in the discharge from the diseased part.

To speak of the solution of tissues in the discharges of ulcers may seem like the revival of an old error long since disproved. But though the expression may be revived, it is with a new meaning. The proof has, truly, been long completed, that healthy tissues, even though they be dead, cannot be dissolved in pus, or any such discharge; but the

---

* Gulstonian Lectures: Medical Gazette, 1847.

tissues that bound or form the walls of a spreading ulcer are not healthy; they are inflamed, and, as I have been just saying, their elements, and the products of inflammation in and among them, are degenerate, so that they may be now minutely divided, or even soluble in fluids that could not dissolve them while they were sound. Insolubility is as great an obstacle to absorption as to ejection in discharges; no tissue can be absorbed without being first so far changed as to be soluble in fluids with which it was before in contact and unharmed. Therefore, whether we hold the ordinary spreading of an ulcer to be by absorption of its boundaries, or ascribe it to their ejection, we must in either case, admit that they are first made soluble. And if this be admitted, then it is most consistent with analogy, and most probable, that the extension of an ulcer, independently of sloughing, is accomplished by the gradual degeneration of the tissues that form its walls, and by their being either disintegrated and cast off in minute molecular matter, or else dissolved and ejected in solution in the discharges from the ulcer.

The solution here spoken of is such as may be effected by the fluid discharged from any spreading ulcers; but we may doubt whether all discharges from ulcers possess a *corroding* property, such as Rokitansky seems to ascribe to them, and such as he considers to be the chief cause of the extension of all ulcers. We may doubt, I say, whether all ulceration can be described as a corrosion or erosion of the tissues by ichor; but, on the other side, we cannot well doubt that the properties of the discharge from an ulcer, or a sloughing sore, may have a great influence in accelerating the degeneration and decomposition, and thereby the solution, of the tissues that form its walls or boundaries. Many ichorous discharges from ulcers inflame and excoriate the parts over which they flow, and thus inflaming them, they promote their degeneration, and lead them more readily to enter into the ulcerative process. Many such discharges, also, are in an active state of decomposition; and their contact with the inflamed tissues cannot but have some tendency to excite decomposition in them; a tendency which the tissues will be the less able to resist, in the same proportion as they are already feebly maintaining themselves, or as they have been moved by inflammation from their normal conditions, and their normal tenacity of composition.

On the whole, then, we may conclude, respecting the process of ulceration, that its beginning is usually the detachment of a slough, or portion of dead tissue, by the removal of the layer of living tissue that bounded it; that the spreading of an ulcer, independent of such visible sloughing, is effected by the inflamed tissues that bound it becoming degenerate, and being detached in minute particles, or molecular matter, or being decomposed and dissolved in the fluid discharge or ichor; and that this spreading may be accelerated by the influence of the discharge itself, which may inflame the healthy tissues that it rests on, and may exercise a decomposing "catalytic" action on those that are inflamed already.

I need hardly say that we have no knowledge by which to explain the peculiar and characteristic form of certain ulcers. We seem wholly without a guide to such knowledge; but the existence of such specific form is conclusive against the supposition that the extension of an ulcer is entirely due to corrosion by an exuded fluid. Such a fluid would act uniformily, unless the various effects of disease on the tissues bounding the ulcer should make them variously amenable to its influence.

We have as little knowledge of the nature and real differences of the various fluids discharged from ulcerating surfaces,—the various kinds of ichor* that they yield. They consist, generally, of fluid exuded from the surface as an inflammatory product, and holding in suspension or solution the disintegrated materials of the ulcerating tissue, and of the lymph infiltrated in them. The inflammatory product exuded on a spreading ulcer has, indeed, the constituents of lymph or pus; but they appear immature or degenerate, consisting of abundant molecular matter, with flakes of soft, dotted fibrine, and ill-formed lymph or pus-cells, floating in an excess of liquid. Such a substance is, probably, always incapable of organization, both because of its own defect, and because of the inflamed state of the parts it is in contact with. The differences that may, from the first, exist in the several examples of ichor are moreover quickly increased by the various chemical transformations that they undergo. Rokitansky alone has endeavored to enumerate the varieties of properties that may hence issue, and the influences they may exercise in the maintenance of the disease.†

As from other inflammatory processes, so, from observation, we may trace the transitions to the healing process. In the case of ulcerated cartilage, Dr. Redfern's researches show that the healing is accomplished, mainly, by the complete transformation of the remaining cartilage-substance into fibrous tissue. Here is no proper process of exudation, for here are no interstitial blood-vessels; the materials of the tissue itself, by transformation, form the scar.

But in the vascular tissues, the reparative material is the lymph infiltrated in them at and near the boundaries of the ulcer. As the inflammation subsides (for here, as in other cases, the inflammation that produced the lymph must cease for its development) the lymph passes through changes like those described in the abscess-wall, and the tissues in which it was infiltrated may, perhaps, recover from their degeneration. Part of the lymph, increased by fresh exudation, assumes the characters of

* I think it would be useful to employ the term exclusively for those discharges mixed with exudation that take place from ulcerating, i. e. from progressively ulcerating or sloughing surfaces. For, although it may be often impossible to distinguish, by any manifest properties, such ichor from some of the thinner kinds of pus, yet, if the account of suppuration and of ulceration be true, a constant difference between pus and ichor will be, that the latter contains disintegrated materials of the ulcerating tissue, the former does not.

† Pathologische Anatomie, B. i. p. 213.

granulations, which, as we watch the progress of an improving ulcer, assume daily more of the characters of those on healing open wounds. We cannot, indeed, mark the very act, or tell the hour, at which the inflammatory process was changed for the reparative; at which the degeneration ceased, and development began; there are no hard boundary lines here, or in any passage from disease to health; but the change is gradually accomplished, and is manifest both in the organizing material of the granulations, and in the pus which takes the place of the ichor, and exactly resembles that of the healing granulating wound. The ulcer is no longer ulcerating, but healing; and the histories of the healing ulcer, and of the healing wound, might be told in the same words.

LECTURE XVIII.

NATURE AND CAUSES OF INFLAMMATION.

THE several parts of the inflammatory process have been now considered. They are—increased fullness of the blood-vessels, with retarded movement of the blood; swelling; pain, or other morbid exalted sensation; increased heat; exudation of lymph from the blood-vessels; defective nutrition of the proper elements of the affected part. The first five are often spoken of as the signs of inflammation, the last two as its effects; but these terms have reference only to the former being more transitory phenomena than the latter: they are all, when they concur, constituent parts of the disease; but the latter are less quickly recovered from than the former.

It would not be judicious, I think, to refuse to call that process inflammation, in which any one of the conditions just enumerated is absent or unobserved. Swelling, or pain, or much oftener, increased heat, may be inappreciable in tissues that we may still rightly call inflamed, while the other evidences of the disease are present. The same may be said of increased or altered exudation from the blood-vessels. No such exudation is observed in the diseased cornea or articular cartilages; but it would be unreasonable, in the case of an inflamed eye, to say that the changes are due to inflammation in every part but the cornea; and to call the process leading to the ulceration or leucoma of the cornea by a name different from that which we give to the coincident and similarly excited process in the other tissues. So, during the inflammation of a joint, it would be, at the least, inconvenient, to say that all the tissues are inflamed except the softening or ulcerating cartilages. The progressive degeneration of tissue is, probably, never absent when the other parts of the inflammatory process exist; but, in quickly transitory cases, it is often inappreciable. The altered state of the circulation may be unobserved: but it is, probably, always present; for in the case of the parts that have no interstitial blood-vessels, inflammation may still be attended by enlargement of those of adjacent parts, on which their ordinary nutrition depends.

The conclusion, then, may be, that in what may be regarded as well-marked or typical examples of inflammation, all the characters I have enumerated are present as concurrent parts of the disease; but that the same name should not be refused to diseases in which any one of these parts is absent or unobserved, especially when its absence may be explained, as in the case of inflamed cartilages, by some peculiarity of tissue or other condition of the disease. I think it would not be right to call any process inflammation in which there is neither an exudation of lymph (*i. e.* of material capable of such developments or degenerations as I have described), nor a deterioration of the proper tissue of the affected part; even though the other characters of the disease might be present. But, really, whatever rule of nomenclature be adopted, we may expect to meet with many cases in which we shall doubt what name to give to the processes which we watch, or of which we see the results. There is neither here, nor in any other part of pathology, anything like the unity, or circumscription, of species by which the zoologist, whose nomenclature pathologists are prone to imitate, is justified in attaching to each specific name the idea of several constant and unalterable characters in the beings to which it is assigned.

An examination of the very nature of the process of inflammation may best be made in the form of a comparison of its effects with those of the normal process of nutrition. And this comparison may be drawn with two principal views; namely, to determine—1st, how the effects of inflammation differ, in respect of *quantity*, from those of the normal process; and 2d, how they differ from the same, in respect of *quality* or *method*.

The decision on the first of these points may seem to be given in the term "increased action," which is commonly used as synonymous with inflammation. As used by Mr. Hunter, this term was meant to imply that the small vessels of an inflamed part are more than naturally active, in formation or absorption, or in both these processes. This is, probably, the meaning still generally attached to the term by some; while, as employed by those who believe the vessels are only accessories in the work of nutrition, the expression "increased action" may be used to imply merely increased formation, or increased absorption. In either, or in any, meaning, however, the term seems to involve the idea of an increased exercise of vital forces, *i. e.* of those forces through the operation of which the various acts of organic formation are accomplished. But, if "increased action" is to imply this, the description of the process and effects of inflammation shows that the term cannot be properly used, without some limit or qualification.

If we consider the quantity of organic formation effected during the inflammatory process, in the proper substance of the inflamed part, it is evidently less than in health. All the changes described in the last lecture are examples of diminished or suspended nutrition in the tissues of the inflamed part: they are all characteristic of atrophy, degeneration, or death. The tissues become soft, or quite disorganized; they are relaxed and weakened; they degenerate, and remain lowered at once in structure, chemical composition, and functional power; or else, after degeneration, they are absorbed, or are disintegrated, or dissolved, and cast out; they die in particles or in the mass. During all the process of inflammation, there is no such thing as an increased formation of the natural structures of the inflamed part; they are not even maintained: their nutrition is always impaired, or quite suspended. It is only after the inflammation has ceased that there is an increased formation in some of the lowly organized tissues, as the bones and cellular tissue.

So far, then, as the proper substance of the inflamed part is concerned, there appears to be decreased action; that is, decreased formation. There may be, indeed, an increased absorption; but this is also, in one sense, characteristic of decreased exercise of vital force; since all absorption implies a previous degeneration of the part absorbed. Nor can we justly call this, in any sense, "increased action," till we can show how absorption is an action of vessels.

Thus far, one of the constituents of the inflammatory process, one of the characters in which it differs, in respect of quantity, from normal nutrition, is a defect in the nutrition of the proper substance of the inflamed part.

But it is characteristic of the complete process of inflammation, that, while the inflamed structure itself suffers deterioration, there is a production of material which may be peculiarly organized. Here, therefore, may be an evidence of increased formation, of increased action.

Doubtless, in relation to the productive part of the inflammatory process, the expression "increased action" may be in some sense justly used; for the weight of an inflamed part, or of the material separated from it, may be much increased by the formation of organized matter. But the quantity of organized matter formed in an inflammation must not be unconditionally taken as a measure of increase in the exercise of the vital forces: for it is to be observed, that the material formed presents only the lowest grades of organization, and that it is not capable of development, but rather tends to degeneration, so long as the inflammation lasts.

It may be but a vague estimate that we can make of the amount of force exercised in any act of formation; yet we may be sure that a comparatively small amount is sufficient for the production of low organisms, such as are the fibrinous and corpuscular lymphs of inflammation. The abundant production of lowly organized structures is one of the features of the life of the lowest creatures, in both the vegetable and animal kingdoms. And, in our own cases, a corresponding abundant production is often noticed in the lowest states of vital force; witness the final inflammations, so frequent in the last stages of granular degeneration of the kidneys, of phthisis, of cancer, and other exhausting diseases. In all these, even large quantities of the lowly organized cells of inflammatory lymph may be formed, when life is at its last ebb. And with these cases those correspond which show the most rapid increase of tubercle and cancer, and of lowly organized tumors, when the health is most enfeebled, and when the blood and all the natural structures are wasting.

From these considerations we may conclude that the productive part of the inflammatory process is not declaratory of the exercise of a large amount of formative or organizing force; and this conclusion is confirmed by observing that development, which always requires the highest and most favored exercise of the powers of organic life, does not occur while inflammation lasts. The general conclusions, therefore, may be, as well from the productive as from the destructive effects of the inflammatory process, that it is accomplished with small expenditure of vital force; and that even when large quantities of lymph are lowly organized, such an expression as "increased action" cannot be rightly used, unless we can be sure that the defect of the formative power, exercised in the proper tissue of the inflamed part, is more than counterbalanced by the excess employed in the production and low organization of lymph.

It may be said that the signs of inflammation are signs of increased action. But these are fallacious, if, again, by increased action be meant any increased exercise of vital force. The redness and the swelling of the inflamed part declare the presence of more blood; but this blood moves slowly; and it is a quick renewal of blood, rather than a large quantity at any time in a part, that is significant of active life. An abundance of blood, with slow movement of it, is not characteristic of activity in a part; it often implies the contrary, as in the erectile tissues, and the cancellous tissue of bones.

The local increase of heat is too inconstant to afford ground for judging of the nature of inflammation.* When manifest, it is not, I think, to be exactly compared with that of an actively growing part, or of one which is the seat of "determination" of blood, or of "active congestion." In these cases, the heat is high chiefly because the blood, brought quickly from the heart, is quickly renewed; but, in an inflamed part, the blood is not so renewed; it moves more slowly. The heat may, indeed, be in some measure ascribed to this condition; for the quickly moving blood around the inflamed part may communicate its heat to that which is moving more slowly. But the proper heat of inflammation (I mean that which is measurable by the thermometer) cannot, I think, be wholly thus explained.

* See, especially, v. Barensprüng, in Müller's Archiv, 1852, p. 268.

Some of it is, probably, due to the oxidation of the degenerating tissues; a process which we might safely assume to be rapidly going on in the more destructive inflammations, and which is, indeed, nearly proved by some of the evidences of the increased excretion of oxidized substances in inflammations, especially by the increase of phosphates in the urine during inflammation of the brain.* It is far from proved, indeed, that this source of heat is sufficient for the explanation of the increase in an inflamed part; and it may be at once objected that we have no evidence that the hottest inflamed parts are those in which the most destructive processes are going on. Still, in relation to the question, how far the increased heat is a sign of the quantity of formative force that is being exercised, we may argue that, as the general supply of heat in our bodies is derived from oxidation or combustion of wasted tissues or of surplus food, so, in these local augmentations of heat, the source is rather from some similar destruction of organized substances, than from increased formation of them. If it be so, the increased heat will give no ground for regarding the inflammatory process as the result of a greater exercise of formative force than is employed in ordinary nutrition; none for speaking of it as increased nutrition, or increased action. Rather, this sign may be added to the evidences, that the inflammatory process presents, of diminished formative force, and of a premature and rapid degeneration, in the affected part.

In thus endeavoring to estimate the difference between the normal and the inflammatory modes of nutrition, in regard to the quantity of formative or other vital force exercised in them respectively, I have also stated the chief differences in relation to the quality or method of nutrition.

The most general peculiarity of the inflammatory method is the concurrence of the two distinct, though usually coincident, events of which I have spoken at such length; namely, 1st, the impairment or suspension of the nutrition of the proper substance of the inflamed part; and, 2d, the exudation, from the blood, of a material more than sufficient in quantity for the nutrition of the part, but less than sufficient in its capacity of development.

By these concurring, it is plainly distinguished from the normal method of nutrition. The same combination of events establishes the chief differences between the inflammatory and every other mode of nutrition in a part. Thus, from all the forms of mere atrophy or degeneration, the inflammatory process, at least in the typical examples, is distinguished by the production of the lymph, which may be organizing, even while the proper tissue of the inflamed part is in process of atrophy, degeneration, or absorption. So far as the tissues inflamed are con-

* Dr. Bence Jones: On the Contrast between Delirium Tremens and Inflammation of the Brain, Med. Chir. Trans., vol. xxx., p. 37; and Virchow, B. iv., H. 1.

cerned, some inflammations might be classed with atrophies or degenerations; but the concurrent production of lymph is distinctive of them.

On the other side, the inflammatory mode of nutrition is distinguished from hypertrophy by the failure of the nutrition of the inflamed part itself. So far as mere production and formation of organisms are concerned, some inflammations might be paralleled with hypertrophies; but the organization of the lymph commonly falls short of that proper to the part in which it is exuded; and the substance of the part, instead of being augmented, is only replaced by one of lower organization.

And, lastly, from the production of new growths, such as tumors, the inflammatory process is distinguished by this,—that its organized products, though like natural tissues of the body, are usually infiltrated, fused, and interwoven into the textures of the inflamed parts; and that, when once their development is achieved, they have no tendency to increase in a greater ratio than the rest of the body.

I am well aware that these can be accepted as only the generally distinguishing characters of the complete inflammatory process. Cases might be easily adduced in which the border-lines are obscured; inflammations confounded on one side with atrophies, on another with hypertrophies, on a third with tumors, and, on others, with yet other local phenomena of disease. But the same difficulties are in every department of our science; yet we must acknowledge the value of general distinctions among diseases even more alike than these are.

The case that I have chosen for illustrating the general nature of the inflammatory process is one representing the disease in its simplest form and earliest stage, manifesting only the formation of lymph, and such a change as the softening or absorption of the inflamed part. This is but the beginning of the history: but, if the inflammation continues, or increases in severity, all that follows is consistent with this beginning; all displays the same double series of events, the same defective nutrition of the part, and the same production of low organisms. But these additions are observed: the part is more and more deteriorated, and perishes in the mass, or in minute fragments; the newly-organized products, not finding the necessary conditions of nutrition, partake in the degenerative process, and, instead of being developed, are degenerated into pus, or some yet lower forms, or perish with the tissues in which they are imbedded.

Respecting, now, the cause of inflammation, I shall not say more of its exciting causes than that, from the external ones, which alone we can at all appreciate, we may derive a confirmation of the opinion I have expressed concerning the nature of the process. They are such as would be apt to produce depression of the vital forces in a part; all being, I think, such as, when applied with more severity, or for a longer time, lead, not to inflammation, but to the death of the part. If a certain excess of heat will inflame, a certain yet greater heat will kill: if some violence will inflame, a greater violence will kill; if a diluted chemical agent will only irritate, the same concentrated will destroy the part. The same may be said, I think, of cold, and all the other external exciting causes of inflammation. I am aware that other explanations of their actions are given; but none seem to me so simple or so consistent with the nature of the process that follows them, as this, which assumes that they all tend (as it may be said) to depress the vital forces exercised in the affected part. They may be stimulants or excitants of the sensitive nerves of the part, but they lead to the opposite of activity in its nutritive process. In the reaction which follows the application of some of them, they may seem to have been the excitants of nutritive action; but if the inflammatory state ensues, the formative process, we have seen, is really diminished.

The proximate causes, or immediately preceding conditions, of inflammation appear to be various perversions of the necessary conditions of healthy nutrition in a part; that is, morbid changes in either the supply of blood, the composition of the blood, the influence of the nervous force, or the condition of the proper substance of the inflamed part. Any one or more of these four conditions of nutrition being changed in quality may initiate an inflammation. A change of quantity more usually produces either an excess or deficiency of nutrition in the part, or some process different from inflammation. Thus, a diminution or withdrawal of the blood without alteration of its quality is usually followed by atrophy, degeneration, or death: a mere increase of blood in a part may produce hypertrophy, or something more nearly resembling inflammation, yet falling short of it. Similar effects may ensue from a mere increase or decrease, or abstraction, of nervous force. Change in the quality, whether with or without one in the quantity, of the conditions of nutrition, appears essential to the production of the phenomena of inflammation.

I will endeavor now to show that inflammation may follow such perversion or qualitative change in each of the conditions of nutrition, even though all the rest of them remain for a time in their normal state: selecting, for this purpose, such cases of inflammation as we may trace, proceeding, in the first instance, from the uncomplicated error of a single condition of nutrition.

I. Inflammation may perhaps be produced—it certainly may be commenced, and in some measure imitated—by changes in the blood-vessels; changes attended with alteration of their size, or their permeability, or the other qualities by which they affect the supply of blood to a part. This may be concluded from the similarity to some of the phenomena of inflammation which may be observed in certain cases of mechanical obstruction to the venous circulation. In a case of ascites from diseased heart or liver, the peritoneum often contains coagula of fibrine floating free in the serum, though no organ may present appearances of having been inflamed. In such a case, moreover, I have found the fibrine developing itself in the form of nucleated blastema, even while floating free. I another case of mechanical dropsy, I have found the fluid of anasarca in the scrotum containing both fibrine and abundant lymph-corpuscles, like those in the fluid of an inflammatory exudation. In like manner, an apparently uncomplicated obstruction at the left side of the heart may produce many of the phenomena of bronchitis. Such as these are the cases through which mechanical congestions of blood connect themselves with inflammation. And if to these we add the constancy of increased vascularity among the phenomena of inflammation, they may be sufficient to make us believe, that disturbances in the circulation of a part may produce some of the principal phenomena of inflammation, even though all the other conditions of nutrition are, in the first instance, unchanged. But I know no other good evidence for the belief; and I think we should not lay much stress on these cases, since they display an imitation of only some parts of the process of inflammation; namely, the fullness of the vessels, the retarded blood, and the exudation of organizable matter. The nutrition of the proper tissues of a part with merely obstructed circulation suffers but a trivial loss or disturbance, in comparison with that which would accompany an inflammation with an equal amount of retardation in the movement of the blood. So far as the exudation in an inflamed part depends on the altered mechanical relations of the blood and vessels, so far may similar alterations alone produce effects imitating those of inflammation; they may also be the beginning of the more complete process; but I believe that the mere mechanical disturbances of the circulation are no more adequate alone to the explanation of the whole process of inflammation, than the normal movements of the blood are adequate to the explanation of the ordinary process of nutrition.

II. We may speak much less equivocally of the influence of the state of the blood itself in causing inflammations; for there can be little doubt that a very great majority of the so-called spontaneous or constitutional as distinguised from traumatic, inflammations, have herein their origin. We might anticipate this from the consideration that, in normal nutrition, the principal factors are the tissues and the blood in their mutual relations: but we have better evidence than this, in cases of local inflammations occurring in consequence of general diseases of the blood. Some instances of this are clearly proved, as e. g. in the cases of eruptive fevers, when the presence of morbid materials in the blood is proved by the effects of their transference in inoculation. Scarcely less thoroughly demonstrated are the cases of rheumatism and gout, of lepra, psoriasis, herpes, eczema, erysipelas, and other such affections, whose constitutional nature—in other words, whose primary seat in the blood—all readily acknowledge in practice, if not in theory.

Now, in all these cases, local inflammations are the external signs of the general affection of the blood: and I apprehend, that if any difficulty be felt in receiving these as evidences, that the morbid condition of the blood is the cause of the local inflammation, it will be through doubt whether a general disease of the blood—a disease affecting the blood sent to every part—can produce peculiar phenomena of disease in only certain small parts of organs. But this local effect of a general disease of blood, has its illustration in some of the sure principles of physiology; especially in one which I have fully illustrated in a former lecture (p. 33 et seq. and p. 54); namely, that the presence of certain materials in the blood may determine the formation of appropriate organisms, in which they may be incorporated.

It is in exact parallel with the facts in physiology which I then adduced, that in certain general diseases of the blood, organs are formed, as the products of inflammation, within which the specific morbid material is incorporated. Thus, in small-pox, cow-pox, primary syphilis, and whatever other diseases may be transferred by inoculation, the morbid material from the blood is incorporated in the products of inflammation, which are enclosed within the characteristic vesicle or pustule, or infiltrated lymph, just as, in the cases already cited, the constituents of urine or of medicines are incorporated in the renal cells, which are formed within the substance of the kidney; or just as the constituents of sap are incorporated in fruit.

In the cases of disease produced by a demonstrable virus, we have all the evidence that can be necessary to prove the principle, that a general disease of the blood may be the cause of a local inflammation in one or more circumscribed portions of a tissue. And the analogy is so close, that I think we need not hesitate to receive the same explanation of other inflammations, which I have cited as occurring during morbid conditions of the blood. For although we cannot, by inoculation, prove that a specific morbid material of such a disease as herpes or eczema, gout or rheumatism, has been incorporated in the inflammatory products, yet we find great probability hereof in the many analogies which these diseases present to the inoculable diseases, in their whole history, and, especially, in the decrease or modification of general illness which ensues on the full manifestation of the local inflammation.

If it be asked why a morbid material is determined to one part or tissue rather than another, or why, for example, the skin is the normal seat of inflammation in small-pox, the joints in rheumatism, and so on, I believe we must say that we are, on this point, in the same ignorance as we are concerning the reason why the materials of sweat are discharged at the skin, those of urine at the kidneys, of bile at the liver, or why the greater part of the albuminous principles are incorporated in the muscles, and of the gelatinous in the bones. We cannot tell why these things are so, but they are familiar facts, and parallel with what I here assume of the incorporation of morbid materials derived from the blood.

Again, it may be said that we need some explanation of the fact that the morbid condition of the blood does not influence the whole extent of any given tissue, but only portions of it.   In the secretion of urine, it may be believed that the whole kidney is affected and works alike; but in the assumed separation of the virus of small-pox, only patches of the skin are the seats of pustules; in vaccinia and primary syphilis, only a single point; in secondary and tertiary syphilis, a certain, but sometimes disorderly, succession of various parts; and so on.

It must be admitted that many of the facts here referred to cannot yet be explained.   In some cases, however, we can assign, with much probability, the conditions that determine the locality in which a general disease of the blood will manifest itself by inflammation.   In some instances, it is evident that the localization is determined by such as we may call a weakened or depressed condition, a state of already impaired nutrition, in some one part.   For instance, when a stream of cold air is impelled on some part, say the shoulder, of a person disposed to rheumatism, it determines, as a more general exposure to cold might do in the same person, the rheumatic state of the blood, with all its general symptoms; but it determines, besides, the part in which that rheumatic state shall manifest itself first or alone.   The depressed nutrition of the chilled shoulder makes it more liable than any other part to be the seat of inflammation excited by the diseased blood.

Or, again, when a virus is inserted, as in all cases of poisoned wounds, the local inflammation produced by the disease with which the whole blood is infected will commonly have its seat in the wounded part.   The virus must have produced some change in the place in which it was inserted, as well as in the whole mass of the blood.   The change is not merely that of a wound; for a simple wound made in the same person, at the same time, will not similarly inflame; it is a change due to the direct influence of the virus.   And the part thus changed may long remain in a peculiar morbid state, and peculiarly prone to inflammation from diseased blood.   Thus, an infant was vaccinated in the middle of June, and the disease had its usual course; six ordinary vesicles formed in the punctures in the left arm, and common cicatrices remained, and all appeared well.   In the middle of July, inflammation of the left axillary glands ensued.   When I saw the child on August 21st, the glands were very large, and partially suppurated, and there was extensive inflammation of the skin of the upper arm.   On August 30th, the pus having been partially discharged by incision, the glands had subsided, but superficial inflammation of the integuments existed still, and now there was, on the middle of each vaccine cicatrix, a distinct circular low vesicle, not unlike that of the true vaccine eruption, except that it was not umbilicated, and appeared to have an undivided cavity.

Such cases are, probably, only examples of a general rule, that a part whose natural force of nutrition is in any way depressed, is, more than a healthy part, liable to become the seat of chief manifestation of a general blood-disease. A part that has been the seat of former disease or injury, and that has never recovered its vigor of nutrition, is always so liable; it is *a weak part.* Thus, the old gouty or rheumatic joint is apt to receive the brunt of the new attack. And the same may happen in a more general way. A man was under my care with chronic inflammation of the synovial membrane of his knee, and general swelling about it: he was attacked with measles, and the eruption over the diseased knee was a diffused bright scarlet rash. A patient under Dr. Budd's care had small-pox soon after a fall on the nates: the pustules were thinly scattered everywhere, except in the seat of former injury, and on this they were crowded as thickly as possible. Thus, too, when a part has been injured, and, it may be, is healing, a disease having begun in the blood will manifest itself in this part. Impetigo appears about blows and scratches in unhealthy children; erysipelas about the same in men with unhealthy blood.

Such are some of the cases in which we seem able to explain the apparent choice of locality for inflammation, made by a morbid material which is diffused through all the blood. Many remain unexplained; if it were not so, this portion of pathology would be a singular exception to the general condition of the science. But these difficulties afford no warrant for the rejection of a theory, of which the general probability is affirmed by so many analogies, by the sufficiency of its terms for the expression of the facts, and, it may be added, by nearly every particular in the constitutional treatment of local inflammation. For, I suppose there are few parts of the medicinal treatment of local inflammation, for which any reason can be shown, unless it be assumed that the medicine corrects some morbid condition of the blood.

Let it be added that the state of the blood may, in part, or chiefly, determine, not only the locality, but also the degree and form of the inflammation. It may, as Dr. Ormerod has well expressed it, "imprint on the morbid product (of inflammation) certain tendencies which take effect after the morbid products have entered upon a condition of comparatively independent existence."* But on this point I need not dwell; for a large portion of Lecture XIV. is devoted to it, and it will be again considered in the Lecture on Specific Diseases.

To test the influence of a disturbance of the nervous force in engendering the inflammatory process, we must not, as is commonly done, take cases of the effects of external injury. Such an injury, or the presence

* In his Lectures on the Pathology and Treatment of Valvular Disease of the Heart, in the Medical Gazette, 1851. These should have been cited before, as containing the fullest demonstration of the principle referred to here; and at p. 219.

of a foreign body, is supposed to excite inflammation by stimulating the nerves of the part, and by changing, through their influence, the state or action of the blood-vessels. This may be true; but we should remember that when a common injury is inflicted, it acts not only on the nerves of the part, but also on its proper tissues; and it may so affect the state of these tissues, that the changes produced in them may be the excitant of inflammation, independent of the affection of the nerves. All such cases as these are, thus, ambiguous.

For a better test, we must select cases in which the excitant of inflammation acts (at least in the first instance) on the nervous system alone. Such cases are those already referred to (p. 208). When the conjunctiva is inflamed after over-working of the eye, we cannot suppose that the light, by its direct contact, has affected the vessels, or the nutritive act, in the conjunctiva: it can, probably, affect either of these only through an influence reflected from the retina. So, when irritation of the urethra excites inflammation in the testicle; when the irritation of teething excites it in any distant part; when, as in a case quoted from Lallemand, by Dr. Williams, inflammation of the brain followed the application of a ligature to part of the brachial plexus; in these and the like cases we cannot but refer to the disturbance of the nervous force as the initiator of the phenomena of inflammation.

Now, for the explanation of such cases as these, there appear to be two chief theories: 1. It may be that the nerves distributed to the minute blood-vessels of a part may be so affected that these vessels may dilate, and their dilatation may produce the other phenomena of inflammation; or, 2. The disturbance of the nervous force may more directly interfere with the process of nutrition, inasmuch as this force exercises always some influence in the nutrition of each part, and is (as one may say) one among the plasturgic forces (p. 40).

The first of these theories has lately acquired a dominant place in systems of pathology, especially in those of Germany. The principal form of it, which has been maintained most prominently by Henle, has enlisted the approval of even Rokitansky, and is largely received, professing to explain all inflammations, and passing by the name of "neuro-pathological," to distinguish it from the "humoral," and all other theories of inflammation. This theory may be thus briefly stated. The exciting cause of inflammation, whether an external cause, such as an injury of a part, or an internal one, such as diseased blood, acts, in the first instance, on the sensitive, centripetal, or afferent nerves of the part. These it affects as a stimulant, producing in them an excited state, which state, being conveyed to some nervous centre, is thence reflected on the centrifugal or motor nerves of the blood-vessels of the same, or some other related part. This reflection, however, is supposed to bring about a kind of antagonistic sympathy, such that, instead of exciting the motor forces of the blood-vessels to make them contract, it paralyzes them, and is followed by their dilitation or relaxation. This dilitation being established, the exudation and other phenomena of inflammation are assumed to follow as natural, and most of them as mechanical, consequences.

The eminence of those who have supported this hypothesis makes one hesitate in rejecting it; and yet I cannot help believing it to be groundless. If we remember that parts may present some of the chief phenomena of inflammation, though they have no nerves, as the firmest tendons and articular cartilages; that the degrees of inflammation in parts bear no proportion to the amounts of pain in them when inflamed; that the severest pains may endure for very long periods with only trivial, if any, phenomena of inflammation; that the phenomena of the so-called reflex paralysis are rare, equivocal, and altogether insufficient for the foundation of a law or general principle; we may well think that there can be no sufficient ground for the invention of such an hypothesis as this. And, if we add that, even admitting the dilatation of blood-vessels as a possible consequence of the stimulus of sensitive nerves, yet the phenomena of even simple inflammation would be no necessary consequences thereof; that the varieties of inflammations would be quite unintelligible as results of similar mechanical disturbances of the circulation; and that the dilatation of blood-vessels, in any mechanical way produced, is followed by only feeble imitations of a part of the inflammatory process; then we may think that the hypothesis, if all its postulates be granted, will yet be insufficient for the explanation of the facts.

I believe that, if we would have any clear thoughts respecting the influence of the nerves in initiating inflammations, we must first receive the theory already referred to (p. 40 and 208), that a certain exercise of the nervous force is habitually and directly engaged in the act of normal nutrition. If we admit this, there can be no difficulty in believing, whatever there may be in explaining, that the perturbations of the nervous force may engender the inflammatory mode of nutrition more directly, than by first paralysing the blood-vessels of a part. We attain nearly to a proof of this in the instances of altered nutrition adduced in a former lecture (p. 41), and in those of secretions altered, not in quantity alone, but in quality, by affections of the nervous system. It is almost inconceivable that any of the essential properties of a secretion should be changed by an alteration in the quantity or movement of the blood in a gland: yet such changes are frequently manifest in the milk, tears, urine, and sweat, under the influence of mental affections of the nervous force; and the analogies of secretion and nutrition give these cases nearly the weight of proof, in the question of the influence of the disturbed nervous force in causing inflammations.

IV. The last of the necessary conditions of normal nutrition in a part is the healthy state of the part itself; and it appears highly probable that a disturbance of this may initiate, and, in this sense, be the cause of, inflammation. This is probable for many reasons; and, first, from analogy with normal nutrition. Generally, the principal conditions of nutrition are in the relative and mutual influences of the elements of the tissues and the blood. More particularly, the state of the tissues determines, at least in great measure, both the quantity and the rate of movement of the blood supplied to them; the changes of the tissues, whether in growth or decrease, usually just preceding the adapted changes in the supply of blood (p. 58). So, we may believe, a change in a part anyhow engendered may, by altering its relation to the blood, alter its mode of nutrition; and some of the changes may produce the inflammatory mode of nutrition, together with the altered supply of blood, and other characteristic signs. I am disposed to think such changes would be especially effective, as causes of inflammation, when they ensue in the rudimental and still developing elements of the tissue; for, as it seems to be chiefly these which determine the normal supply of blood in a part, so, probably, the abnormal state of them would most affect that supply.

Secondly, we may judge the same from the analogy between inflammation and the process of repair. Certainly it is the state of the injured part, i. e. of its proper tissues, not of its nerves and blood-vessels, which initiates the processes of repair. Now some of these are so like those of inflammation, that they are commonly identified, and are not capable of even a refined distinction. This is, especially, the case with the articular cartilages, and the cornea.*

And thirdly, the influence of the condition of the proper tissues of a part in initiating inflammation in it, is illustrated by more direct facts; such as, that injuries of parts that have no vessels or nerves are followed by altered modes of nutrition, which are more or less exact resemblances of inflammation. Thus e. g. it is in the cornea, lens, vitreous humor, and the like, after injury. In all of these, it is difficult to imagine any other cause of inflammation than the altered relations between the tissue and the blood or the materials derived from it.

On the whole, therefore, I think we may conclude that inflammation may have its origin in disturbance of the normal condition of the proper tissues of a part; in such a disturbance as may be produced by injury, or by the proximity of disease. To this source, indeed, I should be disposed to refer nearly all inflammations that originate in the direct application of local stimuli, whether mechanical or chemical. It is true, that in most cases, the stimulus affects at once the proper elements of the part, its nerves, and its blood-vessels, so that we cannot say how much of the disease is to be ascribed to the affection of each; but the fact that a process, resembling, so far as it goes, that of inflammation, may ensue after injury in parts that have neither vessels nor nerves, may make

* See Dr. Redfern's researches, l. c., and compare Mr. Bowman's account of the healing of wounds in the cornea, in his Lectures on the Parts concerned in Operations on the Eye, p. 29, with the observations already quoted from Virchow.

one believe that, in parts that have both, the inflammation depends mainly on injury, or other affection, of the proper tissue.

I have thus endeavored to show that inflammation may take its rise, may have its proximate cause, in a disturbance of any one of the conditions of nutrition. In the examination of different cases, we find that, even while any three of the four chief conditions may be normal, yet a qualitative error of the fourth may bring in the phenomena of the inflammatory process. In the necessity of choosing pointed cases, I may seem to have implied that it is usual for inflammation not only to begin, but to be maintained, by an error in one of the conditions of nutrition: but this is improbable. Rather we may believe, that many of the excitants of inflammation may affect at once more than one of these conditions; and, as I stated in the first lecture on the subject, it is nearly certain that in every inflammation, after a short continuance, all the conditions of the nutritive process are alike involved in error.

The following are references to some of the recent essays on inflammation, from which the reader, if he have learned the main principles concerning the disease from some of the classical works upon it,—such as those of Hunter, Thomson, Alison, or Gendrin,—may gather the best facts and guidance for future inquiry.

J. Hughes Bennett: On Inflammation as an Anormal Process of Nutrition. Edinburgh, 1844.—And in the first of a Series of Clinical Lectures published in the Monthly Journal of Medical Sciences, from 1850, onwards.

Bruecke (as quoted by Lebert): Bemerkungen über Entzundung; in the Sitzungsberichte der Weiner Akademie. June and July, 1849.

Carpenter: In an article in the British and Foreign Medical Review, vol. xviii. p. 91. July, 1844.

Andrew Clark: In the Medical Gazette, vol. xlii. p. 286; and in subsequent numbers.

Gluge: Pathologische Histologie, 4to. Jena, 1850.

Henle: Rationelle Pathologie, B. i. And in his Zeitschrift, especially the 2d volume.

G. W. Humphrey: Lectures on Surgery; in the Provincial Medical and Surgical Journal 1849, and following years.

Wharton Jones: On the State of the Blood and the Blood-vessels in Inflammation; in Guy's Hospital Reports, vol. vii. 1851.

Kliss (as often quoted by Lebert and Virchow): De la Vascularité et de l'Inflammation. 1846.

Lebert: Physiologie Pathologique, t. i. 8vo. 1845.—And in later works; especially in papers communicated to the Gazette Medicale: Juillet 15 et 22, 1852. In these he speaks of a large work on Inflammation which he is preparing for the press.

Redfern: Anormal Nutrition in Articular Cartilages. Edinburgh, 1850. And, especially in an Appendix to a Paper in the Monthly Journal of Medical Science, Sept. 1851.

Reinhardt: Ueber die Genesis der mikrosk, Elemente in den Entzündungsproducten; in Traübe's Beiträge, H. ii. 1846.

Rokitansky: Pathologische Anatomie, B. i.

Simon: Lectures on General Pathology. In the Lancet, 1850; and, collected, 8vo. London, 1850.

Travers: Physiology of Inflammation and the Healing Process, 8vo. 1844.

Virchow: Essays in the 1st and 3d, and especially in the 5th volumes of his Archiv für Pathologische Anatomie. And in the 1st volume of the Verhandlungen der phys.-med. Gesellschaft in Würzburg.

H. Weber: Experimente über die Stase in der Froschschwimmhaut, in Muller's Archiv, H. iv. 1852. In this essay, which I did not receive till this sheet was in the press, the

19

author relates experiments showing that all the essential phenomena of the stagnation of blood in the capillaries and small vessels of the frog's web, after the application of stimuli, may be produced as well when the circulation has been stopped by ligature round the limb, as when the circulation is free. His observations, with others that he promises, appear likely to elucidate that phenomena of the movement of blood in inflamed parts for which, as I have said (p. 204), the usual mechanical explanations seem insufficient.

C. J. B. Williams: Principles of Medicine, 8vo. 1843 and 1848.

The process of inflammation, so far as it can be illustrated by specimens, may be fully studied in the Museum of the College, in the preparations Nos. 71 to 129, and in those which are referred to after the descriptions of those in the 1st volume of the Pathological Catalogue. Many of the facts relating to the state of the blood-vessels, also, are illustrated by the microscopic specimens in the same Museum. All the best illustrations of the process, in the Museum of St. Bartholomew's, may be studied by the references in the Catalogue, vol. i. p. xii.

LECTURE XIX.

MORTIFICATION.

By Mortification, or Sphacelus, is meant the death of any portion of the body, while the rest remains living. The term "gangrene" is commonly used in the same sense; "necrosis" for similar death of portions of bone or cartilage, or, in some recent writers, of any other tissue; "necræmia" for a corresponding death of the blood. The dead piece of tissue is called a "slough," or, if it be bone, a "sequestrum." The process of progressive dying is commonly called "sloughing," a term which is, however, also applied to the process by which a slough is separated, with the same meaning as "exfoliation" is used for the process of separating a "sequestrum" or dead piece of bone. None of these terms, however, are used unless the portions of dead tissue be visible to the naked eye. It is probable that what is ejected from the tissues in the ulcerative process is quite dead; but, so long as it is in the form of minute particles, visible only with the microscope, we speak of the disease as ulceration, not sloughing or mortification. The two processes are, however, often mingled, and can be only in general terms, and in well-marked examples, distinguished (p. 272).

It might, also, be difficult to define, in precise terms, this death of parts from some examples of their degeneration. We may doubt, sometimes, whether the degenerative changes, imitated, as certain of them are, by chemical changes in the tissues after death, are not consequences of the total cessation of the influence of vital forces; and it seems nearly certain that degeneration of a part may proceed to its death, and is very apt to do so when, during progress, many of the conditions of nutrition are at once interfered with. In a general view we may distinguish the degeneration of a part from its death by this—that the degenerate part never becomes putrid, and that no process ensues for its separation or isolation, such as we can see in the case of a dead part. However degenerate a tissue may be, it either remains in continuity with those around it, or is absorbed. If the same tissue were dead, those around it would separate from it, and it would be ejected from them.

Still, it may not be pretended that degeneration and death are separated by a strong border-line. Rather, many of the instances of mortification to which I am about to refer may be read as histories of the transition of one of these conditions to the other. It will appear that a part may degenerate even to death while the rest of the body remains alive; that, as a certain diminution of the supply of arterial blood may lead to degeneration, so a greater diminution may lead to death; that, as a certain amount of inflammation has always in it a defective nutrition of the inflamed part, so, in a greater amount, the death of the same part ensues; and that the same agent may kill one portion of a tissue and inflame the portions around it. Of all such cases we might say that the local death is the extreme of degeneration.

A convenient method of studying the causes of mortification may be to divide those among them that are explicable into the direct and the indirect; i. e. into such as disorganize and kill the tissues at once, and directly, though sometimes slowly, and such as do so indirectly, by depriving them of some or all of the conditions of their nutrition. Such a division, however, must not lead us to forget that, in many cases, mortification is the result of many concurring causes of both kinds.

I. In the first class we may reckon the mortifications that are the extremes of degeneration. But these can rarely be observed in unmixed examples. The more evident instances are those which result from great heat, rapidly decomposing chemical agents, and severe mechanical injury. The appearances of the dead tissues are, in these cases, modified by the presence of blood in those that are vascular, and by the blood being killed in and with them: but the state of the blood is no cause of their death; the tissues and the contained blood are killed together; and the same mode and consequences of mortification would be manifested in the non-vascular tissues.

Now, as I just suggested, it may be observed of all these destructive agents, that when they are applied in smaller measure, the effect of the injury is not to kill the part at once, but to excite an inflammation in it; and the inflammatory degeneration, thus added to the damage the part sustained from the direct effect of the injury, may lead to an indirect or secondary mortification. To this mixed origin, probably, many of the cases of traumatic grangrene may be ascribed, which are not manifest very speedily after the injury; in these we may say that a severe injury has so nearly disorganized a part, that the subsequent inflammation, with the concurrent defective nutrition, has completed · its death. But, mechanical violence, heat, or chemical action, may kill a tissue at once, without the intervention of inflammation; and although, in the case of the vascular tissues, it is scarcely possible to separate the influence of the injury on their proper elements, from that which is, at the same time, inflicted on their blood and vessels, yet we must consider the phenomena of mortification as having their seat, essentially, in the elements of the tissues. Whatever we understand as the life of a part, that life may cease; and as the life of a part is its own property, maintained, indeed, by the blood and other conditions of nutrition, yet not derived from them, so may that life cease, or, as it is said, be destroyed, without interference of the blood or any other exterior conditions of nutrition.

The immediateness of such death of a part is shown by the rapidity with which it is manifested. It is nearly instantaneous on the application of extreme heat or the strongest mechanical agents; slower after mechanical injury: but within twelve hours of the infliction of a blow the struck or crushed part may be evidently dead; there may be little or no ecchymosis, no sign of inflammation, no pain, except that which directly followed the injury, and, in the case of a bone, no apparent change of texture; but the piece of tissue is killed in the midst of the living parts; its recovery, by the re-establishment of its relations with the blood, is not possible: it cannot even be absorbed.

II. Among the instances of indirect mortification of parts, the most numerous are those in which nutrition is made impossible by some defect either (1) in the quantity, or (2), in the movement of the blood.

Defects in the quantity of blood have been already noticed as leading to death of parts (p. 37). The following are the chief general methods of the events:—

The main artery of a part may be closed by pressure, or by some internal obstruction. Thus, sometimes, sloughing of the foot or leg follows ligature of the femoral artery for popliteal aneurism; or sloughing of part of the brain may follow ligature of the common carotid artery; and in this case, the difference, and yet the close relation, between the death of a part and its degeneration, are well shown (compare p. 37 and 103). Thus, also, through equal internal obstruction of main arteries, sloughing may follow blows which crack the internal and middle coats, and let them fold inwards across the stream of blood: * or, the blocking of masses of fibrine, washed from the left valves of the heart, and arrested in the iliac or some other artery: † or the closure of inflamed arteries.

Portions of tissue may similarly perish when, by injury, or by progressive ulceration or absorption, all their minute blood-vessels are destroyed, and their supply of blood cut off. Thus necrosis may follow

---

* Two such specimens are in the Museum of St. Bartholomew's.
† See Dr. Kirkes's essay in Med.-Chir. Trans., vol. xxxv.

the separation of periosteum from the surface of a bone; when it is either violently stripped off, or raised by effused blood, or by suppuration beneath it. Thus, also, sometimes, as an abscess approaches the surface, the thinned skin dies; and, not like an inflamed part, but as one deprived of nutriment, it shrivels and is dried. Such sloughing is more common in perforating ulcers of the stomach or intestines; in the course of which, when ulceration has destroyed a portion of the subperitoneal tissue and its blood-vessels, the peritoneum, hitherto fed by them, perishes, and is separated as a grayish or yellowish-white slough. In like manner, ulceration, in its progress, may so undermine or intrench a part, that at length it dies through defect of blood: thus, often, small fragments of bone are detached in strumuous disease of the tarsus and other parts. And, similarly, through mere defect of blood, the centre of a tumor may slough: and here, again, is manifest the relation between the death, and the more frequent degeneration, of an imperfectly nourished part.

The effect of pressure constantly maintained on a part may be a similarly produced mortification; the part may die because its blood is pressed from it and not renewed; but more commonly, as we see in bed sores, inflammation ensues, and the death of the part has a double or mixed origin.

Senile grangrene, also, is, without doubt, in many cases, due, in a measure, to defective quantity of blood: but it is a more complicated example of mortification than any of the foregoing, and I shall therefore again refer to it.

I have said that parts may die through defective movement of blood. It may be present in sufficient or excessive quantity; but it may be fatally stagnant. So far as the proper elements of the tissue are concerned, there may be little difference in their modes of death, or in their subsequent changes, in these two sets of cases; but, as seen in the mass, the tissue dead through defect of blood is very different from that dead through stagnation of blood. In the former, we find little more than its own structures dried and shrunken or disorganized; in the latter, the materials of abundant blood, and often of substances exuded from the congested vessels, lie mingled with the proper structures, having died with them. Hence, mainly, the differences between the mortifications distinguished as the dry and moist grangrenes; or as the cold and hot, the white and the black, gangrenes; these being, respectively, the technical terms for parts dead through defect, or through stagnation, of blood.

This stagnation of blood may ensue in many ways. The simplest is when a part is strangulated; as the contents of a hernial sac may be. If the strangulation is sudden and complete, the stagnation is equally so, and the death of the part follows very quickly, with little excess of blood in it. But, if the strangulation be less in degree, or be more slowly completed, the veins suffer more in the gradual compression than the arteries do: the vessels of the part thus become gorged with blood, admitted into them in larger quantity than it can leave them, and so mortification ensues after intense congestion or inflammation of all the tissues.*

Mere passive congestion of the vessels of a part may, in enfeebled persons, lead to mortification: but this is a rare event, for unless a part be injured, or of itself already degenerate, it may be maintained by a very slow movement of the blood.

The congestion which more commonly leads to mortification is that which forms part of the inflammatory process. It is, perhaps, to be regretted that the cases of this class should have been taken as if they were the simplest types of the process of mortification, and that the process should have been studied as an appendage, a so-called termination, of inflammation : for, in truth, the death of an inflamed part is a very complex matter ; and in certain examples of it, all the more simple causes of mortification may be involved. Thus (1) the inflammatory congestion may end in stagnation of the blood, and this, as an indirect cause of mortification, may lead to the death of the blood, and that of the tissues that need moving blood for their support. But (2) a degeneration of the proper textures is a constant part of the inflammatory process; and this degeneration may itself proceed to death, while it is concurrent with defects in the conditions of nutrition. And (3) the exudation of fluid in some inflamed parts may so compress, and by the swelling so elongate, the blood-vessels, as to diminish materially the influx of fresh blood, even when little of that already in the part is stagnant.

All these, and perhaps other, conditions may concur in the mortification of an inflamed part; and their united force is commonly the more effective, by being exercised in a previously defective or degenerate condition of the inflamed tissue. The second of them, I think, has been too little considered ; for by it, more than by any other event, we may understand the sloughing that ensues in the inflamed parts of enfeebled persons. The intensity of an inflammation is not, alone, a measure of the probability of mortification ensuing in its course: neither is mere debility; for we daily see inflammation without death of parts in the feeblest patients with phthisis and other diseases : rather when mortification happens in an inflamed part, it seems to be through the occurrence of the disease in those that have degenerate tissues because of old age or defective food or other materials for life, or through habitual intemperance. It is as if the death of the part were the consequence of the defective nutrition, which concurs with the rest of the inflammatory process, being superadded to that previously existing in the part. To the same occurrence we may, in some measure, ascribe the mortification of parts after comparatively slight injuries in the aged and intemperate: already degenerate, they perish through the addition of what, in heal-

* This difference in the effects of constrictions of parts is particularly described by Sir B. C. Brodie : Lectures on Surgery and Pathology, p. 304.

thier persons, would have led to only some degeneration, or to the inflammatory process, in the injured part. Such cases as these, also, stand in no distant relation to those of the mortification that ensues in inflammations after injuries. And with these we may probably class the similar effects of intense cold. Cold alone does not, in general, directly kill a part, whether in cold or in warm-blooded animals: the death that ensues appears to be the result of inflammation in the part that was cold or frozen.

Such may be the explanations of the local death that may occur in inflammation; but, in many more cases of what appear as mortifications in inflamed parts, the death is the first event in the process, and the inflammation appears as its consequence; or else the death and the inflammation are coincident in different parts of the same tissue. To these cases I shall again refer.

In senile gangrene we commonly find a very large number of conditions ministering to the death of the affected part. First, occurring, as its name implies, in the old, and often in those that are old in structure rather than in years, it affects tissues already degenerate, and at the very extremity and most feebly nourished part of the body. I think that, in some cases, its beginning may be when the progressive degeneration of the part has arrived at death. But, if this do not happen, some injury or disease, even a very trivial one, kills that which was already nearly dead; as a severe injury might kill any part, however actively alive. Now, when death has thus commenced, it may in the same manner extend more widely and deeply, with little or no sign of attendant disease; the parts may successively die, blacken, and become dry and shriveled; in this case, the senile gangrene is a dry one. But, more commonly, when a portion of a toe or of the foot has thus died, the parts around or within it become inflamed: and in these, degenerate as they were already, the further degeneration of the inflammatory process is destructive; and thus, or in this extent, by progressive inflammation and death, the gangrene, moist, though senile, spreads. In either case, the extension of the gangrene is favored by many other things; especially by the defective muscular and elastic power, and by the narrowing or obstruction, of the degenerate arteries of the part; by the defective movement of the blood, readily inducing a passive congestion or stagnation in the parts of its course; by an enfeebled heart; by the blood being, like the tissues, old, and doubtless, like them, defective; and by the aptness of the slow-moving blood to coagulate in the vessels. All these favor the occurrence and extension of the senile gangrene: one or more of them may, sometimes, be the efficient cause of it: but my impression is, that it is essentially, and in the first instance, due, either to senile degeneration having reached its end in local death, or to the fatal superaddition of an inflammatory degeneration in a part already scarcely living.

III. In the foregoing cases, we seem able, in some measure, to explain the occurrence of mortification. But there are yet many cases in which explanation, except in the most general and vague terms, is far more difficult. In some, the local death is to be ascribed to defective quality of the blood, or to morbid materials in it. Among these, the instances of sloughing of the cornea observed in animals, and more rarely in men, whose food is deficient in nitrogen; and those of mortifications of the extremities that have ensued after eating rye with ergot, may prove the general principle,—that certain parts, even small and circumscribed parts, may die through defects or errors of the blood, which yet do not quite hinder its maintaining the rest of the body. They may, thus, be types of a large class of cases, in all of which the death of a portion of tissue seems to ensue through some wrong in the blood by which their mutual influence is destroyed; of which cases, therefore, we may say that, as there are morbid conditions of the whole blood in which local inflammations may have their origin, so are there others in which local deaths have theirs.

Boils and carbuncles, for example, are of this kind. The sloughs, so often separated from them, are pale and bloodless; they are not portions of the tissue that have died in consequence of stagnation of blood in them: they are white sloughs in the midst of inflamed parts. In boils, the first event of the disease may appear in the small central slough; in such cases, the surrounding inflammation may appear to be the consequence of the slough; but, much more probably, it is the result of a lesser influence of the same morbid condition of the blood. In the idiopathic sloughing of the cellular tissue of the scrotum, the local death is evidently, in some cases, the first event of the disease. To this class, also, of mortifications in consequence of morbid conditions of the blood, we must refer, I presume, the cases of hospital gangrene; those of the most severe and most rapidly extending traumatic kind; those of the sloughings of mucous membranes and other parts, that sometimes ensue in typhus, scarlet fever, and other allied diseases, when they deviate from their ordinary course; the sloughing of syphilitic sores, and many others.

Lastly, we may enumerate among the causes of death of parts, the defect of nervous force: but the examples of this have been related in a former lecture (p. 42);* and it only needs, perhaps, to be said here that this defect may mingle its influence with many other more obvious causes of mortification. When a part is severely injured, its nerves suffer proportionate violence, and their defective force may add to the danger of mortification; in the old, not the blood, of the tissues alone, are degenerate, but the nervous structures also; and defective nervous force may be, in them, counted among the many conditions favorable to the senile

* There are yet many cases which I can neither explain nor classify; such as those from the effects of animal poisons, malignant pustule, peculiar gangrenes of the skin, and many others. On all these, and, indeed, on the whole subject of mortifications, the reader will find no work that he can study with so much profit as the lectures of Sir B. C. Brodie.

gangrene; and so, yet more evidently, the sloughing of compressed parts is peculiarly rapid and severe when those parts are deprived of nervous force by injury of the spinal cord, or otherwise.

While the causes of mortification are so manifold; while it is in fact, the end of so many different affections, it is not strange that the appearances of the dying and dead parts should be extremely various. The changes in them (independent of those produced by great heat, caustics, and other such disorganizing agents) may be referred to three chief sources: namely, (1) those that ensue in the dying and dead tissues; (2) those in the blood, dying with the tissues, and often accumulated in them in unnatural abundance; (3) those which are due to the inflammation or other disease or injury, which has preceded the death of the part, and of which the products die with the tissue and the blood, and change with them after death.

But though we may thus classify the morbid changes in mortified parts, yet we can hardly enumerate the varieties which, in each class, are due to the previous diseases of the part, or to external conditions; such as differences of temperature, of moisture, and others. All the chemical changes which, in life, are repaired and unobserved, are here cumulative; all those external forces are now submitted to, which, while the parts were living, they seemed to disregard; so exactly were they adjusted in counter-action. It is, therefore, only in typical examples that mortifications can be well described. The technical terms applied to them have been already mentioned; and "dry" and "moist" signify the chief differences dependent on the quantity of blood and of inflammatory products in the dead parts. "Dry gangrene" is usually preceded by diminished supply of blood to the part; "moist or humid gangrene" by increased supply, and often by inflammation; the former, more slowly progressive, is usually a "chronic," or, as some have called it, "cold gangrene;" the latter an "acute or hot gangrene."

Among the examples of mortification due to defective supply of blood, and therefore classed as dry gangrenes, great differences of appearance are due to the degrees in which the dead parts can be tried. As it may be observed in the integuments of the leg, for example, it may be noticed that, in the first instance, the part about to die appears livid, or mottled with various dusky shades of purple, brown, or indigo, through which it seems to pass as its colors change from the dull ruddiness of stagnant or tardy blood towards the blackness of complete death. It becomes colder, and gradually insensible; its cuticle separates, and is raised in blisters by a serous or more or less blood-colored or brownish fluid. Then, as the cuticle breaks and is removed, the subjacent integument, hitherto kept moist, being now exposed to the air, gradually becomes drier; withering, mummifying, becoming dark brown and black, having a mouldy rather than a putrid smell; it is changed, as Rokitansky says,*

* Pathologische Anatomie, i. p. 237.

like organic substances decomposed with insufficient moisture and with separation of free carbon. Such are the changes often seen in the dry senile gangrene, and in that which may follow obstruction of the main arteries in young persons: but, very generally, as the interior parts of the limb cannot be dried so quickly as the exterior, and are, perhaps, less completely deprived as their supply of blood, they, or portions of them, become soft and putrid, while the integuments become dry and musty.

In other cases of mortification similarly caused, the dead parts, though deprived of blood, cannot become dry; either they are not exposed to air, or they are soaked with fluid exuded near them. In these instances the sloughs may be dark; but they are commonly nearly white; and hence one of the grounds for the technical distinction of white and black gangrene. Such white sloughs are commonly seen when the peritoneum mortifies, after being deprived of blood by ulceration gradually deepening in the walls of the digestive canal; and, sometimes, in the integuments over an abscess, when the cuticle has not previously separated. If this have happened, the dead and undermined integument may become dry and horny; but if the cuticle remain, it is commonly white, soft, and putrid.

The typical examples of the moist gangrene are those which occur in inflamed parts, and chiefly in consequence of inflammation, and to which, therefore, the names of "acute" and "hot" gangrene have been applied.

We must not reckon among these the cases in which the death of the part precedes, or has a common origin with, the inflammation; for in these, as in boils, carbuncles, and hospital gangrene, the slough is commonly bloodless, white or yellowish, or grayish-white, and, if it were not immersed in fluid, would probably be dry and shriveled. The mortification that occurs during inflammation, and as in part a consequence of it, finds the tissues full of blood, and often of exuded lymph and serum, which all perish with them.

If such a process be watched in an inflammation involving the integuments, or in senile gangrene rapidly progressive with inflammation, or, as in the most striking instance, in the traumatic gangrene following a severe injury of a limb, the parts that were swollen, full red, and hot, and perhaps very tense and painful, become mottled with overspreading shades of dusky brown, green, blue, and black. These tints, in mortification after injuries, may, sometimes, seem at first like the effects of ecchymoses; and often, after fractures of the leg, a further likeness between the two is produced by the rising of the cuticle in blisters filled with serous or blood-colored fluids at the most injured parts. But the coincident or quickly following signs of mortification leave no doubt of what is happening. The discolored parts become cold and insensible, and more and more dark, except at their borders, which are dusky red; a thin, brownish, stinking fluid issues from the exposed integuments; gas is evolved from similar fluids decomposing in the deeper seated tissues, and its bubbles crepitate as we press them; the limb retains its size or enlarges, but its tissues are no longer tense; they soften as in inflammation, but both more rapidly and more thoroughly, for they become utterly rotten. At the borders of the dying and dead tissues, if the mortification be still extending, these changes are gradually lost; the colors fade into the dusky red of the inflamed but still living parts; and the tint of these parts may afford the earliest and best sign of the progress towards death, or the return to a more perfect life. Their becoming more dark and dull, with a browner red, is the sure precursor of their death; their brightening and assuming a more florid hue is as sure a sign that they are more actively alive. Doubtless the varieties of color indicate, respectively, the stagnation and the movement of the blood in the parts which, thus situated, may, according to the progress of their inflammation, be added to the dead, or become the apparatus of repair.

The interior of a part thus mortified corresponds with the foregoing description. All the softer tissues are, like the integuments, rotten, soft, putrid, soaked with serum and decomposed exuded fluid; ash-colored, green, or brown; more rarely blue or black; crackling with various gases extricated in decomposition. The tendons and articular cartilages in a mortified limb may seem but little changed; at the most they may be softened, and deprived of lustre. The bones appear dry, bloodless, and often like such as have been macerated and bleached; their periosteum is usually separated from them, or may be easily and cleanly stripped off. But these harder and interior parts of a limb either die more slowly, or more slowly manifest the signs of death, than do those around them; for, not only do they appear comparatively little changed, but, often, when all the dead soft parts are completely separated from the living, the bone remains continuous, and its medullary vessels bleed when it is sawn off. Usually, also, after complete spontaneous separation of the mortified part of a limb, the stump is conical; the outer parts of it having died higher up than the parts in its axis.

Another appearance of mortified parts, characteristic of a class, is presented after they have been strangulated. I have mentioned the difference which in these cases depends on whether the strangulation have been suddenly complete, or have been gradually made perfect (p. 293). In the former case, the slough is very quickly formed, and may be ash-colored, gray, or whitish, and apt to shrivel and become dry before its separation. In the latter case, as best exemplified in strangulated hernia, the blood-vessels become gradually more and more full, and the blood more dark, till the walls of the intestine, passing through the deepest tints of blood-color and of crimson, become completely black. Commonly, by partial extravasation of blood, and by inflammatory exudation, they become also thick, firm, and leathery, a condition which materially adds to the difficulty of reducing the hernia, but which is generally an evidence that the tissues are not dead; for when they are dead, they become not only duller to the eye, but softer, more flaccid and yielding, and easily torn, like the rotten tissue of other mortified parts. The canal, which was before cylindrical, may now collapse; and now, commonly, the odor of the intestinal contents penetrates its walls.

I have spoken of the death of the blood as coinciding with that of the part in whose vessel it is enclosed. Very commonly, when this happens, coagulation of blood ensues in the vessels for some distance above, *i. e.* nearer to the heart than, the mortified parts. Hence, as it has been often observed, no bleeding may appear from even large arteries divided in amputations above the dead parts of sloughing limbs.

It remains now to speak of the phenomena which ensue when gangrene ceases, and of which the end is, that the dead parts are separated from the living.

As for the dead parts, they only continue to decompose while, if exposed to a dry atmosphere, they gradually shrivel, become drier and darker. But more important changes ensue in the living parts that border them. The first change that occurs in this process (the whole of which may be studied as the most remarkable instance of the adaptation of disease for the recovery of health,) the first indication of the coming reparative process, is a more decided limitation and contrast of color at the border of the dying part. As we watch it in the integuments, the dusky redness of the surrounding skin becomes more bright, and paler, as if mingled with pink rather than with brown; and the contrast reaches its height when, as the redness of the living part brightens, the dead whiteness or blackness of the slough becomes more perfect. The touch may detect a corresponding contrast: the living part, turgid with moving blood, feels tense and warm; the dead part is soft, or inelastic, cold, and often a little sunken below the level of the living. These contrasts mark out the limits of the two parts: they constitute the " line of demarcation" between them.

The separation of the dead and living parts, which remain continuous for various periods after the mortification has ceased and the line of demarcation is formed, is accomplished by the ulceration of the portions of the living tissues which are immediately contiguous to the dead. At this border, and (in parts that are exposed) commencing at the surface, a groove is formed by ulceration, which circumscribes and intrenches the dead part, and then, gradually deepening and converging, undermines it, till, reaching its centre, the separation is completed, and the slough falls or is dislodged by the discharge from the surface of the ulcerated living part. Commonly, before the borders of the integuments ulcerates, it becomes white and very soft; so that, for a time, a dull white line appears to divide the dead and living parts.

Closely following in the wake of this process of ulceration is one more definitely directed towards repair. As the ulcerated groove deepens day by day around and beneath the dead part, so do granulations rise from its surface; so that, as one might say, that which was yesterday ulcerating is to-day granulating; and thus, very soon after the slough is separated, the whole surface of the living part, from which it was detached, is covered with granulations, and proceeds, like an ordinary ulcer, towards healing.

There is, I believe, nothing in the method of thus separating a dead part, thus "casting off a slough," which is not in conformity with the general process of ulceration. When a portion of the very interior substance of an organ dies, and is separated, there may be doubt, as in some nearly corresponding cases of ulceration (p. 270), whether the clearing away of the living tissue adjacent to it be effected by absorption or by disintegration, and mingling with the fluid in which, after separation, the dead piece lies. We may have this doubt in such cases as the sloughing of subcutaneous tissue in carbuncles not yet open, or in phlegmonous erysipelas, or in the cases of internal necrosis; in which, without any external discharge, pieces of dead tissue are completely detached from the living tissue around them: and I do not know how such doubt can be solved. But the separation of superficial or exposed dead parts might be studied as the type of the ulcerative process, of which, indeed, it is in disease the usual beginning (see p. 272), and with the more advantage, because the sloughing of parts of limbs affords illustrations of the process in tissues in which it very rarely happens otherwise. Especially, it shows the times at which, in different tissues, ulceration may ensue, and hereby the times during which, under similar conditions of hindered nutrition, the tissues may severally maintain life.

The process which I have exemplified by the mortification of soft parts has an exact and instructive parallel in necrosis or mortification of bone; but there are in the phenomena of necrosis some things which deserve a brief mention because of their clearly illustrating the general nature of the process following the death of a part.

Thus (1) we find in bones a permanent evidence of the increase of vascularity of the tissues around a dead part; for, in specimens of necrosis, the bone at the border of the dead piece has always very numerous and enlarged Haversion canals. (2) We may often see that the reparative process, on the borders of the living part, keeps pace with or rather precedes by some short interval, the process by which the living and the dead are separated: for new bone is always formed in and beneath the periosteum at the border of the living bone, while the groove around the dead piece is being deepened, or even before its formation has commenced. (3) Instances of necrosis show some of the progressive changes that lead to the formation of the groove of separation. The bone at the very junction of the living and the dead becomes, first, soft and ruddy, as an inflamed bone does. Its earthy matter, as Mr. Hunter described, is first (by absorption, as we must suppose) removed in larger proportion than its animal basis. This basis remains, for a time, connecting the dead and the living bone, both of which, retaining their natural hardness, appear in strong contrast with it; but soon this also is removed, and the separation is completed. (4) From some cases of necrosis, also, we obtain evidence on a question about the removal of dead tissue. It is asked whether dead tissue may not be absorbed, and so removed. Examples of necrosis show that in the large majority of cases, the separation of dead bone is accomplished entirely by the ulceration or absorption of the living bone around it; but that, in certain cases, especially in those in which pieces of bone, though dead, remain continuous with the living, the dead bone may be in part absorbed, or otherwise removed, not indeed in mass but after being disintegrated or dissolved.* (5) In cases of necrosis we find the best examples in which, apparently through want of vital force, the dead and living parts remain long united and continuous. A piece of dead bone, proved to be dead by its blackness, insensibility, and total absence of change, may remain even for months connected with living bone: and no process for its separation is established till the patients general health improves. (6) Lastly, in the death of bone, we may see a simpler process for the separation of the living tissues than that which is accomplished by ulceration. In superficial necrosis, the periosteum, at least in those parts in which its own tissue does not penetrate, so as to be continuous with, that of the bone, separates cleanly from the surface of the dead bone, retaining its own integrity and smoothness, and leaving the bone equally entire and smooth. No observations have yet been made, I believe, which show how this retirement of one tissue from another is effected, or how the blood-vessels that pass from one to another are disposed of. Another method of separation without the ulcerative process is observed when teeth die, especially in old persons. Their sockets enlarge, apparently by mere atrophy or absorption of the walls and margins; so that the teeth-fangs are no longer tightly grasped by them, but become loose, and project further from the jaw.

---

* Such cases are recorded by Mr. Stanley, in whose Treatise on Diseases of the Bones I need hardly say that all the phenomena of necrosis are much more fully described than they are here. The possibility of the absorption of the dead bone seems amply proved by cases (one of which I watched while it was under his care) in which portions of pegs of ivory, driven like nails into bones, to excite inflammation for the repair of ununited fractures have been removed. The absorption, I say, seems amply proved; but the method of it is made, by the same observations, more difficult than ever to explain; for only those portions of the ivory that were imbedded in the bone were absorbed; the portions that were not in contact with bone, though imbedded in granulations or pus, were unchanged.

LECTURE XX.

SPECIFIC DISEASES.

It would be far beyond the design of these lectures, intended only for the illustration of the General Principles of Pathology, in its relations with Surgery, if I were to enter largely on the consideration of the diseases named specific. It will be sufficient, I hope, and certainly will more nearly correspond with the rest of my plan, if I describe the general features of specific diseases, and their general import; and if I point out, though only in suggestions, how we may more effectually study them; how many things relating to them, which we are apt to dismiss with words, may be subjects of deeper, and perhaps useful, thought.

The term "specific disease," as employed in common usage and in its most general sense, means something distinct from common or simple disease. Thus, when a "specific inflammation" or a "specific ulcer" is spoken of, we understand that these present certain features in which they differ from what the same person would call a "common" or a "simple inflammation" or "ulcer." The specific characters of any disease, whether syphilis or hydrophobia, gout or rheumatism, typhus, small pox, or any other, are those in which it constantly deviates from the characters of a common or simple disease of the same general kind.* Our first inquiry, therefore, must be,—what are these common diseases, which we seem to be agreed to take as the standard by which to measure the specific characters of others.

I believe that, in relation to inflammatory diseases and their consequences, our chief thoughts concerning such standards for comparison are derived from the affections which follow injuries by violence, or by inorganic chemical agents, by heat, or any other commonly applied causes of disease. When such a blow is inflicted as kills a portion of the body, its consequences afford a standard with which we may compare all other instances of mortification and sloughing: and when, among these, we fine a certain number of examples which differ, in some constant characters, from this standard, we place them, as it were, in a separate group, as examples of a specific disease. Or, again, when a part is submitted to such pressure as leads to its ulceration, we regard the disease as a common, simple, or standard ulcer; and by their several

---

* It may not be unnecessary to guard some students at once from the suspicion, which the terms in common use may suggest, that there is a correspondence between the species of diseases and those of living creatures as studied in natural history. There is really no likeness, correspondence, or true analogy between them; and if nosological systems, framed after the pattern of those of zoology, lead to the belief that they have any other resemblance than that of the modes of briefly describing, and of grouping double names they had better be disused.

constant differences from it, and from one another, we judge of the various ulcers which we name specific. In like manner, our standard of common or simple inflammation seems to be derived from the processes which follow violence, the application of heat, the lodgment of foreign bodies, or the application of certain chemical stimulants. And the standard of common or simple fever is that which ensues in a previously healthy man, soon after he has received some such local injury as any of these agents might produce. Now, it is very resonable that we should take these as the best examples of common or simple disease; the best, I mean, for comparison with those that may be called specific. For not only can we produce some of these common diseases when we will, and study them experimentally, but they manifestly present disease in its least complicated form: least specified by peculiarities either in its cause or in its subject. Only, in adjusting our standards of disease from them, it is necessary that we should take the characters presented by all or by the great majority of instances; since the consequences of even the simplest mechanical injuries are apt to vary according to the peculiar constitution of the person injured.

The terms simple and specific are sometimes applied, in equal contradistinction, to tumors. Here we have no such standard of accidental or experimental disease; but that which seems to be taken as the measure of simplicity in a tumor, is the conformity of its structure with some of the natural parts of the body. The more a tumor is like a mere overgrowth of some natural structure, the more "simple" is it considered; and the specific characters of a tumor are chiefly those in which, whether in texture or in mode of life, it differs from the natural parts. When, however, a tumor is diseased,—for instance, when a cancer ulcerates,— the specific characters of the ulcer are estimated by comparison with the characters of common or simple ulcers.

Such are, in the most general terms, the standards of common or simple diseases. The title "common" applied to them is, in another sense, justified by the features which they present being, for the most part, common to them and to the specific diseases. For, in the specific diseases, we do not find morbid processes altogether different from those which are taken as standards, but only such processes as are conformed with them in all general and common features, but differ from them by some modification or addition. In other words, no specific disease is entirely peculiar or specific; each consists of a common morbid process, whether an inflammation, an ulceration, a gangrene, or any other, and of a specific modification or plan in some part thereof.

Let us now see what these modifications, these specific characters, are; and here, the history of tumors being reserved to the next volume, let me almost limit the inquiry to a comparison of the inflammatory affections of the two kinds, and select examples from only such as are, by the most general consent, called specific; as syphilis, gout, rheumatism, the eruptive fevers, and the like.

1. Each specific disease constantly observes a certain plan or construction in its morbid process; each, as I just said, presents the phenomena of a common or simple disease, but either there is some addition to these, or, else, one or more of these is so modified as to constitute a specific character; a peculiarity by which each is distinguished at once from all common, and from all other specific, diseases. Thus, we see a patient with, say, two or three annular or crescentic ulcers on his legs; and, if we can watch these, they are, perhaps, healing at their concave borders at the same time as they are extending at their convex borders. Now, here are all the conditions that belong to common ulcers; and, in different instances, we might find these ulcers liable to the variations of common ones, as being more or less inflamed or congested, acute or chronic, progressive or stationary; but we look beyond these characters, and see, in the shape and mode of extension of these ulcers, properties which are not observed in common ones; we recognize these as specific characters; we may call the ulcers specific; or, because we know how commonly such ulcers occur in syphilis, and how rarely in any other disease, we call them syphilitic ulcers, and treat them with iodide of potassium, or some other specific; that is, specially curative medicines. Another patient has, say, numerous small, round, dusky, or light brownish-red, slightly elevated patches of inflammation of the surface of his skin; on many of them there are small, dry, white scales; and some of them may be arranged in a ring. Here, again, are the common characters of inflammation: but they are peculiarized in plan and tint of redness, and in general aspect; and because of these we regard the disease as specific, and call it psoriasis, and, because of the additional peculiarity of dusky or coppery redness, and of the annular or some other figurate arrangement, we suspect that it is syphilitic psoriasis. Or, we look through a series of preparations of ulcerated intestines; and we call one ulcer simple or catarrhal, another typhous, another dysenteric, a fourth tuberculous: all have the common characters of ulcers; but these are, in each, peculiarly or specifically modified in some respect of plan; and the modifications are so constant that, without hearing any history of the specimens, we may be sure of all the chief events of the disease by which each ulcer was preceded. Or, among a heap of diseased bones, we can select those whose possessors were strumous, rheumatic, syphilitic, or cancerous; finding in them specific modifications of the results of some common disease, such as new bone, *i. e.* ossified inflammatory deposits, arranged in peculiar methods of construction, or at particular parts; or ulcers of peculiar shape and peculiar method of extension.

I need not cite more examples of the thousand varieties in which the common phenomena of disease are modified in specific diseases. In some, the most evident specific characteristics are peculiar affections of the

20

movement of the blood, as in the cutaneous erythemata; in some, affections of certain parts of the nervous centres, as in tetanus, hydrophobia, and hooping-cough; in some, peculiar exudations from the blood, as in gout and the inoculable diseases; in some, peculiar structures formed by the exuded materials, as in variola, vaccina, and other cutaneous pustular eruptions; in some, destruction of tissues, as in the ulcers of syphilis, the sloughs of boils and carbuncles; in some, peculiar growths, as in cancer; in some, or indeed in nearly all, peculiar methods of febrile general disturbance; but, in each of all the number, phenomena admit of distinction into those of common disease, and those in which such disease is peculiarly modified, or by which, if I may so say, it is specificated.

The morbid process thus modified may be local or general. Usually, in specific diseases, both local and general morbid processes are concurrent, and both are, in a measure, specific; but, although we can scarcely doubt that there is in every case an exact and specific correspondence between the two, yet, at present, the general or constitutional affections of many different specific diseases appear so alike, that we derive our evidence of specific characters almost entirely from the local part of the disease. The premonitory general disturbances of the exanthemata, or the slighter disorders preceding cutaneous eruptions, are, severally, so alike, that, except by collateral evidence, we could seldom do more than guess what they portend; their specific modifications of common general disturbance are too slight for us to recognize them with our present knowledge and means of observation.

2. Observing the causes of specific diseases, we find that some, and these the most striking examples of the whole class, are due to the introduction of peculiar organic compounds,—morbid poisons, as they are generally called,—into the blood. Such are all the diseases that can be transmitted by inoculation, contagion, or infection. All these are essentially specific diseases; each of them is produced by a distinct substance, and each produces the same substance, and by a morbid process separates it from the blood. In most of these, also, as well as in many of which the causes are internal and less evident, the local phenomena are preceded by some affection of the whole economy: the whole blood seems diseased, and nearly every function and sensation is more or less disturbed from its health; the patient feels "ill all over," before the local disease appears; i. e. before the more distinct and specific morbid process is manifest in the place of inoculation or in some other part. Herein is a very general ground of distinction between the specific and the simple or common diseases: in the latter, the local phenomena precede the general or constitutional; in the former, the order is reversed. We might, indeed, expect this to be a constant difference between the two; and perhaps it is so; for though many exceptions to any rule founded on it might be adduced, yet these may be ascribed to the unavoidable sources of fallacy in our observations. Thus, every severe injury, every long-continued irritation, excites at once both local and general disease;

and the latter may be evident before the former, and may not only modify it, but may seem to produce it. On the other hand, the insertion of certain specific poisons, *e. g.* that of the venom of a serpent or an insect, gives rise so rapidly to specific local disease that this seems to precede all constitutional affection.

Notwithstanding such exceptions as these are, or seem to be, this contrast between specific and common diseases, in regard to the order in which the local and the constitutional symptoms arise, is so usual that the terms specific and constitutional are often employed as convertible terms in relation to disease. But this is not convenient; for some specific diseases are, or become, local; and some constitutional diseases are not specific.

3. A character very generally observed in specific diseases is an apparent want of proportion between the cause and the effect. In common disease, one might say that, on the whole, the quantity of local disease is in direct proportion to the cause exciting it,—whether violent injury, heat, poison, or any other. Numerous exceptions might be found, but this is, on the whole, the rule.* In specific diseases there is no appearance of such a rule: we cannot doubt its existence, but it is lost sight of. Thus, in small-pox, measles, hydrophobia, or syphilis, the severity of the disease is not, evidently, proportionate to the cause applied: a minimum of inoculated virus engenders as vast a disease as any larger quantity might.

4. I have said that there is generally a correspondence between the local and the constitutional characters of a specific disease: but this is only in respect of quality: in respect of quantity there is often such a want of correspondence between the two as we rarely or never see in common diseases. In general, the amount of common inflammatory fever after an operation bears a direct proportion to the injury, and the amount of hectic fever to the quantity of local disease (here, again, are numerous exceptions, but this is the rule); but in specific diseases it is far otherwise. In syphilis and cancer, the severest defects or disturbances in the whole economy may co-exist with the smallest amounts of specific local disease; and, as Dr. Robert Williams† has well said, "It may be laid down as a general law, that when a morbid poison acts with its greatest intensity, and produces its severest forms of disease, fewer traces of organic alterations of structure will be found than when the disorder has been of a milder character."

5. To specific diseases belong all that was said, in former lectures

---

* I am tempted to say here, that in pathology, we must admit the existence of many rules or laws the apparent exceptions to which are more numerous than the plain examples of them. This, however, is not enough to invalidate the truth of the laws; it could scarcely be otherwise in the case of laws, the exact observance of which requires the concurrence of so many conditions as are engaged in nearly all the phenomena studied in pathology.

† Elements of Medicine, vol. i. p. 12.

(p. 27, e. s.), of the symmetrical diseases, and of seats of election: such phenomena occur in degenerations, but, I think, in no common diseases.

6. The local process of a specific disease of nutrition is less apt than that of a common one to be nearly limited to the area in which, in the first instance, the cause of disease was applied. Specific diseases are peculiarly prone to spread, that is, to extend their area. They also, among the diseases of nutrition, are alone capable of being erratic, i. e. of disappearing from the part in which they were first manifest, while extending thence through other parts continuous with it; and they alone are capable of metastasis, i. e. of suddenly ceasing in one locality, and manifesting themselves, with similar local phenomena, in another.

7. In all the particulars mentioned in the last preceding, and in some of the earlier paragraphs, specific diseases manifest a peculiar character in that they seem capable of self-augmentation; no evident fresh cause is applied, and yet the disease increases: witness the seemingly spontaneous increase of manifest local disease in secondary and tertiary syphilis, or in the increasing eruption of eczema or of herpes, or the extension of a carbuncle, or the multiplication of secondary cancers.

8. Specific diseases alone are capable of transformation or metamorphosis. As we watch a common disease, its changes seem to be only those of degree; it appears increasing or declining, but is always the same and a continuous disease. But in many specific diseases we see changes in quality or kind, as well as in quantity. In syphilis, for example, a long series of diseases may occur as the successive consequences of one primary disease different from them all. They are all, in one sense, the same disease, as having a single origin: but it is a disease susceptible of change in so far as it manifests itself, at different times, not only in different parts, but in different forms in each, and in forms which are not wholly determined by the nature of the tissue affected. The successive phenomena of measles, scarlet fever, and many others, may, I think, be similarly expressed as metamorphoses or transformations of disease.

9. A similar transformation of specific disease may take place in their transference from one person to another, whether by inheritance,[*] or by infection, or contagion. A parent with one form of secondary syphilis may have a child with another form; the child of a parent with scirrhous cancer may have an epithelial, a colloid, or a medullary cancer: the inoculation of several persons with the matter from one primary syphilitic sore may produce different forms of the primary disease and different consecutive phenomena; the same contagion of small-pox, measles, or scarlet fever may produce in different subjects all the modifications of which those diseases are severally capable; the puerperal

---

* It might seem as if none but specific diseases could be hereditary; but many tumors are so which we cannot well call specific: such as the cutaneous cysts or wens, and fatty and cartilaginous tumors.

woman, or the patient who has sustained a severe accidental or surgical injury, may modify, or, as it were, color with the peculiarities of her own condition, whatever epidemic or other zymotic disease she may incur.*

10. Lastly, time is a peculiarly important condition in many of the specific diseases. If we except the period of calm or incubation, which usually occurs between the infliction of an injury and the beginning of an evident reparative process, a period of which the length is, in general, proportionate to the severity of the injury, there are few of the events of common diseases that are periodic or measurable in time; there are none that are regularly intermittent or remittent; none that can be compared, for regularity, with the set times of latency of the morbid poisons of the eruptive fevers, or the periods in which they run their course, or change their plan or chief place of action. Neither are there, in common diseases, any periods of latency so long as those which elapse between the application of the specific cause, and the appearance of its specific effect in the eruptive fevers, tetanus, or hydrophobia.

Such, briefly, are the chief general characters of the diseases which are commonly named specific, or described as having something specific in their action. In some of them, chiefly such as depend on distinct morbid poisons, whether miasma, or virus, or matter of contagion, all these characters may be observed; and these are the best types of the class. In others, part only of the same characters concur. I do not pretend to define the exact boundary of what should be called specific, and what common, in diseases; but it seems reasonable that any disease, in which the majority of the characters just enumerated are found, should be studied as one of the class, and that its phenomena should be interpreted, if possible, by the rules, or by the theory, derived from the more typical members of the same class.

The theory of specific diseases, in its most general terms, is, that each of them depends on a definite and specific morbid condition of the blood; that the local process in which each is manifested is due to the disorder produced by the morbid blood in the nutrition of one or more tissues; and that, generally, this disorder is attended with the accumulation, and leads to the discharge, or transformation, of some morbid constituents of the blood in the disordered part. It is held, also, that in some specific diseases, the morbid condition of the blood consists in undue proportions of one or more of its normal constituents; and that in others, some new morbid substance is added to or formed in the blood. In either case, the theory is, that the phenomena of each specific disease depend chiefly, and in the first instance, on certain corresponding specific materials in the blood: and that if characteristic morbid struc-

* See Carpenter; Br. and For. Med.-Chir. Review, Jan. 1853, quoting from Simpson, in Monthly Journ. of Med. Sc. vol. xi. and xiii.

tures be formed in the local process, they are organs in which these morbid materials are incorporated.

Now in regard to certain diseases, such as some of those that can be communicated by inoculation, these terms are scarcely theoretical; they may rather be taken as the simplest expressions of facts. For example (as I have already said, p. 283), in either syphilis, vaccinia, glanders, or small-pox, especially when produced by inoculation, we have demonstration (1) of a morbid condition of the blood; (2) of the definite and specific nature of that condition, in that it is, and may be at will, produced by the introduction of a definite substance into the blood, and manifests itself into a local disease which, within certain limits, has constant characters; and (3) of the same substance being accumulated and discharged, or for a time incorporated in the morbid structures, at the seat of the local disease. And it seems important to mark, that all which is thus seen in some specific diseases, and is assumed for the explanation of others, is consistent with facts of physiology; especially with those referred to in a former Lecture (p. 33, e. s.), as evidences, that certain normal organs of the body are formed in consequence of the presence of materials in the blood, which in relation to them, might be called specific, and which they, in their formation, take from the blood and incorporate in their own structures.*

The proof of the theory of specific diseases is scarcely less complete for all those that are infectious or contagious, but cannot be communicated by inoculation—such as typhus, measles, erysipelas; and scarcely less for those which are neither infectious nor contagious, but depend, like cholera and ague, on certain materials which are introduced into the blood, and produce uniform results, though they are not proved to exist in the products of the morbid processes. For other diseases, classed or usually regarded as specific, such as gout, rheumatism, carbuncle, boil, the various definite, but not communicable, cutaneous eruptions, hydrophobia, tetanus, and many more, the evidences of the theory are less complete. Yet they seem not insufficient; while we have, in many of these affections, proofs of the accumulation and separation of morbid substances at the seats of local disease, and while, in all, the chief phenomena are in close conformity with those of the diseases which are typically specific. Relying on the similarity of all members of the group of specific diseases, on the sufficiency of the terms of the theory

---

* Abundant illustrations of the same general laws, of both healthy and morbid formation of structures incorporating specific materials from the blood, are supplied by the action of medicines whose operation ensues in only certain organs. Dr. Robert Williams (l. c. p. 8) has justly said, "The general laws observable in the actions of morbid poisons are, for the most part, precisely similar to those which govern medicinal substances, or only differ on a few minor points." The subject is too extensive for discussion here. It is admirably treated by Mr. Simon in his Lectures on Pathology; the work, which, together with that of Dr. Robert Williams, may be studied with more profit, in relation to all the subjects of this Lecture, than any I have yet read.

for the expression of the facts concerning them all, and on the evidences mose or less complete which each of them supplies for its truth, we seem justified in adopting the same theory for them all.

But now, if we may hold this theory to be true for some specific diseases, and not unreasonable for the rest, let us see how, in its terms, we can explain or express the chief characters of these diseases; such as their periodicity, metastases, and metamorphoses, the apparent increase of the specific substance in the blood, and the others just enumerated. This may be done while tracing the probable history, or, as I would call it, the life, of the morbid material in the blood, and in the tissues.*

Specific morbid materials, or at least their chief constituents, may enter the body from without, by inoculation, contagion, or infection; or they may be formed in the blood, or added to it, within the body: in other words, some morbid materials are inserted, others are imbred, in the blood; with some, probably, both modes of introduction are possible. Doubtless, an important difference is thus marked between two chief groups of the specific diseases: but it is not within my present purpose to dwell on it; for only one general history can as yet be written for the whole class of morbid materials on which the specific diseases depend; and, although this may be best drawn from the instances of those that are derived from without, i. e. from such as are called morbid poisons, yet it would probably be as true, in all essential features, for those that are inbred.

When a morbid poison is inoculated,—for example, when the matter from a syphilitic sore, or from a vaccine vesicle, is inserted in the skin, —it produces a specific effect both on the tissue at the place of insertion, and on the blood, as soon as it, or any part of it is absorbed; in other words, it produces both a local and a constitutional change; and in both these effects its history must be traced.

I. First, respecting the local change: of which, with another design, I have already spoken (p. 284). It is not proved by anything that can be seen immediately, or even within one or two days after the inoculation. The place of inoculation remains, for a time, apparently unaffected; and yet that a peculiar change is being wrought in it is clear, for it presently becomes the seat of specific disease, the materials of which disease are supplied by blood that nourishes healthily all other parts, even such parts as may have received common injuries at or near the time of inoculation. The inoculated part, therefore, is not merely injured, but is peculiarly altered in its relation to the blood, which now nourishes it differently from all the rest of the body. The change of the blood is proved, if not by general fibrile or other disturbance, yet

* Several of the characters of specific diseases are already explained, in the terms of this theory, in the earlier Lectures: namely, their specific forms and construction (pp. 33, 37, 54); symmetry and seats of election (pp. 27, 29, 283, e. s.) extension and errantry (p. 29, note).

by the specific character of the presently ensuing disease, and by the consecutive secondary disease, or by the consecutive immunity from later disease of the same kind.

If further proof be needed of the specific local change produced in the inoculated part, it may be furnished by the analogy of the more visible effects of certain animal poisons,—such as those of venomous serpents and insects. None of these appear to be simple irritants; the consequences of their insertion are not like simple inflammations, but are peculiar, and constant in their peculiarities. The bite of a bug or a flea will not, I hope, be thought too trivial for an illustration.

In less than a minute after the bite, the bitten part begins to itch; and quickly after this, a wheal or circumscribed pale swelling, with a nearly level surface and a defined border, gradually rises and extends in the skin. It seems to be produced by an œdema of a small portion of the cutis at and around the bite; it is not a simple inflammatory swelling; it is, from the first, paler than the surrounding skin, which may be healthy or slightly reddened by afflux of blood; and the contrast between them becomes more striking, as the surrounding skin becomes gradually redder, as if with a more augmented fullness of the blood-vessels. Thus, for some minutes, the wheal appears raised on a more general, and less defined, vascular swelling of the surrounding and subjacent tissues; but after these minutes, and as the itching subsides, the wheal, or paler swelling becomes less defined, and the more general swelling appears gradually to encroach on it and involve it. Then all subsides: but only for a time; for in about twenty-four hours a papule, or some form of secondary inflammation appears, with renewed itching, at the seat of the puncture, and this after one, two, or sometimes more days, gradually subsides.*

Now, the first pale and circumscribed swelling at any of these bites may serve to illustrate the immediate effects of a morbid poison on the tissues at and around the seat of inoculation. In the area of such a swelling the tissues are, by the direct contact and influence of the venom, altered in their nutritive relation to the blood. So, I believe, immediately after the insertion of syphilitic, vaccine, or other virus, there ensues a corresponding specific alteration of those parts of the surrounding tissues which afterwards become seats of the specific local disease.†

* Some persons are so happily constituted, that they do not thus, or with any other discomfort, suffer the consequences of insect-bites; but I think the description I have given will be found generally true for cases in which the bitten part is left undisturbed. The fortunate exempt may illustrate the rarer exceptions from the usual influence of the severer morbid poisons.

† The direct influence of animal poisons on the tissues appears to be well shown in the effects of the bites of the viper and rattlesnake. Sir B. C. Brodie particularly noticed this in a man bitten by a rattlesnake (Lectures on Pathology and Surgery, p. 345). The primary local, though widely extended, effect of the poison was a sloughing of the cellular mem-

I will not venture to say that the secondary inflammation, which usually appears on the day after any of these bites, is to be ascribed in some measure to an influence exercised by the virus on the blood; though, indeed, this will not seem impossible to those who are considerate of the effect of the minutest portion of vaccine virus, and of the intense constitutional disturbance excited by the other venoms. But, whatever be thought on this point, the occurrence of a new and different inflammation in the bitten part proves that it did not return to perfect health when its first affection subsided; it proves that some altered material of the virus, or some changing trace of its effects upon the tissues, remained, altering their relation to the blood, and making them alone, of all the parts of the body, prone to specific disease. The bitten part thus, in its interval of apparent health, instructively illustrates the state of parts after inoculation with syphilitic or vaccine virus. In them, as in it, we must suppose that some virus, or some specific effect produced by it on the tissues, remains during all that period of latency, or incubation, as it is called, which intervenes between the inoculation and the appearance of the specific disease.

Whatever be the state thus indirectly induced in the inoculated or bitten part, let it be noted as one constantly changing. The tissues of the part, like the rest of the body, are engaged in the constant mutations of nutrition; and the morbid material in the part is probably, like every organic matter, in constant process of transformation. Some of the local phenomena of specific diseases indicate these progressive changes in the part itself; but they can scarcely be traced separately from those that are occurring in the morbid material absorbed into the blood.

The local and peculiar change produced by the direct effect of the morbid poison is essential to the complete manifestation of some specific diseases. In many others, as in typhus, variola, acute rheumatism, and gout, the morbid condition of the blood is sufficient to determine the local disease in tissues previously healthy. But it is, perhaps, true for all, that the existence of some part whose nutrition is depressed, whether through simple or specific injury, is very favorable to the manifestation of the constitutional disease (see p. 284). Thus, I shall have to mention cases of cancer in which the constitutional condition, or diathesis, seems to have been latent till some local injury brought a certain part into a state apt for the cancerous growth,—the diathesis, as one may say, waited for the necessary local condition. In like manner, cases sometimes occur

brane, which began "immediately after the injury was received." The poison "seemed to operate on the cellular membrane, neither in the direction of the nerves, nor in that of the absorbents, nor in that of the blood-vessels." His account has been recently confirmed in a more quickly fatal case. Many years ago, one of my brethren was stung by a Weever-fish (Trachinus Draco); and I remember that next day, though no severe inflammation had intervened, there was a little black slough at the puncture, as if the venom had completely killed a piece of the skin.

in which constitutional syphilis is justly presumed to exist, but in which it has no local manifestation till some part is appropriated for it by the effects of injury. I know a gentleman, who, for not less than five years after a syphilitic affection of the testicle, had no sign of syphilis, except that of generally feeble health; but he accidentally struck his nose severely, and at once a well-marked syphilitic disease of its bones ensued. In another case, syphilitic disease of the skull followed an injury of the head. In similar cases, ulcers like those of tertiary syphilis have appeared in healing operation-wounds. I lately saw a gentleman who had long suffered with diabetes, a condition with which, as is well known, boils often coincide. He, however, had none till he accidentally struck his leg, and the injury was quickly followed by a succession of more than twenty boils near the injured part. And, in like manner, as I have stated in a former lecture (p. 285), even variola and measles may have their intensest local manifestations in injured parts.

I need not dwell on the importance of cases such as these, for caution against supposing that the diseases which seem to originate in local injury are only local processes. The most intense constitutional affections may appear, almost irrespective of locality, able to manifest themselves in nearly every part; but the less intense may abide unobserved, so long as all the tissues are being maintained without external hinderance or interference; they may be able to manifest themselves only in some part whose normal power of maintenance is disturbed by injury or other disease. It may, generally also, be noticed that the more intense the constitutional affection, and the less the need for preparation of a locality for its manifestation, the less tenacious is it of its primary seat. Contrast, for example, in this respect, the fugacity of acute rheumatism or gout with the tenacity of chronic rheumatism in some locality of old disease or injury.*

II. Respecting, secondly, the changes which a morbid material, inoculated and absorbed, may undergo in the blood, these may be enumerated as the chief;—increase, transformation, combination, and separation or excretion. Here, again, one assumes for an example such a morbid material as may be inoculated; but it will be plain that most of what is said, in the following illustrations, might also be said of those that are otherwise introduced into the blood; and further, that the particulars of the life of these morbid materials are generally consistent with those of ordinary constituents of the blood.

(a) The *increase* of the morbid material in the blood is illustrated in syphilis, small-pox, vaccinia, glanders. In any of these, the inoculation of the minutest portion of the virus is followed by the formation of one or more suppurating structures, from which virus, similarly and equally

* Dr. Carpenter (l. c.) has clearly traced that epidemic and other zymotic influences bear, with peculiar force, on those in whose blood there is "an accumulation of disintegrating azotized compounds in a state of change." Is it not a similar degenerate condition which makes an injured part peculiarly amenable to the influence of specific morbid materials in the blood?

potent, is produced in million-fold quantity. So, the matter of any contagion working in one person may render his exhalation capable of similarly affecting a thousand others.

The increase is thus evident. The effect of the inoculated morbid poison may be compared· with that of a ferment introduced into some azotized compound, in some of the materials of which it excites such changes as issue in the production of material like itself. What are the materials of the blood thus changed and converted to the likeness of the morbid poison we cannot tell. The observations of Dr. Carpenter,* showing how peculiarly liable to all contagious and other zymotic influences they are whose blood is surcharged with decomposing azotized materials, may well lead us to believe that it is among these materials that many of the morbid poisons find the means of their increase. And, as Mr. Simon† argues, it seems nearly sure that certain of these poisons in their increase, so convert some material of the blood, that they wholly exhaust it, and leave the blood for a long time, or for life, incapable of being again affected by the same morbid poison.

' The increase of the morbid material, however effected, explains these characters of specific diseases:—the apparent disproportion between the specific cause and its effect (p. 307); the want of correspondence, in respect of quantity, between the local and the constitutional phenomena (p. 307); the seeming capacity of self-augmentation (p. 308).

(b) The *transformation* of a morbid material is indicated by the diversity of the successive manifestations of a single and continuous specific disease. Thus, in syphilis, the primary disease, if left to its unhindered course, is followed, with general regularity, by a series of secondary and tertiary diseases. The terms often used would imply that these diseases are due to a morbid poison which is, all along, one and the same. But, identity of causes should be manifested in identity of effects; the succession of morbid processes proves a succession of changes, either in the agent poison, or in the patient. They may be in the latter; but, regularly, they are in the former: for, on the whole, the succession of secondary and tertiary syphilitic diseases is uniform in even a great variety of patients. We may, therefore, believe that the regular syphilitic phenomena depend on the transformation of the morbid poison: their irregularities, on the peculiarities of the patient, whether natural or acquired from treatment.

The transformation here assumed is self-probable, seeing the analogy of successive transformations in all organic living materials. It is nearly proved by the different properties, in regard to communicability, of the syphilitic poison at different periods: in the primary disease communicable by inoculation, but not through the maternal blood to the fœtus; in the secondary, having these relations reversed; in the tertiary, not at all communicable. In like manner, such facts as that the material found

* Loc. cit. p. 159.   † Lectures on Surgical Pathology, p. 262.

in the vaccine vesicle, on the eighth day, is better for fresh vaccinations than that taken earlier or later, prove successive transformations,— periods, we may say, of development, maturity, and degeneration, in the material of the virus.

Many similar phenomena of transformations in the morbid poisons may be cited; and if it may be accepted as a general occurrence, it will explain many of the phenomena of specific diseases. The period of incubation or latency of a disease (p. 309) may correspond with the transformation preceding the effective state of the morbid poison, with its periods of development. The prodromata, the precursive constitutional affections, and the successive stages of the disease, indicate the continuous transformations and varying influences of the same : just as every difference of organic construction indicates a difference in the yet unformed materials used in it. The increasing disturbance of the general health probably implies that the morbid poison increases while being transformed; that it grows with its development. The periodicity of all these events (p. 309) is a sign that the transformations of morbid poisons, like those of all other materials in the living body, are, in ordinary circumstances, accomplished in definite times. The sequelæ of specific diseases indicate yet further transformations, or, more probably, that the changes of the morbid poison have left the blood in a morbid state, through the exhaustion of some of its natural constituents, or through the presence of some complemental material.

(c) The *combination* of a morbid poison with one or more of the normal materials of the blood is indicated by the fact, that when the same specific disease, produced even by the inoculation of the same matter, affects many persons, it may present in each of them certain peculiar features. And these personal peculiarities, as they might be called, indicate modified qualities of the disease; not merely such differences of quantity as might be explained by assuming that each person has, in his blood, a different quantity of such material as may be convertible into the morbid poison. Difference of quantity may explain (as Mr. Simon and Dr. Carpenter have shown) difference of intensity of specific disease, and difference of liability to epidemic influence ; but it does not explain the varied method of the same disease in different persons. For this, I believe, we must assume that the specific material of each disease may be, in some measure, modified by its combination with one or more of those normal materials of the blood which have, in each person, a peculiar or personal character (see p. 26, e. s.)

By such combination, we may best explain those characters of specific disease, which appear in its changes in transmission from one person to another (p. 308): such as the varieties of syphilitic sores, and the varieties of their consequences in different persons inoculated from the same source ; the change in the form of secondary syphilis or of cancer in transmission from parent to offspring ; the several peculiarities in the results of the same miasm when affecting ordinary persons, or puerperal women, or those who have survived injuries.

A remarkable instance, exemplifying, I think, as well the changes in the morbid poison itself, as its various effects on different persons, has been told me by my friend Mr. Huxley. One of the crew of H. M. S. Rattlesnake, after slightly wounding his hand with a beef-bone, had suppuration of the axillary lymphatic glands, with which typhoid symptoms and delirium were associated, and proved fatal. His illness began the day after the ship left Sydney, where all the crew had been remarkably healthy. A few days after his death, the sailor who washed his clothes had similar symptoms of disease in the axilla, and, for four or five months, he suffered with sloughings of portions of the cellular tissue of the axilla, arm, and trunk on the same side. Near the same time, a third sailor had diffuse inflammation and sloughing in the axilla: and after this "the disease ran, in various forms, through the ship's company, between thirty and forty of whom were sometimes on the sick-list at once." Some had diffuse cellular inflammation; some had inflammation of the lymphatic glands of the head, axilla, or lower extremities; one had severe idiopathic erysipelas of the head and neck; another had phlegmonous erysipelas of the hand and arm after an accidental wound; others had low fever with or without enlargement of glands. "Finally the disease took the form of mumps, which affected almost everybody on board." The epidemic lasted from May to July. The ship was at sea the whole time, and in the greater part of it, in the intense cold of a southern winter.

(d) The *separation* of the material of a specific disease may, probably, be accomplished in many different ways, and may be regarded as the final purpose (if we may venture to trace one) of the greater part of the morbid process. It is evident in the inoculable products of sores and pustules; in the infectious exhalations of the skin, pulmonary, and other surfaces in the exanthematous and other fevers; in the deposits in and near gouty joints. Analogy with these cases makes it, also, probable that the specific materials of several other diseases are separated from the blood accumulated at the seats of the local morbid process; whence, if no organisms incorporating them be constructed, they may be reabsorbed after transformation. And it is nearly certain that the materials of most specific diseases may be excreted with the natural evacuations in the course of the disease, and this, either in their mature state, or after transformation, or in combination with the constituents of specific medicines.

The results of such separation or excretion are, also, various. Sometimes, it seems as if the whole of the morbid material were (after various transformations) removed, and the blood left healthy: as in small-pox, vaccina, cured primary syphilis. Sometimes, part of the morbid material, transformed or combined, so as to be incapable of excretion, remains in the blood, and produces secondary phenomena or sequelæ of the disease.   Sometimes, the production of the morbid material continues, notwithstanding the separation of what is already formed: as in the increase of the cancerous diathesis during the growth of cancers.   Generally, in whatever manner the separation be accomplished, it is attended by such disturbance of the natural functions of parts, that serious disease is superadded to that which is the more direct consequence of the presence of the morbid material in the blood.   And lastly, a local disease which owes its origin, and for a time, its maintenance, to a specific morbid condition of the blood, may persist after that condition has ceased; the blood may regain its health by the separation of the morbid material, but the part diseased in the process of separation may so continue. Now, however, the disease may be wholly local, and curable by local treatment.

Thus may the theory of specific diseases be applied in explanation of their phenomena.   I will only add that in assuming all this of the changes occurring in morbid materials in the blood, we really assume little more than we believe of the organizable materials introduced, as nutriment, into the blood.   If we could trace these, in their changes, first in the chyle and blood, and then in some complex tissue, then in the lymph and blood again, and again through the tissues of some excretory gland, we should trace a career of changes not less numerous, not less definite in method and in time, not less influential in the economy, than those which I have assumed for morbid materials in the blood. Only, the increase of the morbid material, and the apparent independence of its changes, are not imitated in the normal events of life.

LECTURE XXI.

CLASSIFICATION OF TUMORS.

THE class of diseases which includes the tumors may be reckoned as a part of the great division named Hypertrophies or Overgrowths.   All its members consist in additions to the organized materials of the body, and appear to be expressions of a morbid excess of formative force; but, in the case of each hypertrophy, the mode is peculiar in which this excess is manifested.   If we compare any tumor with one of the hypertrophies that are least morbid, with one of those, for instance, in which the excessive growth is adapted to some emergency of disease, as an hypertrophy of the heart is adapted to some emergency of the circulation, we shall, I believe, always see between them this chief difference: that, to whatever extent the adapted hypertrophy may proceed, the overgrown part maintains itself in the normal type of shape and structure; while a tumor is essentially a deviation from the normal type of the body in which it grows, and, in general, the longer it exists the wider is the deviation. A striking illustration of this contrast may be found in some of the cases of fibrous tumors that grow in the cavity of the uterus.* Such a tumor may resemble in its tissues the substance of the uterus itself, having well-formed muscular and fibrous tissues; and, so far as the structures formed in excess are concerned, we might regard the tumor as the result of an hypertrophy not essentially different from that which, at the same time and rate, may take place in the uterine walls around it. But an essential difference is in this: the uterus, in its growth around the tumor, maintains a normal type, though excited to its growth, if we may so speak, by an abnormal stimulus: it exactly imitates, in vascularity and muscular development, the pregnant uterus, and may even acquire the like power; and at length, by contractions, like those of parturition, may expel the tumor, spontaneously separated. But the tumor imitates in its growth no natural shape or construction: the longer it continues the greater is its deformity. Neither may we overlook the contrast in respect of purpose, or adaptation to the general welfare of the body, which is as manifest in the increase of the uterus as it is improbable in that of the tumor.

Herein we seem to discern an essential difference between the overgrowth of tumors, and those accomplished by any exercise of the normal power of nutrition in a part. This power, capable of augmented exercise in any emergency, is yet not a mere capacity of production; neither is it dependent upon circumstances for the fashion of its products; identical with that which effected the development of the germ, it is equally bound to conformity with the proper type of the part or species in which it is exercised.

An equal contrast may, in general, be drawn between the class of diseases that includes tumors, and all the others that issue in a morbid excess of nutritive formation. We may take, as the examples of these, the inflammatory diseases attended with exudation, and say (reserving certain conditions†) that in these there is an excessive exercise of formative force, an hypertrophy. But between such diseases and tumors we shall rarely fail to observe the following differences :—1st, The accumulation and increase of lymph in inflammation appears chiefly due to the morbid state of the parts at or adjacent to the place of exudation. We have, I think, no evidence that the lymph of inflammation increases, by any adherent force, any attraction of self-organizing matter, or any multiplication of its own cells; but the increase of all, or nearly all,

* Such as (e. g.) No. 2682 in the College Museum. Respecting the conditions in which the changes in the uterus here described are likely to occur, see Rokitansky, Pathologische Anatomie, iii. 546.
† See p. 277.

tumors, is "of themselves:" they grow as part of the body, but by their own inherent force, and depend on the surrounding parts for little more than the supply of blood, from which they may appropriate materials. A tumor, therefore, as a general rule, increases constantly; an inflammatory exudation generally increases only so long as the disease in the adjacent parts continues.

2d. The materials severally produced in excess, in these two cases, have different capacities of development. The inflammatory exudation, in whatever part it lies, has scarcely more than the single capacity to form, in the first instance, fibro-cellular or fibrous tissue: the material that begins or is added to a tumor may, indeed, assume either of these forms, but it may assume any one of several other forms.

But, 3dly, the most striking contrast is in the events subsequent to the first organizing of the two materials. The later course of organized inflammatory exudations, like that of the organized material for repair after injuries, is usually one of constant approximation to the healthy state. As newly-formed parts, they gradually assimilate themselves to the shape and purpose, if not to the tissue, of the parts among which they lie; or they are apt to waste, degenerate, and be removed. Their changes tend ever towards a better state; so that, in the whole course of exudative inflammatory diseases, some can see nothing but an "effort of nature" to avert or repair some greater evil.* It is very different with the class of diseases to which tumors belong: it is in their very nature to proceed to further and further deviation from the proper type of the body. The structure of tumors may indeed be like that of some of the natural parts; it may be identical with that of the part in which they lie: in this respect they may be called homologous; but, considered in their life, they are not so; for, commonly, they are growing while the tissues far and near around them are only maintaining their integrity, or are even degenerating, or yielding themselves to the anormal growth.

I think that it is only in the consideration of this activity and partial independence of the life of tumors, and of the diseases allied to them, that we shall ever discern their true nature. We too much limit the grounds of pathology when, examining a tumor after removal, we only now compare it with the natural tissues. The knowledge of all its present properties may leave us ignorant of the property which it alone, of all the components of the body, had some time ago—the property of growing. And so, if we can ever attain the knowledge of the origin of a tumor, it may avail little, unless it supply also the explanation of its progress. If, for example, what is very improbable could be proved, namely, that tumors have their origin in the organization of extravasated blood, or of an inflammatory exudation, still this greater problem would

* There are, indeed, cases in which organized lymph and scars continue to grow; but these are quite exceptional, and are to be regarded as diseases of the same class as tumors, peculiar only in respect of the materials in which they are manifested.

remain unsolved :—How or why is it, that, in ordinary cases, these materials, when organized, gradually decrease, and assimilate themselves to the adjacent parts; while, in the assumed formation of tumors, they gradually increase, and pursue, in many cases, a peculiar method of development and growth? Why is it that, assuming even a similarity of origin, the new-formed part manifests, in the one class of cases, a continuous tendency towards conformity with the type of the body; in the other, a continuous deviation from it in shape and volume, if not in texture? How is it that, to take an extreme case, we can never find, as in a specimen * at St. George's Hospital, fatty tumors of considerable size in the mesentery of a patient from whom, in the extremest emaciation of phthisis, nearly all the natural fat was removed; or, as in a case related by Schuh,† huge lumps of fat, on the head, throat, and chest of a man whose abdomen and legs were extremely thin?

I do not pretend to answer these questions; but I think that in them is the touchstone by which we may tell the value of a pathology of this great class of diseases. It is not in the likeness or in the unlikeness to the natural tissues that we can express the true nature of tumors: it is not enough to consider their anatomy; their physiology, also, must be studied: as dead masses, or as growths achieved, they may be called like or unlike the rest of a part; but, as things growing, they are unlike it. It is, therefore, not enough to think of them as hypertrophies or overgrowths: they must be considered as parts overgrowing with appearance of inherent power, irrespective of the growing or maintenance of the rest of the body, discordant from its normal type, and with no seeming purpose.

To all this, I know, it may be objected that tumors, and other like growths, may cease to grow, or grow unequally, and yet are tumors still. But this is only in appearance opposed to what I have said, which is no more than that the best or only time, in which we may discern the true difference of these from other growths, is the time of their active increase. As we can have no complete idea of any living thing, unless it include the recognition of its origin, and of its passage through certain phases of development and growth; so must our thoughts of these abnormities be imperfect and untrue, unless we have regard to their development, and growth, and maintenance, as independent parts. But, indeed, the cessation of growth in tumors and the allied diseases often affords evidences of their peculiar nature, confirmatory of that deduced from their increase. Such cessation may occur when they have attained a certain regular size; as in the painful subcutaneous tumors, the osseous tumors on the phalanges of great toes, and some others, which, perhaps always, cease to grow when they have reached a limit of dimensions that appears as natural and constant for them as the average stature is for the individuals of any

* Y. 71, Museum of St. George's Hospital.
† Die Erkenntniss der Pseudoplasmen, p. 101. Wein, 1851.
21

species. Or, the cessation of growth may occur when the tumor degenerates or wastes; as when a fibrous tumor calcifies, or when a mammary
glandular tumor is absorbed. But it is to be observed that these events
are, or may be, as irrespective of the nutrition of all the rest of the
body, as the development and growth of the tumor were; and that,
except in the comparatively rare event of the absorption of a tumor,
there is, in no case, an indication of return to the normal type or condition of the body: there is no improvement, as in the organized lymph
exuded in the inflammatory process, no adaptation to purpose, no assumption of a more natural shape. In all these events, therefore, as well as
in their growth, the nearly independent nature of the tumor is shown:
while forming part of the body, and borrowing from it the apparatus
and the materials necessary to its life, the tumor grows or maintains
itself, or degenerates, according to peculiar laws.

The characters of which I have been speaking belong to a larger number of abnormities than are usually called tumors: they belong, indeed,
to a large class, of which tumors form one part or section, while the
other is composed of certain morbid enlargements of organs, by what is
regarded as merely hypertrophy; such as that of the prostate, the thyroid gland and others.* Now the distinction between these two divisions
of the class must, I believe, be an arbitrary one; for the two are so little
unlike, that, really, it is in these hypertrophies of glands that we may
hope to find the truest guidance to an insight into the nature of tumors.
In speaking of cysts from the walls of which vascular growths may
spring and fill their cavities, I shall have to describe that these intra-
cystic growths are, in their best state of structure, close imitations of
the gland in which they occur. In relation to tumors, the most instructive examples of this fact are in the cystic tumors of the breast, of which
the general structure has been especially illustrated by Dr. Hodgkin and
Sir B. C. Brodie, and the microscopic characters by M. Lebert and Mr.
Birkett. Among these, a series of specimens in the Museum,† may illustrate every stage of the transition, from the simple cyst, to the cyst so

---

* The class may seem to include, also, those abnormal states of the fœtus which are attended with excessive growth or development of organs or members, yet cannot be ascribed
to a fusion of two germs; and, indeed, in the case of certain bony growths the line cannot
be drawn, without artifice, between monstrosities by excess and tumors (see Lectures XXVII).
But, in the large majority, there are sufficient characters of distinction between them;
for, 1st, the congenital excesses of development present a more complex structure, and are
more conformed to the plan and construction of the body, than anything that can be reasonably called a tumor. And, if it be said that this higher organization is no more than is
consistent with the period of formation, which is in embryo-life, when the force of development is greatest, then, 2dly, we may note this difference; that the congenital excesses
are usually limited for their increase to the period of natural growth of the body. They
commonly cease to grow when or before the body has attained its full stature: they con-
conform to its methods and times of development, growth, and decay.

† Mus. Coll. Surg., Nos. 168, 169, 170, 172, &c.

filled with gland substance as to form a solid tumor,—the chronic mammary, or mammary glandular tumor. Now a near parallel with the history of these mammary tumors is presented by the observations of Frerichs[*] and Rokitansky[†] on the intra-cystic growths which occur within the substance of enlarging thyroid glands, *i. e.* of increasing bronchoceles. In these, masses of new-formed thyroid gland-tissue are found imbedded and inclosed in fibro-cellular coverings or capsules, within the proper though increased substance of the gland.   In like manner, as Rokitansky has shown, it is not unsual in enlargements of the prostate gland, to find distinct masses of new structure imitating that of the prostate, which lie imbedded and incapsuled in the proper substance of the gland. Moreover (and here is a closer contact between these hypertrophies and tumors), these growths of new gland-tissue may appear, not only in the substance of the enlarging thyroid and prostate glands, but external to and detached from the glands.   Such outlying masses of thyroid gland are not rare near bronchoceles ; lying by them like the little spleens one often sees near the larger mass.   Near the enlarged prostate, similar detached outlying masses of new substance, like tumors in their shape and relations, and like prostate gland in tissue, may be sometimes found. A very large and remarkable specimen of the kind was sent to me by Mr. Wyman.[‡]   It was taken from a man, 64 years old, who, for the last four years of his life, was unable to pass his urine without the help of the catheter.   He died with bronchitis ; and a tumor, measuring $2\frac{1}{4}$ inches by $1\frac{1}{2}$, was found, as Mr. Wyman described it, "lying loose in the bladder, only connected to it by a pedicle, moving on this like a hinge, and when pressed forwards, obstructing the orifice of the urethra." Now, both in general aspect and in microscopic structure, this tumor is so like a portion of enlarged prostate gland, that I know no character by which to distinguish them.[§]

The relation of these new-formed isolated portions of thyroid or prostate gland is so intimate, on the one side, to admitted tumors, such as the chronic mammary, and, on the other side, to the general hypertrophies of the glands, that we cannot dissociate these diseases without great violence to nature.   Clearly these are all essentially the same kind of disease : yet, to call them all "tumors" would be to do as much violence to the conventional use of terms which have become not merely the expressions, but the guides, of our thoughts.   The best course seems to be to make an arbitrary division of this group.   In accordance, then, with the arbitration of custom, we may assign the name of tumors to such

* Ueber Gallert-oder Colloidgeschwülste. Göttingen, 1847.
† Zur Anatomie des Kropfes ; and Ueber die Cyste, in the Denkschr. der k. Akademie der Wissenschaften, Wien, 1849.
‡ The specimen is in the Museum of St. Bartholomew's Hospital. A remarkable tumor of the same kind, but imbedded in the substance of the prostate, is in the Museum of the Middlesex Hospital.
§ Such tumors will be further described in the twenty-eighth lecture.

examples of these morbid growths or growing parts, as, 1st, are isolated from the surrounding parts by distinct investing layers of tissue; or, 2dly, though continuous with the natural parts, are abruptly circumscribed in the greater part of their extent; or, 3dly, are formed of new materials infiltrated and growing in the interstices of natural parts.

If the group of what are to be called tumors may be thus inclosed, we may next proceed to divide it into smaller parts. And, first, it seems proper to divide tumors according as they may be named innocent or malignant. I would employ these terms still, because, though not free from objections, they imply a more natural and a less untrue division than any yet invented to replace them. The distinction between innocent and malignant tumors is probably one, not of mere visible structure, but of origin and vital properties; it is, therefore, less falsely expressed by terms implying quality of nature, than by such as refer to structure alone.

The chief distinctions are to be traced in certain characters which, in the malignant tumors or cancers (for these terms are synonymous) are superadded to those already cited as belonging to the whole class.

And, first, the intimate structure of malignant tumors is, usually, not like that of any of the fully developed natural parts of the body, nor like that which is formed in a natural process of repair or degeneration.

Many of the cells of cancers, for example, may be somewhat like gland-cells or like epithelium-cells; yet a practised eye can distinguish them, even singly. And much more plainly their grouping distinguishes them: they are heaped together disorderly, and seldom have any lobular or laminar arrangement, such as exists in the natural glands and epithelia, or in the innocent glandular or epithelial or epidermal tumors. These innocent tumors are really imitations, so far as their structure is concerned, of the natural parts; and the existence of such imitations in any tumors make the diversity—the heterology, as it is called—of the malignant tumors, appear more evident.

Still, this rule of dissimilarity of structure in malignant tumors is only general. The other properties of malignancy may be sometimes observed in tumors that have, apparently, the same structure as those that are generally innocent. I shall have to refer to cases of fibrous tumors which, in every respect of structure, were like common fibrous tumors, and yet returned after removal, and ulcerated, with infection of adjacent parts, and appeared in internal organs. These, with some others, must be regarded as malignant, though in structure resembling innocent tumors and natural tissues. On the other hand there are some innocent cartilaginous tumors, with structures as different from those that exist in our natural tissues, as cancer-cells are from gland-cells or from epithelial-cells. The two sets of cases, though both be exceptional, supply sufficient grounds for not preferring such terms as "homologous" and "heterologous" before "innocent" and "malignant," if the former are meant, as they commonly are, to apply to the structure of the several growths.

Secondly, malignant growths may have the character of infiltration; *i. e.* their elementary structures may be inserted, infiltrated, or diffused in the interspaces and cavities of the tissues in which they lie. Thus, in its early state a malignant tumor may comprise, with its own proper elements, those of the organ in which it is formed; and it is only in its later life that the elements of the tissue or organ disappear from it, gradually degenerating and being absorbed, or, possibly, yielding themselves as materials for its growth.*

Thus, a hard cancer of the mammary gland includes in its mass a part, or even the whole, of the gland itself, as if they were only a conversion of the gland-tissue: and one may find, within the very substance of the cancer, the remains of the lactiferous tubes involved in it, and with the microscope, may trace in it the fibro-cellular tissues that separated the gland-lobes, and the degenerate elements of the epithelial contents of the tubes and acini. But among all these lie the proper cells of the cancerous growth, and these usually increase while the original structures of the gland decrease. So, too, in medullary cancerous disease of the uterus, the uterus itself, or part of it, is in the tumor, and gradually wastes, while the medullary matter, diffused or infiltrated in it, is growing.

The malignant growths may, I say, thus appear in infiltrations; but they are not always so. Thus, though the hard cancer of the breast is, commonly, or always, an infiltration of cancerous substance in and among the proper structures of the gland, yet the hard cancer of the bones is often a distinct tumor, such as has no mixture of bone in it, but may be enucleated from the cavity or shell of bone in which it lies. So, too, while the medullary cancer of the uterus plainly consists in an infiltration or insertion of new material in the substance of the organ, that of the breast is usually a separate tumor, and altogether discontinuous from the surrounding parts.†

Many other instances of similar contrast might be cited; still the fact that their elemental structures may be thus infiltrated in the tissues they affect is a characteristic feature of malignant tumors. I think it is rarely imitated in cases of innocent tumors.

3d. It is, also, generally characteristic of malignant tumors that they have a peculiar tendency to ulcerate, their ulceration being com-

---

* See, on this last-mentioned point, Rokitansky, Pathol. Anatomie, i. 121. If, in such a case, the removal of the original textures be quicker or more considerable than the production of the new morbid substance, there may be no swelling or visible tumor: yet, since the new material increases, the essential character of a growth is observed. Such growth without swelling is often noticed in hard cancers of the breast and of the bones.

† Nos. 2787, 2796, and others in the College Museum; and Nos. 15 in Ser. 32, and 28 in Ser. 35, or that of St. Bartholomew's, illustrate these contrasts. On the difference between *infiltrations and outgrowths*, see p. 331.

monly preceded by softening. One can, indeed, in this particular, only observe a graduated difference between the innocent and the malignant diseases; for certain innocent tumors, if they grow very rapidly, are apt very rapidly to decay; and they may suppurate and discharge their ichor and débris with foul and dangerous ulceration. Thus the quickly-growing cartilaginous tumors may imitate, in these respects, malignant growths; so may large fibrous tumors when they soften or decay. Or, again, when an innocent tumor grows more rapidly than the parts over it can yield, they may waste and ulcerate, and allow it to protrude; and it may now itself ulcerate and look very like malignant disease. This may be seen in the protruding fibrous tumors that ulcerate and bleed; or, in a more striking manner, in the protruding vascular growths that have sprung up in the cystic tumors of the breast. Or, once more, the characters of readiness to ulcerate may be imitated by innocent tumors after injuries, or in exposure to continued irritation; for they resist these things with less force than the similar natural parts do. Hence, sloughing and ulcerating fibrous, erectile, and other tumors have been often thought cancerous, and so described.

The respective tendencies to ulcerate can, therefore, be counted only as constituting differences of degree between the innocent and the malignant tumors. We may speak of a liability in the one case, of a proneness in the other.

4th. The softening that often precedes the ulceration of malignant growths can hardly be considered separately from the minute account of their structure. I therefore pass it by, and proceed to their fourth distinctive character, which is to be noticed in the modes of their ulceration.

This is, that the ulcer which forms in, or succeeds, a malignant growth, has no apparent disposition to heal; but a morbid substance, like that of which the original growth was composed, forms the walls or boundaries of the ulcer; and as this substance passes through the same process of ulceration which the primary growth passes through, so the malignant ulcer spreads and makes its way through tissues of all kinds.

In contrast with this character of malignant growths, it is observable that beneath and around an ordinary ulcer of the natural tissues, or of an innocent tumor, we find the proper tissues unchanged; or, perhaps, infiltrated and succulent with recent lymph, or the materials for repair; or somewhat indurated with lymph already organized. The base and margins of a cancerous ulcer are themselves also cancerous; those of a common ulcer are infiltrated with only reparative or inflammatory material. In like manner, if ulceration extend through an innocent growth, it may destroy it all, and no similar growth will form in the adjacent parts, replacing that which has been destroyed: but in the ulceration of cancer, while the cancerous matter is being constantly discharged, by sloughing or ulceration, from the surface, new matter of the same kind, and in more abundance, is being formed at some distance from the surface; so that, in a section through an ulcerated cancer, one does not arrive at healthy tissues till after passing through a stratum of cancer.

5th. Malignant tumors are, again, characterized by this: that they not only enlarge, but apparently multiply or propagate themselves; so that, after one has existed for some time, or has been extirpated, others like it grow, either in widening circles round its seat, or in parts more remote.

Mere multiplicity is not a distinctive character of malignant diseases; for many innocent tumors may be found in the same person. But in the conditions and circumstances of the multiplicity there are characteristic differences. Thus, when many innocent tumors exist in the same person, they are commonly, or always, all in one tissue. A man may have a hundred fatty tumors, but they shall all be in his subcutaneous fat: many fibrous tumors may exist in the same uterus, but it is so rare, that we may call it chance, if one be found in any other part in the same patient; so, many cartilaginous tumors may be in the bones of the hands and feet, but to these, or to these and the adjacent bones, they are limited.

There is no such limitation in the case of multiplicity of malignant tumors. They tend especially to affect the lymphatics connected with the part in which they first arise; but they are not limited to these. The breast, the lymphatics, the skin and muscles, the liver, the lungs, may be all and at once, the seats of tumors. Indeed (and here is the chief contrast), it is more common to find the many malignant tumors scattered through several organs or tissues than to find them limited to one.

Moreover if there be a multiplicity of innocent tumors, they have generally a contemporary origin, and all seem to make (at least for a time) a commensurate progress. But the more ordinary course of malignant tumors is, that one first appears, and then, after a clear interval of progress in it, others appear; and these are followed by others, which with an accelerating succession, spring up in distant parts.

6th. A sixth distinctive character of malignant tumors is that, in their multiplication, as well as in their progress of ulceration, there is scarcely a tissue or an organ which they may not invade.

In regard to their multiplicity, I have just illustrated their contrast in this point with the innocent tumors; and a similar contrast is as obvious in the characters of the ulcers. It is seldom that a common ulcer extends, without sloughing, from the tissues it has first affected into any other; rather, as a new tissue is approached, it is thickened and indurated, as if to resist the progress of the ulcer. But before a cancerous ulcer the tissues in succession all give way, becoming first infiltrated, then, layer after layer degenerating and ulcerating away with the cancerous matter.

One may see this very well in bones. Specimens are to be found in nearly all the Museums, of tibiæ (for example) on the front surfaces of which new bone is formed, in a circumscribed round or oval layer, a line or two in thickness. This bone, which is compact, hard, smooth, and closely united with the shaft beneath it, was formed under an old ulcer of the integuments of the shin. But, on the other side, specimens are found, which show that when a cancerous ulcer reaches bone, at once the bone clears away before it; and a cavity with abrupt, jagged, eaten-out edges, tells the rapid work of destruction.* Neither are specimens rare, showing the progressive destruction of more various tissues; such as a cancer of the scalp making way by ulceration through the pericranium, skull, and dura mater, and then penetrating deeply into the brain;† or one in the integuments of the shin going right through the tibia, and deep into the muscles of the calf.‡

Such are the general characters of malignant tumors. Those of innocent ones are their opposites or negatives. Thus: innocent tumors have not a structure widely different from that of a natural tissue: they do not appear as infiltrations displacing or overwhelming the original tissues of their seat: they do not show a natural proneness to ulceration; nor is the ulceration, which may happen in one through injury or disease, prone to extend into the adjacent parts: they do not appear capable of multiplying or propagating themselves in distant parts: they do not grow at the same time in many different tissues.

Now, the distinctive value of each of these characteristics of malignant disease may be appreciated: indeed, I have myself lowered it, by showing that each of them may be absent in tumors having all the other features of malignancy, and that certain of them may be observed occasionally in tumors that in other respects appear non-malignant. But objections against each character separated from the rest are of little weight against the total value of all these characters of malignancy, or of a majority of them, concurrent in one case. Similar objections might be made against even the classifications of natural history: and none but such as are disposed to cavil at all nosology, could fail, in watching a series of cases of tumors through many years, to observe that the great majority of them could be classed according as, in their course, they did or did not present the characters that I have enumerated. Some cases would be found in which one or two of the signs might be wanting, or, if I may so speak, misplaced; but, putting these aside, as exceptions to be regulated by future inquiry; and looking broadly at the whole subject, no one could doubt that this division of tumors into innocent and malignant may be justly made, and that the outward marks by which they are discriminated are expressions of real difference in their properties and import.

* In the College Museum, Nos. 3082-3-3 A; 3267-8, and many others, illustrate these points.
† Museum of St. Bartholomew's, vi. 57.
‡ Museum of the College of Surgeons, 232.

In what these differences may consist I shall not discuss till I have completed my account of each kind of tumor. For the present I will say only, that I think malignant tumors are local manifestations of some specific morbid states of the blood; and that in them are incorporated peculiar morbid materials which accumulate in the blood, and which their growth may tend to increase. All their distinctive characters are, I think, consistent with this view; and the absence of the same characters in innocent tumors may lead us to believe that they are usually local diseases, the result of some inexplicable error of nutrition in the part that they affect, and only in the same measure dependent on the state of the blood as are the natural tissues, which require, and may be favored by, the presence of their appropriate materials of nutrition. Or, when, as sometimes happens, an innocent tumor begins its growth during, or soon after, some general disease, we may suppose that it owes its first formation to an abnormal condition of the blood: but that, when the blood recovers its health, the tumor subsists or grows on the nourishment supplied by the normal materials of the blood. Instances of tumors thus constitutional in their origin, but subsisting as local diseases, will be mentioned in the general history of cancers.

It may be best to speculate no further, either on this point, or on the origin or determining causes of tumors. I could speak certainly of very little connected with these points, unless it were of the error or insufficiency of all the hypotheses concerning them that I have proposed to myself, or have read in the works of others. One of these alone seems to need disproof: namely, that tumors, whether innocent or malignant, are due to the organization of effused blood, or of some inflammatory exudation, or of the material of repair. The great objections to this view are as follows: 1. It is an almost infinitely small proportion of injuries that are followed by the growth of tumors. 2. In a large majority of cases of tumor, no injury or previous local disease is assigned, even by the patients, as the cause of the growth. In 200 cases, taken indiscriminately from those I have lately recorded, no local cause whatever could be assigned for the growth of 155 tumors, of which 64 were innocent and 91 malignant: of the remaining 45, referred by the patients to previous injury or disease of the part, 15 were innocent and 30 malignant tumors. 3. Blood extravasated, and the products of the inflammatory and reparative processes, are not indifferent materials, such as would pursue this or that direction or development, according to chance, or some imaginary influence exercised on them. They have a proper tendency to assume the form of fibro-cellular, fibrous, or osseous tissue. They do not become, when their history can be traced, either fatty, or perfectly cartilaginous, or glandular tissue, such as we find in tumors. 4. No intermediate conditions have been yet found between blood or lymph and a tumor. And, lastly, all the facts relating to injuries, as favoring or determining the growth of tumors, are explicable on the supposition that the injury impairs for a time the nutrition of a part, and diminishes its power of excluding abnormal methods of nutrition.

Narrowing now the objects of consideration to the innocent tumors alone, I will speak very briefly of their classification.

A first subdivision of them may be made, according to the usual arrangement, into the cysts or cystic tumors, and the solid tumors. There are, indeed, not a few instances in which the two divisions overlap or are confused. Thus, on the one side, in cases to which I have already referred, a solid growth may spring from the inner walls of a cyst, and, enlarging more rapidly than the walls do, may fill the cavity, and come in contact and unite with the walls; and thus may be traced a complete series of gradations from the cystic to the solid tumor. On the other hand, cysts may be formed within solid tumors, and increasing more rapidly than the solid structure, may reduce it to scarcely more than a congeries of cysts, or to one great cyst. Such changes are illustrated sometimes in fibrous tumors of the uterus: and I think, also, in the tumors which Sir Astley Cooper called "hydatid disease" of the testicle.

But though there are these instances of confusion, yet the division is very convenient, and is probably deeply and well founded.

Next, among cysts, some are filled with a simple fluid, containing no organized matter, and resembling one or other of the fluids of serous cavities. These may be called simple or barren, or in most instances, serous cysts.

Other cysts contain organized substances, and may be named, as a group, proliferous; and the several members of the group may be described, according to their contents, as glandular, cutaneous, sebaceous, dental, and the like.

Of the solid innocent tumors, no method of arrangement at present appears reasonable but the old one, which is founded on their likeness to the natural tissues. On this ground they may be arranged in the following divisions, with names, as specific names, expressing their several resemblances—viz., fatty, fibro-cellular, fibrous, fibroid, and fibro-nucleated, cartilaginous, myeloid, osseous, glandular, and vascular or erectile. And, again, under each of these may be arranged certain varieties, including instances that, in some uniform manner, deviate, without quite departing, from the usual characters; as the fibro-cystic, fibro-calcareous, and other varieties of the fibrous tumors.

In each assumed kind or group of these solid tumors, moreover, we must make a division, according to their modes of growth, and of connection with the adjacent parts. Some among them are only intermediately connected with the adjacent parts; a layer of tissue at once separates and combines them, and, by division of this layer, such a tumor may be cleanly and alone removed from the surrounding parts; it may be enucleated or shelled out from them. Thus, with a common fatty tumor, or a fibrous tumor of the uterus, if we cut along one part of its surface, we may, with a blunt instrument, detach the whole mass, by splitting the layer of fibro-cellular tissue which, like a capsule, incloses and isolates it.

These are what we commonly accept as the proper or typical tumors, these which are "discontinuous hypertrophies."

Other growths resemble these in every character, except in that they are connected with the adjacent parts by continuity of similar tissue, and thus appear as growths, not in, but of, the parts. Thus we cannot exactly isolate a polypus of the nose or of the uterus: the overgrown part cannot be enucleated, because the proper tissue of the nasal mucous membrane, or of the uterine wall, is continued into it; the tissue of the growth is here not only uniform, but continuous, with that of the adjacent parts. So, too, with epulis: the gum itself, or the periosteum of the jaw together with the gum, seems, by its own excessive growth, to form the tumor; and in other fibrous tumors on bones, the fibres of the periosteum appear to be in the growth, and to form part of it.

Such growths as these might be named "continuous hypertrophies," or "outgrowths;" and I will, in general, observe this distinction wherever the same tissue is, in different cases, found in both forms of growth; calling the discontinuous masses tumors, the continuous ones, outgrowths. Thus, answering to the common fatty tumor, we find the pendulous and continuous fatty outgrowths of the neck or the abdominal walls; answering to the fibro-cellular tumor that grows, as a discontinuous mass in the scrotum or beneath the labia, we have the cutaneous outgrowths or enlargements of these parts; to the fibrous tumors of the uterus answer the fibrous polypi or continuous outgrowths of its substance. All these instances of clear distinction might lead us to think that a strong definition line might be drawn to divide the whole class of innocent overgrowths into tumors and outgrowths. But when we come to the tumors of bone and periosteum, and to the erectile tumors, we find the distinctions vanishing, and in many instances no longer possible.

It may seem as if these "outgrowths" needed distinction from the "infiltrations" which were spoken of as peculiar to malignant diseases. The distinctions between them are well marked. In the outgrowth the new material is like that with which it is connected, or like its normal rudiment, so that it is as if the tissue were itself outgrown; but, in the infiltration, the new material is dissimilar from that in the interstices of which it is placed. And in the outgrowth the materials of the original part appear to be at least maintained, if they are not increased; but in the infiltration they degenerate and waste. We may compare, for this contrast, the cancerous diseases of the skin, with the cutaneous outgrowths of the labia, nymphæ, prepuce, or scrotum.

In thus briefly indicating that which appears still the most reasonable method of classifying tumors, I have referred to difficulties which have appeared to be insuperable objections to any attempt at an arrangement of these diseases. I will therefore state, so far as I can, what is the real weight of these objections.*

First, it is said, such classifications cannot be well made, because, between each two assumed kinds or groups of tumors, intermediate examples may be found transitional, as it were, from one species to the other: the one, it is said, "runs into" the other; or, as Mr. Abernethy expressed it, "diseases resemble colors in this respect—that a few of the primary ones only can be discriminated and expressed, whilst the intermediate shades, though distinguishable by close attention and comparative observation, do not admit of description and denomination."†

This is exactly true; but Mr. Abernethy seems to have felt that his sentence supplied the answer to the objection against classification by structure, which it expressed; for, as he did not, because of the intermediate tints, refuse to name and arrange the primary colors, so neither did he, nor need we, hesitate to name and classify diseases, and among them the principal forms of tumors.

Moreover, the objection that structures may be found intermediate between those belonging to the chief forms of tumors, may be as well made against the use of names and systems for the natural tissues. There are no strongly outlined characters defining any of the natural tissues that are ever imitated in tumors; intermediate and confusing forms are found everywhere. The various forms of fibro-cartilage, for instance, fill up every possible gradation from cartilage to fibrous tissue: between fibro-cellular and fibrous tissues, between tendons, aponeuroses, and fasciæ, between epithelium and simple membrane, there are, in the natural tissues, the narrowest gradations. Yet we name and arrange the natural tissues with some truth and much utility; and so we may the tumors that resemble them.

Another objection against this classification of tumors is made on the ground that there are some in which two or more different tissues are mingled. Thus, tumors may be often found, in which fat and fibro-cellular tissue, or fibrous tissue and organic muscle, or cartilage and glandular tissue, or other combinations, meet together. But, among these, some are imitations of natural combinations of tissues, as the fibrous and organic muscular tissues of the uterus are imitated by the so-called fibrous tumors in its walls; and of the others, it need only be remembered that such combinations do occur, and these may be put aside from any interference with arrangement, by making a series of mixed tumors, or by adding to the description of each species the combinations into which it may enter.

---

* The best statement of these objections is by Vogel; but he has well answered his own arguments by disregarding them in his nomenclature of tumors.

† An attempt to form a Classification of Tumors according to their Anatomical Structure. Surgical Works, vol. ii. ed. 1815.

Yet another objection is made, that the characters of tumors are not constant, and that many must be reckoned as examples of one species, which are not much, if at all, like one another.

The diversity of characters is, indeed, the great difficulty with which the pathology of tumors has to contend; but the diversity is not to be called inconstancy: it is due to the fact that each tumor has, like each natural tissue, its phases of development, of degeneration, and of disease. Now we have scarcely yet begun the study of the variations to which, in each of these phases, the several tumors are liable. We may have learned, for example, the general characters of cartilaginous tumors, as they grow in the most favorable conditions; but how little do we know of the various aspects these may present when they fail of due development, or fall into various diseases, or variously degenerate! Yet all these changes have to be studied in the history of every tumor; and it would be as reasonable to charge any natural tissue with inconstancy, because it is altered in development and disease, as to hold that the similar diversity of tumors is an objection to their classification according to their structure.

However, while I put this aside as an objection against classification, let me not be thought to underrate it as a great difficulty; it is the great difficulty with which we have to contend. The work we have to do is not only to distinguish each kind of tumor from all other kinds, but, and in order to this end, to distinguish, as I may say, each kind from itself, by learning in each all the changes occurring in the various stages of its life. The difficulty of such a task cannot be exaggerated, while we consider the rarity of the objects to be studied; but it must be overcome before we can cease to speak of "anomalous tumors," and of "strange distempered masses," or, which is more important, before we can, even after the removal of a tumor, speak with certainty of the issue of a case.

LECTURE XXII.

SIMPLE OR BARREN CYSTS.

THE *Cysts*, or *Cystic Tumors*, to which I shall devote this lecture and the next, form a very numerous group, and have only or barely these characters in common; namely, that each of them is essentially a cyst, sac, or bag, filled with some substance which may be regarded as entirely, or for the most part, its product, whether as a secretion, or as an endogenous growth.

We may conveniently arrange cysts under the titles "simple" or "barren," and "compound" or "proliferous;" the former containing fluid or unorganized matter, the latter containing variously organized bodies.

Among the simple or barren cysts, we find that some contain a fluid like that of one of the serous membranes; such are certain mammary cysts, and those of the choroid plexus: some are full of synovia-like fluid, as the enlarged bursæ: others are full of blood, or of colloid, or some peculiar abnormal, fluid: while others, forming the transition between the barren and the proliferous cysts, contain more highly organic secretions, such as milk, or mucous, or salivary or seminal fluid. These several forms we may arrange with names appropriate to their contents; as serous, synovial, mucous, sanguineous, colloid, salivary, seminal, and others.

Among the cysts, whether barren or proliferous, it is probable that at least three modes of origin may obtain. 1st. Some are formed by the enlargement and fusion of the spaces or areolæ in fibro-cellular, areolar, or other tissues. In these spaces fluids collect and accumulate ; the tissue becomes rarified ; and, gradually, the boundaries of the spaces are leveled down and walled in, till a perfect sac or cyst is formed, the walls of which continue to secrete. Thus are produced the bursæ over the patella, and others ; and to this we may refer, at least in some cases, the formation of cysts in tumors, and, perhaps, in other parts.

2dly. Some cysts are formed by dilatation and growth of natural ducts or sacculi ; as are those sebaceous or epidermal cysts which, formed by enlarged hair-follicles, have permanent openings. Such, also, are certain cysts containing milk, that are formed of enlarged portions of lactiferous tubes : such the ovarian cysts formed by distended and overgrown Grafian vesicles; and such appear to be certain cysts formed of dilated portions of blood-vessels shut off from the main streams.

3dly. Many, and perhaps the great majority of cysts, such as those of the kidney, the choroid plexuses, the chorion, and the thyroid gland, are formed by the enormous growth of new-formed elementary structures having the characters of cells or nuclei, which pursue a morbid course from their origin, or from a very early period of their development.

It might, on some grounds, be desirable to classify the cysts according to their respective modes of formation ; separating the " secondary cysts," as those have been called which are derived by growth or expansion of normal parts, from the "primary," or, as they might be called, the "autogenous" cysts, But, at present, I believe, such a division cannot be made ; for of some cysts it is impossible to say in which method they originate, and, in some instances, either method may lead to an apparently similar result. Thus, some sebaceous or epidermal cysts are clearly formed of overgrown hair follicles ; others are of distinct autogenous origin. Some ranulæ are probably formed by dilatation of the submaxillary duct obstructed by calculi or otherwise; others by anormal development of distinct cysts, or possibly of a bursa between the muscles of the tongue.* Some cysts in the mammary gland are certainly dilated portions of ducts; others are, from their origin, anormal transformations of the elementary structures of the gland. But in each of these cases it may be impossible, when the cyst is fully formed, to decide what was its mode of origin: whether by growth of parts once normally formed, or by transformation of elementary and rudimental structures.

Of the three modes of the formation of cysts to which I have referred, the first two, namely, that which is accomplished by expansion of areolar spaces, and that by dilatation and growth of ducts or vesicles, scarcely need an explanation.

Indeed, if it were not for some convenience in surgical practice, we should not retain most of the cysts thus formed in the list of tumors; for their growth appears, in most instances, to be due only to the accumulation of the contents of the obstructed tube or sacculus, and to be exactly adjusted to this accumulation, and commensurate with it. Thus it is in the cases of ranula with obstruction of the submaxillary duct, and the similar dilatations of the pancreatic duct; in the cystiform dilatation of the obstructed Fallopian tube; in the dilated hair-follicles; in bursæ; and in some others. These are all conventionally reckoned among cysts, and arranged with tumors: but several of the like kind are never so reckoned: such as the cyst-like gall-bladder, dilated with thin mucus, when the cystic duct is completely obstructed; the dilatation of the uterus, filled with serum after closure of its external orifice; the distended sheath of a tendon; and others. Convenience and common usage have decided what cysts may be grouped with those which alone, we may anticipate, will be classed with tumors when pathology becomes more accurate and strict. Convenience alone, also, decides for the omission, from so vague a class as this, of the sacs or capsules that are formed round foreign bodies and solid tumors, and of the sacs that may be formed on the free surfaces of extravasated blood or inflammatory exudation.

For the third method of formation enumerated above, a more detailed account is required; and this I will now endeavor to give.

The general structures of the cysts thus formed may be best studied in those that are so commonly found in the kidneys, or the mammary or thyroid gland, or in any instance of an ordinary serous cyst. Such a cyst, when large enough for naked-eye examination, is usually constructed of fine, well-formed, fibro-cellular tissue, of which the filaments are commonly mingled with nuclei, or nucleus-fibres, and are variously interwoven in a single layer, or in many that are separable. The membranous walls thus formed, are, in general, rather firmly connected with the adjacent parts, so that the cyst cannot easily be removed entire; and from

* See Fleischman, in Schmidt's Jahrbucher, 1841, B. 32, and Frerichs, Ueber-Gallert- oder Colloidgeschwülste, Göttingen, 1847, p. 37.

these parts they derive the blood-vessels that usually ramify copiously upon them. They are usually, also, lined with epithelium, which is generally of the tessellated form, and may consist, according to Rokitansky, of either nuclei or nucleated cells.*

I am not aware that minute examinations have been made of the modes of earliest formation of any of the cysts of this kind, that are common subjects of surgical consideration; but there can be little doubt that, in their formation, they resemble the cysts of the kidney and other internal organs. In these organs the origin and progress of cysts have been profoundly studied by Rokitansky;† and I shall best describe them by giving an abstract of some of his observations, in illustration of a copy of one of his outline sketches of the minute structure of the cystic disease of the kidney. (Fig. 44.) They confirm and greatly extend the results obtained by their similar investigations of Frerichs,‡ and they fully establish the accuracy of the observations on the cystic degeneration of the kidney, which were made by Mr. Simon,§ to whom pathology is indebted for the first sure step in this rich path of inquiry. They may be repeated in almost any portion of a granular kidney containing cysts, or in a choroid plexus with cysts; but, I believe, the process may be best traced in the cystic disease of the embryonic chorion—the hydatid mole, as it has been called.|| To this I shall again refer in the next lecture.

In a portion of a granular and cystic kidney, nests, as Rokitansky calls them, of delicate vesicles, from a size just visible to that of a millet-seed, may be seen imbedded in a reddish-gray or whitish substance. These differ in size alone from the larger cysts to which one's attention would be sooner attracted; and on the other side, it is only in size that they differ from many much smaller. For if a portion of such a nest be examined with a microscope, one finds, together with the débris of the kidney, variously diseased it may be, a vast number of vesicles or cysts that were invisible to the naked eye.

The most striking of these have a wall consisting of layers of fibres scattered over with curved nuclei (a), and are filled with granulated nuclei, or, more rarely, with round or polyhedral cells, some of which may contain a molecular or granular pigmental matter, (d.) In many of these cysts, the nuclei or cells are reduced to an epithelial lining of the

* Rokitansky says (Uber die Cyste, p. 4) there is often no epithelium in the larger cysts, and their "inner layer is a nucleated, structureless, or striated blastema, externally splitting into fibres in the direction of the long axis of the oval nuclei it contains." Epithelial cells, apparently altered so as to resemble very large cells of inflammatory lymph, are commonly found in the tenacious contents of bursæ. M. Giraldès tells me that the cysts which so often occur in the antrum are commonly lined with ciliary epithelium.

† Uber die Cyste. Wien, 1850.

‡ Uber Gallert-oder Colloidgeschwülste.

§ On Subacute Inflammation of the Kidney, in the Medico-Chirurgical Transactions, vol. XXX.

|| Mettenheimer, in Müller's Archiv, 1850.

cyst; and in some even this is absent, and the "barren" cyst is filled with a clear or opaline adhesive fluid.

From the size just visible to the naked eye, such cysts vary to $\frac{1}{100}$ of an inch in diameter; and, together with these, are cysts whose walls (though their contents are like those of the others) consist of a structureless hyaline membrane: and these lie in a stroma which is equally simple, but seems to develop itself gradually into a fibrous structure circumscribing the cysts.

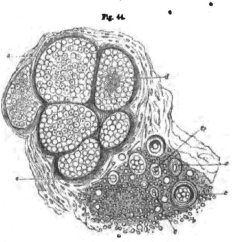

Fig. 44.

Moreover, one finds, in the same specimens (as in the lower part of Fig. 44), structures of the most various sizes, which, except in size, agree completely with the last-mentioned simple and structureless vesicles, and show every grade of size down to that which is just larger than a nucleus. The smallest of these contain a clear fluid, or are slightly granulated: in the larger there is a central nucleus, and to this are added a second, a third, and a fourth nucleus, and so on till there appear several, which fill up the commensurately enlarged vesicle (e, e, e, &c.) Now, in such a nucleus seem to lie the nucleus of the history of development of those autogenous cysts, not in the kidney alone, but in any part in which they may occur. A nucleus grows to be a cyst, whether a simple or barren one, or one that has an endogenous production of nuclei or cells, or any other structures. And, perhaps, in the same specimen, the early history of the nucleus itself may be traced; for one sees (as in the same figure), together with the nuclei, still smaller corpuscles of all sizes, down to that of the elementary granule so-called; and these, the larger they grow, the more are they like nuclei; so that, perhaps, the progress of the disease is from these granules, enlarging to the formation of nuclei, and thence pursuing some abnormal course.

It would be tedious now to trace, from this general sketch of their origin, all the phases through which such cysts may pass. Rokitansky has done it amply. We have here the elementary constituents. But the simple cyst-wall is capable, not only of growing, but of acquiring, by appropriation and development of surrounding blastema, the laminar and nucleated fibrous tissue which we find in its full estate; acquiring

22

these we may presume, just as more normally, the simple membranous
wall of a new blood-vessel acquires, as it grows, the nuclei and fibrous
tissue that belongs to its more perfect state. Such might be the least
abnormal course of any cyst: but from this it may deviate; thickening,
acquiring continually new layers, calcifying, and in other ways showing
the signs of degeneration or disease. The contents, also, of the cyst
may assume even yet more various forms: to name only the extremes—
they may retain the simple state of liquid; or with liquid there may be
a simple, or a specially secreting, epithelial layer; or, a series of successively enclosed nuclei or cells may be formed within that which first
enlarges; or, the contents may acquire the structure of well-organised
glands, or of cancer, or some other tissue; and between these extremes,
according to conditions which we have no power to trace or explain, they
may pass in any of the manifold ways of wrong, the ends of which I shall
have to describe.

Important as the history of cysts may be in its direct bearings, yet
these are not all that we may observe in it. In their history I cannot
but think we may discern an image of the first form and early progress
of many innocent solid tumors also. For, as the cyst is traced from
the mere nucleus, or even from the granule, onwards to its extreme size
or complexity of structure or contents, so, it is very probable, from the
numerous correspondences between them, that these solid tumors also
have a similar beginning in some detached element, or tissue-germ, or in
some group of such germs, which in their development and growth, may
coalesce, and then may appropriate, or exclude for absorption, the intervening substance.

Thus, in the form of erring nuclei, we may, I think, almost apprehend
the structural origin of these cysts and tumors: yet, if we may, the
question still remains whether the elementary structures in which they
begin be some new and special morbid elements, or some natural rudimental structure perverted from their normal course. Mr. Simon, speaking of the cysts of the kidney, regards them as "vesicular transformations of the ultimate structure of the gland;" and to this view, without
adopting some ingenious suppositions which he has connected with it, I
would adhere. For, unless a cyst or a solid tumor (assuming this mode
of their origin to be correct) were really a transformation of the nucleus,
or a cell, in the part in which it grows, we could not understand the very
general similarity that we find between the contents of certain cysts and
the secretions or structures of the glands in or near which they occur;
nor yet the likeness which commonly exists between the solid tumor and
the tissue in which it is imbedded. These things are as if the first beginning of the abnormal growth were in some detached element of the
natural tissue, which element, being perverted from its normal course,
thenceforward multiplies and grows, conforming with the type in minute

structure and composition, but more and more widely deviating from it in shape and size.

Such are the facts, and such the speculations that we may entertain, respecting the origin, or, at least, the smallest visible beginning, of a cyst or an innocent solid tumor. Need I add that if even this be true, we are yet far from the explanation of the cardinal point in the pathology of tumors—their continual growing. Why should these detached tissue-germs, or any less minute and less isolated portion of an organ, grow while all other germs and parts that are most like them remain unchanged? I have already confessed my ignorance.

I will endeavor now to illustrate the histories of particular forms of the simple or barren cysts.

1. The first that, may be enumerated are GASEOUS CYSTS. I know indeed, concerning them only the specimens placed by Hunter in his museum ;* but these should be admired, or almost venerated; for their histories include the honorable names of Hunter, of Jenner, and of Cavendish. Mr. Hunter says of them—"I have a piece of the intestine of a hog, which has a number of air-bladders in it. . . . . "It was sent to me by my friend Mr. Jenner, Surgeon, at Berkley, who informed me that this appearance is found very frequently upon the intestines of hogs that are killed in the summer months." . . . . . "Mr. Cavendish was so kind as to examine a little of this air; and he found 'it contained a little fixed air, and the remainder not at all inflammable, and almost completely phlogisticated.' "†

What a relic have we here! Surely, never, on an object so mean to common apprehensions, did such rays of intellectual light converge, as on these to which were addressed the frequent and inquiring observation of Jenner, the keen analysis by Cavendish, and the vast comprehension and deep reflection of John Hunter! Surely, never were the elements of an inductive process combined in such perfection! Jenner to observe; Cavendish to analyse; Hunter to compare and reflect.

2. The SEROUS CYSTS, or Hygromata, are of all the order, the most abundant. The term includes nearly all such as have thinly liquid, or honey-like contents, of yellow, brown, or other tint. Their most frequent seats are, by a hundred-fold majority, in or near the secreting glands or membranes, or the so-called vascular glands; but there is scarcely a part in which they may not be found. Their frequency in connection with secreting structures has led some to hold that they are all examples of perverted epithelial or gland-cells; but their occurrence in such parts as bones and nerves, among deep-seated muscles, and in fibrous tumors, makes it sure that they may originate independently of

* Museum of the Coll. of Surg., No. 153–4.
† See Hunter's Works, vol. iv. p. 98, and description of Pl. xxxvii.

gland-cells;* though why any element of a solid tissue should retain the vesicular form which it has in its germ-state, and in that form grow, we cannot tell.

Of this numerous group of serous cysts, however, I will speak at present of only such as may best illustrate their general pathology, and are of most importance in surgical practice; and I will, to these ends, refer chiefly to the cysts in the neck, the mammary gland, and the gums.

Single serous cysts in the neck form what have been called "hydroceles of the neck," and are well exemplified by a specimen in the Museum of the College.† This is a single oval cyst, with thin, flaccid, membranous walls, which even now, after shrinking, measures more than six inches in its chief diameter. It was successfully removed by Mr. Thomas Blizard* from between the platysma and sterno-mastoid muscles; and a part of it is said to have passed behind the clavicle. It was filled with a clear brownish fluid.

Such cysts, but various in size and other characters, are more apt to occur in the neck than in any other part of the body. Many are single cysts like this; but others are complex, having many cavities, whether separate or communicating; and some consist of very numerous cysts, even of hundreds, clustered in one comparatively firm mass.

In situation, too, they are various. In some cases they lie in the front of the neck; in others, at one or both sides: they may lie by the lower jaw, over the parotid, by the clavicle, or anywhere and everywhere in the mid spaces. And in any of these situations they may extend very deeply among the structures of the neck, and may adhere to them so closely, and may so thinly cover them, as scarcely to conceal them when laid open. Their date of origin is often obscure. In many, perhaps in the majority of cases, they appear to be congenital; but they may be first observed at any later period of life. Last year Mr. Lawrence removed a collection of four large cysts from over the parotid gland and mastoid region of a man, twenty-eight years old, who had observed their beginning only seven years previously. Three of these were filled with serum, and one with pus.

Of course, in such a variety of forms, there must be more than one

---

* Some very interesting specimens of serous cysts in bones are in the Museum of St. George's Hospital. They are described by Mr. Cæsar Hawkins, in his Lectures on Tumors, in the Medical Gazette, vols. xxi. xxii.; and in the Clinical Lecture in the same, vol. xxv. p. 472. See also a remarkable case by Vanzetti, in Schuh (Pseudoplasmen, 175). There are some remarkable specimens of cysts in the antrum, in the museum of St. Thomas's Hospital, prepared by Mr. Wm. Adams, who showed them to me. M. Giraldès considers all such as these to be formed by cystic disease of the gland-structures discovered by him in the mucous membrane of the antrum.

† Mus. Coll. Surg. 146. Many well-marked examples of the disease in all its forms are recorded by Dr. O'Beirne (Dublin Jour. of Med. and Chem. Sc. vol. vi. p. 834); Mr. Lawrence (Med.-Chir. Trans. vol. xxii. p. 44); Mr. Cæsar Hawkins (Med.-Chir. Trans. vol. xxii. p. 231); Mr. Liston (Practical Surgery, p. 330, ed. 1846); and others. A monograph by Wernher (Die angeborenen Cysten-Hygrome, Giessen, 1843) is referred to by Bruch, l. c., but I have not been able to see it.

kind, in the group of cysts that are thus, for mere convenience, placed together. The variety of origins, indeed, to which cysts in the neck may be traced, gives them peculiar interest in relation to the general pathology of cysts.

Some are evidently connected with the thyroid gland; though, being singly developed, and growing to a very large size, their relation to it may be at length obscured, and they may appear, during life, quite isolated. A woman, forty-eight years old, was under Mr. Vincent's care, in St. Bartholomew's Hospital, in July, 1841, with a tumor in the front of her neck as large as the head of a child two years old. The tumor contained fluid, which was twice withdrawn with a trocar. At the first time the fluid looked like serum, but coagulated spontaneously; at the second, it was mixed with blood. After the second operation the cyst inflamed and discharged grumous and sanious pus: but it also enlarged quickly, and the patient died unexpectedly, and rather suddenly, suffocated.

The preparation* displays a cyst occupying nearly the whole right lobe of the thyroid gland: its walls are nearly two lines in thickness; its cavity was full of lymph, pus, and blood: and the sudden death was due to a discharge of a great part of its contents into the pharynx and larynx, through an ulcerated aperture into the former.

Besides these cysts which lie within the thyroid gland, some that lie near to it are very probably of the same nature; cysts formed in some outlying portion of the gland, such as I referred to in the last lecture. But of this mode of origin we can scarcely have a proof when the cyst is fully formed and largely grown.

Other of these cysts in the neck appear to be transformations of vascular tumors; *i. e.* of erectile vascular growths or nævi. I shall refer to this point again: it is made probable by the close connection which some of these cysts have with large deep-seated veins; by the occasional opening of blood-vessels into their cavities; and by their sometimes distinctly forming portions of vascular nævi. A girl, three and a half years old, was under Mr. Lawrence's care, in 1849, in St. Bartholomew's Hospital, with a large soft and obscurely fluctuating tumor covering the greater part of the left side of the neck, and the lower part of the cheek. Such a swelling had existed from birth, but it had of late enlarged very much. It was composed of a cluster of close-set cysts, containing spontaneously coagulable fluid; but at its upper part a firmer portion of its mass consisted of a collection of tortuous and dilated blood-vessels, like those of a nævus. The examination made of it, by Mr. Coote,† after its removal, was such as to leave little doubt in his mind that it had origin in or with a nævous growth; and other cases,

* Museum of St. Bartholomew's Hospital, Ser. xxii. No. 16.
† Lecture, by Mr. Lawrence, in the Medical Times, November 30, 1850.

to which I shall refer in speaking of erectile tumors, have confirmed this view, especially some of those which are published by Mr. Hawkins.

But when we have separated all the serous cysts in the neck that may be referred to these two sources, there will probably still remain many that we can assign to no such mode of origin, and which at present we must class among primary or autogenous cysts, independent of any secreting structure.

Among these are some with fluid contents of peculiar viscidity, ropy, or honey-like, and deriving a peculiar aspect from including abundant crystals of cholestearine. Such contents may occur, perhaps, in any cyst in the neck or elsewhere; but they appear to be comparatively frequent at or near the front of the larynx. In the College Museum there is such a cyst,* attached to the hyoid bone of a sailor, who was between fifty and sixty years old, and in whom it had existed nearly as long as he could remember. It contained a brownish-yellow, grumous, honey-like fluid, with abundant crystals of cholestearine.

In 1849, Mr. Lawrence had, at St. Bartholomew's Hospital, a patient, thirty-five years old, on the left side of whose neck, directly over and closely attached to the thyro-hyoid membrane, was a smooth oval tumor, about an inch in length. He had observed a regular increase of this tumor for five or six years; but its bulk and deformity alone were inconvenient. Mr. Lawrence freely cut into it, and let out a thick honey-like fluid, in which large groups of crystals of cholestearine were visible even with the naked eye. The cyst, after the incision, suppurated, and then the wound healed, and the patient left the hospital quite well: but I have lately seen him with an appearance as if some remains of the cyst were again filling.

Cysts like the last-described are not uncommon in or near the gums, lying usually behind the reflection of the mucous membrane from the gum to the cheek. Their occasional large size, and their thick tough walls obscuring the sense of fluctuation, may make them at first look formidable. A woman, thirty-eight years old, was under my care in 1849, in whom, at first sight, I could not but suppose something was distending the antrum, so closely was the deformity of the face due to such diseases imitated. But the swelling was soft and elastic, and projected the thin mucous membrane of the gum of the upper jaw, like a half-empty sac. I cut into the sac, and let out nearly an ounce of turbid brownish fluid, sparkling with crystals of cholestearine. The posterior wall of the cyst rested in a deep excavation on the surface of the alveolar border of the upper jaw; an adaptation of shape attained, I suppose, as the result of the long-continued pressure of the cyst, which had existed six years.

* Mus. Coll. Surg. 148. These, I presume, are examples of Meliceris. The cysts which Müller describes under the name of cholesteatoma are quite different from these, and will be noticed with the cutaneous cysts in the next lecture.

At nearly the same time a young man was under my care with a similar swelling of large size, which he ascribed to an injury of the gum
or alveolar border of the upper jaw only six months previously. In
neither of the cases could I find any disease of the maxillary bone; but
it sometimes exists in intimate connection with these cysts, and sometimes
the fang or socket of the nearest tooth appears diseased. I lately saw a
lady in whom a small cyst of this kind had existed twenty-seven years,
almost daily discharging and refilling. It had its origin in a blow by
which the two median upper incisors were loosened. One of them was
again firmly fixed; the other had remained slightly loose, and its crown
was dark.

In no organ is the formation of cysts so important than in the mammary gland. Every variety of them will be found here: but I will speak
at present of only the serous cysts.

Some of these cysts are dilated ducts, or portions of ducts grown into
the cyst-form. During lactation, cysts thus derived may fill with milk,
and may attain an enormous size, so as to hold, for example, a pint or
more of milk.* In other cases they may retain the remains of milk, as
fatty matter, epithelial scales, &c.; or they may be filled with transparent
watery fluid, without coagulable matter; † but much more commonly they
contain serous fluid, pure, or variously tinged with blood or its altered
coloring matter, or various green, or brown, or nearly black fluids.‡

The complete proof of the origin of some of these cysts as dilated
portions of ducts is, that by pressure they may be emptied through the
nipple, or that bristles may be passed into them from the orifices of tubes.
But although these facts may be often observed, yet I agree with Mr.
Birkett in thinking that the majority of cysts in the mammary gland are
formed in the manner of the renal cysts, to which, indeed, they present
many points of resemblance.

The most notable instances of mammary cysts are those in which the
whole of the gland is found beset with them. This may occur while the
proper substance of the gland appears quite healthy;§ but I think it
more commonly concurrent with a contracted and partially indurated
state of the gland; a state which, independent of the cysts, appears
similar to cirrhosis of the liver, and has, I think, been named cirrhosis of
the mammary gland. Its coincidence with cysts proves its nearer rela-

* See a case by M. Jobert de Lambelle, in the Med. Times, Jan. 4, 11, 1845; and a collection of cases by Mr. Birkett, in one of which ten pints of milk were evacuated (Diseases
of the Breast, p. 201).

† Brodie, Lectures on Pathology and Surgery, p. 155.

‡ Their various contents are well shown in Cooper's Illustrations of Diseases of the
Breast, Pl. i.; and a full account of all the diseases of this class is given by Mr. Birkett in
his work already cited.

§ Two such cases are described by Sir B. C. Brodie (Lectures on Pathology and Surgery,
p. 139).

tion to that shriveled and contracted state of the glandular kidney with which the renal cysts are so commonly connected; or (when the cysts are formed by partial dilatation of the ducts), to the shriveled, indurated state of the lung that may coincide with dilatation of the bronchi.

The cysts in these cases are usually of small size, thin-walled, full of yellow, brown, green, and variously deep-colored fluids; fluids that are usually turbid, various in tinge and density, but not usually much denser than serum. They do not lie in groups, but are scattered through, it may be, the whole extent of the gland; and their walls, though thin, are tough and tense, and very closely adherent to the surrounding gland-substance. Similar small cysts are sometimes found in connection with hard cancer of the breast; and in this case they have been called by Mr. Hunter and others "cancerous hydatids:" but their proper relation in such cases appears to be, not with the cancer, but with the coincidently shriveled gland.

In this disease of the mammary gland there is no reason to believe a malignant nature, though the coincidence with cancer appears not rare, yet the diagnosis between it and cancer is not always clear, and many breasts have been removed in this uncertainty. I once saw such a case, and it ended fatally. A woman, fifty years old, had, in her left breast, just below the surface of the mammary gland, a small, smooth, oval, and movable tumor. It felt firm, but not hard; but, external to it, in a line extending towards the axilla, were two or three small round "knots," scarcely as large as peas, and quite hard. In the axilla was an enlarged gland. The breast was soft, flaccid, and pendulous. The tumor was sometimes painful, and a serous and bloody fluid often flowed from the nipple. The patient's youngest child was sixteen years old, and the tumor had been noticed six months, having arisen without evident cause. There was doubt enough about the diagnosis of this case to suggest that the tumor should first be cut into. An incision exposed the cavity of a cyst full of dark, turbid, greenish fluid, and near it many more cysts. Similar cysts pervaded the whole extent of the gland, and the whole breast was therefore removed. Many of the cysts communicated with lactiferous tubes, from which bristles could be passed through the nipple.*

In this case one comparatively large cyst existed, with many of much smaller size. In more usual cases one cyst has a yet greater predominance over the others, or even exists alone. Sometimes, in such instances, the removal or laying open one large cyst has been sufficient; but in some, smaller cysts neglected have enlarged, and the disease has appeared to recur.†

The single cysts of the mammary gland may become enormous. I

---

* In the Museum of the Middlesex Hospital is a breast from a woman in which both mammary glands were thus diseased. In the College Museum, Nos. 151 and 152 best illustrate the disease.

† Sir B. C. Brodie, loc. cit. p. 146, note.

know not what boundary may be set to their possible size; but I find one case in which nine pounds of limpid "serosity" were produced in three months in the breast of a woman thirty years old.* In this case the walls of the cyst were thin, and the fluid serous; and the fact illustrates a general rule, that the cysts which contain the simplest fluids, and which have the simplest walls, are apt to grow to the largest size: thickening of cyst-walls, and, much more, their calcification,† are here, as elsewhere, signs of degeneracy, and loss of productive power.

It would appear as if any cyst of the mammary gland might, after some time of existence in the barren state, become prolific, and bear on its inner surface growths of glandular or other tissue. But of these proliferous cysts I will speak in the next lecture.‡

3. Of SYNOVIAL CYSTS I need say very little. Under the name may be included all the anormal bursæ, or ganglions, as they are called. In these, again, two methods of formation probably obtain. Some, of which the best example is the bursa over the patella and its ligament, are merely enlargements, with various transformations, of bursæ naturally existing. Not materially different from these are the bursæ which form anew in parts subjected to occasional localized pressure, and which appear to arise, essentially, from the widening of spaces in areolar or fibro-cellular tissue, and the subsequent leveling or smoothing of the boundaries of these spaces. But others, such as the bursæ or ganglions which form about the sheaths of the tendons at the wrist, appear to be the cystic transformations of the cells inclosed in the fringe-like processes of the synovial membrane of the sheaths. The opportunities of dissecting these are rare; but I believe there is a close resemblance, in mode of formation, between them and the cysts of the choroid plexus. Rokitansky has shown that these are due to cystic growth in the villi appended to the margins of the plexus, which villi are very similar, in their constituent structures, to the processes of the synovial fringes. And the probability of similar origin is enhanced by the likeness of the contents of the cysts, in both cases, to the fluids secreted by the fringes in the normal state.

4. Under the name of MUCOUS CYSTS we may include all such as are

---

* Case by M. Marini, cited by M. Bérard, "Diagnostic differentiel des Tumeurs du Sein," p. 86.

† For a case in which the walls of a cyst in the breast were calcified, and crackled like those of ossified arteries when pressed, see Bérard, loc. cit. p. 56.

‡ Having in view only the illustration of the more general pathology of these cysts, I have not referred to more special instances of them. Examples enough are to be found in all the works here quoted. Neither have I mentioned any analysis of the contents of serous cysts: for few have been made, and these few were made on such various materials, that no general account of them can be rendered. Several are cited in Simon's Medical Chemistry; and in Frerichs, Ueber Gallert-oder Colloidgeschwülste, p. 7–9, &c.; and by Virchow, in the Verhandlungen der med.-phys. Gesellsch. in Würzburg, B. ii., p. 281. See, also, on the contents of ovarian cysts, Dr. Tilt's papers in the Lancet, June, 1850.

formed in connection with simple mucous membranes, or with glandular
structures which we call mucous, while we know no other or peculiar
office served by their secretions.

There may be many cysts of this kind; but the best examples appear
to be those that may be named *Nabothian* and *Cowperian* cysts. The
former probably originated in cystic degeneration of the glands of the
mucous membrane about the cervix uteri. Protruding, either alone, or
with polypoid outgrowths of the mucous membrane, they are observed
successively enlarging, then bursting and discharging their mucous contents, and then replaced by others following the same morbid course. Or,
instead of clusters of such cysts, one alone of larger size and simpler
structure may be found.

The Cowperian cysts appear to be connected with the Cowper's or
Duvernoy's glands in the female. Whether arising from dilatation of
the duct, or from cystic transformation of the elementary structures of
the gland, cannot be yet stated; but, in the exact position of the Cowper's gland, and projecting into the vagina near its orifice, a cyst is often
found, of regular oval shape, thin-walled, of uncertain size, but growing
sometimes to the capacity of a pint. Commonly the contents of such a
cyst are a colorless, pellucid, or opaline ropy fluid, like that found in
the closed-up gall-bladder. But from this they often vary. I have seen
the contents of such cysts like the ink of the cuttle-fish, like the fluid of
melanotic tumors, and like thick turbid coffee; or, to the sight, they
may exactly resemble fluid fæcal matter.† Moreover these cysts are
very apt to inflame and suppurate. Many abscesses projecting into the
vagina have in these their origin; and the treatment these abscesses receive, by free incision, is, I believe, appropriate for the cysts under all
conditions.

It is not apparent upon what the varieties in the contents of these cysts
depend. The only instances that I could minutely examine were the two
following:—In the first, a woman, 25 years old, under the care of Dr.
West, had a smooth oval swelling in the lower and fore part of the right
labium, projecting on its inner surface, and nearly an inch in diameter.
This had been observed slowly increasing for six years, and had commenced three months after parturition. It was not painful. I punctured
it, and let out about three drachms of pellucid fluid, like mucus, or the
white of egg. The cyst had a polished white internal surface, and the
fluid contained numerous corpuscles, like very large white blood-corpuscles,
and like such as are commonly found in the tenacious fluid of bursæ. The
cyst closed on the healing of the wound: but two years afterwards either
it, or some other part of the gland similarly diseased, appeared again.

* A remarkable example of a cyst thus, I suppose, originating, is in the Museum of the
Middlesex Hospital.
† As in a case related by Mr. Cæsar Hawkins in his Lectures, Medical Gazette, vol. xxii.,
and in two cases by Lebert, Abhandlungen, p. 109.

In the other case, the patient was forty-five years old, and under the care of Mr. Stanley. The tumor was nearly regularly oval, occupying the whole length of the right labium, and obstructing the vagina. She had observed it increasing for four years: it was painless, but had been often struck. A free incision gave issue to about fourteen ounces of thick, inodorous, dark brown fluid,.like turbid coffee. The walls of the cyst were about one-third of a line thick, tough, compact, and closely connected with the surrounding tissues. Mr. Abernethy Kingdon, who examined the contents, found abundant molecular matter, and granule-masses, together with groups of cells, apparently resembling epithelial cells of various sizes.

5. The SANGUINEOUS CYSTS, or cysts containing blood, are, probably, in many instances, very nearly related to the serous. Some may be explained by an accidental hemorrhage into the cavity of a serous cyst; an event corresponding with the transformation of a common hydrocele into an hematocele. The contents of some of these cysts, are, indeed, just like those of a hematocele, with fluid and coagulated and variously decolorized blood.* But some cysts appear, from their origin, to contain blood; and this blood, I think, always remains fluid till it is let out, while that which collects by hemorrhage into a serous cyst is generally partially or wholly coagulated. Some of these cysts with blood are found in the same positions and circumstances as the serous. Thus, in the neck, a series of cases of blood-cysts might be collected, exactly corresponding with the serous cysts in that part, and like them, probably derived from various origins, some lying in the thyroid gland, some near it, some traceable to connection with vascular naevi, some of proper origin.

Of the last class one appeared to be, which was in St. Bartholomew's Hospital several years ago. A lad, about sixteen years old, was under Mr. Stanley's care, with a large, oval, and somewhat pendulous swelling in the left side of the neck, which had existed many years, and appeared merely subcutaneous. It was punctured, and about sixteen ounces of fluid blood escaped, which soon coagulated. After this the cyst closed: a result more favorable than may generally be anticipated from such simple treatment: for usually these like other cysts, are not obliterated unless after free incision.

In the parotid gland, also, cysts containing fluid blood have peculiar interest. In 1848, I assisted Mr. Stanley in the removal of one which lay quite within the parotid of a gentleman about forty years old. It had been for some years increasing in size, and lay beneath some branches of the facial nerve, from which the need of separating it with-

---

* Such hemorrhages are frequent in cysts of the thyroid gland (Ferichs; Rokitansky; Museum of the College of Surgeons, 1502). Thus, also, we may explain the hematocles of the spermatic cord, as in Mus. Coll. Surg. 2460; and Mus. St. Bartholomew's, Ser. xxviii. 11.

out injury made its removal very difficult. This, however, was safely accomplished, and the patient remains well.

At nearly the same time, a man, 25 years old, was under my care with a similar cyst, which had been increasing without pain for two years. It lay in the parotid, but very near its surface. I punctured it, and evacuated two or three drachms of bloody-looking fluid, with some grumous and flocculent paler substance intermingled. This fluid coagulated like blood, and contained blood-cells, much free granular matter, crystals of cholestearine, and what appeared to be white corpuscles of blood acquiring the character of granule-cells. The cyst filled again with similar fluid after being thus evacuated : I therefore dissected it from the parotid gland, and the patient recovered.

Occasionally, one meets with sanguineous cysts, which derive a peculiar aspect from a columnar or fasciculated structure of their interior, making them look like the right auricle of the heart. This was singularly the case in one which I assisted Mr. Macilwain in removing from over the lower angle of the scapula of a lad 15 years old. It had existed more than eight years, and grew rapidly, while in the last year, he was actively at work. It was now also painful. It felt like a fatty tumor, but proved to be a cyst thus fasciculated like an auricle, with a finely polished internal surface, and containing about an ounce and a half of liquid blood. Its walls were from one to two lines in thickness, and seemed in great part made up of small cells, such as one sees in a bronchocele, full of serous and bloody fluids. No trouble followed the operation, and the patient remains well twelve years after it.*

A cyst presenting the same peculiarity of internal surface was removed by Mr. Stanley, in October, 1848, from over the pubes of a boy 13 years old. It was observed increasing for nine months, and a part of it, consisting of a simple thin-walled serous cyst, was transparent; but behind, and projecting into this, was a more thickly walled cyst, containing about a drachm of dark liquid blood, and on its surface fasciculate and polished like an auricle. Its walls were well-defined, formed of fibro-cellular tissue imperfectly filamentous and nucleated, and I could find no epithelium lining it. The operation was successful.

It is not improbable, I think, that both these cases may have had their origin in vascular nævi, like other cysts containing blood, to which I shall refer in speaking of erectile tumors. I will now only refer to certain cysts which, without any erectile formation, appear to be derived from portions of veins dilated, and obstructed, and shut-off from the stream of blood. Such an one was removed by Mr. Lloyd, many years ago, from a man's thigh. It lay in the course of the saphena vein; but neither that, nor any other considerable vein, was divided in the operation, or could be traced into this cyst. This cyst† was of spherical

* The cyst is in the Museum of St. Bartholomew's, Ser. xxxv. 38.
† Museum of St. Bartholomew's Hospital, Appendix, 10.

form, about an inch and a half in diameter, closed on all sides: its walls were tough, and polished on their inner surface; it was full of dark fluid blood, and its venous character was manifested by two valves, like those of veins, placed on its inner surface. On one of these a soft lobed mass, like an intra-cystic growth, is seated.*

6. CYSTS containing OIL or fatty matter, without any more highly organized substance, are very rare. Many contain fatty matters mingled with serous, epithelial, and other substances; but in these the fatty constituent is probably the result of the degeneration of the other contents. Some, however, appear to contain fatty matter alone. Mr. Hunter preserved a specimen† of what he marked as "oil from an adipose encysted tumor." It was taken, I believe, from a cyst that grew "between the bony orbit and the upper eyelid" of a young gentleman. When recent, it was described as "pure oil, perfectly clear and sweet, which burnt with a very clear light, and did not mix with aqueous fluids, and when exposed to cold, became as solid as the human fat."

In 1850, Mr. Wormald removed a small cyst from a woman's breast, the contents of which appeared to be pure oily matter, that congealed into a substance like lard, and contained crystals of margarine, but no organized corpuscles. The patient remains well. Schuh‡ relates two cases of cysts under the brow, which contained similar oily matter, and whose walls had all the structures of skin, with implanted hairs.

7. COLLOID CYSTS are, at present, a very ill-defined group; the term "colloid" being used by Frerichs,§ and other recent German writers, for all those morbid materials that are pellucid, jelly-like, flickering, half-solid, or more or less closely resembling the material found in gelatiniform, alveolar, or colloid cancer. Such a material is common in the cysts of bronchoceles, and in those of the kidney; especially, I think, in those which are not associated with contraction of the renal substance, and which Baillie, and other writers of his time, described as hydatid disease of the kidney.

The contents of these cysts may present the most diverse conditions; may be of all densities, from that of dilute serum to that of a firm jelly; may range between pellucidity and the thickest turbidness; may be of all hues of yellow, olive-green, orange, brown, pink, and nearly black. The thick and pellucid contents of such renal cysts are enumerated as examples of colloid matter; so are the contents of ranulæ, and of many bursæ; but the type is the material of the so-called colloid

* In the Museum of King's College is a large cyst removed from a thigh, into which it is said the saphena vein opened.
† Mus. Coll. Surg., 181: Pathological Catalogue, vol. iv. p. 177.
‡ Ueber . . . Pseudoplasmen, p. 144.
§ Ueber Gallert-oder Colloidgeschwülste.

cancer. This, however, is beyond my present range; and I pass by it, referring only to the already cited works of Frerichs and Rokitansky, and to that of Bruch,* for the best information yet supplied.

8. The last group of cysts of which I shall now speak includes such as contain secreted fluids, like those of the glands, by the dilated ducts or transformed elements of which they are formed. Such are the cysts in the breast that contain milk, and probably many instances of ranula. The origin of the former is, probably, in dilatation of lactiferous ducts: that of the latter is uncertain. But the examples of this group, of which I wish more particularly to speak, are the SEMINAL CYSTS, including under this name those that are usually called encysted hydroceles, or hydroceles of the spermatic cord. Their various forms are fully described by Mr. Curling,† and are well illustrated by specimens in the Museum of the College.‡ They are usually thin-walled spherical or oval cysts, imbedded in, and loosely connected with, the tissue of the cord. They may occur singly, or in a group. Their most frequent seat is just above the epididymis, but they may be found in any part of the spermatic cord. Their walls are formed of fibro-cellular tissue, and they may be lined with delicate tesselated epithelium. Their contents are usually a colorless, slightly opaline fluid, like water, with which a little milk has been mingled.

The discovery was made at the same time, and independently, by Mr. Lloyd and Mr. Liston,§ that the fluid obtained from these cysts usually contains the seminal filaments or spermatozoa. Repeated observations have confirmed their discovery; and both the existence of these bodies, and the usual characters of the fluid, justify the speaking of it as a diluted or imperfect seminal fluid, and, therefore, of the cysts, as "seminal cysts."

It was my lot, I believe, first to dissect some of these cysts;|| and I found that they had no open communication or other connection with any part of the secretory apparatus of the testicle, and that their relation to the epididymus, on which they lay, was such as to forbid the supposition of the seminal secretion being transmitted to them from the tubes. I suggested, therefore, that these cysts were formed quite independently of the tubes; and that being seated near the organ that naturally secretes the semen, they possessed a power of secreting a similar fluid; just as cysts beneath the hairy parts of the body may produce hair and epidermis, and the ordinary products of the skin. The explanation was, I believe, deemed unsatisfactory; but it is supported by the later investigations of other cysts, especially of those to which I have already referred,

* Ueber Carcinoma alveolare und den alveolären Gewebsty pus; in Henle and Pfeufer's Zeitschrift, vii. 1849.

† Treatise on Diseases of the Testis, &c.

‡ Especially Nos. 2456 to 2459.

§ Medico-Chirurgical Trans., vol. xxvi. pp. 216 and 368. See, also, a paper by Mr. Curling, in the Monthly Journal of Medical Science, x. p. 1023.

|| Medico-Chirurgical Transactions, vol. xxvii. p. 398.

growing in the thyroid and mammary glands. While we find in these that perfect gland-substance may grow from the cyst-walls, it cannot seem singular if, in a cyst lying near the testicle or its duct, materials like the secretion of the testicle should be formed. The growth and nutrition of gland tissue, and the formation of gland-secretion, are so truly parts of one process, that the truth of the former occurring in one group of cysts removes all improbability from the belief that the latter may occur in another group.

If, then, we may regard these seminal cysts as autogenous, and may arrange them with those of the kidney and other glands, which are derived from the transformation and overgrowth of isolated nuclei or cells, they may supply some facts of interest to the general pathology of cysts. Especially, we may observe that in different specimens of these "hydroceles of the cord," or in the same at different times, the contents may be either a seminal fluid or an ordinary serous fluid. In one of the cases in which I dissected a seminal cyst, there existed, besides that which contained seminal fluid, another large cyst, above and separate from the testicle and tunica vaginalis; but this contained only serous fluid like that of a common hydrocele. Now this diversity is common among cysts. Those in the kidney may contain the materials of urine, but they more commonly do not; those of the lactiferous tubes may contain either milk or some form of serous fluid; ovarian cysts may at one period produce hair and the other growths and secretions from skin, and then, casting off these, they may produce only serous or some other fluid.

In different cysts, this diversity of contents may sometimes depend on difference of origin or of early construction. But when it happens in different periods of the same cyst, it illustrates the general rule that, in the course of time, cysts are apt to degenerate, and to produce less and less highly organized substances or secretions. This degeneration does not take place in any certain time; but generally, the larger a cyst grows, the less organized are its products; as if nearly all the formative force were expended in growth, and little remained available for secretion. Generally, also, the longer a cyst has lived, the less organized are its products. However, both these rules are only general. I met with a remarkable exception to them in a seminal cyst, which had existed for seven or eight years in a man more than 70 years old. I withdrew from it eighteen ounces of fluid laden with seminal filaments; and no fresh accumulation took place in the two years following the operation. In another case of four years' duration, Mr. Stanley removed from a cyst on the right side of the scrotum 25 ounces of such fluid, and from one on the left side 46 ounces.

I have spoken of these seminal cysts as separate from the testicle and tunica vaginalis. Mr. Lloyd believed that, in some cases, he obtained fluid containing spermatoza from hydroceles of the tunica vaginalis; and his belief was lately confirmed by the examination of a case after death. The specimen presents the ordinary appearances of a common hydrocele, except that the inner surface of the tunica vaginalis is uneven, with a few small depressions or pouches from it. This hydrocele has been repeatedly tapped; the fluid had always the ordinary serous appearance of that of common hydrocele; but it always contained abundant seminal filaments. Can we suppose, then, that the tunica vaginalis has the power of secreting seminal fluid? or, were there in this case minute secreting cysts, which, by dehiscence, discharged their seminal fluid into the cavity of the tunica vaginalis, as sometimes ovarian cysts by spontaneous openings discharge their contents into one another, or into the cavity of a parent cyst? I am disposed to think this latter explanation the more probable; but as yet the facts are too few to justify any conclusion.

LECTURE XXIII.

COMPOUND OR PROLIFEROUS CYSTS.

IN the last lecture I traced and illustrated the formation of simple or barren cysts,—the cysts that have only liquid contents. Among these, the instances of the highest productive power appear to be in the cysts that secrete a seminal fluid, and those that are lined with a complete secreting epithelium. In the present lecture I propose to describe the cysts that appear to have the power of producing more highly organized, and even vascular, structures; or, as they may be generally named, proliferous cysts.*

These include such as are often called "compound cysts," or "compound cystoid growths;" but I would avoid these terms, because they do

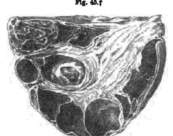

Fig. 45.†

not suggest the difference between the cysts with endogenous growths, and those that may appear equally compound, though they are only simple cysts clustered or grouped together. This difference should be clearly marked in names, for it generally is so in nature. In an ovary, for example, such as is drawn in Fig. 45, from a specimen in St. Bartholomew's Museum, it is not unfrequent to find many small cysts, formed, apparently, by the coincident

---

* Under this name are here included the sero-cystic sarcomata of Sir B. C. Brodie (Lectures on Pathology and Surgery); most of the specimens of Cysto-sarcoma phyllodes and proliferum of Müller (On Cancer); and most of the tuberous cystic tumors of Mr. Cæsar Hawkins (Medical Gazette, vol. xxi., p. 951).

† Section of an ovary with many closely-placed cysts formed by enlargement of Graafian vesicles: natural size.

enlargement of separate Graafian vesicles. These lie close and mutually compressed; and, as they all enlarge together, and, sometimes, by the wasting of their partition walls, come into communication, they may at length look like a single many-chambered cyst, having its one proper wall formed by the extended fibrous covering of the ovary. Many multilocular cysts, as they are named, are only groups of close-packed single cysts; though, when examined in late periods of their growth, and, especially, when one of the group of cysts enlarges much more than the rest, it may be difficult to distinguish them from some of the proliferous cysts.

Of the first formation of cysts that may be proliferous I need not speak; for, so far as is at present known, they may be formed exactly as the barren cysts are. A cyst may be proliferous in whichever of the plans described in the last lecture it may have had its origin. Thus, 1. Bursæ formed by expansion and rarefying of areolar spaces may be found with organised, pendulous, or loose growths from their walls.* 2. Among the cysts formed by growth of natural cavities or obstructed ducts, we have instances of surpassing proliferous power in the ovarian cysts from Graafian vesicles, and of less power in some cases of dilated lactiferous tubes and dilated veins.† And 3. Among the autogenous cysts we find, in the breast and other glands, some of the principal examples from which the following history of proliferous cysts will be derived.

The account given in the last lecture of the modes of origin of barren cysts may therefore, so far as the cyst is concerned, suffice for the proliferous; and I shall now need to speak of only the intra-cystic productions, the differences of which may decide the grouping of the whole division of proliferous cysts.

1. The first group includes the cysts which have others growing in or upon their walls. Of these, two chief examples are presented, in the complex ovarian cysts, and in the cystic disease of the chorion or "hydatid mole."

The principal varieties of the complex ovarian cysts have been described to the very life of Dr. Hodgkin, to whom we are indebted for the first knowledge of their true pathology.‡ But, since his minute description of them is, or should be, well known, I will more briefly say that according to his arrangement, we may find in these proliferous ovarian cysts two principal or extreme forms of endogenous cysts; namely, those that are broad-based and spheroidal, imitating more or less the characters of the parent cyst, and those that are slender, pedunculated, clustered, and thin-walled. Between these forms, indeed, many

* Museum Coll. Surg., 367, &c. See also a case, by Mr. Cæsar Hawkins (Medical Gazette vol. xxi. p. 951). Perhaps, also, the case may be here referred to, in which Mr. Hunter found loose bodies in a cavity formed round the ends of the bones in an ununited fracture (Museum Coll. Surg., Nos. 469, 470).

† Museum of St. Bartholomew's Hospital, Appendix 10; and see last lecture, p. 348.

‡ Med.-Chir. Trans. xv. 256; and Lectures on the Morbid Anatomy of Serous Membranes, p. 221, et. seq.

23

transitional and many mixed forms may be found; yet it is convenient to distinguish the two extremes.

A typical example of the first is in the College Museum,* and is sketched in fig. 46. It is an Hunterian specimen; and the mode of preparation shows that Mr. Hunter had clearly apprehended the peculiarities of its structure. It is a large cyst, with tough, compact, and laminated walls, polished on both their surfaces. On its inner surface there project, with broad bases, many smaller cysts, of various sizes, and variously grouped and accumulated. These nearly fill the cavity of the parent cyst; many of them are globular; many deviate from the globular form through mutual compression; and within many of them are similar but more thinly-walled cysts of a third order.

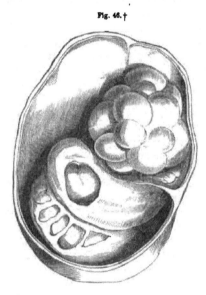

Fig. 46.†

Here the endogenous cysts, projecting inwards, appear to have nearly filled the cavity of the principal or parent cyst; and this filling up is complete in another specimen, in which there remains, in the middle of the parent cyst, only a narrow space bounded by the endogenous cysts converging in their growth from all parts of the parent walls.‡

For a typical example of the slender, thin-walled, pedunculated, and clustered form of endogenous cysts, I may adduce the specimen from the Museum of St. Bartholomew's Hospital,§ which is drawn in fig. 47. It shows part of the thick laminated wall of an ovarian cyst, the inner surface of which is thickly covered with crowds of pyriform and leaflike pellucid vesicles, heaped together, and one above another. This is a comparatively simple specimen of the kind: in the more complex, the endogenous cysts or vesicles are multiplied a thousand-fold. and clustered in large-lobed and warty-looking masses, that nearly fill the cavity of the cyst. Specimens of this kind are among the most valuable possessions of the Museum of Guy's Hospital.

The College Museum furnishes specimens of the forms intermediate

* No. 166.

† Fig. 46, section of a proliferous ovarian cyst, described in the text: about one-third of the natural size.

‡ Mus. Coll. Surg., No. 2622.

§ Series xxxi. 18.

between these extremes,* in which the edogeneous cysts of the second and third orders have walls that are not pellucid, yet are thin and vascular, and are attached by pedicles rather than by broad bases. Mixed forms are also found,‡ in which the parent cyst-wall bears, at one part, oval and spherical membranous cysts developed beneath its lining membrane, which they raise in low convex projections into its cavity; and at another part, groups of small leaf-like, narrowly pedunculated, and pendulous cysts. And again, the same prolific power which is shown in these endogenous converging cysts, is often, in the same specimens shown in exogenous growths; similar cysts, singly or in clusters, projecting from the exterior walls of the parent.§

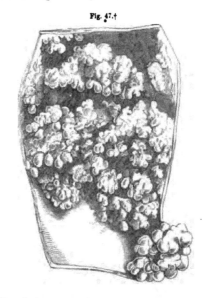

Fig. 47.†

But a lecture would not suffice to describe, even briefly, the variety of forms into which these ovarian proliferous cysts may deviate. Whether we regard their walls, the arrangement and shape of the endogenous cysts, their seats and modes of origin, their various contents, and the yet greater differences engendered by disease, they are so multiform, that even imagination could hardly pass the boundaries of their diversity. It must suffice to refer to Dr. Hodgkin's works for an elaborate account of the structure and arrangement of the cysts; and to the essays of Dr. Tilt‖ for descriptions of their contents.

The foregoing account of the structure of these cyst-bearing cysts in the ovaries is derived entirely from naked-eye observations. Respecting the mode of generation of the endogenous cysts, it could only be supposed that they are derived from germs developed in the parent cyst-walls, and thence, as they grow into secondary cysts, projecting into the parent cavity; or, disparting the mid-layers of the walls, and remaining quite enclosed between them; or, more rarely growing outwards, and projecting into the cavity of the peritoneum.

* Nos. 165 A, and 165 B.

† Fig. 47, part of the wall of a proliferous ovarian cyst, described above: natural size.

‡ No. 2621.

§ No. 2622 in the College Museum presents an instance of the endogeneous and exogenous modes of growth in the same specimen.

‖ Lancet, 1849.

But a more complete illustration of the origin of such secondary cysts,

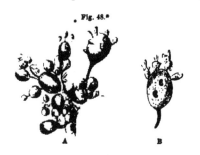

Fig. 48.*

and a good confirmation of what I have been describing, may be drawn from Dr. Mettenheimer's investigations on the microscopic structure of the cystic disease of the chorion.† Some of his illustrations are copied in fig. 49.

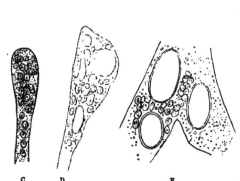

The general characters of this disease, constituting the hydatid mole, are well known. A part, or even the whole, of the chorion is covered with pellucid vesicles with limpid contents, borne on long, slender, and often branching pedicles (A). The cysts are usually oval or pyriform; their walls are clear, or have minute, opaque dots (B); they may be simple, or may bear others projecting from their walls.

Dr. Mettenheimer has found that the minute dots besetting these cysts are villous processes, exactly resembling those of the natural chorion, and growing from the walls of the cysts, either outwardly or into their cavities. In these villi he traced the development of cysts. In their natural state the villi may be described as filiform or clavate processes, often branching and bearing bud-like projections, and composed of dimly-granular substance, in which are imbedded minute nucleated cells (c). In this cystic disease, vesicular bodies may be seen (as in D and E) scattered among the cells in the villi, which bodies are distinguished from the cells by their pellucidity, their larger size, and, when largest, by double contours; but, from the cells to these, every gradation may be so traced as to leave scarcely a doubt that the vesicles are derived from cells deviating from their normal characters. Thus, in some of the cells,

* Fig. 48, cystic disease of the chorion, as described above: A and B, natural size; c, D, E, magnified 250 times.

† Müller's Archiv, 1850, H. v. p. 417. His account, though different in interpretation, is consistent, as to facts, with one by Gierse and H. Meckel, in the Verhandl. der Gesellsch. für Geburtshülfe in Berlin, 1847.

the contents are seen lighter and less granular; in some they have entirely disappeared without increase of size; and then, when their contents are thus become uniformly pellucid, and they have acquired the character of vesicles, the cells appear to grow, while their walls become stronger, and they acquire such a size that they are recognized as very small cysts, similar in all but their size, to those which are visible to the naked eye.

Now, though this method of formation of cysts has been traced by Mettenheimer only in the villi which grow in the cysts themselves, and therefore, so to speak, only in the production of cysts of the second and later generations, yet there can be little doubt that the first cysts in the diseased chorion are formed in its own villi after the same manner. For the villi which are borne on the cysts, and which to the naked eye appear like little dots, are, in all essential characters, like those natural to the chorion; and the cysts of all generations are equally like. The whole process may, therefore, be probably thus described:—Certain of the cells in the proper villi of the chorion, deviating in their cell-form, and increasing disproportionately in size, form cysts, which remain connected by the gradually elongated and hypertrophied tissue of the villi. "On the outer surface of the new-formed cysts, each of which would, as it were, repeat the chorion, and surpass its powers, a new vegetation of villi sprouts out, of the same structure as the proper villi of the chorion. In these begins again a similar development of cysts; and so on *ad infinitum*." Each cyst, as it enlarges, seems to lead to the wasting of the cells around it; and then, moving away from the villus in which it was formed, it draws out the base of the villus, which strengthens itself, and forms the pedicle on which the cyst remains suspended.

Such is the account of the minute structure and formation of the cystic disease of the chorion; and perhaps no instance could afford a better confirmation of the production of cysts by the enormous growth of elementary cells, or a better type of the capacity of cysts thus formed to produce structures resembling those in the abnormities of which themselves originated. A similar capacity is among the characters of all the cysts of which I shall next have to speak.

2. I pass now to the consideration of the cysts that are proliferous with vascular growths from their internal surfaces.*

* It may be well to refer to the fact that abnormal growths upon natural free surfaces commonly affect the same forms as will be described in the following account of the vascular growths in cysts. The chief forms are three: namely, 1st, groups of slender, small, and pedunculated bodies; 2d, larger round pendulous masses; 3d, nearly level, slightly elevated layers, such as granulations. Now groups of pedunculated leaflike processes occur on natural free surfaces, in the growths that are so frequent in chronic rheumatic diseases of joints, from some of which Müller draws his account of *lipoma arborescens;* in certain warty cancerous growths on the skin, which appear like cancerous overgrowths of the papillæ; and in similar growths in the larynx about the vocal cords. Of the larger, round, pedunculated masses growing on natural free surfaces, instances exist in the medullary cancers of the urinary bladder, the polypi of the intestines and stomach, the pendulous

The first group of them may include those that bear glandular growths —the "glandular proliferous cysts," as we may call them, because the minute structure of the substance growing into them is, in its perfect state, exactly comparable with that of a secreting or vascular gland.

Such cysts form part of the group to which the name of "sero-cystic sarcoma" was given by Sir B. C. Brodie, who first clearly distinguished them.* They are also part of those which furnished to Dr. Hodgkin the chief grounds for his well-known theory of the formation of solid tumors—a theory which, in regard to at least these growths, has good foundation.

The chief seats of the formation of glandular proliferous cysts are the mammary and thyroid glands. Their history in the thyroid, in which their formation scarcely passes the bounds of health, is amply illustrated in the often cited works of Frerichs and Rokitansky, to which, as well as to the essay by Mr. Simon† on the natural structure of the gland, I must, for brevity's sake, refer.

A series of preparations,‡ such as are represented in figs. 49, 50, 51, may clearly illustrate the corresponding process in the mammary gland;§ but here the conditions are far more remote from the normal type. If we may believe that a series of specimens may be read as the continuous history of one case, because they seem to present successive phases of the same disease, then, we may suppose, first, the existence of a cyst (fig. 49), or of a collection of cysts (fig. 51), in the mammary gland. Such cysts may be formed by the dilatation of parts of ducts; but, much more commonly, the cysts that bear vascular growths are derived through transformation and enormous growth of some elementary structure of the gland.‖ So far as I know, there is nothing peculiar in the structure of the mammary cysts that may be proliferous. They are usually ovoid or spherical, unless changed by mutual compression, as in fig. 51: they usually appear formed of thin fibro-cellular tissue, with or without elastic fibres: they have abundant blood-vessels, and are closely adherent to the surrounding parts: their walls are peculiarly apt, in disease, to become œdematous, succulent, and almost gelatinous. They may grow to an enormous size. A specimen is in the Museum of St. George's Hospital, in which a cyst that would contain more than two pints of fluid, has

outgrowths of the skin; and of the flatter, and more nearly level layers, the condylomatous outgrowths of skin, the epithelial cancers of the stomach and intestines, and the cheloid growths, often afford examples. There is in all these resemblances a good illustration of the tendency of the growths in cysts to imitate those on natural parts. (See the sixth note under the heading of Villous Cancer, in Lecture xxxiii.)

* The disease is admirably illustrated by the specimens in the Museum of the College and in those of St. George's, Guy's, and St. Bartholomew's Hospitals.

† Philosophical Transactions, 1844, Part ii.

‡ Such as those in the College Museum, Nos. 168 to 172, &c.

§ All the cases recorded have occurred in the female breast, except two: one by M'Arnott; Medical Gazette, xxii. 378: and one by Müller; "On Cancer," p. 180.

‖ On the difference between the solid contents of dilated ducts, and those of the proper or autogenous cysts, see Mr. Birkett's account in his Essay on the Diseases of the Breast

some lowly lobed growths from one portion of its inner surface; one in the College Museum, removed by Mr. Liston, weighed twelve pounds; and Dr. Warren relates a case in which he removed a tumor of this kind of thirteen pounds weight. The cysts may contain any of the varieties of serous or bloody fluid, clear or turbid, that I described in the last lecture.

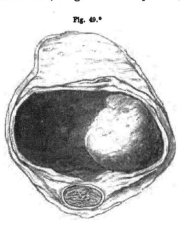

Fig. 49.*

Now, from some part of the inner surface of such a cyst, a vascular growth may spring (fig. 49); and, as this gradually increases at a rate beyond that of the increase of the cyst, it fills more and more of the cavity. At length, the growth wholly excludes the fluid contents of the cyst, and its surfaces come in contact with the remainder of the cyst-walls (figs. 50, 51). The growth may now coalesce with the walls of the cyst, and form one solid tumor, enclosed in and connected with them, just as ordinary solid tumors are invested and connected with their fibro-cellular capsules. Or, growing yet further and more rapidly, the growth, hitherto intra-cystic, may protrude through its cyst-walls and the superjacent integuments; protruding through them as a hernia of the brain does through the skull, growing exuberantly over the adjacent skin (fig. 51), and, like such a hernia, reproduced when cut away.

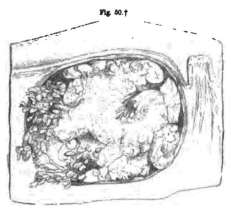

Fig. 50.†

The time in which these changes may be accomplished is extremely various. Usually, the increase of the intra-cystic growth appears to be painless, and it may be very slow: ten years or more may pass with little change; but the increase is generally faster,

* Fig. 49, a cyst in a mammary gland, to part of the inner surface of which a vascular growth is attached. Below it a smaller cyst is nearly filled with a similar growth. Mus. St. Bartholomew's: three-fourths of the natural size.

† Fig. 50, a cyst in the mammary gland filled with a vascular growth bearing clusters of pedunculated processes. Mus. Coll. Surg. Natural size.

and it often shows an accelerating rate; so that, late in the disease, the progress is extremely quick, even quicker than that of most cancerous growths.

The characters of the intra-cystic mammary growths are various, not only according to our observations of them at different periods of their existence, but, apparently, even from their very origin. In looking through a large series of them while they are still in early periods of their development, we may reduce them to these chief forms; namely, low, broad-based, convex layers, like coarse granulations; spheroidal, lobed, and nodulated masses, cauliflower-like, attached by narrower bases (fig. 49): masses or clusters of pedunculated leaf-like processes, slender, single or variously branched, and interlaced in all possible forms (fig. 50); masses of firmer and much paler substance, appearing as if formed of close-packed lobes, or fimbriated processes, or involuted layers (fig. 51).

In apparent structure, also, the varieties of these growths are scarcely less numerous. Some of them are opaque, yellow, and soft, yet elastic,

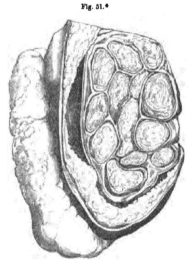

Fig. 51.*

and rather tough, so as to be separable in laminæ like fibrine-clot; others are more vascular, succulent and spongy, like granulations; others are like layers and masses, or heaped-up layers, of gelatine, not firmer than size, or even like vitreous humor, yielding a tenacious synovia-like fluid: others are firm, compact, nearly pure white, imitating the mammary gland, but not succulent.

To these varieties of appearance we might add yet more, due either to diverse shades of yellow, pink, gray, or purple; or to the various clustering and incomplete fulness of the cysts; or to the increasing firmness of the growths, and their fusion with the cell-walls; or to the development of new barren or proliferous cysts: in the solid growths that now fill the cysts of a former generation; or to various changes of decay or disease ensuing in either the cyst-walls or their contents.

It would be too tedious to describe all these varieties, especially while we do not yet know whether, or in what degree, these forms are related

* Fig. 51. collection of cysts filled with glandular growths in and protruding from the mammary gland: described p. 361. Half the natural size.

to one another, or to any one typical condition of the intra-cystic growths.

Respecting their minute structure, we have good guidance in the probability, which will be supported in the twenty-eighth lecture, that the proper mammary glandular tumors—the chronic mammary tumors of Sir A. Cooper—have their origin in intra-cystic growths, transformed into solid tumors in the manner just described. The mammary glandular tumors are composed of minute structures closely imitating those of the gland itself. They present microscopic lobes, and fine tubules, lined or filled with nuclei and nucleated cells, like those of secreting organs; these, inclosed within pellucid membrane, form a pseudo-glandular substance, such as, we might suppose, needs only a main duct to enable it to discharge the office of a mammary gland. In the like manner and degree, in some specimens in which the cysts and their contained growths are still easily separable, we can discern in the growths a likeness to the mammary gland itself in their minute structure.

These facts have been observed especially by Mr. Birkett, and were very well marked in a case in which I was recently able to examine, and of which fig. 51 represents a section. It was a very large protruding tumor of the breast removed by Mr. Lawrence from a lady 55 years old. It had been observed for thirty years, remaining like a small knot for twenty-six years, and then slowly increasing, till, at the end of five years, a red, fungous mass protruded from the breast, bled freely sometimes, and discharged profusely. This, too, increased quickly, and was painful. The whole breast was removed, and the patient recovered.

The tumor (fig. 51) measured nearly seven inches by five. The part which did not protrude beyond the level of the skin was imbedded in the substance of the gland. It consisted of numerous lobes of various sizes and shapes, and variously divided into smaller lobes; all being evidently formed of distinct cysts closely packed and compressed together. Most of these cysts were filled with intra-cystic growths; yet in many of them it was easy to pass a probe between their walls and the surfaces of their contained growths, which were fixed to only one part of the cyst-walls. In the protruding part, of which the overhanging outer border is shown in the sketch (fig. 51), the same general plan of structure could be discerned, but less distinctly.

Among the solid growths that filled the cysts, some showed clavate, close-packed lobes; some were nearly simple; nearly all were pale, white, grayish, or yellowish, and smooth and shining; a few were spotted with yellow, from degeneration of their tissue. Repeated examinations showed that all these consisted essentially of a tissue imitating that of a gland, and such as will be described in the twenty-ninth lecture. The edges and surfaces of the examined portions were minutely lobed or acinous, like terminations of gland-tubes. These were inclosed by well-defined, pellucid membrane; and their cavities were full of nuclei and nucleated cells, like

mammary gland-cells, with some granular matter.   Except in that these
acini led to no distinct ducts, but seemed confusedly heaped together, the
imitation of gland-structure was complete.

Now the glandular nature of these growths in the best-marked cases of
proliferous mammary cysts, and the probably constant relation of the
mammary glandular tumors to them, as well as the analogy of the intra-
cystic thyroid growths, may seem to make it probable that, in all cases,
the growths within the mammary cysts are essentially of the same glandular nature, and that their various appearances are due to their being in
rudimental, or degenerate, or diseased states.   But we cannot be sure of
this.   In three cases, in which I have minutely examined soft intra-cystic
growths, I could not recognise a glandular structure.   In all, I found a
basis-substance, which was pellucid, soft, and in one case diffluent; it had
little or no appearance of fibrous structure, and no distinct fibres, but,
rather, presented the uniformity as well as the consistence of soft gelatine.   In it, as in a blastema, were imbedded nuclei and cells, which
chiefly presented the forms of developing fibro-cellular tissue, like those
in granulations, or of inflammatory lymph: or their forms might be
explained, I think, by the disorderly conditions of their production and
development.   Nearly similar, and equally indecisive results appear from
an accurate observation of such a growth by Dr. Mettenheimer,* and
from two cases related by Bruch.†

Perhaps we may conclude that, in these specimens, the intra-cystic
growths were in a rudimental, or in a morbid state; that the general
destiny of such growths is towards a grandular stucture, but that in these
and the like instances they fell short of it, or swerved from the right
course.   But I would rather not form any conclusion at present.   These
are just the cases of which, as yet, the interpretation is scarcely possible,
while we are ignorant of the changes that may ensue during development,
degeneration, and disease.

I have said that the mammary and thyroid glands might be regarded
as the elected seats for cysts having glandular growths; but they are sometimes met with in other parts, as in the prostate, and, I believe, also in
the lip.   In the Museum at St. George's Hospital is a tumor removed
from a man's upper lip, in which it had been growing, without pain, for
8¼ years.   One half of it is a cyst that was filled with a thin flaky fluid,
and was thought to be a dilated labial gland-duct; the other half is a
solid tumor, just like a glandular tumor of the lip which I shall describe in a future lecture.   I have lately seen another case with nearly
the same characters: and the combination of a barren cyst with a proliferous one, which they seem to illustrate, is not rare in the mammary gland.

* Müller's Archiv, 1850, p. 207.
† Die Diagnose der bösartigen Geschwülste, p. 185, 191.

In the same Museum is a cyst, with a broad vascular growth, like granulations, from its walls, which was taken from a girl's labium by Mr. Cutler. It has a small external opening, suggesting that it may have had its origin in a cystic mucous or sebaceous gland.* In the College Museum, No. 167, is a thick-walled cyst, from the cheek of an old woman, which contains two large, lobed, and pedunculated masses, so like some of those found in the mammary cysts that we can hardly doubt their glandular nature.

All these specimens, however, need more minute examination; at present they only make it probable that any cyst originating in or near a secreting gland may be the parent, or the habitation, of an endogenous glandular growth.

To this account of glanduliferous cysts it must be added, that their characters may be closely imitated by cysts formed in parts altogether unconnected with secreting glands. It is not, indeed, probable that the contained growths in such cysts are glandular; yet they present characters like the softer growths that are found in the mammary cysts.

I found one of these proliferous cysts beneath the gracilis and adductor longus muscles of a woman 25 years old. It was a large spheroidal mass, which felt as if held down tightly on the front of the pelvis, and had pushed the femoral vessels a little outwards. It lay too deep to form a clear diagnosis of its nature; it was assigned to no distinct cause; it had been noticed for only seven months, but when first seen was "as large as a tea-cup." I removed it without much difficulty; for it was not closely adherent to the parts, except to a small portion of the front of the pubes, where it rested on the adductor brevis. The patient has since remained well for more than three years.

The tumor was spheroidal, about four inches in diameter, and consisted chiefly of cysts, from two of which six or eight ounces of turbid serous fluid escaped when they were cut across. One of these cysts was thickly lined with pale, brownish, fibrinous substance, like that which one finds in old hæmatoceles; and this appeared as fibrine on minute examination. Another was nearly filled with a ruddy mass, in most part soft and succulent, like blood-stained gelatine. Much of this mass was also like fibrine-clot, with abundant corpuscles; but the layers of it next the cyst-walls were firmer than the central parts, and contained all the forms that one finds in common granulations developing into fibro-cellular tissue. The microscopic likeness to granulations was, in these parts, exact. The rest of the tumor, including some large portions between the cysts, consisted of fibro-cellular tissue more or less perfectly developed.†

* See also an account of a specimen in the same Museum, by Dr. Hawkins: Medical Gazette, xxi. p. 951; and Proc. of Pathol. Soc. ii. p. 340. I suppose there is some relation between these and the subcutaneous warts and condylomata described by Hauck and Krämer; but I have not seen what they refer to. (See Simon: Hautkrankheiten, p 225.)

† The tumor is in the Museum of St. Bartholomew's Hospital.

A similar tumor was removed by Mr. Lawrence from the exactly corresponding part of a woman, 50 years old, in whom it had grown slowly, and without pain, for nine or ten years. It gave the sensation of a firm, fatty tumor, as large as an egg, but when removed was found to be a bilocular cyst. Each cavity contained, together with serous fluid, a soft, reddish, gelatinous looking mass, like a polypus in one, and solid and folded in the other. The cyst-walls were tough, pure white, formed of fibro-cellular tissue, and polished on their inner surface. The intracystic growths consisted of a structureless or dimly-granular or fibrilating blastema, with abundant oily molecules, granule-cells, and corpuscles, like nuclei or cytoblasts, imbedded in it.

And to these two instances, since the disease seems very rare, I may add a third. A girl, twenty-three years old, under the care of Mr. Lawrence, had a pyriform pendulous tumor in her neck, about 2¼ inches long. Its surface was ulcerated, livid, and painful, and bled occasionally. Its history was doubtful; but it had existed for at least a year. On removal, it appeared to have grown in the subcutaneous tissue, and to be composed of a collection of cysts, closely and irregularly packed, and, for the most part, filled with lobed, soft, cauliflower-like growths from parts of their walls. It closely resembled, in its general aspect, the collections of proliferous cysts, with soft intra-cystic growths, in the mammary gland. In microscopic structure the intra-cystic growths appeared composed entirely of corpuscles, like those of lymph or granulations: but my record of the examination, made several years ago, is too incomplete for a clear account of them.

I believe that all the cysts that I spoke of, before these that contain vascular growths, may be regarded as completely void of the characters of malignant disease; at least, I have met with no evidence contrary to this statement, except in certain cases of proliferous ovarian cysts, to which I shall presently refer. And, in general, the reputation of innocency is deserved by the glanduliferous cysts also. Yet there are cases which show that such tumors may have an exceeding tendency to recur after removal.

A healthy, robust woman, 37 years old, was under Mr. Lawrence's care with a very large protruding tumor in her right breast. This had been slowly increasing for ten years, but, till lately, had given little uneasiness, except by its bulk, and had not hindered her nursing. Mr. Lawrence removed the greater part of the breast and the tumor in 1844. It weighed 7¼ pounds, and was a well-marked example of that form of "sero-cystic sarcoma," in which the cyst-walls, if altered by inflammation, or imperfectly formed, are soft, succulent, and glistening, with solid growths of similar substance, lobed and fissured. Many cysts in it still contained serous fluid. Its appearance when recent, and even now as preserved,* leaves no room for doubt as to its nature.

* In the Museum of St Bartholomew's, Ser. 34, Nos. 19 and 20.

The patient remained well for fifteen months; then a tumor began to grow under the scar, and quickly increased. After nine months' growth Mr. Lawrence removed this also, with all the surrounding tissues. It was a pale, pinkish, and yellowish mass, like soft size or jelly. It was lobed and folded, and included some irregular spaces, containing a fluid like mucus or half-melted jelly. It was like the solid parts of the tumor last removed, and consisted of a -pellucid dimly-fibrillated blastema or basis-substance, in which were imbedded nuclei and abundant granule-cells, of various forms. The sketches and account of these, which I drew at the time, make me still sure that they had none of the characters of cancer-cells, but were like nuclei or cytoblasts of ordinary form, or elongated, many of which were changed by fatty or granular degeneration.

After this second operation, the patient remained well for seven months, and fully regained her stout, robust appearance. But now a third tumor appeared; a fourth soon after; and both grew rapidly, till, after two months, Mr. Lawrence removed them, and all the parts bounding them. They were, in every respect, exactly like those removed in the last operation, and near them lay another not discerned before the removal. Erysipelas following this operation proved fatal, and no post-mortem examination could be obtained.

Now in the first of these operations some portion of the mammary gland was left. It is possible that some cysts already existed in this portion, and were subsequently developed into the second tumor, which, therefore, might not deserve to be called a recurring tumor, although, indeed, it appeared under the scar of the former operation, and not in the place where the gland was left. But, after the second operation, there is little probability that any gland remained, and we may, with as little doubt, regard the third tumor as an instance of recurrence or repetition; i. e. of reappearance of the disease in an entirely new-growth.

Sir B. C. Brodie* has related two cases of single recurrence of tumors very closely resembling that just now described; and the liability to recurrence which Mr. Lawrence's case presented is surpassed by one recorded by M. Lesauvages,† whose description of the tumors he removed accords so closely with what was observed in the foregoing case, that I can have very little doubt they were of the same nature. The patient was 63 years old. The first tumor of the breast, which was of great size, was removed in February, 1832; a second appeared, and was removed before the healing of the first wound; a third in May; a fourth in September of the same year; a fifth sprang up, and was removed in February, 1833; a sixth in May; in a seventh operation, in June of the same year, three tumors were removed; but from the same spot two more arose, and these grew rapidly, and the patient died.

* Lectures on Pathology and Surgery, p. 145.
† Archives Gén. de Médecine, Février 1844, p. 186.

Now, if, as I believe, all these cases were examples of the proliferous cystic disease of the breast, they prove such an inveterate tendency to recurrence in this disease, as is scarcely surpassed by any even of the well-marked malignant tumors. Unfortunately no examination of either case was made after death; so that it is not possible to say whether the more characteristic features of malignant disease existed, such as the concurrence of similar disease in internal organs. The same defect does not exist in a most remarkable case related by Dr. Cooke.* The patient was about 40 years old when, in April, 1847, six ounces of a glairy brown fluid was drawn from a cyst in her breast, which formed part of a large tumor that had been growing for seven months, and felt in some parts firm, in others soft and fluctuating. Occasional tappings were subsequently employed; but after five or six weeks the integuments inflamed and sloughed over the cyst, and a profuse discharge of a similar glairy fluid ensued. "Fungoid masses" soon protruded, and in July, 1847, Dr. Cooke removed the whole disease. It weighed 3½ pounds, and consisted of fungoid masses of various degrees of firmness, with a central cavity lined by a vascular membrane. In December of the same year, a small enlargement on the scar was removed. In March and in October of the next year (1848), renewed growths were again removed. In 1849, the disease again returned, and was extirpated in June, 1850. This was "a miniature representation of the tumor removed at first:" and it was examined by Mr. Birkett, who reported of it, that, "in a stroma of fibrous tissue cysts appeared, containing a yellow tenacious fluid. The follicular terminations of ducts of glands were very distinctly seen in the fibrous tissue, and nucleated corpuscles: within these follicles were clearly seen the elements of the epithelium glands." The patient recovered rapidly from this last operation, and no recurrence of the disease in the breast again ensued; but in June, 1351, she began to suffer with what proved to be cancer of the peritoneum, liver, pleura, pelvic organs, and lumbar of the thoracic lymphatic glands. When she died, in November, 1851, abundant cancerous disease was found in all these parts: but the seat of former disease in the breast was healthy, and, as Mr. Birkett especially remarks, all the lymphatic glands connected with the breast were, as they always had been, unaffected, while all those connected with the cancerous parts in the pelvis and elsewhere were the seats of cancer.

The fact last mentioned makes it improbable that the cancerous disease with which this patient died was continuous with, or a part of, the disease which had been manifested in the breast. Rather, we may believe that the two affections were essentially distinct, and that the first was, like the others I have related, an example of recurring proliferous cystic disease. But farther inquiries are necessary to elucidate these cases; at present, they are obscure in all but their practical import, and in their proof

* Medical Times and Gazette, August 7, 1852.

that the cystic disease of the breast, though generally a completely innocent disease, is, in certain cases, peculiarly prone to recur after removal.
Such inquiries, I may add, would be likely to obtain knowledge on
several important but unsettled points in relation to the whole class of
tumors; such as (1) whether any, and what, tumors may be regarded as
transitional, or intermediate, between the innocent and the malignant;
(2) whether tumors which, though having the general characters of
innocent tumors, are yet apt to recur, may not in their successive recurrences, assume more and more of both the structure and other properties
of cancers; (3) whether tumors, like such as are generally innocent, are
not peculiarly prone thus to recur in persons who are members of cancerous families; (4) whether there is not peculiarly near affinity between
some forms of these proliferous cysts, and the alveolar or gelatiniform
cancer. Such an affinity is made probable by some of the diseases of
the ovary. In some of these, it is difficult to decide to which of the two
affections they should be referred: in some, what seems to be a complex cystic disease of the ovary is coincident with medullary cancer of
the same or other parts;* and in some, medullary or alveolar cancer
seems to be developed in the interior or portions of the complex cysts.
I shall consider these questions more fully in the lectures on the general
pathology of cancers.

8. It may be inserted here, that the mode of growth observed in the
glandular proliferous cysts may be imitated by genuine cancerous
diseases.

Cancerous growths may be found in cysts under at least two conditions; namely, in cysts that of themselves appear innocent, and in cysts
produced within cancers.

Of the former mode of growth we have the examples in ovarian cysts,
to which I just referred; and herein are, perhaps, the only unexceptionable instances of the transformation of an innocent into a malignant
tumor.

The second mode of production of intra-cystic cancers is best shown
in some examples of medullary tumors of the testicle. In these† we
may see a repetition, so far as the plan is concerned, of the intra-cystic
production of thyroid gland. The great mass of the medullary disease
includes smaller masses, incapsuled with fibro-cellular tissue, and commonly presenting a lobed and laminated form, at once reminding us of
the intra-cystic glandular growths, and justifying the application to them
of the principles of Dr. Hodgkin's theory of the growth of cancers.

In these medullary testicles the intra-cystic medullary growths have
usually filled the cysts and coalesced with their walls. In rare cases one

* This was the case in the patient whose history was last mentioned, and the same fact
has been frequently observed.
† As in Mus. Coll. Surg., No. 2396.

can discern how the growths spring up as spheroidal, or as pedunculated, branching, and grouped processes from the interior of the cysts. This condition was peculiarly well shown in a case of cancer of the clitoris, in which the whole of that organ was occupied or concealed by a cancerous mass inclosing several distinctly walled cysts, which were half-filled with small, soft, and lobed cancerous intra-cystic growths.*

4. I proceed to the consideration of the *cutaneous proliferous cysts;* *i. e.* of cysts within which, in the typical examples, a tissue grows, having more or less the structure and the productive properties of the skin.

Instances of these in a perfect or typical state are rare. In the large majority of cases the cutaneous structure, if it were ever present, has degenerated or disappeared; and we recognise the relations and import of the cysts only through their containing epidermal and sebaceous materials, of which the natural production is a peculiar attribute of the tissues of the skin.

Among the parts in which these skin-bearing cysts may be found are some that have no natural connection with the skin.

1. They are frequent in the ovaries; one or more Graafian vesicles enlarge and grow, and then, apparently, produce on their inner surface a growth of skin, with its layer of cutis, subcutaneous fat, epidermis, and all the minute appended organs of the proper hairy integument of the body. The general likeness of the interior of these cysts to ordinary skin had been often noticed; but the first minute demonstration of it was by Kohlrausch,† whose observations have been fully confirmed by others as well as by myself. Among the specimens in the College Museum, one (No. 164 A) presents all the textures of a hairy piece of skin growing on the interior of one of the cavities of a large multilocular ovarian cyst. Of the other divisions of the same cyst, some contained

---

* Museum of St. Bartholomew's Ser. xxxii. 39. Rokitansky gives to cases of this kind the name of cysto-carcinoma, and draws a just parallel between them and the instances of cysto-sarcoma. (Pathol. Anat. i. p. 390.) Cysto-sarcoma he regards, nearly following Müller herein, as a combination of sarcoma with cyst-formation. The cases included by him and Müller (On Cancer, p. 170) under the name, cannot be all inclosed in the groups which I have brought near together. (1.) Some are cases in which simple cysts are found within solid tumors: these are named Cysto-sarcoma simplex, and such as these will be mentioned or referred to as varieties of fatty, fibrous, fibro-plastic, and cartilaginous tumors, in all of which the formation of cysts may ensue. (2.) The Cysto-sarcoma proliferum, if it be correctly described as constructed of cysts contained in a solid tumor, and *containing younger cysts* in their interior, I have never seen. The case to which Müller refers as exemplifying it, and which is figured by Sir. A. Cooper (Illustrations, p. 41, pl. iii.), was, I believe, an instance of proliferous glandular cyst in the mammary gland. (3.) The Cysto-sarcoma phyllodes is a proliferous glandular cyst of the breast, and is especially exemplified by the cases in which the intra-cystic growths are firm, lobed, pedunculated, and clustered, and in which many cysts are close-set in the breast. But in this disease there is, I think, no solid tumor in which the cysts are set: they appear to be themselves the primary disease, the solid growths within them being secondary formations; and if this be true, they cannot properly be grouped with the examples of Müller's Cysto-sarcoma simplex.

† Müller's Archiv, 1843, p. 365.

fatty matter and loose hair; others, various fluids; others, secondary and tertiary cysts: and this is commonly the case. Another specimen in the College Museum (No. 2624) shows very well the origin of these skin-bearing cysts. It is an ovary, with a cyst, the small size of which, as well as the structure of its walls, and the mode in which they are connected with the surrounding substance of the ovary, leaves no doubt that it is a simply enlarged Graafian vesicle. Yet it contains some hairs, and a small mass of fat, resembling the subcutaneous fat, with its tough fibro-cellular partitions.

2. Cutaneous proliferous cysts may form in the subcutaneous tissue. They are, indeed, rare in this tissue in man, except in cases of congenital growths. In the little cysts about the brow, or in or near the orbit, the inner surface is often perfectly cutaneous; and Lebert* has detected in such cysts all the minute structures and organs of the skin. Most of these cysts are first observed at or soon after birth. Some similar specimens of cysts lined with skin are in the Museum of the College.† These were taken from the subcutaneous tissue of a cow and of an ox; and, in some of them, the inner surface of the cyst could hardly be distinguished from the outer hairy integument of the animal.

3. Besides these, the common seats of cutaneous cysts, perhaps any part or organ may in rare instances present them; for the records of surgery and pathology would furnish abundant instances of aberrant cysts containing hair and fatty matter, such as we must class with these in which the cutaneous structure and products are more perfect. The most singular and frequent of these rarer examples are in the testicle,‡ the lung,§ the kidney,‖ the bladder;¶ and under the tongue,** and within the skull or brain. Those in the brain are of chief interest. I found one†† many years ago in an elderly man. While he was in St. Bartholomew's Hospital with an ulcerated leg, he suddenly died; and the only probable cause of death appeared to be a mass of granular fatty matter mixed with short stiff hairs, which lay in the tissue of the pia mater under the cerebellum.

A yet more remarkable case is in the Museum of St. George's Hospital, in Mr. Cæsar Hawkins's collection. It exhibits a mass of fatty matter, and a lock of dark hair 1½ or 2 inches long, attached to the inner surface of the dura mater at the torcular Herophili. This was

---

* Abhandlungen, p. 99, e. s. The structure is well shown in No. 158 in the College Museum.

† Nos. 161, 163, &c.

‡ See Goodsir, in Edinb. Monthly Journal, June, 1845.

§ Kölliker, in the Zeitschrift für wissensch. Zoologie, B. ii., p. 281.

‖ Mus. Coll. Surg. 1904.

¶ Mus. Coll. Surg. 2625.

** Schuh, Pseudoplasmen, p. 154; and Mus. St. Bartholomew's, Ser. xxxv. No. 25.

†† Mus. St. Bartholomew's, Ser. vi. 56.

24

found in a child two and a half years old, in whom it appeared to have been congenital.

It is perhaps only during the vigor of the formative forces in the foetal or earliest extra-uterine periods of life, that cysts thus highly organized and productive are ever formed. The *sebaceous, epidermal,* or *cuticular* cysts that grow in later life are imperfect, impotent imitations of these; yet clearly are the same disease, and are, therefore, most naturally classed with the proliferous cysts, needing only to be named according to their contents. We cannot tell, in any advanced case of such a cyst, whether the more complicate structures of the skin ever existed; if they did, they have degenerated before the cyst became of distinct size; yet the retained likeness is sometimes shown in the fact that, when such cysts are laid open to the air, they do not granulate, but assume for their internal surfaces the characters of the adjacent and now continuous skin.*

Of these sebaceous or epidermal cysts it is interesting to notice the frequent hereditary origin. Perhaps, in the majority of cases, the bearers of these have known one or more members of their family similarly endowed. They are certainly more commonly hereditary than are any forms of cancer.

I have already referred to the double mode of origin of the epidermal cysts. Sir Astley Cooper first observed that some among them could be emptied, by pressing their contents through a small aperture in the cutis over them, and hence concluded that they are all examples of hair-follicles distended with their secretions, and overgrown: but probably this conclusion is true for only a minority of these cysts. They are, I think, comparatively few in which an aperture can be found;† the greater part are closed on all sides alike, and must be regarded as cysts new-formed.

The characters of these epidermal cysts may be extremely various, in regard not only to their walls, but to their contents. Their walls may be thin, delicate, and pliant; or laminated, thick, and hard, with tough fibrous tissue; or they may be calcified; and I believe a general rule may be connected with the differences in these, as in other cysts, namely, that the thin-walled are the most productive, grow most rapidly, and are the seats of most active change.

Among the contents of these cysts we may observe extreme varieties. The chief alone need be referred to. And 1st, we find successive productions of epidermis, formed in layers on the inner walls of the cyst, and thence successively shed, and pushed inwards towards its centre. A

---

* See Home, Hunter's Works, vol. iii., p. 635, and a remarkable case by Mr. Green, in the Medical Gazette, vol. ii., p. 346.

† Mr. South especially notices this in his edition of Chelius's Surgery, vol. ii., p. 698. See also Walther, in Vogel's Pathol. Anat., p. 224.

section of such cysts (which were particularly described by Sir Everard Home from the Hunterian specimens) presents layers, of white soft epidermis, like macerated epidermis of the heel or palm. ' The external layers are commonly quite regular, white and flaky; but the internal are more disorderly, as if broken up and mingled with less organized productions.

2dly. A peculiar appearance is given to contents like these, where, among the layers of epidermal scales, abundant crystals of cholestearine are mingled. They hence derive an appearance like that of the masses to which Müller* has given the name of cholesteatoma, or laminated fatty tumor; and, indeed, the few well-marked examples of this disease which I have been able to examine, as well as Müller's own account, make me think that what he named cholesteatoma is only a combination of layers of epidermal scales with crystals of cholestearine.†

The appearance produced by such a combination is quite peculiar. It forms nodular masses of soft and brittle substance, like wax or spermaceti, the surfaces of which present a bright glistening, like that of mother-of-pearl, while their sections are finely laminated. It is a rare disease; the most frequent seats of well-marked specimens appearing to be in ovarian cysts, and in connection with the membranes of the brane. The characters are well shown in the contents of a small ovarian cyst in St. Bartholomew's Hospital; and in the tumor within the occipital part of the cranium, in Mr. Hawkin's collection, to which I have already referred. Striking examples are figured by Cruveilhier;‡ but the want of microscopic examination leaves their constitution uncertain.

3dly. In the opposite extreme to these cysts, in which the cuticular product is most perfect, we find an innumerable variety of contents, of buff and ochre-yellow, and brownish materials, that seem to consist mainly of degenerate cuticle mingled with sebaceous secretions. The microscope finds in them a confused mass of withered scales, of granular and fatty matter, clustered and floating free of cholestearine-crystals, and of earthy matter in free molecules, or enclosed within the cells or scales. And all these may be floating in a turbid liquid, or retained in some soft tenacious mass, or clustered in hard nodular and pointed masses, projecting like stalactites from the old cyst-walls.§

One more phase of this disease deserves especial notice—that in which the cyst ulcerates, and its contents protrude. An inflammation in or about the sac often appears the inducement to this change; and sometimes the inflammation itself can be traced to nothing but disturbance

---

* On Cancer, p. 155.

† See, also, an account of such a case by Mr. W. Adams, in Proc. of Pathol. Soc. 1850–1. Other writers since Müller have applied the name of cholesteatoma more vaguely.

‡ Anatomie Pathol. liv. ii. p. 6.

§ College Museum, 157 A and 2267. A most remarkable specimen is in the Museum of Guy's Hospital, which was removed from an old man's thigh.

of the general health. The probability that it may thus arise makes
the caution very valuable which Mr. Humphry* gives concerning the
removal of all tumors. "It is always well," he says, "to bear in mind
that persons are most likely to consult us respecting these, or other
growths of the like kind, when they are out of health, and consequently
unfit to bear an operation; they do so, because the tumor is then most
productive of pain and annoyance."

A distressing instance of the truth of this occurred to myself five years
ago. A strong but very intemperate man came to me as an out-patient
with an ulcerated sebaceous cyst, about three-quarters of an inch in
diameter, just below and to the right of the umbilicus. He had observed
a tumor here for sixteen years; but he had scarcely thought of it till,
during the last five weeks, it had grown quick, and in the last fortnight
had ulcerated. I saw no reason to be very cautious in such a case; so
slit the tumor and removed it, as well as the thickening and adhesion of
the parts would allow. In the evening, having returned to his work and
some intemperance, hemorrhage ensued from a small cutaneous vessel,
and before he reached the hospital he lost more than a pint of blood. I
tied the artery, and applied solution of alum to the rest of the wound,
for its whole surface was oozing blood, and he was admitted into the hospital. The next day he became very feverish, and he appeared as if he
were going to have typhus, which was then prevalent. But from this
state he partially recovered; and then abscesses formed in his groins,
and discharged profusely. Nothing improved his health, and three
months after the operation he died, apparently exhausted by the continued discharge from the abscesses, and with both external epigastric
veins and parts of the femoral veins full of old clotted blood—the consequence of slow phlebitis.

Cases like this, or ending fatally much sooner than this did, with erysipelas or more acute phlebitis, have occurred to many surgeons. They
need no comment to make them instructive.

I believe the contents thus protruded from cutaneous cysts may become
vascular. I have not seen this event, but it seemed certain in a case
observed by Mr. James Reid. A woman, eighty years old, had numerous
cysts in her scalp. They were like common sebaceous cysts, and three
of her daughters had cysts like them. Two years and a half before her
death, one of the cysts, which had not previously appeared different from
the rest, inflamed. It was opened, and sebaceous matter was discharged
from it. The opening did not heal, but ulcerated, and a small hard lump
remained under the ulcer for a year, when, after erysipelas of the head,
it began to grow, and rather quickly increased to a mass nearly five inches
in diameter, which occasionally bled largely. The mass had the appearance of the firm contents of a cuticular and sebaceous cyst, and contains

* Lectures on Surgery, p. 135; from the Provincial Medical and Surgical Journal.

abundant epidermal cells;[*] so that there can be scarcely a doubt that it had its origin in the contents of such a cyst.

5. Concerning cysts containing teeth, a few words must suffice. They are of two kinds. Some, occurring in the ovaries, and more rarely in other parts, bear, with one or more teeth, the products of skin, as hair, epidermis, &c.[†] These may be regarded as diseases of the same general group with the cutaneous proliferous cysts; and the great formative power which they manifest is consistent with their occurring only in embryonic or fœtal life, and in the ovaries, in which, even independently of impregnation, one discovers so many signs of great capacity of development.

Other dentigerous cysts occur within the jaws. In some cases, cysts are hollowed out in the substance of the upper or lower jaw, and are lined with a distinct membrane, to some part of which a tooth is attached. I believe these are examples of tooth-capsules, from which the teeth, though perfectly formed, at least in their crown, are not extruded, and which therefore remain, becoming filled with fluid, and growing larger.[‡] In other cases, that which appears as a cyst is the antrum, distended with fluid, and having a tooth imbedded in some part of its wall, and projecting into its cavity.[§] In the most remarkable case of the kind, Professor Baum removed a tooth from each antrum of a woman thirty-eight years old. The distension of the antra, with excessive thickening of their lining membranes, and thinning of their osseous walls, and with accumulations of purulent fluid, had been in progress for thirty years, and produced horrible deformity of the face. The operation was completely curative.

[*] Museum of St. Bartholomew's Hospital, Series xxxv. No. 57. Probably the case was similar which was related by Mr. Abernethy in his Essay on Tumors, p. 117. Such cases have peculiar interest in relation to the question of the possible origin of certain epithelial cancers in these cysts. This will be referred to in Lecture XXXII.

[†] A very remarkable specimen is in the Museum of St. Bartholomew's Hospital (Malformations, A. 177). It was presented by Mr. Kingdon, and is described by Mr. Gordon in the Med.-Chir. Trans., vol. xiii. In the anterior mediastinum of a woman twenty-one years old, a tumor, probably of congenital origin, contained portions of skin and fat, serous fluid, and sebaceous matter, and two pieces of bone like parts of upper jaws, in which seven well-formed teeth were imbedded. In an ovarian tumor more than 300 teeth were once found: in another case, a piece of bone, like part of an upper jaw, with 44 teeth. See Lang, in the essay cited below, p. 11.

[‡] Two such cases are in the Museum of St. Bartholomew's, Series i. 119, 119 A. I saw a third cured by Mr. Wormald by cutting away part of the cyst, and removing the tooth.

[§] The principal cases are collected in two essays, for which I have to thank Professor Baum, namely, Lang, Ueber das Vorkommen Von Zähnen im Sinus Maxillare; Tübingen, 1844; and Glasewald, De Tumore quodam utriusque Antri Highmori; Gryphiæ, 1844.

LECTURE XXIV.

FATTY AND FIBRO-CELLULAR TUMORS: PAINFUL SUBCUTANEOUS TUMORS.

AMONG the solid tumors, the first that may be considered is the fatty or adipose tumor, the Lipoma of some, the Steatoma of others; the most simple in its texture, the most like the natural parts, the least liable to variations; a morbid growth so well known, that I can scarcely hope to impart any interest to an account of it.

Among the growths commonly included as fatty tumors, we find examples of both the forms of morbid hypertrophies of which I spoke in the first lecture. There are both continuous and discontinuous morbid hypertrophies of fat; both fatty outgrowths and fatty tumors, more properly so called.*

The *Fatty Outgrowth* is thus described by Sir B. C. Brodie, in his well known lecture upon fatty tumors. He says, "there is no distinct boundary to it, and you cannot say where the natural adipose structure ends, and the morbid growth begins. . . . . These tumors feel like fat, but they may be distinguished from the common fatty tumors by their having no well-defined boundary, and by their being less soft and elastic. Such deposits may take place in any part of the body; but I have seen them more frequently in the neck than anywhere else."† Doubtless the case will be familiar to you by which Sir B. Brodie illustrates this account —the case of a footman, with an enormous double chin, and a great mass of fat extending from ear to ear, who was cured by the *liquor potassæ*. The case already cited from Schuh's essay (p. 321), was of the same kind.

I can add nothing to this account, except the mention of a singular case of fatty growth connected with the heart of a sheep.‡ The right ventricle is nearly filled with a lobulated mass of fat, distending it, and pressing back the tricuspid valve. The left auricle and ventricle are similarly nearly filled with fatty growths, and fat is accumulated on the exterior of the heart, adding altogether about twenty-five ounces to its weight. The textures of the heart itself appear healthy, though it is the seat of all these fatty growths.

The discontinuous *Fatty Tumors*, of which alone I shall now speak, present a tissue exactly or very nearly resembling the normal fatty or adipose tissue of the animal in which they grow. Certain differences may, indeed, be sometimes found between the fat of a tumor and that of

* M. Lebert (Abhandlungen, p. 112) distinguishes the fatty tumors according to their degrees of isolation, as Lipoma circumscriptum and L. diffusum. A diagram illustrating the general differences of the two modes of growth is given in the twenty-fifth lecture.
† Lectures on Pathology and Surgery, p. 275.
‡ Mus. Coll. Surg., 1529.

the part in which it lies; such as the larger size of the tumor's cells, its less or greater firmness at the same temperature, and the usual crystalizing of the margarine; but I believe there are no greater differences than may be found in the natural fat of different parts of the same person.

It would be superfluous to describe or delineate the minute characters of this well-known tissue: it is only in its arrangement that the tumors have any peculiarity worth notice. It is, in all, composed essentially of clustered oil-cells; but these are, in some tumors, placed in a uniform mass, smooth on its surface, and only obscurely partitioned; in others, arranged in oval or pyriform lobes, projecting on the surface, easily separable by splitting their fibro-cellular partitions; and in some of these it may be dissected into thin layers, which are wrapped in each lobe, one within the other, like the leaflets of a bud. Moreover, any of these forms, whether "simple," or "lobed," or "involuted," may be either deeply imbedded in the tissues, or "pendulous."

Fatty tumors are, I believe, always invested with a capsule or covering of fibro-cellular tissue; and of these capsules, since they exist with most of the innocent tumors, I may speak now once for all. The capsule, then, of such a tumor is usually a layer of fibro-cellular, areolar, or connective tissue, well organized, dry, and containing blood-vessels proportioned to the size of the tumor. It appears to be formed of the fibro-cellular tissue of the part in which the tumor grows, increased, and often strengthened, in adaptation to the bulk and other conditions of what it encloses. It grows with the tumor, invests it, and at once connects it with the adjacent tissues, and separates it from them; just as, e. g., similar fibro-cellular tissue does each muscle in a limb. Its adhesion to both the tumor and the parts around it is more intimate than that of its layers or portions to one another; so that when such a tumor is cut into, it may be dislodged by splitting its capsule, and leaving some of it on the tumor, and some in the cavity from which the tumor is extracted. This, at least, can be easily done unless the tumor has been the seat of inflammation, which may thicken the capsule and make all its parts adherent to one another, and to the tissues on either side of it. As Schuh observes, when a fatty tumor is just under the skin its capsule is usually more closely connected with the skin in the interspaces between the lobes than in any other part, so that the skin appears dimpled over it, especially if one squeezes the tumor at its base, and presses it up to make the skin tense.

In the capsule, the blood-vessels that supply the tumor usually first ramify. One principal artery, indeed, commonly passes straightway into the tumor at its deepest part, but the rest branch in the capsule, especially in any thicker parts of it that lie in the spaces between projecting lobes of the tumor Hence, with the partitions of the tumor that are derived from the capsule, the blood-vessels pass into its substance.

The capsules of these fatty tumors may vary somewhat in thickness and toughness; and so may the partitions that proceed from them into

the mass.   They are usually very delicate ; but they are sometimes thick
and strong, and give a density and toughness which approach to the characters of a fibrous tumor.   To such examples of fatty tumors deviating
from the common type, Müller* has assigned the name of Lipoma mix-
tum; and Vogel,† Gluge,‡ Rokitansky,§ and some others, call them
"Steatoma," and "lardaceous tumor" (Speckgeschwülst).||

Fatty tumors usually occur singly; but there are many exceptions to
this rule.   Two or three in the same person are not rarely seen, and a
hundred or more may exist.   Sir B. C. Brodie mentions such cases; and
I am acquainted with a gentleman, who has borne, for nearly twenty
years, firm tumors, feeling like fatty masses, in the subcutaneous tissue
of his trunk and all his limbs.   They are usually stationary, but sometimes one grows a little, or one diminishes, or a new one appears.   Lately,
I have seen a woman, 50 years old, in whom a large number of similar
tumors had been growing for about ten years in the subcutaneous tissue
of the arms, thighs, and haunches.   They were all small and firm, and
felt like tumors of mixed fatty and tough cellular tissue.

The most frequent seats of fatty tumors are the trunk, and the parts
of the neck and limbs that are nearest to it; but they may occur in any
part where fat naturally exists, and they are not limited even to these.¶
It is, perhaps, impossible to say why they should affect one locality of fat
rather than another.   Their rarity in the human mesentery and omentum,
and the fat about the internal organs is remarkable.   I have never seen
one in the recent state in any of these parts; and I know only two or
three specimens in museums.**   In the College Museum (No. 194) is a
bilobed mass of fat, enclosed in a thick capsule, and attached by a long
pedicle to the intestine of an ox.   In the trunk and limbs, they appear
least frequent in-the parts in which the natural fat, though abundant, is
subject to least variations in its quantity; such as the palms and soles,
and the bones; and they are rarely, if ever, formed in parts of or near
the trunk where very little fat naturally exists, as the eyelids and the
greater part of the scrotum.   Fatty tumors, have, indeed, been found in

* On Cancer, p. 153.   † Pathologische Anatomie, p. 179.
‡ Pathologische Anatomie.   § Pathologische Anatomie, B. i. p. 283.
|| Müller also gives the name of Lipoma arborescens to the pendulous fatty processes with
synovial membrane that are clustered about chronic diseased joints.   Sir B. C. Brodie (Lectures, i. c.) describes a form of fatty tumor, which I have not yet seen, in which the tumor
is covered with a double layer of membrane, like a serous sac.
¶ Müller (on Cancer, p. 153) describes one between the optic nerves and corpora albi-
cantia; and Rokitansky (B. i. p. 282), including both the tumors and the outgrowths, refers
to examples of Lipoma in the submucous tissue of the stomach, intestines, and bronchi
in the subserous tissue of the pleura, peritoneum, dura mater, and cerebral ventricles; and
in the lungs, liver, and kidneys.
** One, referred to in Lecture xxi., is in the Museum of St. George's Hospital.   Other cases
are related by Vogel (Path. Anat. tab. xxii. fig. 1); Gluge (l. c. Lief. viii.); Lebert (Phys.
Pathol. ii. p. 105.)   They are not rare in the corresponding parts of horses and other domes-
tic mammalia.   (Fürstenburg: Die Fettgeschwülste und ihrer Metamorphose: Berlin, 1851.

the scrotum ;* and one very remarkable case is related by Mr. Lawrence and Sir B. C. Brodie: but, perhaps, such tumors have not begun to grow in the part in which they were at length found ; they may have grown or shifted into it.

This shifting of fatty tumors is worth notice ; for the fact may be used in the diagnosis of them when they occur in the groin or scrotum, or other unusual place.

A patient was under Mr. Lloyd's care, in St. Bartholomew's Hospital, with a strange-looking pendulous fatty tumor in the perineum. It hung like a pocket-flask between his scrotum and thigh: but he was quite clear that it was in his groin ten years before, and that it had gradually shifted downwards. It was removed, and no pedicle or other trace of it remained in the groin.

I find, also, a case by Mr. Lyford,† in which a large fatty tumor began to grow in the abdominal wall, midway between the spine of the ilium and the pubes, and thence, as it increased, gradually moved downwards, and was excised from the upper and inner part of the thigh. And thus, in Mr. Lawrence's case, the tumor began to grow in the spermatic cord, and thence had partly extended and partly shifted into the scrotum behind the testicle, where it was extremely difficult to decide its nature.

The fatty tumors usually lie in the subcutaneous tissue, extending in it between the skin and the deeper fascia: but they may extend more deeply. Mr. Wormald removed one, from which distinct lobes or prolongations passed between the fasciculi of the trapezius muscle, and, expanding below them, were constricted by them. In the case of a great fatty tumor‡ of the neck, removed by Mr. Liston, the operation was made formidable by the lobes of fat extending deeply to the trachea and œsophagus. In rare cases, fatty tumors may be altogether deeply seated: I found one resting on the lesser trochanter of the femur, growing up by the side of the pectineus muscle, but not prominent externally. Vogel mentions the case of a woman who had several fatty tumors, one of which was so closely connected with the nasal bone and the nasal process of the superior maxillary bone, that it was necessary to remove these with it. Mr. Abernethy also refers to a fatty tumor removed by Mr. Cline, which adhered to the capsule of the hip-joint.§ In the Museum of the Middlesex Hospital is a fatty tumor one and a half inches long, which was removed from beneath the tongue, where it looked like a ranula; and in the College Museum‖ is one taken from the substance of the tongue.

Such are some of the chief facts respecting the structure of this kind of tumors. Of their life, I need say little.

There development is, probably, like that of the natural fat.

---

* Gluge mentions one in the labium of a woman seventy years old, It was pyriform, and looked liked a hernia (Path. Anat. Lief. viii. Taf. i. fig. 1.)

† Med. Gaz., iv. 348.　　　　　　　　　　　　　　‡ Mus. Col. Surg., No. 190.

‡ See also Brodie, l. c.; Simon, Lectures on Pathology; and others.　　　‖ No. 1065.

Their growth is usually slow, and without pain or any affection of the adjacent parts; but they often grow capriciously, having uncertain periods of acceleration and arrest, of which no explanation can be given. The extent of growth cannot well be measured; for fatty tumors have been cut out that weighed between fifty and sixty pounds, and such as these, after twenty or even fifty years, were still growing, and might have continued to do so as long as the patient lived. I believe the largest in London is that in the Museum of St. Thomas's Hospital, which was removed from a man's abdomen by Sir Astley Cooper, and weighed 37 lbs. 10 oz.* One of the most formidable is that in the College Museum, removed by Mr. Liston from a man's neck,† where it had been growing for twenty-two years. A parallel to it is drawn in the splendid work of Auvert.‡

What degenerations the fatty tumors may be liable to are not known; their diseases have some points of interest.

They may be partially indurated. The chief mass of a tumor may be found with the characteristic softness, pliancy, and inelasticity of fat; but in its substance one or more lumps, like hard knots, may be imbedded. So far as I have seen, these depend on induration, contraction, and a proportionate increase, of the fibro-cellular tissue of the fat; and the change is probably due to slow inflammation of the tumor. It may be sometimes traced to frequent pressure. A laundress had a fatty tumor, as large as a fœtal head, above her ilium, and portions of it were as hard to the touch as cartilage, and appeared to move so freely in the soft fat-tissue about them, that one might have thought them loose bodies, or fluid within cysts. Where these were, the patient had been in the habit of resting her linen-basket.

The indurated parts of a fatty tumor may be the seats of bone-like formations. This is, I believe, very rare; and I have seen only the single specimen in the Museum of St. Bartholomew's Hospital:§ but Auvert describes the same change.||

Cysts, also, may form in fatty tumors. In the case with partial indurations just mentioned, I found in another part of the tumor, a cyst with thin and partially calcified walls, which contained a glutinous and greenish oily fluid. I presume it is to tumors of this kind that Gluge gives the name of Lipoma collodies.

Suppuration and sloughing may occur in these tumors: but they are on the whole very rare events, except in large pendulous tumors, which have grown too large to be effectively nourished through their bases of attachment. Pathologically these changes have little interest; but in practice they are more important, as being almost the only way in which external fatty tumors are likely to lead to death. Even in these cases,

* Medico-Chirurg. Trans. vol. xi. p. 440.   † No. 190.
‡ Obs. Med.-Chir. Tab. li. See, for a list of the largest elsewhere recorded, Mr. South's edition of Chelius's Surgery, ii. p. 691-2.
§ Ser. xxxv. 11. || Tab. xvi.

however, they show no real imitation of malignant disease.* I once, indeed, saw a case in which the end of a pendulous fatty tumor in a woman's perineum was so ulcerated that it looked like cancerous disease ; but after a week's rest in bed, during which the patient menstruated, it lost its malignant aspect. It now acquired (what the ulcers over and in fatty tumors commonly present) clean, inverted and overhanging, wedge-shaped, granulating edges.

Lastly, respecting the causes of these tumors few things can be more obscure. Nearly all knowledge on this point is negative. The growth may have followed an injury, and we may call this the cause of its formation ; but we can give no explanation why such an event as an injury, which usually produces only a transitory impairment of nutrition, or a trivial inflammation, should, in these cases, give rise to the production of a new and constantly growing mass of fat.

FIBRO-CELLULAR TUMORS.

Under this name I propose to consider the tumors which, in their minute structure and their general aspect, resemble the fibro-cellular, areolar, or connective tissue of the body. So far as I know, no general account of them is published. The first distinction of them was made, I believe, by Mr. Lawrence,† who described an admirable example in his paper on Tumors ; and they are briefly but accurately described by Mr. Cæsar Hawkins,‡ as a softer and more elastic form of the fibrous tumor. Müller,§ also, refers to them by the name of Cellulo-fibrous tumor ; Vogel‖ by that of Connective-tissue tumor (Bindegewebgeschwülste), comparing their tissue with that of the cutis ; and Rokitansky¶ points to them as a variety of " gelatinous sarcoma." But these passing references have not obtained for this kind of tumor a general recognition, and in many works it is altogether overlooked.

As in the last kind, so in this, we find instances of both outgrowths and tumors ; i. e. of both continuous and discontinuous overgrowths. The former are, indeed, abundant and often described ; for, among them, as being formed chiefly of overgrowing fibro-cellular tissue, are the most

---

* On the possible conjunction of fatty tumors and malignant disease, see Sir B. C. Brodie's Lectures, p. 282 ; and the same on the combination of fatty and mammary glandular tumors.

† Medico-Chirurg. Trans., vol. xvii. p. 14.

‡ Medical Gazette, vol. xxi. p. 925.

§ On Cancer, p. 14.

‖ Pathologische Anatomie, p. 185.

¶ Path. Anat. i. p. 336. Müller and others describe under the name of "Collonema" a tumor such as I have not seen, unless it be an example of very soft, fibro-cellular tumor. Rokitansky (i. 335) describes it as a very soft, tolerably clear, flickering substance, like gelatine, of grayish-yellow color. He briefly describes four specimens observed by himself. Bruch describes as a genuine example of Collonema what I can scarcely doubt was a very soft fibro-cellular tumor. (Ueber Carcinoma alveolare ; in Henle and Pfeufer's Zeitschrift, 1849, p. 356.)

frequent forms of polypi of mucous membranes, and of hypertrophies of skin or cutaneous outgrowths.

1. Nearly all the softer kinds of POLYPI, growing from mucous membranes, consist of rudimental or more nearly perfect fibro-cellular tissue, made succulent by serous or synovia-like fluid infiltrated in its meshes: the firmer kinds of polypi are formed of a tougher, more compact, dryer, and more fibrous or fascia-like tissue. Of the softer kind, the best examples are the common polypi of the nose: mucous, gelatinous, or vesicular polypi, as they have been called. These are pale, pellucid, or opaque-whitish, pendulous outgrowths of the mucous membrane of the nose,—most frequently of that which covers the middle of its outer wall. They are soft and easily crushed, and in their growth they adapt themselves to the shape of the nasal cavity, or, when of large size, project beyond it into the pharynx, or more rarely, dilate it. As they increase in size, so, in general, does the part by which they are continuous with the natural or slightly thickened membrane become comparatively thinner, or flatter; their surfaces may be simple and smooth, or lobed; they often hang in clusters, and thus make up a great mass, though none of them singly may be large. A clear ropy fluid is diffused through the substance of such polypi, and the quantity of this fluid, which is generally enough to make them soft and hyaline, appears to be increased when evaporation is hindered; for in damp weather the polypi are always larger. Blood-vessels enter their bases, and ramify with wide-extending branches through their substance, accompanying usually the larger and more opaque bundles of fibro-cellular tissue. Cysts full of synovia-like fluid sometimes exist within them.

To the microscopic examination these polypi present delicate fibro-cellular tissue, in fine undulating and interlacing bundles of filaments. In the interstitial liquid or half-liquid substance, nucleated cells appear, imbedded in a clear or dimly-granular substance; and these cells may be spherical or elongated, or stellate: imitating all the forms of such as occur in the natural embryonic fibro-cellular tissue: or, the mass may be more completely formed of fibro-cellular tissue, in which, on adding acetic acid, abundant nuclei appear. In general, the firmer the polypus is, the more perfect, as well as the more abundant, is the fibro-cellular tissue. The surface is covered with ciliary epithelium exactly similar to that which invests the healthy nasal mucous membrane, and supplies the most convenient specimens for the examination of active ciliary movement in human tissues.

The soft polypi that grow, very rarely, in the antrum, and other cavities communicating with the nose, are, I believe, just like these.* And those of the external auditory passage are, in structure not essentially different. All that I have been able to examine appeared composed of

---

* See Schuh, Pseudoplasmen, p. 75; the best account of polypi I have yet read.

rudimental fibro-cellular* tissue; but they are generally more vascular, firmer, and less succulent than the nasal mucous polypi; they are also much more prone to inflammation and to superficial ulceration, perhaps through being so often connected with disease of the tympanum or its membrane. The mucous polypi of the uterus, are also, I believe, like those of the nose.

A large, deeply lobed, soft, and nearly clear polypus in the urinary bladder, the only specimen I have seen in the recent state,† was composed, in part, of very fine filamentous fibro-cellular tissue, and, in greater part, of granular, or dim, homogeneous substance, with imbedded nuclei. Over the substance which these formed, there was an immense quantity of tessellated epithelium, with large scales, like those of the epithelium of the mouth: indeed, so abundant was this, that it formed the chief constituent of the smaller lobes of the polypus. Once, also, I have been able to examine a polypus of the rectum, which, being soft and succulent, might have been classed with these; but it was composed almost entirely of gland-textures. It was like a disorderly mass of such tubular glands, lined with cylindriform epithelium, as are found in the mucous membrane of the rectum. These were heaped together with some intersecting fibro-cellular tissue, and with abundant viscid fluid like synovia or thin mucus. The polypus was spheroidal, about two-thirds of an inch in diameter, and attached by a pedicle nearly an inch long to the anterior wall of the rectum: it received so abundant a supply of blood through the pedicle that I think excision would have been very unsafe, unless I had first tied the base of the pedicle.

2. The best examples of CUTANEOUS OUTGROWTHS of which, as I have said, a second division of the fibro-cellular outgrowths is composed, are those which occur in the scrotum, prepuce, labia, nymphæ, clitoris and its prepuce.‡ These, which reach their maximum of growth in the huge "elephantiasis scroti" of tropical countries, consist mainly of overgrowing fibro-cellular tissue, which, mingled with elastic tissue, and with more or less fat, imitates in general structure the outer compact layer of the cutis. Their tissue is always closely woven, very tough, and elastic; in some cases it is compressible and succulent, as if anasarcous, and it yields, on section, a large quantity of serous-looking fluid; in others, it is much denser, interlaced with strong, shining bands, like those of a fascia; in others, it is meshed with intervening lobes of fat; and in others, it is uniformly solid and glistening, yellowish, or with an ochre tinge, and like udder. The minute textures are, however, I believe, essentially the same

* M. Lebert says the specimens he has observed were composed of fibro-plastic tissue. Professor Baum tells me he has generally found the surfaces of aural as well as of nasal polypi covered with ciliary epithelium.

† It is in the Museum of St. Bartholomew's, and is described by Mr. Savory in the Medical Times, July 31, 1852.

‡ I suppose that the disease named Molluscum simplex should be classed with these; but I have never seen an instance of it. The best accounts that I have read are by G. Simon; "Die Hautkrankheiten," p. 50 and 219, and Jacobovics; Du Molluscum.

among these diversities of general aspect; they are, in various proportions, the usual textures of the cutis and subcutaneous tissue, excepting (so far at least as present observation extends) the smooth muscular fibres. The diversities of external form are more numerous. In some, as, most commonly, on the nymphæ and prepuce of the clitoris, the masses are suspended by comparatively narrow pedicles; thus, also, are suspended most of the small cutaneous outgrowths that are common on the trunk and limbs; in some the bases are very broad, as in the nose, in which, moreover, the growth of the skin is generally associated with acne and dilatation of its minute blood-vessels; in some, as in the elephantiasis scroti, a large extent of skin appears uniformly affected. Again, in different instances, they are lobed, or less deeply subdivided, or smooth or warty on their surfaces; healthy or darkened epidermis covers them; and the sebaceous glands and hair follicles sinking beneath their surfaces, as in the healthy skin, are not unfrequently considerably enlarged. In the elephantiasis, of the extremities and of the scrotum, not only the isolation, but even the circumscribed appearance, of a tumor is lost; the affection is classed with the diseases of the skin rather than with tumors, and, in morbid anatomy, is, perhaps, not to be distinguished from the consequences of chronic or repeated inflammations of the integuments. In all cases, however, let the external form be what it may, there is such uninterrupted continuity between the several tissues of the overgrowth and those of the healthy cutis that the disease might be taken as the type of the "continuous overgrowths."*

FIBRO-CELLULAR TUMORS, properly so-called, are much rarer than the outgrowths of the same texture which I have just described. They are also rare, in comparison with other tumors; and this is singular, considering the abundance of the fibro-cellular tissue naturally existing, its general diffusion, its easy formation after injuries, in disease, and even in and about other tumors. I can in no wise explain the fact; but it is certain that for ten tumors formed of fat or cartilage (tissues which are rarely produced in other diseases), we do not find more than one formed of fibro-cellular tissue.

The form in which the fibro-cellular tumors are most frequently seen is that of oval or round masses of soft, elastic, close and pliant tissue, smooth and uniform, or, when they grow among yielding parts, deeply and variously lobed. Their exterior surface is connected with the adjacent parts by a capsule of fibro-cellular tissue, which generally splits readily. When handled they feel peculiarly tense and elastic; their

---

* Well-marked specimens of cutaneous outgrowths are in the Museum of the College: Nos. 2283 to 2290, 2466–7; 2708 to 2714; and in that of St. Bartholomew's, Ser. xi., 18, 19; Ser. xxviii., 18; and Ser. xxxii., 36, 37. I lately cut one from a man's nates (a very unusual place of growth), which weighed upwards of eight pounds. It had been growing for twenty years, and formed a great pendulous mass, on which he used to sit: its base covered the whole region of the glutei muscles.

outer surface may shine like a thin sac full of fluid. On their sections
we see opaque white bands, intersecting a shining succulent basis-substance of serous-yellow or greenish-yellow tint. Through this basis the
bands course in circles or wavy lines, or form complete partitions; or,
in the smaller lobes of the tumor, they run without order, only forming
white marks on the yellow ground-color, but giving no appearance of
grain, or of regularly fibrous structure.

The peculiar yellow color of the basis-substance of these tumors makes
them look at first like fat; it is due, however, not to fat, but to a serous,
or synovia-like, or very viscid fluid, which is infiltrated through the
substance of the tumor. The mass is just like anasarcous cellular tissue;
most of all like the subcutaneous cellular tissue of the back, as one sees
it dissected in a dropsical body. When such a tumor is cut through or
sliced, the clear yellow fluid oozes from it, or may be abundantly pressed
out; in alcohol the same fluid coagulates; in both cases, the filamentous
tissue contracting, becomes denser and more compact, and more uniformly
opaque white, like that of the softer varieties of fibrous tumor. It is to
these last-named tumors, indeed, that the fibro-cellular have the nearest
relations, and into them that they "pass" through gradational specimens,
but there is just the same difference, as well as just the same relation
between these kinds of tumors, as there is between the natural fibro-
cellular and fibrous tissues; and there is a similar propriety in distinguishing them.

Examined with the microscope, the fibro-cellular tumors display the
filamentous tissue or appearance characteristic of that after which they
are named. In many cases, or in many parts, parallel, soft, undulating
filaments are found
collected in fasciculi,
which interlace, and
from which single
filaments can often
be traced out (fig.
52); or, where this
is not seen, the tex-
ture looks filament-
ous, through mark-
ings or wrinkles of
the surface of a more
homogeneous sub-
stance. The best
developed and most

Fig. 52.*

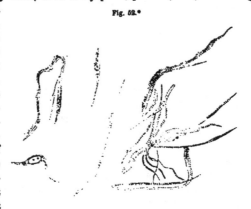

filamentous tissue is in the intersecting white bands: but similar tissue
is usually present everywhere. In many instances abundant nuclei

* Microscopic elements of a fibro-cellular tumor, with cells in various stages of elongation and attenuation into filaments. Magnified about 450 times.

appear among the filaments, or imbedded in the more homogeneous substance, and acetic acid rarely fails to bring into view such nuclei in
crowds. In many, also, cells like those of granulations, and others
elongated and attenuated, appear as if in process of development into
filaments.

The homology of these tumors, in respect of tissue, is thus as perfect
as that of the fatty tumors. In chemical analysis they may yield gelatine from the well-formed fibro-cellular tissue ; but I believe they yield
much more albuminous mat-
ter from their imperfectly
developed tissue, and from
the serous fluid that is soaked in them.

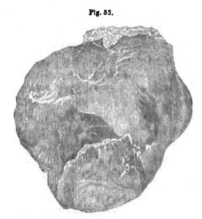

Fig. 53.

In general, there is nearly
complete uniformity through
the whole mass of one of
these tumors. Oftentimes,
however, different portions
are more or less œdematous
(if I may so call them) ; and,
which is more remarkable,
portions of cartilage, sometimes partially ossified, may
be found in or over them.
I have thrice seen this. In
the first case nodules of cartilage were imbedded in a fibro-cellular tumor
that grew in the ball of the great toe : in the second (a similar tumor
from the thigh) (fig. 53), a portion of its surface, and one of its chief
partitions, were formed with cartilage partially ossified ; in the third, a
similar tumor from the thigh was thinly, but completely, encased with
bone.[†] Moreover, besides the differences dependent on mixtures of
other tissues with those proper to the tumors, some may be found which
are due to parts of the tumor being immature or imperfectly developed,
and from this imperfect state degenerate. I have lately seen two such
specimens, of which one was removed from the inner and deeper part
of a gentleman's ham by Mr. Lawrence ; and the other, seated between
the superficial and deep muscles of a woman's forearm, was removed by
Mr. Gay. The former was of three years', the latter of two years',
growth. Both were of oval form, deeply lobed, very soft, loosely connected by a thin capsule with the adjacent healthy parts, and about eight
inches in chief diameter. Partitions, proceeding from the capsule, and
including large blood-vessels, intersected the tumors, which were mainly

* Section of a fibro-cellular tumor intersected with cartilage and partially encased with
bone : reduced one-half. Described above, and p. 389.

† All these specimens are in the Museum of St. Bartholomew's Hospital.

composed of a bright serous-yellow, flickering, but tenacious substance, half pellucid, like size-gelatine. Opaque-white lines traversing this substance gave it the general appearance of the softest and most succulent fibro-cellular tumors, or the common mucous polypus of the nose.

These characters, which were common to large portions of both tumors, were, however, in some lobes of each, widely deviated from. In the tumor from the ham, some lobes were suffused and traced over with bright crimson and vermilion tints, and looked like lumps of size and vermilion ill-mixed for an injection. Other lobes had patches of buff-colored or ochery soft shreddy substance, or consisted almost wholly of such a substance. In the tumor in the forearm there was less appearance of vascularity, but the ochrey substance was more abundant, and parts of some lobes seemed liquified in a turbid thick fluid of ochre or buff-yellow tint. In some portions it had a greenish-yellow hue, as if infiltrated with dried-up pus; in others, it was nearly white and brain-like; in others, it had mingled shades of pink and gray. But various as were the aspects of these tumors, so that with the naked eye it would have been extremely difficult or impossible to discern their kind, yet, in all parts, they showed microscopic structures characteristic of the fibro-cellular tissue in an immature state. Serous or synovia-like fluid oozed from them, but none that was pulpy or cream-like. The serous-colored parts consisted mainly of well-formed fibro-cellular tissue, or of a clear imperfectly fibrillated blastema, with closely imbedded corpuscles, like nuclei. Many of the corpuscles were clear, but many were granular, as if with fatty degeneration, or appeared changed into small granule-masses. In the buff and ochre-colored parts, similar tissue or blastema was sprinkled over, or was quite obscured, with minute shining black-edged molecules, like oil-particles, and with drops of oil. In other parts, some nuclei appeared like those of very soft cartilage; in others, crystals of cholestearine were mingled with the oily matter. In the greenish yellow parts, also, were corpuscles, like shriveled pus-cells, mixed with fatty particles and debris; and again, in other parts, cells elongated like those of granulations.

No specimens could illustrate better than such as these the necessity of learning, as I have already said, to distinguish, in each tumor, the exceeding varieties presented in the phases of development of premature degeneration and of disease.

The most frequent seats of fibro-cellular tumors appear to be the scrotum, the labium or the tissues by the side of the vagina, and the deep-seated intermuscular spaces in the thigh and arm. They may occur, probably, in many other parts; but either they particulary affect these, or else a singular chance has shown them to me in these situations with usual frequency.

In the scrotum I have been able to examine two cases, and have found

25

records or notices of many more. The first case is represented in a large specimen in the Museum of St. Bartholomew's, and in a drawing made shortly after the parts were removed. The patient was a carpenter, 74 years old; and, when he was under Mr. Stanley's care, the tumor had existed four years. It was a huge mass, about a foot long, and six or seven inches wide, filling the scrotum, and drawing over it all the adjacent integuments. A collection of fluid, like a hydrocele, was at its lower part, a large hernial sac was above it, and the scrotum was thick and œdematous. The obscurities these complications threw upon the diagnosis of the tumor, the doubt how far the hernial sac might extend, the patient's age, and his aversion from any operation, were sufficient to dissuade from active interference.

The patient died about half a year after leaving the hospital. The tumor had attained the weight of twenty-four pounds; the testicle, with a distended tunica vaginalis, lay pressed-down below it, and the hernial sac was quite clear of it above. It was easily separable from the surrounding tissues, into which many lobes extended far from the chief mass, and on section appeared partitioned into lobes of various sizes and shapes. It had all the characters which I have described as belonging generally to these tumors, varied only by the unequal collections of blood or of serum, or by its various firmness of texture in its several portions.

A similar case was brought to St. Bartholomew's by Mr. C. R. Thompson, to whom I am indebted for the history. The patient was a parish clerk, 70 years old, a sickly-looking man, and the tumor had been nine years in progress before his death. It was first noticed as a hardness just above the testicle; but, as it constantly increased in size, it filled the whole scrotum, displacing the adjacent integuments, and looking at first sight like an enormous hydrocele. Its surface was uneven and lobed, in some parts feeling hard and brawny, in some soft and fluctuating. For many years it was inconvenient only by its size and weight; but, about a month before death, one of its prominent parts sloughed, and hemorrhage took place from it. After this, more extensive sloughing took place, and more considerable hemorrhage, and the patient sank.

The tumor had the same characters as the last, except in the part that was sloughing, which was denser and more compact, and of dark, blood-stained color, like congested liver. This might have been thought cancerous; but with the microscope I found only fibro-cellular tissue infiltrated with inflammatory exudation and blood; in other portions, unmixed fibro-cellular tissue.*

To these cases I might add one related by M. Lesauvages,† in which

* The two foregoing cases are published by Mr. Thompson in the Medical Gazette, May 30, 1851.

† Archives Gén. de Med. t. ix. p. 212, 1845. M. Lesauvages refers to another very probable case in which Bayle removed the tumor. It was of three or four years' growth, and as large as a head. The patient died, without return of the disease, seven or eight years afterwards.

the tumor, in a man 70 years old, weighed at least 44 pounds, and was of such size that, as the patient sat with it resting on his thighs, it reached to his sternum and beyond his knees. And another of the same kind is related by Dr. O'Ferrall, which he removed successfully; but, excellent as the surgery of this case was, its pathological completeness is marred by the suspicion that a small portion of it was of cancerous structure, and by the finding of a "solitary, hard, circumscribed tuber" in the patient's liver, when, some months after complete recovery from the operation, he died with phthisis.*

Of the similar tumors growing by the vagina, the best instance that I know is that recorded by Mr. Lawrence.† A portion of the tumor is in the Museum of St. Bartholomew's Hospital; and, though altered from its first condition, it proves the identity of the disease with that of which I have been speaking.

The patient was a lady, 28 years old, and the tumor, suspended from the labium and buttock as far as the coccyx, reached near to her knees, was as broad as her two thighs, and measured 32 inches in its greatest circumference. It had been growing four years, and produced no inconvenience except by its weight and bulk. It was soft and lobed, and the skin was loosely connected with it. Mr. Lawrence removed the greater part of this tumor; but a portion which advanced into the labium and along the side of the vagina could not be eradicated: this was therefore cut across; and, when it had grown again, was removed in a second operation two years afterwards. The patient then recovered perfectly, and is still living, without any return of the disease, more than twenty years after the operation. Mr. Lawrence's account of the tumor, and its present appearance, leave no doubt that it was of this fibro-cellular kind.

A similar specimen, weighing more than 10 pounds, was removed by Mr. Liston from a patient 80 years old, in whom it had been growing many years, and a portion of it is in the Museum of the College (No. 2715). Many of smaller size have been removed from the same part;‡

---

* I am indebted for these particulars, beyond what were published in the Dublin Journal of Medical and Chemical Science, vol. i. 1846, to the kindness of Dr. O'Ferrall. Mr. Curling (On Diseases of the Testis, p. 51) refers to two cases of small "fibrous" tumors removed from the scrotum, in one of which the tumor was supposed to be a third testicle. These were probably of the kind here described. So, probably, were those referred to by Schuh (Pseudoplasmen, p. 69), in one of which a fatty tumor was combined with one of several "fibroid" tumors in a scrotum.

† Medico-Chirurgical Transactions, vol. xvii. p. 11.

‡ Mr. Lawrence, l. c., refers to one by Mr. Earle. Cases are also described by Sir B. C. Brodie, Med. Gaz., vol. i. p. 484; Mr. Cæsar Hawkins, Med. Gaz., vol. xxi. p. 925; Mr. Curling, Proceedings of the Pathological Society, Part ii. p. 301; and (probably) by Dr. O'Ferrall, Dublin Journal, vol. i. p. 520, and vol. iv. p. 337. A specimen from a case by Mr. Keate is in the Museum of St. George's Hospital.

and I have met with two which have presented the same disease in another phase.

A woman, 34 years old, had a tumor pendulous from the right wall of the vagina and the right nympha. It was a large flask-shaped mass, about five inches in diameter, attached by a pedicle about one inch and a half in length and thickness, over the.upper part of which the orifice of the urethra was arched. All the lower part of the tumor was slough-ing, and discharging an offensive ichorous fluid. The upper half was covered with healthy mucous membrane, and felt uniformly tough, pliant, and elastic.

The patient had noticed this disease for three or four years. It began as a tumor, projecting into the vagina from beneath its right wall, and in this situation acquired a large size before it protuded externally. It was punctured, and then grew more rapidly; but the protrusion did not take place till about ten days before I saw the patient. After this pro-trusion it enlarged very quickly, and, with the sloughing, the general health suffered severely. I removed the tumor eighteen months ago, dissecting it out with little difficulty, and the patient, I believe, remains well.

It presented a well-marked instance of a very œdematous and sloughing fibro-cellular tumor, and microscopic examination found abundant inflam-matory exudation mingled with the rudimental fibro-cellular tissue.

At nearly the same time I saw a case essentially similar to this; but the tumor was suspended from the labium, and the patient was about 60 years old. And this last fact is, perhaps, worth notice; inasmuch as, with this exception, all the cases of the fibro-cellular tumor by the vagina that I have met with have occurred in young women, while all the similar tumors in the scrotum have been in old men.

The occurrence of such tumors as these in the scrotum and labium may make it necessary that I should particularly say they are not the same disease as are the cutaneous growths which form the pendulous tumors—the elephantiasis, as it is sometimes called—of the same parts, and which I have already briefly described. The main differences are:—1st. That these fibro-cellular tumors may be separated or enucleated from the tissues among which they lie; whereas the cutaneous growths have no definite boundary, but are continuous with the proper tissue of the scro-tum, or labium, or nympha; the two diseases have the common diffe-rences between tumors and outgrowths. 2d. In the growth of the fibro-cellular tumors, the surrounding parts, including the skin, or the mucous membrane, grow in adaptation to the tumor, but often defectively, or, at the most, only normally; but in the cutaneous outgrowths, all the tissues take part, and the proper tissue and appended organs of the cutis are nearly as much exaggerated as the fibro-cellular substance. And 3dly. In the tumors, fibro-cellular tissue is the highest form attained, or, at most, a small quantity of elastic tissue is mingled with it; but, in the outgrowths, all the component structures of the skin and subcutaneous tissue are increased.

The two diseases are thus different. Still, the fact is significant, that the parts most liable to the cutaneous outgrowths are also those in or near which the fibro-cellular tumors most frequently occur; and it may be noted that, among those parts in which fatty tumors are most rare, the fibro-cellular are the most common.

For examples of fibro-cellular tumors removed from deep intermuscular spaces, I may refer to two specimens already described, and to two others in the Museum of St. Bartholomew's Hospital. One of these was removed twelve years ago, by Mr. Stanley, from an elderly man: it lay under the vastus internus muscle, and was easily dislodged from the cavity in which it was imbedded: it was a smooth, spheroidal mass, thinly incapsuled, and the bright yellowish color of its surface made it to be regarded as a firm-textured fatty tumor; but the microscope found little or no fat in it, and its present aspect leaves no doubt of its nature. The patient died after the operation, and had no similar disease in other parts.

The second of these specimens was removed by Mr. Savory from beneath the tensor vaginæ femoris of a man 38 years old. It was of uncertain date, but had been observed about five months: it was firm, elastic, smooth, movable, and painless. In the operation it was easily removed from its resting-place on the rectus muscle and the inferior spine of the ilium; the patient recovered perfectly, and has remained well for nearly two years.

This tumor was a smooth oval mass, measuring about 5 inches by 3½. Both in general aspect and in microscopic characters it might have been taken for a type of the species, except for the peculiarity of its being at one end capped with a layer of cartilage and cancellous bone, and having nodules of cartilage set along the course of one of the chief partitions between its lobes (fig. 53).

To these specimens I may add another, in the College Museum, of which Mr. Hunter has left the record that it was taken from the thigh, and had been supposed to be an aneurism.

These seem to be the most common seats of the fibro-cellular tumors, but I have preserved specimens from other parts. One was removed by Mr. Stanley from the sole of the foot, where, surely, we might have expected a fatty, rather than any other tumor. The patient was a healthy man, 41 years old, and the deeply-bilobed and very prominent tumor lay in the subcutaneous tissue over the metatarsal bones, with small lobular prolongations extending among the deeper-seated tissues. It was of eight years' growth, and nodules of cartilage were imbedded in the pliant and œdamatous fibro-cellular tissue of many of its lobules.

Another of these specimens was removed by Mr. John Lawrence, with the testicle, within the tunica albuginea of which it appears to be entirely enclosed. The patient was a healthy-looking man, 37 years old, and the tumor had, in seven years, grown to a measurement of nearly six inches by four. When first removed, it was to the eye exactly like a fatty tumor, but it contained no fat, and was a typical specimen of fibro-cellular tumor in a very œdematous or anasarcous state.

A third was removed from over the upper part of a girl's saphena vein, by Mr. Skey. It was completely encased in bone; but its mass was perfect soft and elastic fibro-cellular tissue.

A fourth specimen is a tumor which I removed from the orbit of a man 40 years old, in whom it had been growing for about eighteen months. It has the general and microscopic characters of the species, but is very soft, and is composed of a cluster of small masses, looking almost like a bunch of small gelatinous polypi of the nose.*

A fifth is an oval bilobed tumor, about half an inch in diameter, which I removed from a young man's tongue, in the very substance of which, near its apex, it had been growing for three years. It was firmer than most of the others; yet succulent, and formed an obscurely filamentous tissue, abundantly nucleated.

The specimens to which I have now referred will be sufficient, I think, to justify the giving a distinct name to the kind of tumor of which they are examples. There may be found, indeed, many specimens that will connect these with fibrous tumors; but, as I have already said, if we may, among the natural tissues, distinguish the fibro-cellular from the fibrous or tendinous, so should we make a corresponding distinction of the tumors that are respectively like them.

I need only add a few words respecting the general history of these tumors. They have been found, I believe, only in or after the adult period of life, and in persons with apparently good general health. Their causes are wholly unknown. Their development appears to be, in most cases, like that of many examples of natural fibro-cellular tissue, through nucleated blastema; but I have often found in them abundant cells lengthening and attenuating themselves into fibres, as in the organizing of lymph or granulations. These may have been formed from exuded lymph: yet I am more disposed to think them proper rudimental parts of the growth; for they are peculiarly well marked, and have no appearance of being produced in disease.

* Three cases of tumor in the orbit, which, I think, must have been like this, are described by Schuh (p. 63) under the names "Zellgewebsschwamm," "Fungus Cellulosus." Besides the specimens above described, which are all in the Museum of St. Bartholomew's, I have seen two removed from the scalp, both of which, before removal, were supposed to be cutaneous cysts. A tumor removed by Mr. Humphrey (Lectures on Surgery, p. 187) from a finger, and one described by Lebert (Phys. Pathol., p. 173) as a fibrous tumor of the neck, were probably of this kind.

The growth of these tumors is quick, in comparison with the average rate (so far as we can roughly estimate it) of innocent tumors. They often enlarge very quickly; but this enlargement is probably not growth, but swelling, through increase of the œdematous effusion: (and this difference between growth and swelling may be usefully remembered in the diagnosis of many tumors.) The growth is usually painless; but about the vagina is apt to be too rapid for the superjacent tissues. Its possible extent is very great. I have mentioned one tumor of 44 pounds weight, and another of 24 pounds, which was still growing.

Of the diseases of these tumors, nothing has been yet observed, except the sloughing and suppuration that occurred in one of the cases I have mentioned. As to their nature, all that has been said implies that they are completely innocent; and I have seen no sufficient reason to doubt that they generally, or always, are so. Once, indeed, I think such a tumor recurred after removal; and once, in the testicle, a small growth of medullary cancer existed near, but separate from, a large fibro-cellular tumor: but these are the only suspicious cases I have known.

PAINFUL SUBCUTANEOUS TUMORS.

A group of tumors peculiar for the pain with which they are connected, are thus named, and are so remarkable as to justify giving a description of them separate from that of the fibro-cellular and fibrous tumors, with which, considering their other characters, the chief examples of them might be placed.

The painful subcutaneous tumor, or tubercle, has been often well described in relation to its general characters. Its intense painfulness was too striking to escape observation. It was described by A. Petit, Cheselden, Camper, and others; but the first, and to this time the best general account of the disease, drawn from many instances, was given by Mr. William Wood, in 1812.* Dupuytren added many instances to those which he copied from Mr. Wood's paper, and made the disease much more widely known.†

The especial seat of growth of these little tumors is, as their name implies, in the subcutaneous cellular and adipose tissue. They are most frequent in the extremities, especially the lower: very rarely they occur on the trunk, or the face.‡ They are about four times more frequent in women than in men; they rarely, if ever, begin to form before adult life, or after the commencement of old age. It is seldom that local injury, or any other cause, can be assigned for their occurrence. The tumor usually lies just beneath the skin, scarcely prominent; it has a capsule loosely connected with all the surrounding parts, unless it be to

* Edinburgh Med. and Surg. Journal, viii. 1812. Mr. Wood first gave these tumors the appropriate name which they have since borne.

† Leçons Orales, i. 530. He named them fibro-cellular encysted tumors.

‡ One is mentioned by Mr. Cæsar Hawkins, as removed from the cheek by Sir B. C. Brodie (Medical Gazette, vol. xxi., p. 926); and one by Dupuytren.

the cutis, to which it may be tightly fixed, and which, in such cases, is generally thin, tense, polished, and like a superficial scar. Sometimes the small blood-vessels of the skin over and around the tumor are enlarged and tortuous, like those near a cutaneous nævus; but, else, all the adjacent parts appear healthy.

Tumors of this kind rarely exceed half an inch in diameter; they are usually spheroidal, oval, or cylindriform; they are firm, nearly hard, tense, and very elastic. Their outer surface is usually smooth, bright, yellowish, or grayish, or pure white; and their sections have the same aspect and consistence, or are varied by an obscure appearance of pure white fibres traversing a grayish basis.*

Among the painful subcutaneous tumors that I have been able to examine microscopically, one was composed of dense fibrous tissue, with filaments laid inseparably close in their fasciculi, and compactly interwoven. These appeared to have been formed in or from a nucleated blastema; for thick-set, oval, and elongated nuclei were displayed when acetic acid was added. Another was composed of well-formed fibro-cellular tissue, with bundles of parallel undulating filaments, matted or closely interwoven. With these were elongated fibro-cells, the products, perhaps, of inflammation, to which the tumor appeared to have been subject. The substance between the filaments, and that from which they were probably developed, was here, also, a nucleated blastema. A third specimen presented obscure appearances of a filamentous structure, but no separable filaments; it seemed composed wholly of such nucleated blastema as was exposed by the action of acetic acid on the former specimens. In some parts, also, this presented appearances of filaments and nuclei arranged in concentric circles around small cavities.† A fourth, which had existed for many years at the end of a woman's thumb, consisted of large clear nuclei in a dimly-shaded homogeneous substance.

From these examples, or, at least, from the first three, we may believe that the painful subcutaneous tumors may be formed of either fibro-cellular or fibrous tissue, in either a rudimental or a perfect state. They may, also, I believe, be fibro-cartilaginous, as described by Professor Miller,‡ and by many other writers. But whatever such slight diversity of tissue they may present, the characteristic of all these tumors is their pain; pain which may precede all notice of the tumor, or may not commence till much later, or may be cotemporary with it, but which, when

* Sometimes the tumor has a central cavity filled with fluid, as in two cases by Mr. Caruthers, in Edin. Med. and Surg. Journ., vol. xxxiii.; but it is observable that in one of these, occurring in a man, a visible nerve was connected with the tumor. Perhaps this was a neuroma; for in these the cystic character is not unfrequent.

† Like those drawn from a fibrous tumor of the uterus by Prof. Bennet (On Cancerous and Cancroid Growths, p. 189).

‡ Principles of Surgery, p. 630. An engraving, from the sketch by Prof. Bennet, makes this the only sure instance of fibro-cartilaginous structure. In the other recorded case the microscope was not used; and the naked eye cannot discern between fibrous cartilage fibrous tissue.

once it has set in, may rise to very agony, such as I suppose is not equalled by any other morbid growth. It is not often constant; but, generally, without evident cause, or with only a slight touch of the tumor, a paroxysm of pain begins, and, gradually increasing, soon reaches a terrible severity. Beginning at or near the tumor, it gradually extends into all the adjacent parts, often flashing, like electric shocks, from one part of the limb to another, or to the whole trunk. Such a paroxysm may continue for a few minutes, or for several hours; then it gradually subsides, leaving the parts sore and tender. While it lasts, the tumor, whatever may be its condition at other times, is always exquisitely sensitive: the muscles of the limb may act with irregular spasms; or general convulsions, like those of an epileptic seizure, may ensue; or, the patient falls as if sunk by the intolerable pain, and faints. Sometimes, too, the tumor itself swells, the blood-vessels around it become larger and more tortuous, and the skin becomes œdematous or congested, imitating the change which sometimes ensues in a neuralgic part. There are many diversities in the characters and modes of the pain; but this belongs to all the instances of it,—that its intensity is altogether disproportionate to its apparent cause, and that it cannot be explained by anything that can be seen in the structure or relations of the tumor.

This pain suggests interesting questions in relation to the pathology of all tumors; but, before considering it, let me add some facts to complete the history of these. They appear usually to be of a very slow growth. One, which I removed from the end of a thumb, had existed fourteen years, and was less than a quarter of an inch in diameter. Another, which I removed from the leg of an elderly woman, had gradually increased, for ten years; yet, at last it was less than half an inch in diameter. In other cases they may more quickly attain the same size; but this seems their limit; and, for any number of years, they may remain sources of intense pain, and yet undergo no apparent change of size or structure. They are usually single. I have found only one case in which more than one existed: in this case three lay close together over the great gluteal muscle.* When excised, they are not apt to recur. I removed one from the back of the leg of a lady 28 years old, from whom, two years previously, a similar growth was excised from the same part. After the first operation the pain was scarcely changed; after the second it ceased, and never returned. Sir Astley Cooper† removed two painful tumors, at an interval of a year, from a young lady's leg; but these are the only instances of apparent recurrence that I have found. I believe that they have no tendency to ulcerate, or to assume any of the peculiar characters of malignant disease.‡

* W. Wood, l. c.

† Illustr. of Disease of the Breast, p. 84.

‡ Dr. Warren (On Tumors, p. 60) speaks of a malignant form of the disease in which the lymphatics are affected, but relates no case of it. The case requiring amputation, which he relates, appears to have owed its severity to the treatment. Dupuytren (Leçon Orales,

In considering, now, the painfulness of these tumors, the first question is their relation to nerves : are nerves involved in them ? and do they, as Velpeau* seems to hold, differ from neuromata, *i. e.* from the fibrous or fibro-cellular tumors within the sheaths of the nerves, only in their position ? are they only tumors within the superficial or subcutaneous nerves ?

The general opinion is against this supposition. Dupuytren says that he dissected several of these tumors with minute care, and never saw even the smallest nervous filaments adhering to their surface. I have sought them with as little success with the microscope. Of course, I may have overlooked nerve-fibres that really existed. It is very hard to prove a negative in such cases ; and cases of genuine neuroma, *i. e.* of a fibrous tumor within the sheath of a nerve, do sometimes occur which exactly imitate the cases of painful subcutaneous tumor. Such a case was under Mr. Stanley's care two years ago. An elderly gentleman had for two years observed a small subcutaneous tumor over the lower part of the semi-membranosus muscle. It was easily movable, and, till within the last three months, had not been inconvenient ; but at this time it became the seat and source of pain exactly like that of a painful sub-cutaneous tumor. It was removed ; and I was able to trace, with the microscope, an exceedingly slender nerve, the filaments of which were spread out over one part of the tumor. The tumor was within the neuri-lemma, and was uniformly firm, elastic, yellowish, and composed of well-formed fibrous tissue.

Many that have been called painful subcutaneous tumors may have been such neuromata as this was. Still, I am disposed to think that most of them are only so connected with nerves as ordinary innocent tumors are, that received a few nerve-fibres in their substance. For (1) the connection of the nerves with even very small neuromata is not so difficult to demonstrate, but that it should have been found, if it had existed, in some of the many painful tumors that have been examined. (2) The neuromata often occur in large numbers in the same patient ; the painful subcutaneous tumor is nearly always single. (3) The neuro-mata usually grow constantly, and seem to have no limit of size ; even when subcutaneous, they commonly exceed the size of the painful tumors, which generally grow to a certain small size, and in it remain stationary. (4) Neuromata are most frequent in the male, the painful subcutaneous tumors in the female sex. An analysis of 26 cases of neuroma taken promiscuously, showed that 19 had occurred in men, and 7 in women ; while in 28 cases of painful subcutaneous tumors 28 were in women, and 5 in men ; evidence which is almost conclusive for the different natures of the two diseases.

---

i. 542) says they have or may acquire a scirrhous nature, and then end with cancerous softening ; but he refers to only one case justifying such expressions, and this case is imper-fectly described.

  * Médecine Opératoire, tom. iii. p. 101.

However, even if it could be proved that these painful tumors are within nerves, the question respecting the source of pain would not be fully answered. We cannot ascribe the pain to merely the altered mechanical condition of the nerve-fibres; for tumors that are evidently within nerves are not always, nor even usually, painful. It is remarkable that, in nearly all the cases in which large tumors have existed in the trunks of nerves, there has been little or no pain. The facts collected by Mr. Smith* are clear on this point. Moreover, the subcutaneous tumors themselves often remain long painless, and then become, without any other apparent change, extremely painful; and there are instances of tumors, exactly resembling them, except in that pain has never been felt in them. I removed such an one from a lady's forehead. It was about as large as a pea, had been two years growing in the subcutaneous tissue, and had never given pain except once, when it was severely struck. It had all the apparent characters of structure of the painful subcutaneous tumor. I repeat, therefore, that we cannot assign the pain in these cases entirely to altered mechanical condition of nerve-fibres in or near the tumor. We must admit, though it be a vague expression, that the pain is of the nature of that morbid state of nerve-force which we call *neuralgic*.

Of the exact nature of this neuralgic state, indeed we know nothing; but of its existence as a morbid state of nerve-force, or nervous action, we are aware in many cases in which we can as yet trace no organic change, and in many more in which the sensible organic change of the nerves is inadequate to the explanation of the pain felt through them. In both these sets of cases we assign the pain (speaking vaguely) to a functional, rather than to an organic, disorder of the nerves; to a disorder commencing in the nerves of the part which is the focus of the pain, but transmitted from them to others which, in the nervous centres, are connected with them.

With this view of the neuralgic nature of the pain in the subcutaneous tumors many of their characters and circumstances agree. The pain is commonly paroxysmal, and sometimes regularly periodical; it is diffuse, or flashing, electric, and most intense: it often excites reflex spasmodic movements, or more severe and general convulsions; though not peculiarly frequent in persons of extreme sensibility, yet it is often aggravated by mental emotions, and the other excitants of neuralgic pains; it is sometimes increased, or first felt, about the time of the cessation of the menstrual discharge; it sometimes remains at or about the seat of disease for a long time after the removal of the tumor; it is sometimes attended with what is regarded as reflex vascular fulness, but it precedes no organic change.

The consideration of the probably neuralgic nature of the pain in and about these tumors is of interest in relation to the pathology of many

* Treatise on Neuroma.

others. The pains of many other tumors are probably, in greater or less measure, of the same nature.

The irritable tumor of the breast may be called a neuralgic tumor. Sir Astley Cooper's plates show, indeed, that some which he thus called were like the painful subcutaneous tumors; but the more frequent are, I believe, mammary glandular tumors, imitating in their structure the mammary gland itself. I derive this belief from the general appearance and description of several specimens, and from what I found in two cases with the microscope. A woman, 45 years old, was under my care with a small tumor lying deep in her breast, which felt hard and not movable, except with the tissue around it. She had been aware of this tumor for a month, and during all the time had been the source of intense "darting and dragging" pain, which often extended from it through the chest to the shoulders, and along the neck and arms. The pain was described as so like that commonly assigned to cancer of the breast, that, judging from it, and from the age and other circumstances of the patient, one could not but fear she had cancer. The doubt rendered it proper to make an exploratory incision at the commencement of the operation. This was done, and the tumor, having no cancerous aspect, was alone removed. It proved to be a perfect example of mammary glandular tumor, such as I shall more fully describe in a future lecture. Thus the case seemed to be one of mere neuralgia in a glandular tumor of the breast; and it may be added, that it was only a striking instance of an ordinary fact; for such tumors are often at times extremely painful.

Similar instances might be found, I believe, in tumors of other structures; but, without entering further on their history, I would suggest that the account of all these painful tumors makes it probable that the pain the patients feels is, in great measure, neuralgic or subjective; that it has the tumor, indeed, for an exciting cause; but that it owns, besides, some morbid condition inherent or cumulative in the nerves themselves, so that at times they respond, with a morbid exaggeration, to an habitual or slightly increased stimulus. And if this be true of the most painful tumors, it is probably true, in various measures, of many others.

LECTURE XXV.

FIBROUS TUMORS.

THE name of "fibrous tumor" appears the best, among the sixteen or more, by which different writers have described the tumors whose chief characteristic is their likeness to the natural fibrous or tendinous tissue of the body. This, at least, seems the best for a general designation; and to those among them which are constructed of more than one elementary tissue we may give such names as "fibro-muscular," "fibro-elastic," "fibro-cartilaginous," &c.

The most frequent and notorious examples of the species are the fibrous tumors, or fibrous bodies, of the uterus; the "hard, fleshy tubercle of the uterus," as it was described by Dr. Baillie. From these, chiefly, the general, though not all the microscopic, characters of the species may be described.

First, however, the usual distinction must be drawn between the tumors and the outgrowths of the same structure. The uterus presents examples of both.

The FIBROUS POLYPI of the uterus, more properly so-called, are continuous outgrowths of and from the substance of the uterus; the mucous membrane and the muscular and fibrous tissues of the uterus, growing, in variety of proportions, into its cavity and that of the vagina. The fibrous tumors are discontinuous growths of similar tissue in or near, not of, the substance of the uterus.*

The distinction is often difficult to make during life: for the pendulous, polypoid, and narrow-stemmed outgrowth may be imitated, in all its external characters, by a tumor growing near the surface of the uterus, and projecting into its cavity, with a gradually thinning investment of its muscular and mucous tissues. On dissection, however, or in such a section as the adjoining diagram (fig. 54) may represent, the continuity of the polypus or outgrowth, A, and the discontinuity of the more commonly occurring tumor, B, may generally be discerned, even in specimens which, like two in the Museum of St. Bartholomew's Hospital, are, in external appearance, exactly alike (xxxii. 12 and 34).

Similar differences exist among what are classed together as fibrous tumors of bone or periosteum: some, as we shall see, are tumors; some are outgrowths, and the line of distinction cannot be well drawn.

Fibrous outgrowths are also, sometimes, found in the form of polypi suspended in the pharynx, or in the chambers of the nose, or in some of the cavities communicating with them. But I have not been able to examine any of these minutely in the recent state;

* The distinction is expressed by M. Cruveilhier (Anatamie Pathologique) by the terms "corps fibreux implantés," and "corps fibreux non implantés;" but the "corps fibreux" of the breast, which were described by him, and led to the renowned discussion at the French Academy of Medicine, were, for the most part, mammary glandular tumors, and nearly solidified proliferous cysts.

† Fig. 54, diagram-sections of an uterine outgrowth (A) and of an uterine tumor (B). Both are like polypi, but the former is continuous with the substance of the uterus; the latter is discontinuous.

and I have seen so few in any condition, that I cannot tell whether some, or even many, of them are not separate fibrous tumors, projecting the mucous membrane, and pendulous, as fatty tumors often are, when they grow just beneath the cutis. Neither the description by Schuh, accurate as it is in other points, nor any other that I remember, decides this. The same uncertainty exists as to the relations of the extremely rare fibrous polypi of the œsophagus and larynx. The fibrous structure of all these growths is well-marked, but comparatively soft and elastic, and intermediate between the structures proper to the typical examples of the fibro-cellular and the fibrous tumors.

The FIBROUS TUMORS, of which alone I shall now speak, appear to have a natural tendency towards a spherical or oval shape, with a smooth or superficially lobed surface ; but from these marks they often deviate, in adaptation to mutual pressure or the different resistances of surrounding parts. When, for example, a fibrous tumor is pendulous, its more dependent portion usually grows most, or is most swollen ; it tends from the spheroidal to the pyriform shape, but retains a smooth surface : when one grows into a cavity, it is apt to assume the shape of that cavity, whatever it may be, or else to become deeply lobed. Such varieties as these are often seen in the fibrous tumors of the upper jaw, according as they grow into the cavity of the mouth, or in other directions ; and greater diversities occur among many specimens of the fibrous tumors of the uterus.

The fibrous tumors growing in solid organs have usually a complete fibro-cellular capsule ; and in the uterine walls this is peculiarly dry and loose, so that, when one cuts on the tumor, it almost of itself escapes from its cavity. So, too, are covered the fibrous tumors in the subcutaneous tissue and in the nerves, and those parts of the fibrous tumors and outgrowths from bones which are in contact with other tissues than those from which they spring.

To the touch, the fibrous tumors are usually very firm, often extremely so ; they may even be as hard and incompressible as hard cancers. If they are soft, or "fleshy," or succulent, it is, I think, always through œdema or inflammatory softness and infiltration of their substance ; for such characters as these are rare, except in the case of the pendulous or protuding tumors, or in those that are manifestly diseased. Moreover, in all ordinary cases, the fibrous tumors are heavy, very elastic, and very tense, so that their cut surfaces rise in convexities, like those of intervertebral fibrous cartilages.

In the examination of sections, of which fig. 56 may represent an ordinary example, the most usual characters that one sees are, that the tumors present a grayish basis-substance, nearly homogeneous, and intersected with opaque, pure white bands and lines. They have a general resemblance in their aspect to a section of fibrous cartilage, such as that of the semilunar or the intervertebral cartilages. Many varieties, however, appear; the basis-substance tending towards yellow, brown, or blue, and the white lines being variously arranged.

It would be tedious to describe minutely these various arrangements: let it suffice that there are three principal, but often mingled, plans.* In some tumors, the bundles of white fibres tend to construct concentric circles round one or many centres; so that, in the section, we have a vague imitation of the aspect of one or more intervertebral fibro-cartilages, the appearance of concentric curved fibres representing an arrangement of layers successively enclosed, in the same involute manner as I described in one of the varieties of fatty tumors (p. 375). These are generally the hardest and least vascular of the fibrous tumors; usually, too, they are spherical.

In another variety of the tumors, the white bands course in variously sweeping curves and undulations, the components of the larger bundles diverging and interlacing.

In yet another variety, the fibres are less fasciculate, and appear as if closely matted in a nearly uniform white substance; and, in the extreme specimens of this form, which are most commonly found on or in the jaw-bones, a fibrous structure is scarcely to be discerned with the naked eye: they look nearly uniform, glistening, pale or white, and very firm; but the microscope proves their identity with the other varieties.

As on the exterior, so in sections, these tumors present various degrees of lobular arrangement. Some are uniform and scarcely partitioned; while others are formed in distinct and easily separable pieces; and between these are numerous intermediate forms.

As a general rule, the vascularity of a fibrous tumor is in an inverse proportion to its singleness and toughness of construction; for the blood-vessels, as in the natural fibrous structures, are distributed chiefly or exclusively in the fibro-cellular tissue partitioning and investing the denser substance. The tumors thus present various degrees of vascularity.— Some, when the vessels of the uterus are fully injected, appear still quite white; but some appear as highly colored with the injection as the uterus itself.†

In microscopic examination, one finds, among the fibrous tumors, certain varieties of composition which are not always, if at all, expressed in their more manifest characters. In all, I believe, a large portion of the mass consists of tissue resembling the tendinous or fibrous; being composed of exceedingly slender, uniform, pellucid filaments, undulating or crooked, more or less perfectly developed, and variously arranged.‡ This is the case in all parts of the tumor; in the more homogeneous basis-

---

* See Nos. 2666, 2671, 2672, in the Museum of the College of Surgeons.

† Remarkably good specimens illustrating this point are in the Museum of the Middlesex Hospital.

‡ Some of the best examinations are by Valentine, in his report Repertorium; and by Bidder, in Walter, Ueber fibröse Kröper der Gebärmutter, p. 37.

substance as well as in the intersecting bands; the microscopic difference
between these parts consisting, I think, only in the less or more regular
arrangement of the fibrous structure or fibrous appearance of the tissue.
But in different specimens, or even in different parts of the same, the
tissue appears less or more perfectly formed; so that, while in some, distinct filaments or undulating fasciculi may be dissected out, in others
there is rather a fibrous appearance than a fibrous structure. Commonly,
too, one finds nuclei or cytoblasts strewn through the substance of the
tumor; the less abundantly, I think, the more perfect is the fibrous character of the tissue. But in all these respects, there are not, I think, more
or other differences among fibrous tumors than in series of natural fibrous
tissues.

With these constituents other elementary tissues are mingled in certain
fibrous tumors. In those in the uterus (just as in the uterus itself),
smooth or organic muscular fibres are more or less abundant. I have
not, indeed, seen such a specimen as would quite justify the name of

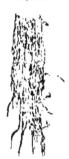

Fig. 54 A.*

"muscular" tumors, assigned by Vogel: but the mingling of muscular fibres, in imitation of the tissue
of the uterus, is usual, if not constant, in these tumors
(fig. 54 A).

In the subcutaneous fibrous tumors, and in some, I
believe, of the uterine tumors also,† elastic fibres, with
all their fully-developed characters, may be intermingled with the more abundant fibrous tissue. The
structure of fascia is thus imitated; and, if we were
to call those last mentioned "muscular" tumors, these
should be named "fascial."

Again, in the fibrous tumors on bones, bone, in small
plates or spicula, is often present; or there may be
mixtures of fibrous and cartilaginous tissue. Possibly,
also, other mixtures of tissues may occur in what we commonly accept as
fibrous tumors; but I suppose that a general statement may be truly
made, to the effect that the common characters of fibrous tumors, such as
I just described, are usually modified towards an imitation of tissues in
or near which they are severally placed.

Their structural homology is thus complete; and I presume they may
be equally similar in chemical properties. They yield gelatine on boiling;
but I am not aware of any examination of their other constituents.

To the varieties of the fibrous tumor already named, two must yet
be added, depending on changes which we may regard as results of disease or degeneration. One consists in the formation of cysts, the other
in the deposit of calcareous and other salts in the substance of the tumor:

---

* Fig. 54 A, Minute structure of an uterine fibrous tumor. Narrow smooth muscular
fibres project from the edges of a fibrous tissue. Magnified about 400 times.

† See Bidder, in Walter, l. c., p. 38. I have found, also, in a subperitoneal fibrous tumor
in the stomach, elastic fibres just corresponding with those of the natural subperitoneal tissue

suggesting, severally, the names of the "fibro-cystic," and the "fibro-calcareous" tumor.

The formation of cysts is not rare in fibrous tumors, especially in such as are more than usually loose-textured. It may be due to a local softening and liquefaction of part of the tumor, with effusion of fluid in the affected part; or to an accumulation of fluid in the interspaces of the intersecting bands; and these are the probable modes of formation of the roughly-bounded cavities that may be found in uterine tumors. But in other cases, and especially in those in which the cysts are of smaller size, and have smooth and polished internal surfaces, it is more probable that their production depends on a process of cyst-formation, corresponding with that traced in the cystic disease of the breast and other organs. The whole subject, however, in relation to the origin of the cyst, needs further consideration; and I will speak only of the general appearance of the fibro-cystic tumors.

First, then, we find certain examples of fibrous tumors thickly beset with numerous well-defined and lined cysts. This appears to be the nature of the "hydatid testis" described by Sir Astley Cooper. The specimens that I have seen of it make me think that it is, essentially, a fibrous or fibrous and cartilaginous tumor in the testicle, with more or less of cyst-formation in the tumor. For, upon or around the tumor, the seminal tubes or their remains may be traced outspread in a thin layer, and without difficulty separable; and the substance of the tumor is a distinct mass of common fibrous tissue with or without imbedded nodules of cartilage, and with a variable number of imbedded cysts, filled with pellucid serous or viscid contents. A similar condition may be found, but is rare, in fibrous tumors of the uterus. It may be found, also, I believe, in fibrous tumors in nerves and other parts.

In another set of cases, we find one large cyst existing alone, or far predominating over all the others in a fibrous tumor. This is most frequent in the tumors in the nerves,* and in the uterus. In the latter organ it has peculiar interest, because the cyst, if it attain a great size, may be mistaken and treated for an ovarian cyst. Several such cases have happened. The preparation from one is in the Museum of the College (No. 2657); the history of which, sent by Sir Edward Home, is, that it is "A portion of an uterus, in which a very large encysted tumor had formed. The patient had been twice tapped, and the cyst emptied. The case was supposed to be ovarian dropsy during life." In another case, Mr. Cæsar Hawkins, suspecting ovarian disease, drew fifteen pints of fluid from a great cyst in a fibrous tumor of the uterus.† The patient died a long time afterwards, and the specimen, which is in the Museum

---

* See Smith on Neuroma, p. 6.

† Medical Gazette, vol. xxxvii. p. 1022. This specimen and others are described by Mr. Prescott Hewett in the London Journal of Medicine. See, also, on suppuration in these cysts, Dr. Robert Lee, in the Med.-Chirurg. Trans. vol. xxxiii. Two remarkable cases of the

of St. George's Hospital, shows an enormous fibrous tumor in the side
wall of the uterus, having one vast cavity, and in its solid part many
small cysts.

With regard to the *fibro-calcareous tumor*, it is to be observed that two
methods of calcification exist; a peripheral, and an interstitial. In the
former, which is the rarer, an ordinary fibrous tumor is coated with a
thin, rough, nodulated layer of chalky or bone-like substance.* In the
latter method, a similar substance is deposited more abundantly throughout the tumor, and is usually so arranged, that by maceration, one obtains a heavy, hard mass, variously knotted and branched like a lump of

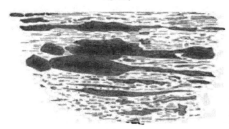

Fig. 55.†

hard coal. Such a speci-
men is in the College Mu-
seum (No. 226): it was
found in a graveyard, and
was sent to Mr. Hunter
as an uninary calculus. It
is an oval, coral-like mass,
about five inches long. On
analysis, it yielded 18·644
per cent. of animal matter,
consisting of gelatine, with
a small proportion of albumen; and its other chief constituents were
found to be phosphate and carbonate of lime, the proportion of carbonate
being greater than in human bone.

A similar, but larger, specimen is in the Museum of St. George's Hospital; and one yet larger in that of the Middlesex Hospital, which has
been described, with a history full of interest, by Mr. Arnott.‡

Now the change which ensues in these cases is not ossification; true
bone, I believe, is not formed in the fibrous tumors of the uterus. The
change is a calcareous degeneration consisting in an amorphous and disorderly deposit of salts of lime and other bases in combination with, or
in the place of, the fibrous tissue.§ It is represented from Dusseau's
plate, in the adjacent figure (fig. 55). The process is important, as
being the manifestation of a loss of formative power in the tumor. The
calcified fibrous tumors probably never grow, and are as inactive as the
calcified arteries of old age.‖

same kind are related by Schuh (Pseudoplasmen, p. 165). In one of them the huge cyst
in the uterine tumor produced the greatest enlargement of the abdomen that he ever saw.

* As in Mus. Coll. Surg. No. 2670.

† Calcareous deposit in a fibrous uterine tumor: copied from Dusseau.

‡ Medico-Chirurgical Transactions, vol. xxiii. p. 199.

§ On the appearance of a crystaline form in the deposits, see Dusseau (Onders. van het
Beenweefsel en van Verbeeningen in zachte Deelen, p. 80).

‖ A remarkable exemplification is in Mr. Arnott's case. In forty years, the calcified tumor
did not more than double its size.

With these degenerations I may mention (though it has probably more of the nature of a disease), a softening of fibrous tumors, in which, quickly, and apparently in connection with increased vascularity and congestion, they become œdematous, and then, as their tissue loosens, become very soft, or even diffluent, or else break up, and appear shreddy and flocculent. In this state the outer and less softened part of the tumor may burst, or they may separate or slough.*

The most frequent seat of fibrous tumors is beyond all comparison, in the uterus. Indeed, we may hold that the fibrous uterine tumors are the most frequent of all innocent tumors, if Bayle's estimate be nearly true, that they are to be found in 20 per cent. of the women who die after 35 years of age. But I shall not dwell on the fibrous tumors in the uterus, fully described as they are by Dr. Robert Lee, and other writers of uterine pathology. I will only say, that such tumors may occur near, as well as in, the uterus; but that, in respect of this nearness, they are probably limited to those parts in which fibrous and smooth muscular tissue, like that of the uterus, extends; namely, to such parts as the utero-rectal and utero-vesical folds and the broad ligaments.†

Next to the uterus, the nerves are the most frequent seats of fibrous tumors. But of these, while I can refer to the splendid monograph by Dr. Smith,‡ I will say only that, among the neuromata, the fibrous tumors reach their climax of multiplicity, existing sometimes in every considerable nerve of the body, and amounting to 1200 or more in the same person.§

So, too, having in view only the general pathology of tumors, and not the study of their local relations or effects, I will but briefly mention the fibrous tumors of bones; referring for a larger account of these to Mr. Stanley's Treatise on the Diseases of the Bones, and to Mr. Cæsar Hawkins's Lectures on their Tumors.||

Leaving these instances of fibrous tumors, the histories of which have been so fully written, I will select, for the general illustration of the whole group, some that are less generally studied; especially those that are found in the subcutaneous tissue, and deeply seated near the periosteum, or other fibrous and tendinous structures.

The *subcutaneous fibrous tumors*, to whose those of the submucous

* The whole of this process is extremely well described in Mr. Humphry's Lectures on Surgery; Lect. xxvii., p. 139.

† It appears, indeed, to be this mixed tissue to which the fibrous tumors particularly attach themselves; for they are in close relation with it in other parts besides the uterus; *e. g.*, in the skin and the submucous tissue of the digestive canal and other parts.

‡ On Neuroma: folio. Numerous cases are also collected by Moleschott in the Nederlandsch Lancet, Nov., 1845.

§ M. Lebert has related a case (Comptes Rendus de la Soc. de Biologie, t. i., p. 3) of a woman, 66 years old, who had several hundreds of fibrous tumors in different parts of her subcutaneous tissue. But these do not seem to have been connected with nerves.

|| Medical Gazette, vols. xxi.–ii.–v.

tissue closely correspond, pass, as I have already said (p. 388), within sensible gradations into the fibro-cellular. Many may be found that might deserve either name, just as there are many examples of natural tissues with the same intermediate characters; but it is not very rare to find specimens with all. the distinctive features ascribed to the fibrous tumors of the uterus. These form firm, nearly hard, and tense, round or oval masses, imbedded, singly or numerously, in the subcutaneous fat, raising and thinning the cutis. They may here attain an immense size, as in a case from the Museum of Mr. Liston.* A tumor, weighing upwards of twelve pounds, was removed from the front of a man's neck, together with a portion of the integuments and platysma that covered it. It was fifteen years in progress, and has an aspect, such as, I think, belongs only to a fibrous tumor. Specimens, however, of this size are very rare; they are commonly removed while less than an inch in diameter.

In microscopic characters the subcutaneous fibrous tumors have the general properties of the species, but they commonly contain elastic tissue, and they are apt, I think, to be lowly developed, having only a fibrous appearance, or even seeming composed of a uniform blastema, with imbedded elongated nuclei, like the material for the formation of new tendons (pages 128 and 178).

A peculiar and important character in these fibrous tumors is, that though they may be completely isolated in every other part, they often adhere closely to the lower surface of the cutis, and that, if in any degree irritated, they soon protrude through it, and form vascular masses —"fungous growths," as they are called. When this happens they may bleed profusely, and in a manner which, I believe, is not imitated by any other innocent tumor.

A woman, 52 years old, was under Mr. Stanley's care with a tumor that projected through the integuments in the inner part of the thigh, its base being imbedded deep in the subcutaneous tissue, and its protruding surface raw and ulcerated. The origin of this tumor was uncertain, but it had existed more than nine years; it had grown quickly, and had begun to protrude within two and a half years. From its ulcerated surface hemorrhage frequently ensued; and the patient stated that at one time two quarts of blood flowed from it. The tumor was excised, and large vessels that entered its base bled freely in the operation. It appeared to be a well-marked specimen of a soft and lowly developed fibrous tumor.

A similar case was under my care in a woman 27 years old. The tumor, of three years' growth, and protruding over the front of the tibia, was similarly ulcerated, and used often to bleed; sometimes it bled largely, and once as much as half a pint of blood flowed from it. This also on removal appeared to be a fibrous tumor.

Through the kindness of Mr. Birkett, I saw a specimen, from a much

* Mus. Coll. Surg. 222.

more formidable example, of the same fact. A woman, 60 years old, had a large pendulous tumor in the front wall of her abdomen, suspended just below the umbilicus, and reaching half-way to her knees. Its surface had a very inflamed appearance, and the separation of a slough from its posterior part gave issue to such hemorrhage as proved quickly fatal.

The tumor is a large, heavy mass, which was attached to the sheath of the rectus. It is everywhere firm and tough, except where its substance appears to have been broken by blood issuing from numerous large vessels that traverse it. Mr. Birkett, who examined it soon after the patient's death, found its texture certainly fibrous.*

The fibrous tumors that occur in or near accumulated fibrous tissues are well exemplified, medically, by some of those of the dura mater, and, surgically, by those which may be found at the tarsus or metatarsus imbedded among the ligaments and other deep-seated parts. Some well-marked specimens are in the Museum of the College. One,[†] from the collection of Mr. Langstaff, is an oval tumor, six inches long, fixed to the periosteum of the tarsal bones and to the adjacent parts, and filling the sole of the foot from the os calcis to the basis of the first phalanges. It was removed, with the foot, from a nobleman, 85 years old, in whom it had been observed gradually increasing for thirty years. It has all the general aspects of the fibrous tumor, as typified in those of the uterus.

A very similar specimen is shown in a tumor growing over the whole length of the dorsal aspect of the metatarsus;[‡] and with these may be mentioned one[§] which has some historic interest, for it was removed from the Hon. William Wyndham, the associate and friend of Pitt, and Fox, and Burke,—"the model of the true English gentleman." When he was 60 years old, and an invalid, he exerted himself very actively one night in saving from fire the library of a friend. During his exertions he fell, and struck his hip; and from that injury the tumor appeared to derive its origin. It grew quickly, and in ten months it seemed necessary to remove it. Mr. Wyndham submitted to the operation, his biographer says, "with neither hope nor fear;" and it would be difficult to describe so briefly a more unfavorable state of mind. The operation was performed by Mr. Lynn. The tumor was attached to the capsule of the hip, and was with difficulty removed. At first all went well; but then, it is said, symptomatic fever came on, and death occurred on the 16th day. The tumor was, by Mr. Wyndham's request, placed in the Museum of this College; and I have had it sketched because it might be signalized as one of the most characteristic examples of its kind.

* This specimen was sent to the Museum of Guy's Hospital by Mr. Nason.
† No. 220. The other half of the same is in the Museum of St. Bartholomew's Hospital Series xxxv., No. 9. ‡ Mus. Coll. Surg., 219. § Mus. Coll. Surg., 218.

I might add several to these cases, but these may suffice for illustra-

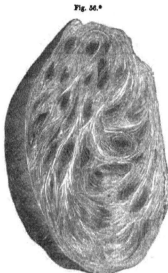

Fig. 56.*

tions of the fibruos tumors connected with the deep-seated fibrous tissues. All the specimens that I have seen have presented the strong white bands intersecting a grayish or dull white basis-substance, the characteristic firmness, heaviness, and tension; all, in microscopic examination, have shown the tough fibrous structure or appearance; all have yielded gelatine in boiling.

The favorite seats of the fibrous tumors of bone and periosteum are about the jaws; on other bones they are very rare. The College Museum is, I suppose, eminently rich in fibrous tumors connected with the jaws, containing as it does the chief of those that were removed by Mr. Liston; a series illustrative at once of his admirable dexterity, and of his sound knowledge of pathology.

These tumors of the jaws may, to both touch and sight, present the ordinary characters of the fibrous tumors, as already described. They usually approach the round or oval shape, but are generally knobbed, or

Fig. 57.†

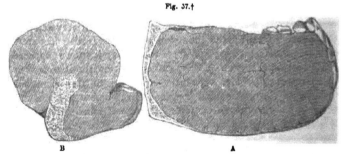

B   A

superficially lobed, or botryoidal, as some have called them. They are firm, dense, and heavy. On section, however, the majority of them, I

---

* Fig. 56 Section of a deep-seated fibrous tumor; from the case described in the text. Natural size.

† Fig. 57, A. Fibrous tumor within the ramus of the lower jaw, disparting and extending its walls. B. A similar tumor outgrowing upon the lower jaw. Both are represented in section, one half of the natural size, from specimens at St. Bartholomew's. Both consisted of perfect and unmixed fibrous tissue.

think, are more uniform than the fibrous tumors of other parts. They are generally almost uniformly white, and scarcely intersected by any distinct fibrous bands, except such as may divide them into lobes. Many of them also present, in their interior, minute spicula of compact, white, bony texture.

As to situation and connection, the fibrous tumors of the jaws may be found isolated and circumscribed, growing within the jaw, divorcing and expanding its walls, and capable of enucleation* (fig. 57 A); but, in a large number of these tumors, the periosteum, with or without the bone itself, is involved or included in the outgrowing mass (fig. 57 B). The difference is illustrated by the sketches (fig. 57). In the case of the upper jaw, either the periosteum, or the fibro-mucous membrane of the antrum or nasal walls, or both of these, may be included in such a tumor. In all cases the tumor lies close upon the bone, and cannot be cleanly or without damage to it separated, except on the outer surface: commonly, indeed, bony growths extend from the involved bone into the tumor; and sometimes the greater part of the bone is as if broken up in the substance of the tumor.

In all these characters of connection, the fibrous tumors on the exterior of the jaws and about other bones resemble outgrowths; they are as if some limited portion of the periosteum were grown into a tumor overlying or surrounding the bone. The character of outgrowth is indeed generally recognized in the epulis, or tumor of the gums and alveoli; but I believe Mr. Hawkins is quite right in the view which he has expressed, that the fibrous epulis should be regarded as a tumor growing, like most of the other fibrous tumors, from the bone and periosteum, and continuous with them.† That it is prominent and lobed is because it grows into the open cavity of the mouth; and it resembles gum only because it carries with it or involves the natural substance of the gum.

I will refer to but one more set of cases of fibrous tumors; those, namely, that occur in the lobules of the ears. These are, indeed, trivial things in comparison with the tumors of the jaws, yet they have points of interest, in that they grow after injuries, and are very apt to recur after removal. They are penalties attached to the barbarism of ear-rings.

---

* For such cases see the Museums of the College of St. Bartholomew's and Guy's Hospitals; Stanley, Illustrations, pl. 16, fig. 8; Ward, Proc. of the Pathol. Soc. Nov, 16, 1846.

† I say *fibrous epulis*, because growths may be found resembling common epulis in many characters, yet differing in some and especially in microscopic structure. M. Lebert classes epulis with fibro-plastic tumors, and I shall refer in the next lecture to specimens presenting the structure to which he gives that name; but more of those which I have examined were of a purely fibrous texture. The difference may be important in surgery; for there is always uncertainty about the operations for epulis; perhaps because among the firm lobed outgrowths from the gums and jaws, to all of which the same name is applied, there are two or more kinds of tumors, with as many different properties. The lecture of Mr. Hawkins (Medical Gazette, vol. xxxvii. p. 1022) is the best study on the subject of epulis. Mr. Birkett tells me he has found the glands of the gum much developed in some instances of tumors thus named.

Shortly after the lobules of the ears have been pierced, it sometimes happens that considerable pain and swelling supervene. These are apt to be followed by a more defined swelling in the track of the puncture; and this swelling presently becomes a well-marked fibrous tumor in the lobule of the ear. There may be, perhaps, some doubt whether the growth be a proper tumor or a cheloid growth of the cicatrix-tissue formed in the track of the wound; but it has the aspect of a distinct fibrous tumor, and the skin appears unaffected.

In one case, of which the specimens were presented to the Museum of St. Bartholomew's Hospital* by Mr. Holberton, a tumor, such as I have described, formed in the lobule of each ear of a young woman, a few months after they were pierced for ear-rings. Both the lobules were cut off with the tumors; but, in or beneath one of the cicatrices, a similar tumor formed shortly afterwards. This was excised; and in the ten years that have since elapsed there has been no return of the disease.

In another case, under the care of Mr. Benjamin Barrow, two such tumors formed in the same ear after puncture. One of these was cut away, the other was left: a third grew, and the excision of the whole lobule was necessary for the complete extirpation of the disease.

Similar instances are recorded by Bruch,† Venzetta,‡ and others; but the histories of the cases are so like these that I need not detail them.

Among tumors so diverse in their seats and relations as the fibrous tumors, there are perhaps few things relating to their life that can be stated as generally true.

In the uterus many may exist at the same time: the whole wall of a uterus may be crammed with them, while others project from it into the peritoneal cavity. As Walter and others have observed, when a fibrous tumor fills the cavity of the uterus, or projects from it into the vagina, it is not usual for another to be found in the walls. Such cases do indeed occur, but they are comparatively rare. It is yet much more rare for fibrous tumors to be found in any other part at the same time as in the uterus. I find but one such case recorded; a case by Dr. Sutherland,§ in which, with several fibrous tumors in the uterus, one was found in the groin of a lunatic 42 years old. But such a case is a most rare exception to the rule; or, indeed, may be more like an example of the rule, if the tumor were connected with the round ligament, and the tissue therein continuous with the uterus.

In the nerves, as in the uterus, a multiplicity of fibrous tumors may be found; but, so far as I know, the rule of singleness generally prevails in every other part liable to be their seat.

* Ser. xxxv. No. 24.   † Die Diagnose der Bösortigen Geschwülste, p. 206.
‡ Annales de Chirurgie, Juillet, 1844.
§ Proceedings of the Pathological Society, vol. ii. p. 87.

The development of fibrous tumors is usually, I believe, through nucleated blastema.

Their growth is generally slow and painless. It is often very slow, so that tumors of thirty or more years' standing are found still far short of the enormous dimensions of some of the last species. But no general rule can be made on this point, especially since the rate of growth is influenced by the resistance offered by the more or less yielding parts around.

The extent of growth appears unlimited; and among the fibrous tumors are the heaviest yet known. They have weighed fifty, sixty and seventy pounds. The tumor that induced Walter to write his admirable essay* weighed seventy-one pounds. He refers, also, to one of seventy-four pounds, and to one described in an American journal as having been estimated at one hundred pounds; but he asks of this, perhaps impertinently, whether it were weighed also (aber auch gewogen?)

In relation to the degeneration and diseases of fibrous tumors, I need add nothing to what has been said concerning the formation of cysts, the calcification, and the process of softening or disintegration.

And respecting their nature, there can be no doubt that, in general, they are completely innocent. Yet there seem to be exceptions to this rule, for occasionally, tumors are found in which both general and microscopic characters exactly resemble, I believe, the ordinary fibrous tumors already described, but which differ from them in that they recur once or more after removal, and form not only in their first locality, but in internal parts remote from it. To these, till their characters are more perfectly known, I would give the name of MALIGNANT FIBROUS TUMORS.

A remarkable instance of these occurred in a poor widow who was under my care twelve years ago. She was 47 years old, and had been crippled with acute rheumatism for ten years before she found a small movable tumor in her right breast. This had increased slowly till seven weeks before I saw her, when, having been struck, it began to grow very rapidly, and became the seat and centre of severe pain. It increased to between two and three inches in diameter, was nearly spherical, very firm, tense, and painful,—even extremely painful. I supposed it to be a large hard cancer, and removed the whole breast. I found the tumor completely separable from the mammary gland, which was pushed aside by it, but was healthy: the cut surface, could not, I think, have been distinguished from that of an ordinary fibrous tumor of the uterus, with undulated white bands, except in that part it had a suffused purplish tinge.† The whole substance of the tumor had the same cha-

---

* Ueber fibröse Körper der Gebärmutter. Dorpat, 4to. 1842.

† One section of it is in the Museum of St. Bartholomew's, Ser. xxxiv. No. 24; another in the College Museum, No. 223.

racters: and in microscopic examination, often and lately repeated, I could find nothing but tough, compact, well-formed fibrous tissue with imbedded elongated nuclei. On boiling, gelatine was freely yielded. In short, I believe it would be impossible to distinguish, by any means but the history, this tumor from a common unmixed fibrous tumor of the jaw or subcutaneous tissue.

Three months after the operation a tumor appeared under the scar. It grew very quickly, and felt just like the former tumor. After two months the thin scar began to ulcerate, and the integuments around sloughed; and shortly the whole of this tumor was separated by slough-ing, and was removed entire. This also had, and, in the Museum of St. Bartholomew's, still retains, every character of the common fibrous tumor.

After the separation of this second tumor, a huge cavity remained, with sloughing walls; then, as the sloughs cleared away, hard knots, like those of a cancerous ulcer, grew up from the walls, and the disease as-sumed all the characters of a vast and deep hard cancerous sore. In two months she died. I found the ulcer nearly a foot in diameter: its walls were formed of a thick nodulated layer of hard, whitish, vascular substance, like the firmest kinds of medullary cancer. Both lungs con-tained between twenty and thirty small masses of similar substance im-bedded or infiltrated in their tissue;* and this substance I have recently again examined, and found to be a complete fibrous tissue, like that of the first tumor removed. I found no similar disease elsewhere.

All the characteristic features of malignant disease were thus super-added to the growth of a tumor which appeared to be, in every struc-tural character, identical with the common innocent fibrous tumor. Nearly the same events were observed in the following case:—In 1835, a man was in St. Bartholomew's Hospital, under the care of Mr. Earle, with a large spheroidal tumor, lying by the base of his scapula, and extending beneath it. It was removed; and I remember that it was easily ena-cleated from the adjacent parts, and was called "albuminous sarcoma;" but it was not preserved. About a year afterwards the man returned with a yet larger tumor in the same situation. Mr. Skey removed this, together with a large portion of the scapula, to both surfaces of which it was closely united. The wound was scarcely healed, when another tumor appeared, and increased rapidly. With this the patient died, and growths of similar substance, white, very firm, and nodulated, were found beneath that part of the pleura which corresponded with the growth on the exterior of the chest. I state these particulars from memory; but I have found, from repeated recent examinations, that the tumor removed by Mr. Skey is of fibrous texture, resembling the common fibrous tumors both in general and in microscopic characters, and, like them, yielding

---

* Mus. St. Bartholomew's, Ser. xiv. No. 43; Mus. Coll. Surg., 224.

gelatine when boiled.* It is lobed, with partitions of fibro-cellular tissue, and its several lobes are intersected with obscure, opaque white fibres: it is tough, compact, and heavy, and tears with an obscure fibrous grain. It is easily dissected for the microscope, tearing into fasciculi, and appears composed wholly of close-placed and nearly parallel undulating filaments. A few shriveled nuclei appear among the fibres, but no cells are distinguishable. Its structure is represented in fig. 58.

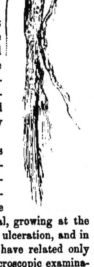

Fig. 58.†

To these cases I may add, though it be an imperfect one, that of a woman from whose back Mr. Lawrence removed a large, well-marked fibrous tumor, which had grown nine months after one of the same appearance had been removed from the same part.‡ Before removal, this was judged by all who saw it to be malignant; but it presented a genuine fibrous structure, and could not, I think, be distinguished from an ordinary fibrous tumor.

Such are the cases which make me believe that tumors occur, resembling in all respects of structure and chemical composition the fibrous tumors of the uterus (excepting their muscular fibres), or of the bones or subcutaneous tissue, yet differing from these in that they pursue a course like that of cancers, recurring after removal, growing at the same time in internal organs, tending to sloughing or ulceration, and in the latter process involving adjacent structures. I have related only cases in which the fibrous structure was proved by microscopic examination; but I have little doubt that others might be added from cases of tumors of the jaws and other bones, which have been believed, from their general appearance, to be fibrous, yet have pursued a malignant course. I will only add that these are not such growths as those which Muller and others have named Carcinoma fibrosum, and of which, I believe, that they are always infiltrations in the substance of the affected organs, that they generally include cancer-cells with their fibrous tissue, and that they have in this tissue such hardness, stiffness, and other peculiarities of structure, as make it easily distinguishable from the normal fibrous tissue and its imitation in the fibrous tumors.

* It is in the Museum of St. Bartholomew's, Series xxxv. No. 51.

† Fig. 58, tissue of a malignant fibrous tumor of the scapula; described above. Magnified about 400 times.

‡ Mus. of St. Bartholomew's, Ser. xxxv. 52.

LECTURE XXVI.

RECURRING FIBROID AND FIBRO-NUCLEATED TUMORS.

THE two groups of tumors, of which I propose to speak in this lecture, have perhaps no near affinity to the fibrous tumors last described; yet they resemble them in general aspect; they have, till within the last few years, been confounded with them; and their component structures resemble those that are rudimental of the fibrous tissue. There will, therefore, be some practical advantage in making the real contrast between them appear, by proximity, more striking.

I have proposed the name "RECURRING FIBROID TUMOR" for a group of which the chief characteristics are that their general aspect very closely resembles that of the common fibrous tumors; their microscopic structure consists of corpuscles caudate and elongated, as if developing into fibres; and the most striking feature in their history is their proneness to return after removal.

A brief account of some cases of this tumor may best illustrate it.

The first I saw was from a gentleman, 60 years old, under the care of Mr. Stanley. In 1846, a tumor was removed by Mr. Cockle from the upper and outer part of his leg. It lay close to the tibia, was as large as a filbert, and was considered fibrous. Some months afterwards another tumor was found in the same place, and, when as large as a walnut, was removed by Mr. Hamilton, of the London Hospital, who considered it "decidedly fibrous." In October, 1847, Mr. Stanley removed from the same place a third tumor; and this I examined minutely. It had the shape, and nearly the size, of a patella; and the note that I made of its general appearance was, that it was "very like those fibrous tumors which are whitest, most homogeneous, and least fasciculate and glistening;" and that "without the microscope I should certainly have called it a fibrous tumor."

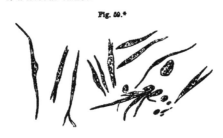

Fig. 59.*

The microscopic examination, however, showed peculiar structures (fig. 59). The tumor was composed almost entirely of very narrow, elongated, caudate, and oat-shaped nucleated cells, many of which had long and subdivided terminal processes. Their contents were dimly shaded; and in many instances the nuclei appeared to swell out the body of the cell, as in the most

* Fig. 59, microscopic elements of a recurring fibroid tumor, described above. Magnified about 400 times.

elongated granulation-cells. With these cells were scattered free nuclei, and grumous or granular matter, such as might have been derived from disintegrated cells. Very little filamentous tissue was contained in any part of the tumor.

Now, in the extirpation of the third tumor, the parts around it were very freely removed, the periostium was scraped from the tibia, and every assurance seemed to exist that the whole disease was cleared away. But, in June, 1848, two small tumors appeared in the subcutaneous tissue, just below the seats of the former operations. These also were removed, and these had the same fibrous appearance, and the same minute texture, as the preceding. Some months only elapsed before in the same place another tumor grew; *i. e.* a sixth tumor. The patient, despairing of remedy by operations, allowed this to grow till November, 1850, by which time it had acquired the diameter of between four and five inches, and protruded as a large soft fungoid mass from the front of the leg. Two profuse hemorrhages occurred from it, and made him earnestly beg that his limb might be removed to relieve him from the extreme misery of his disease. The amputation was performed, and he died in a few days.

The tumor* appeared confused with the thin skin over it. It rested below on the muscles of the leg, but was not mixed with them except at a scar from the former operations. The tumor was milk-white, soft, and brain-like, except where discolored by effused blood, and in the exposed parts was soft, pulpy, and grumous. One would certainly, judging by its general aspect, have called this a brain-like medullary cancer; and yet it had essentially the same microscopic characters as the tumors I first examined from the same patient: only, the narrow, elongated, caudate cells were very generally filled with minute shining molecules, as if from fatty degeneration connected with the protrusion and partial sloughing of the mass. Unfortunately no examination of the body was made after death, and it could only be guessed, from the absence of emaciation, and of all other indication of general loss of health, that no similar disease existed in internal organs.

In another case of the same kind, I assisted Mr. Stanley, in May, 1848, in the removal of a tumor from the shoulder of a gentleman 28 years old. It had been growing under the deltoid for six months, was loosely connected with the surrounding parts, and was about three inches in diameter. It had the general aspect of a common fibrous tumor: firm, tough, white, traversed with irregular bands. It was easily and completely removed, but was not examined with the microscope. The wound of the operation healed well; but, two months afterwards, a second tumor appeared under the cicatrix. This was removed with some of the adjacent muscles, and other tissues. It was like the first, only less tough, and more lobed, and elastic; but under the microscope, instead of appearing fibrous, it was found to be composed almost entirely of elongated

* In the Museum of St. Bartholomew's.

and caudate nucleated cells, very like those described in the last case, and mixed with free nuclei, and granular matter.

In March, 1849, a third tumor was removed from the same part, which had been noticed two months, and again presented the same character; it was indeed grayer, and less firm, and more shining and succulent on its cut surfaces, but the differences to the naked eye were not great, and the microscopic structure was the very same as in the former instances.

In October, 1849, another tumor had formed, and after it had resisted various methods of treatment, Mr. Stanley removed it, by a fourth operation, in December. This had again the same character.

In the course of 1850, a fifth tumor appeared in the same part, and this, after growing slowly for an uncertain time ceased to increase, and has now been for a long time stationary, without in any way interfering with the patient's health. He is pursuing an active occupation, and, but for the tumor, might be thought a healthy man.

In a third case Mr. Syme removed, in 1839, a tumor which, without any known cause, had been growing for a year, over the anterior part of the first right rib of a gentleman 48 years old. Two years after the operation another tumor appeared in or near the same part, and was removed, by Mr. Syme, in 1848. A third was removed by him in 1847; and a fourth in 1849. After another distinct interval of apparent health, a fifth tumor appeared and grew quickly, and was removed by the same gentleman in 1851. In one of these, an account of which was published by Mr. Syme, Dr. Hughes Bennett found microscopic structures similar to those of the fibro-plastic tumors of Lebert;* similar, therefore, I have no doubt, to those described above. The patient recovered from the last operation, as from all the previous ones, quickly and favorably; but the wound had scarcely healed when two more tumors appeared beneath the scar, like the preceding ones, except in that they grew more rapidly.

One of these tumors was so firmly fixed at the clavicle that no further operation could be recommended. In six months' growth the tumors, at first distinct, had formed a single mass, deeply lobed, of oval form, measuring a foot in one direction and about ten inches in the other. It covered, and felt as if tightly fixed to, the middle half of the clavicle, and thence extended downwards over the chest, and outwards towards the axilla. It felt heavy, firm, tense, and elastic. The skin thinly stretched over it, and by its tension appearing as if adherent, was generally florid, but in some parts livid, and over the most prominent lobes ulcerated; but the principal ulcers were superficial, covered with healthy-looking granulations, discharging thick pus, having no cancerous or other specific character: only one of them had a thin slough. Such were the characters of the disease when I saw it in Feb-

* Monthly Journal of Medical Science, vol. x., p. 194   Probably this refers to the elongated cells alone. I have not, in any of these tumors, found the large many-nucleated cells which occur in most of the tumors named fibro-plastic by M. Lebert.

ruary, 1852; and it was very striking, as evincing one of the contrasts between this form of tumor and any rapidly-growing ulcerated cancer, that the patient's general health was scarcely affected. He was still a florid sturdy man; and fed, slept, talked, and moved about as a man in health might do. He suffered scarcely any pain; but, within the last month, the ulcerated surface of the tumor had bled severely. The tumor was now submitted to compression, with Dr. Neil Arnott's apparatus; and with some advantage, insomuch as its growth was retarded, and the hemorrhage was prevented, so long as the pressure was maintained. Twice, however, on the instant of removing the apparatus, I saw arteries, as large as the radial, throw blood in a jet far from the trunk. The bleeding was in this respect such as I have never seen from the proper vessels of any other tumor, and was like that described as occurring in the first of these cases.

It would be useless to tell, at any length, the later history of this case. The tumor increased constantly to the time of the patient's death in July, 1852; but, in the last two months, several small portions of it sloughed away, and it gradually shifted lower down to the chest, leaving the clavicular region, so that at the time of death it lay movable on the muscles, and could be removed, "as a common fatty tumor might be," without dividing any important part: death seemed due to mere exhaustion, consequent on the discharge from the tumor, and the pain to which, as it extended further into the axilla, it gave rise. Dr. Ross, to whom I am indebted for an account of the conclusion of the case, could find no indication of disease in any internal organ. Only the tumor was allowed to be examined after death; and Dr. Ross wrote to me of it, in addition to the account of the absence of any deep connection or infiltration of adjacent tissues, that "its texture was pretty hard, like that of a fibrous tumor, but not nearly so dense or crisp as scirrhus. It scarcely gave out any blood on being cut into; but here and there was to be seen, on the surface of a section, the open mouth of a vessel, just as in a section of liver. All the textures behind, forming the bed of the tumor, appeared quite healthy."

A portion of the tumor, kindly sent to me by Dr. Ross, was, after having lain in spirit, milk-white, firm, elastic, of very close texture, breaking and tearing with a coarse fibrous grain. It had, most nearly, the aspect of a very firm fibro-cellular tumor altered by spirit. When scraped it yielded little or no fluid, but white shreds, in which, together with much that looked like withered tissue or débris, there were abundant slender awn-shaped corpuscles, such as are sketched in fig. 60. They looked dry and shriveled, containing no distinct nuclei, but minute shining particles, as if themselves were outgrown nuclei. With these, also, were numerous broader and shorter corpuscles, of the same general aspect, but enclosing oval nuclei; and yet more numerous smaller bodies, like shrivelled, oval, elongated, free nuclei, dotted, and containing minute shining particles. The whole mass appeared made up of corpuscles of these various shapes, irregularly or lineally imbedded in a substance that

Fig. 60.*

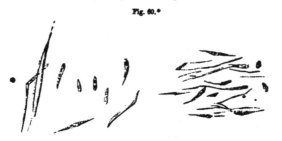

was nearly structureless or imperfectly fibrillated. Only in a few places, perhaps in the partitions of the lobes, there was a very small quantity of fine fibro-cellular tissue.

I think there can be no doubt that this case was essentially of the same kind as the former two; and the constancy of their peculiarities in both history and structure appears sufficient to justify the placing them in a separate group and under a separate title. But these are not the only cases to be cited.

Professor Gluge has given a good general account of the history of such tumors as these, as examples of the forms transitional to cancer. He names them "albuminous sarcoma;" a term one hears frequently used, without, perhaps, any clear meaning; yet, generally, I think, with the suspicion that the growths to which it is applied are not wholly innocent. Among the cases which he cites, one coincides exactly with those I have detailed. A major, 45 years old, fell from his horse in 1843. Six or seven weeks afterwards, a tumor appeared on his scapula. It was removed, but after some months returned. Between 1843 and 1848, four such tumors were removed from the same part. In 1848, the patient was under the care of M. Seutin, who removed the fifth tumor; and Gluge's description of this, including the expression that in color and consistence it was like the muscular tissue of the intestinal canal, leaves little doubt that it was like the less firm of the specimens that I have been describing. In the last of these five operations, and in one previously, the removal of the tumor was followed by free cauterization of the wound; yet the last account published by Professor Gluge was, that in April, 1849, a sixth tumor had appeared in the same part; and he has informed me by letter that in 1850 the patient died.

Lastly, a case which, in its conclusion, is the most instructive of all that have been recorded, is related by Dr. Douglas Maclagan.†

A girl, 22 years old, had a tumor, of three years' growth, on the left

---

* Fig. 60, microscopic structures of the recurring fibroid tumor, described above. Magnified 450 times.

† Edinburgh Medical and Surgical Journal, vol. xlviii.

lumbar region, about an inch from the spine. In 1832, it was about as large as a Jargonelle pear, firm, but elastic and movable, and below it was a portion of indurated skin. The tumor and diseased skin were removed, and the former "possessed most of the characters of a simple fibrous tumor." After about twelve months the disease returned in the scar. Three little tumors formed, and these, with the scar, were removed freely, in February, 1834. "The extirpated mass bore a striking resemblance to that previously removed." Between twelve and eighteen months later, a third growth appeared, which, after increasing for a year and a half, was removed. "It had the same elastic feel and fibrous appearance; and the semi-transparent pinkish-gray color was the same as in the original tumor." After this operation no fresh growth ensued; and Dr. Maclagan informed me, in 1850, that the patient remained perfectly well. The portraits of the several tumors, which he very kindly sent me, made me sure that the disease was, in this case, the same as in those I have before detailed.

Dr. Maclagan has added the account of another case in which the essential features were quite similar; and another, which I believe must be referred to this group, is accurately described and figured by Dr. Hughes Bennett.*

These cases will suffice to prove the existence of a group of tumors having these remarkable characters in common :—1st. A general resemblance to the fibrous tumours in their obvious characters; 2d. A microscopic texture composed, essentially, of elongated and caudate or oatshaped cells, somewhat resembling the elongated cells of granulations or of lymph developing into fibres, yet differing from them enough to be easily distinguished; 3d. An exceeding tendency to local recurrence after removal, and, in the worst extremity, to protrusion and ulceration; 4th. An absence of those events which, in cases of ordinary malignant growths, would coincide with local recurrence: such as cachexia, independent of profuse suppuration, pain, and other ordinary causes of exhaustion; and the absence of all affection of distant parts, or of the lymphatics. 5th. Occasionally, a cessation of the tendency to recurrence, and a complete recovery.

How may we interpret this singular proneness to recur; this tendency which by its existence separates these to some distance from all innocent tumors, and by its existing alone separates them as far from the malignant tumors ?

Two views may be taken of the fact.† The tumors may, from the first, be formed in a cluster or group, and then the removal of one of

* On Cancerous and Cancroid Growths, p. 87.

† Some would add a third, supposing that in all these cases portions of the tumor were left behind in the operations. But this is unreasonable. These tumors are not more difficult to remove wholly than many are which never thus recur, such as the fatty, fibro-cellular, and the like. Besides, in the cases I have cited, the names of the operators are a sufficient guarantee that the whole tumor was every time removed.

27

them only leaves the remainder to continue their growth; or, 2dly, the apparent recurrence may be a real one, such as we suppose occurs in the case of cancers; in which we presume that, in a first operation, every morbid structure already formed in a part is removed, and entirely new growths are produced in the same part.

The former view is supported by whatever of resemblance exists between these and fibrous tumors, whose proneness to multiplicity is remarkable; and by the fact that sometimes, after the removal of one of these, two, or a more numerous group, have appeared in the same part. Yet the objections to this view appear to me more weighty. If we suppose, in any case in which six or seven tumors have been removed in succession from the same part, in as many years, that all began to grow at or about the same time, the last of these ought, according to the rate of growth of the rest, to have come into view much sooner. If the second tumor were not discernible in the first operation, where, or of what size, was the sixth? or why did this sixth require many years to attain the same bulk as the supposed coeval second tumor acquired in one year? It may be added that some of these fibroid tumors appear to have recurred in the substance of a scar left after a former operation; in a tissue, therefore, which did not exist at the time of the previous operations.

We must not overlook, in connection with this apparent aptness to recur, the fact that the later-formed of these tumors may assume more of the characters of thoroughly malignant growths than were observed in the earlier. In the first case I have related, the last tumor was, in general aspect, hardly to be distinguished from brain-like tumor, though, in microscopic characters, essentially like its predecessors. In one of Professor Gluge's cases, the transitions to completely malignant characters appeared yet more sure. Mr. Syme also expresses a similar transition; describing, as the usual course of the cases he has seen, that, after one or two recurrences of the tumor, the next new productions present a degeneration of character, excite pain, proceed to fungous ulceration, and thus in the end prove fatal. And in all cases, unless recovery ensue, the successive tumors increase in rate of growth. So that, although there be cases in which this evil career has not been run, yet I think we may regard these tumors as approximating to characters of malignancy, not only in their proneness to recur after removal, but in their aptness to assume more malignant features the more often they recur. Whatever be the truth concerning the supposed transformation of an innocent into a malignant morbid growth, I think it can hardly be doubted that, in the cases of some recurring growths, such as these, and certain recurring proliferous cysts, the successively later growths acquire more and more of the characters of thoroughly malignant disease.*

---

* See a reference to the same point at p. 364. An illustration is presented by a remarkable case, of which specimens are described in the Catalogue of the Museum of St. Bartholomew's, Ser. xxxv. Nos. 28, 29.

FIBRO-NUCLEATED TUMORS.

Dr. Hughes Bennett* has given the name of *Fibro-nucleated* to certain tumors first described by himself, of which I think that future investigations will prove a very near affinity with those which I have been considering. They are, indeed, of so rare occurrence, that we cannot as yet be sure of many things concerning them; but their most usual characters seem to be, as assigned by Dr. Bennett, a general resemblance to the fibrous tumors; a tendency to return in the part from which one has been excised; an absence of disposition to affect lympathics or more distant parts; and a texture "consisting of filaments infiltrated with oval nuclei." The first three characters are repetitions of those belonging to the recurring fibroid tumors; the last is not so; and yet the difference of structure is such as may consist with a very near natural relationship. For, as we have seen, both cells tending to elongate and attenuate themselves into filaments, and nuclei imbedded in a simple or filamentous blastema, are equally forms through which fibro-cellular or fibrous tissue may be devoloped (see p. 889, &c.). And thus it may be that, in these two groups of tumors, the similarly contrasted forms of elemental structure may be nearly related, in that both alike represent persistently imperfect developments of fibrous masses.

However this may be, the history of these cases is important, especially because, like the last described, they seem to occupy a kind of middle ground between innocent and malignant tumors. They are among the diseases which are often spoken of as "semi-malignant," "locally malignant," or "less malignant than cancer:" terms which are generally used in relation to what are deemed exceptional cases, but which may appear to have a real meaning if ever we can apply them to well-defined groups of tumors.

The most characteristic of the cases described by Dr. Hughes Bennett was that of a lady 25 years old, from whom, when she was 18, a tumor of four years' growth was removed from the left thigh, nearly in front of the great trochanter. After its removal there remained a small hard knot in the scar; but no change ensued in this for six years. Then it began to enlarge and increase, and in a year increased to the size of a small almond-nut. It was superficial, quite movable, and intimately adherent to the skin. It was hard and dense; and its cut surface was smooth, slightly yellowish, and yielded no juice on pressure. It appeared to consist of fine filaments, among which oval bodies, like nuclei with nucleoli, were everywhere infiltrated. Here and there large oval rings appeared, marked by converging irregular lines, and, in a few places, oval spaces, surrounded with concentric marks, like sections of gland-ducts.

The only well-marked case that I have yet seen was that of a boy, 10 years old, on the palmar aspect of whose forearm a small indentation

* On Cancerous and Cancroid Growths, p. 176, &c.

was noticed at birth. This part was slightly wounded when he was two years old, and from that time a tumor began to grow. When he was four, the tumor was removed (of course completely) by Mr. Sands Cox, but the wound did not heal before another growth appeared. This increased at first slowly, but at last quickly; and when the boy came under my care, it formed an oval swelling, rising to nearly an inch and a half above the surrounding skin, and measuring from three to three and a half inches in its diameters. The skin over it was very thin, adherent, tense, and florid, and at the centre ulcerated, and superficially scabbed; the ulcerated surface was granulated, like one slowly healing. The mass felt firm and elastic, and, at its borders, very tough, like the tissue of a cicatrix; little cord-like branching processes extended from its borders outwards in the deeper substance of the cutis; and above the principal mass another, like a small flattened induration of the skin, was felt. The growth was not painful, and the general health appeared good. Some axillary glands were slightly enlarged.

I removed the whole disease, with all the surrounding skin that appeared in any way unhealthy, and large portions of the fascia of the forearm and of the intermusclar scepta, to which the base of the growth adhered intimately, and which were indurated and thickened. The wound very slowly healed; the enlargement of the axillary glands subsided; and I have heard from Mr. Oliver Pemberton, under whose care the recovery ensued, that the patient remained quite well fifteen months after the operation.

The tumor was intitimately adherent to all the parts adjacent to it, yet was distinct and separable from them. Its section was smooth and shining, of stone-gray color, shaded with yellowish tints. It was lobed; but in its several lobes was uniform, and with no appearance of fibrous or other structure; but intersected irregularly by white and buff-yellow branching lines, where the microscope found a fatty degeneration of the tissue. In texture the tumor was firm, but easily breaking and splitting in layers, shell-like: with the microscope it appeared to be composed of two materials; namely, nuclei, and a sparing granular or molecular substance in which they were imbedded. These, as sketched in fig. 60, were so like those represented by Dr. Bennett, as to leave little doubt of the similarity of the two cases; only there was here less appearance of fibrous structure, and less of a texture like that of glands.

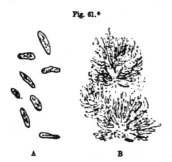

Fig. 61.*

A   B

* Fig. 61, A, nuclei; B, nucleated structure of the tumor described above. A, magnified 450 times; B, about 250 times.

the nuclei were, generally, of regular elongated oval shape, from $\frac{1}{1500}$ to $\frac{1}{1100}$ of an inch in length, and generally bi-nucleolated; comparatively few were broader, or reniform, or irregular. They were very thick-set in a molecular basis-substance, and in many parts (perhaps in all that were not disturbed) they appeared as if arranged in overlying double or triple rows, which radiated to a distance from some point, or from some space of round or elongated oval form. These spaces, if they were such, appeared full of molecular matter.

It would be wrong to endeavor to draw many conclusions from so small experience as yet exists on these tumors. I will only express or repeat my belief (which fully concurs with what Dr. Bennett has stated) that these are examples of a form of tumor different from any others yet classified; and that they will be found most nearly related to the recurring fibroid tumors.

LECTURE XXVII.

CARTILAGINOUS TUMORS.

THE name of Cartilaginous Tumors may be given to those which Müller, in one of the most elaborate portions of his work on Cancer, has named Enchondroma.* Either term will sufficiently imply that the growth is formed, mainly, of a tissue like cartilage; and I would at once point out the singularity of such tumors being formed, and growing to so great a size as I shall have to describe, although cartilage is not commonly formed for the repair of its own injuries, nor, at least in man, in a perfect manner, for the repair of the injuries of bone.

The cartilaginous tumors are found, in the large majority of cases, connected with the bones and joints.† However, they occur not rarely in soft parts, completely detached from bone. Thus, in the pure form, or mixed with other tissues, they are met with in the testicle,‡ mammary

---

* Other names employed are Osteo-chondroma, Chondroma, Benign Osteo-sarcoma. The term osteo-sarcoma cannot be too entirely disused; it has been more vague than even Sarcoma, having been employed indiscriminately for all tumors, of whatever nature, growing in or upon bones, provided only they were not entirely osseous.

† Those referred to as connected with the joints are the cartilaginous masses that are found pendulous or loose in joints. They have sufficient characters in common with these tumors to justify their enumeration in the list; yet they are in so many respects peculiar, that they need and usually receive a separate history. The best account of them, and of their probable origin in the villi of synovial fringes, may be gathered from Bidder, in Henle and Pfeufer's Zeitschr. B. iii.; Rainey, in Proc. Pathol. Soc. ii. p. 140; and Kölliker, Mikrosk. Anat. ii. p. 324.

‡ Mus. Coll. Surg., Nos. 2384-5-6, &c.; Mus. St. Bartholomew's Hosp. Ser. xxviii., No. 17, and Appendix; and several in the Museum of St. Thomas's Hospital. See also Mr. Gamjee's pamphlet, on a Case of Ossifying Enchondroma in the Testicle of a Horse.

gland,[*] subcutaneous tissue,[†] and lungs,[‡] and in the soft parts near bones; but among all the soft parts their favorite seat appears to be the neighborhood of the parotid gland. The greater part of the solid tumors formed in this part have cartilage in them.

Cartilaginous tumors that are connected with bones may, like fibrous tumors (p. 407, fig. 57), occur in two distinct positions; namely, within the walls, or between the walls and the periosteum: rarely they grow in both these positions at once. When they are within the bones, they are isolated and discontinuous, and are surrounded by the bone-walls, which may be extended in a thin shell or capsule around them, or may be wasted and perforated by them. When they grow outside the bones, they are generally fastened to the subjacent bone-wall by outgrowths of new bone; the periosteum, greatly overgrown, invests them, and prolongations from it towards the bone appear to intersect them, and divide them into lobes. When they grow among soft parts, they have a well-formed fibro-cellular or tougher fibrous capsule, which is commonly more dry and glistening than that of most innocent tumors.

In any of these situations, cartilaginous tumors may be either simple or complex, conglobate or conglomerate, if we may adopt such terms; i. e., they may be composed of a single mass without visible partitions, or, of numerous masses or knots clustered, and held together by their several investments of fibro-cellular tissue. According to these conditions they present a less or more knotted or knobbed surface; but in either state they affect the broadly oval or spheroidal shape (fig. 71).

To the touch, cartilaginous tumors may be very firm or hard, especially when they are not nodular and their bases are ossified. In other cases, though firm, they are compressible, and extremely elastic, feeling like thick-walled, tensely-filled sacs. Many a solid cartilaginous tumor has been punctured in the expectation that it would prove to be a cyst.

The knife cuts them crisply and smoothly; and their cut surfaces present, in the best examples, the characters of fœtal cartilage; bright, translucent, grayish, or bluish, or pinkish white, compact, uniform. Usually, each separate mass or lobe is without appearance of fibrous or other compound structure; but, sometimes, the cartilage looks coarsely granular, as if it were made up of clustered granules. This is, I think, especially the case in the cartilaginous tumors inclosed in the bones of the hands and fingers; especially in such of them as are soft. In other cases, when the cartilage is very firm, it may be opaque or milk-white.

In different examples of cartilaginous tumor there are great varieties of consistence or firmness. Some appear almost diffluent, or like vitreous humor; some are like the firmest fœtal cartilage; and all intermediate gradations may be found: but, with the exception of the cartilaginous

* Astley Cooper, Diseases of the Breast, p. 64; Müller, On Cancer, p. 149, No. 13, from a dog; Mus. St. Bartholomew's, Ser. xxxiv., No. 13, from a bitch.

† Rokitansky, Pathol. Anat., B. i. p. 261; Lebert, Abhandlungen, p. 195.

‡ Mus. St. Bartholomew's, Pathol. Appendix; Rokitansky and Lebert, l. c.

growths that are pendulous or loose in joints, I have never seen any present such hardness, dullness, or yellowness, as do the natural adult cartilages of the joints, ribs, or larynx.

As, in all general appearance, the material of these tumors, in its usual and most normal conditions, is identical with fœtal cartilage, so is it, I believe, in its development, and, as Müller has shown, in its chemical characters.* The microscopic characters, also, of cartilaginous tumors agree, speaking generally, with those of fœtal cartilage; yet there are several particulars to be observed concerning them, and, especially, the diversity of form and arrangement, that may be seen in the microscopic constituents of even different parts of the same tumor, needs mention.

This diversity of microscopic forms is enough to baffle any attempt to describe them briefly, or to associate them with any corresponding external characters in the tumors. The most diverse forms may even be seen side by side in the field of the microscope. But this diversity is important. It has its parallel, so far as I know, in no other innocent tumor; and the cartilaginous tumors form perhaps the single exception to a very generally true rule enunciated by Bruch;[†] namely, that it is a characteristic of the cancerous tumors, and a distinction between them and others, that they present, even in one part, a multiformity of elementary shapes.

The diversity of microscopic characters extends to every constituent structure of the cartilage in the tumors. I will state the general and chief results of the examinations of fifteen of the recent specimens,[‡] of which I have made notes, and the drawings from which the annexed figures were copied.

(1) In regard, then, to the basis or intercellular substance:—It is

Fig. 62.[§]   Fig. 63.[‖]

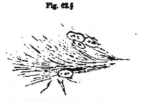 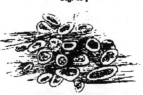

variable in quantity, the cells or nuclei in some specimens lying wide apart (fig. 62), in some closely crowded (fig. 63, &c.): it varies in

* The enchondromata of bones, he says, always yield chondrine; while those of soft parts may yield either gelatine or chondrine (On Cancer, p. 124). The whole account of their analysis is very amply given by him.

† Die Diagnose der bösartige Geschwülste.

‡ These are exclusive of specimens of loose cartilages in joints; of which, indeed, no account will be given in this lecture.

§ Fig. 62. Tufted, pale, filamentous tissue, with a few imbedded cartilage cells. From a tumor over the parotid gland.

‖ Fig. 63. Stronger and denser fibro-cartilaginous tissue; many of the cartilaginous cells having granulated nuclei. From a tumor over the parotid gland, magnified 400 times.

consistence) with all the gradations to which I have already referred: and in texture,—in some specimens, it is pellucid, hyaline, scarcely visible; in some, dim, like glass breathed on; in many more, it is fibrous in texture or in appearance (fig. 62, 63). Most cartilaginous tumors, indeed, might deserve to be called fibro-cartilaginous. It is seldom, and, I think, only in the firmest parts or specimens, that the substance between the cartilage-cells has the strong hard-lined fibrous texture which belongs to the chief natural fibrous cartilages; yet it has generally a fibrous texture. The fibres are, or appear, usually soft, nearly pellucid, and very delicate: sometimes they appear tufted or fasciculate (fig. 62); sometimes they encircle spaces that contain each a large cartilage-cell, or a cluster of cells or nuclei (fig. 64); sometimes they form a fascicu-

Fig. 64.*

Fig. 65.†

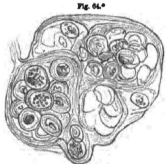

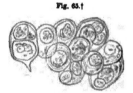

lated tissue in which cartilage-cells lie elongated and imbedded (fig. 63); most commonly of all, I think, they curve among the cells, as if they were derived from a fibrous transformation of an intercellular hyaline substance (fig. 66).

(2) Yet greater varieties may be found in the characters of the cartilage-cells.‡ In plan of arrangement they may be irregularly and widely scattered, or closely placed, or almost regularly clustered with fibrous tissue encircling them (fig. 62, 64, 65). In single cells there are varieties of size from $\frac{1}{710}$th to $\frac{1}{1180}$th of an inch. And there are yet more varieties of shape; some have the typical form of healthy preparatory cartilage-cells, being large, round, or oval, or variously shaped through mutual pressure, faintly outlined, with single nuclei, and clear contents (fig. 66); and some are like normal compound cartilage-cells (fig. 65).

---

* Fig. 64. Groups of cartilage-cells, clustered in a portion of a tumor on the phalanx of a finger. Many of the cells are only drawn in outline; the groups are intersected by bands of tough, fibrous tissue; some of the cells present double or triple contour lines; most of the nuclei are large and granular. Magnified about 400 times.

† Fig. 65. A group of large cartilage-cells from the same; many containing two or three nuclei, of which some have acquired the character of enclosed cells.

‡ I retain this name, although the observations of Bergmann (De Cartilaginibus, 1850) and others show that it is difficult, in some cases, to determine the nature of the cell-contents, and that their nuclei may be more like cells, or, having had the characters and relations of nuclei, may acquire those of included nucleated-cells. Taking, as the type of cartilage-cells, the elements of the chorda dorsalis, I think we shall least often err if we keep the term cell for those elementary structures in other cartilages which are most like the cells of the chorda in their fine clear outline, and the pellucid or dim space just within, or, also, just without it.

But, with various deviations from these more normal characters, some cells have hard dark outlines; and some are bounded by two, three, or

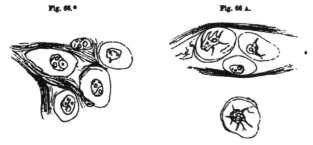

Fig. 66.*   Fig. 66 A.

four dotted or marked concentric circles, as if the cell-walls had become laminated (fig. 64, 65); others appear without any defined cell-walls, as if they were mere cavities hollowed out in the basis-substance; and, in other instances, the cell-walls and their contents, down to the nucleus, appear as if they were completely fused with the basis-substance, so that the nuclei alone appear to be imbedded

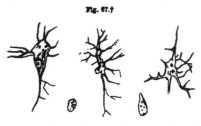

Fig. 67.†

in the hyaline or dimly fibrous material. These last two states appear to be connected with very imperfect development or with degeneration; for I have seen them, I think, in only soft cartilage, or in such as showed other distinct signs of degeneration. In many such cases, also, the nuclei are so loosely connected with the basis-substance, that large numbers of them float free in the field of the microscope.

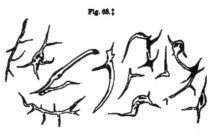

Fig. 68.‡

(3) The varieties of the nuclei in the cartilage of tumors are not less than those of the cells. Some are like those of the normal cartilage;

* Fig. 66. Group of cartilage-cells from a tumor in the tibia. Fine filamentous tissue encircles and intervenes between single cells. Some of the nuclei of the cells contain oil-particles; and some of the same (in fig. 66 A) show, apparently, the process of assuming the stellate or branched form. Magnified 400 times.

† Fig. 67. Free nuclei; some simple, and some enlarged, and variously set with branching processes. From a cartilaginous tumor under the angle of the lower jaw. Magnified 400 times.

‡ Fig. 68. Similar nuclei variously distorted and shriveled. From a mixed cartilaginous tumor over the parotid; similarly magnified.

round or oval, clear, distinctly outlined, with one or two nucleoli (fig. 65). But some appear wrinkled or collapsed, as if shriveled; some containing numerous minute oil-particles, representing all the stages to complete fatty degeneration, and the formation of granular bodies (fig. 63, 66); some are uniformly but palely granular, like large, pale corpuscles of lymph or blood; some are yet larger, nearly filling the cells, pellucid, like large, clear vesicles with one or more oil-particles enclosed; and some have irregularities of outline, which are the first in a series of gradational forms, at the other extremity of which are various stellate, branched, or spicate corpuscles (fig. 66 A, 67, 68).

I have not been able to discern any constant rule of coincidence between these forms of nuclei and the various forms of cells, nor between either and any of the enumerated appearances of the intercellular or basis-substance. All modes of combinations have appeared among them; only, on the whole, the completely developed cells have the best nuclei, and the degenerate or imperfect of both are usually in company.

The last-named nuclei, with irregular outlines, deserve a more particular description, both because they are, so far as I know, found in no normal cartilage in any of the vertebrata, and because their imitating, in some measure, the forms of bone-corpuscles, might wrongly suggest that they have a constant relation to the ossifying process.

They were first described, I think, by Müller; and have since been noticed in cartilaginous tumors by Mr. Quekett, and many others. I have examined them in seven cases; and, to show that they are not peculiar to one form of cartilaginous tumor, I may add that, of these seven, one was a great tumor encircling the upper part of the tibia, one a growth on the last phalanx of the great toe, one a mixed tumor in the anticular end of the fibula, one a very soft tumor in the subcutaneous tissue on the chest, and three were mixed tumors over the parotid or submaxillary gland.

The phases of the transformation by which they are produced appear to be, as represented in fig. 66 A–7–8, that a nucleus of ordinary form, or with one or more oil-particles, enlarges and extends itself in one or several slender, hollow, and crooked processes, which diverge, and sometimes branch as they diverge, towards the circumference of the cell. Such nuclei may be found within the cells (fig. 66 A), or within cavities representing cells whose walls are fused with the intercellular substance; but much more commonly it appears as if, while the nuclei changed their forms, the cells and the rest of their contents were completely fused with the intercellular or basis-substance, so that the nuclei alone appear imbedded in the hyaline or pale fibrous substance. The nuclei thus enlarged may appear like cells, and their nucleoli may be like nuclei. But although at first, as we may suppose, the nuclei, as they send out their processes, may enlarge and retain the round or oval form of their central parts or bodies, yet they afterwards lengthen and attenuate themselves, so as to imitate very closely the shapes of large bone-corpuscles or lacunæ; or they elongate and branch or shrivel up; and in these states, lying in groups, they have the most fantastic appearances (fig. 67, 68). In these various states the nuclei are often loosely connected with the basis-substance; so that they are easily removed from it, or are found floating on the field of the microscope, as nearly as those were which are here drawn.

Now, as I have said, corpuscles like these exist permanently in no normal cartilage yet examined, in man or any of the vertebrata.* If, then, heterology of structure were indicative of malignancy, the tumors that contain these corpuscles should be malignant; but there are no facts to make it probable that they are so; and every presumption is in favor of their being innocent.

As to the meaning of these changes of the nucleus;—they may be, as Mr. Quekett† has shown, preparatory to ossification, and the metamorphosis of the cartilage-nucleus into a bone-corpuscle or lacuna; but in many instances they are unconnected with ossification; for, in most of the cases in which I have found them, the tumor was in no part ossified, and in many of them it was not of a kind in which ossification was likely to ensue. In these cases we may believe the changes of the nuclei to be connected with a process of degeneration. There are many grounds for this; such as the fact, already mentioned, of their likeness to the nuclei of lower cartilages; their likeness in shape to ramified pigment-cells and bone-corpuscles, which have probably lost all power for their own nutrition; the frequent coincidence of more or less fatty degeneration in the nuclei thus changing; the usual conincidence of the fusion of the cell-wall and contents with the basis-substance of the cartilage, and the loosening of the nuclei; and the gradual shriveling or wasting of the nuclei after the assumption of the stellate form.

Such is the anatomy of cartilaginous tumors; and now, in relation to their physiology, several points may deserve notice.

Their rate of growth is singularly uncertain. They may increase very slowly. I have seen one not more than half an inch long, which had been at least four years in progress. Or, after a certain period of increase, they may become stationary; as often happens in the tumors that occur in large numbers on the hands. Or, from beginning to end, their growth may be very rapid. I remember a man, 26 years old, in St. Bartholomew's Hospital, in whom, within three months of his first noticing it, a cartilaginous tumor increased to such an extent that it appeared to occupy nearly the whole length of his thigh, and was as large round as

---

* The only natural cartilage yet known as possessing these corpuscles is, I believe, that of the cuttle-fish (Quekett, in Histol. Catal. of Coll. of Surg. Pl. vi. fig. 7); and it is at least interesting, and may be importantly suggestive, to observe that the morbid structure, deviating from what is natural in its own species, conforms with that of a much lower creature.

† Lectures on Histology, p, 166.

my chest.   He had a pale, unhealthy aspect, and suffered much from the growth; and its size and rapid growth, the tension nearly to ulceration of the skin over it, the enlarged veins, and loss of health, made all suppose it was a great cancerous tumor.   Mr. Vincent, therefore, decided against amputation of the limb, and the patient died exhausted, within six months of the first appearance of the disease.   The examination after death proved that a great cartilaginous tumor, with no appearance of cancerous disease had grown within and around the middle two-thirds of the femur.   The bone, after extension by the growth within it, had been broken, and all the central part of the tumor was soft, nearly liquid, and mixed with fluid blood and decolorised blood-clots.

In another case, under Mr. Lloyd's care, a cartilaginous tumor, surrounding the upper two-thirds of a girl's tibia, grew to a circumference of two feet in about 18 months.   Gluge* also mentions a case in which, in a boy 14 years old, a cartilaginous tumor on a tibia grew in $8\frac{1}{2}$ months to the size of a child's head, and protruded, and caused such pain and hectic, that amputation was necessary.

I need only refer to the importance of these cases in their bearing on the diagnosis of tumors, and as exceptions to the general rule that the malignant grow more rapidly than the innocent.

In extent of growth, the cartilaginous tumors scarcely fall short of the fibrous.   Mr. Frogley† has related two cases of tumors of enormous size. In one, the patient was a young woman 28 years old, and the tumor, of nearly five years' growth, around the shaft of the femur, extended from the knee-joint to within an inch of the trochanters, and measured nearly three feet in circumference.   It was a pure cartilaginous tumor, but its whole central part was soft or liquid, and many of the nodules of which it was composed had the character of cysts, through such central softness as I shall presently have to describe.   The limb was removed near the hip-joint, and the patient has remained in good health for seventeen years since.‡

In the other case by Mr. Frogley, the patient was a lady 37 years old, and the tumor had been growing eleven years; it was $20\frac{1}{2}$ inches in circumference, and exactly resembled that in the former case.   The amputation of the limb was equally successful.

The tumor in Mr. Lloyd's case, to which I have just referred, measured 24 inches in circumference.   But all these are surpassed by an instance related by Sir Philip Crampton, in which a tumor of this kind surrounding the femur, and soft in all its central parts, measured no less than $6\frac{1}{4}$ feet in circumference.

* Pathologische Anatomie, Lief. iv.
† Medico-Chirurgical Transactions, vol. xxvi.
‡ I have to thank Mr. Frogley for affording me this information, and Mr. Lane for an opportunity of exhibiting at the Lecture the remarkable specimen obtained by the operation, and now preserved in his Museum.

The only change of cartilaginous tumors which can be spoken of as a development, is their ossification: and this is, I believe, in all essential and minute characters, an imitation of the ossification of the natural cartilages.

But the more general or larger method of ossification must also be observed. Ossification may ensue, I suppose, in any cartilaginous tumor; but it is rare or imperfect in those that grow within bones, and is yet more imperfect, and is like the deposit of amorphous calcareous matter, in those that lie over the parotid gland. It is best seen in those that lie upon or surround the bones; and in these, two methods of ossification may be noticed.

In one method, the ossification begins at the surface of the bone, where the cartilaginous tumor rests on it, and thence the new-formed bone grows into the cartilage. Thus, the ossification may make progress far into the substance of the cartilage; and the tumor may appear like an outgrowth of bone covered with a layer or outer crust of cartilage, on which the perisoteum is applied. Or, extending yet further, the cartilage may by this method be wholly ossified, and the cartilaginous may be transformed into an osseous tumor.

In the other method of ossification, the new bone is formed in the mid-substance of the cartilage. In a large tumor the process may commence at many points, and, extending from each, the several portions of new bone may coalesce with one another, and with that formed in the first method, like an outgrowth from the surface of the original bone. Indeed, this twofold method of ossification is commonly seen in the large tumors that surround long bones.

The ossification ensuing in several points, and thence extending, is plainly, in these tumors, an imitation of the natural ossification of the skeleton from centres in each of its constituent parts. Sometimes, indeed, this natural process is imitated with singular exactness. Thus, in the College Museum, No. 207 is a portion of a large tumor which was taken from the front of the lumbar vertebræ of a soldier. Half of it is cartilaginous, and half is medullary cancer. The cartilaginous portion consists of numerous small nodules of

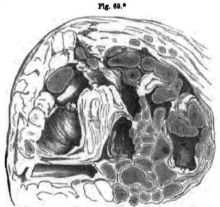

Fig. 69.*

* Fig. 69. Section of the cartilaginous and cancerous tumor described in the text: reduced one-half.

various shapes, each of which is invested with a layer of fibro-cellular tissue, as its perichondrium. In many of these, a single small portion of yellow cancellous bone appears in the very centre, each nodule ossifying from a single nucleus or centre, as orderly as each cartilage of the fœtal skeleton might ossify.

I shall speak in the next lecture of osseous tumors, and among them, of those that are formed by these methods. It may therefore suffice for the present, to say that, in nearly all cases, the bone formed in cartilaginous tumors consists of cancellous tissue, with marrow or medullary substance in its interspaces; and that when the ossification of the tumor is complete, the new cancellous tissue is usually invested with a thin compact layer or outer wall of bone, which, if the tumor have grown on a bone, becomes continuous with the compact tissue of that bone.

The principal defect or degeneration noticeable in cartilaginous tumors is manifested in their boing extremely soft, or even liquid; a clear, yellow, or light pink, jelly-like, or synovia-like material appearing in the place of cartilage. I call it a defect or degeneration, because it is not always certain whether it is the result of cartilage, once well formed, having become soft or liquid, or, whether the soft or liquid material be a blastema, which has failed of gaining the firmness and full organization of cartilage. It is quite probable that the same defective structure would be found in arrests of development as in degeneration; and the history of the cases agree herewith. The conditions in which extreme softness is sometimes found can leave little doubt, I think, that it is in these cases a degeneration,—a liquefaction of that which was once more perfectly nourished; but, in other cases, the softness of structure appears to have characterized the growths from their earliest formation; such, probably, was the case of which the history is told at p. 431; but in many cases we have no guide to the interpretation of the peculiarity.

The soft material of cartilaginous tumor is like melting, transparent, yellowish, or pale pinkish jelly; or like a gum-like substance, or like honey, or synovia, or serum. Such a material may occupy the whole interior of a cartilaginous tumor, one great cavity, filled with it, being found within a wall of solid substance.* Or the whole mass of a tumor,† or its exposed surface‡, may be thus soft or liquid. Often, too, we may trace, in individual nodules of a cartilaginous tumor, a process of what I suppose to be central softening, by which, perhaps, the formation of the great central cavities of the large tumors is best illustrated. Thus, in the tumor of cartilage and medullary cancer, of which I have already spoken, as illustrating the process of ossification from a centre in each

* As in Mr. Frogly's case; and as in many nodules of the tumors, No. 207 and others in the Museum of the College of Surgeons.

† See a drawing of one in the hand, and a specimen in Scr. 1, 115, in the Museum of St. Bartholomew's, and the specimen lately given to the Museum by Mr. Bickersteth, and described in page 432.   ‡ Mus. Col. Surg., No. 200.

nodule, there are many nodules, in the centre of which, instead of bone, small cavities full of fluid are seen. So, too, in a large cartilaginous tumor, growing on the pelvic bones of a man 40 years old, a portion of which was sent to me by Mr. Donald Dalrymple, I found a large number of distinct nodules, each with a central cavity full of honey-like fluid: and the state of the cartilage around these cavities, its softness, the fusion of its cell-walls and their contents with its hyaline basis, and the sparing distribution of nuclei in it, make me believe that the softness and liquefaction were the results of a degenerative process.

When the softening may be safely regarded as degenerative, it is still, often, very difficult to say to what the change is due. In some cases it appears connected with the great bulk of the tumor, and the hinderance to the sufficient penetration of blood to its central parts. Hence it is, I think, proportionally more frequent in the large than in the smaller tumors. In some cases, it may be due to exposure of the tumor, as in the instance of a cartilaginous tumor which grew from the sacro-iliac symphysis and adjacent bones, and projected into the vagina of a woman 34 years old.* But in many more cases we are unable to assign a reason for such softness.

The central softening of single nodules of cartilaginous tumors may extend to the formation of cysts; for when the whole of a nodule is liquefied, the fibro-cellular investment may remain like a cyst enclosing the liquid. This change was shown in the same tumor as illustrated the central ossification and the central softening. And it was not difficult to trace in it what appeared like gradations from central to complete liquefaction, and from a group of cartilaginous nodules to a group of cysts with tenacious fluid contents.

When extensively softened or liquefied, or when almost wholly transformed into cysts with viscid contents, the cartilaginous tumors are very like masses of colloid cancer:† so like, that the diagnosis, without the microscope, might be nearly impossible. Such a tumor was sent to me by Mr. E. Bickersteth. A woman, 45 years old, had two tumors, one on the eminence of the right frontal bone, the other half an inch below the right clavicle. The former was globular, as large as a walnut, and fixed to the bone. It felt soft and doughy, but at its base and around its margins it was hard. The latter was about twice as large, subcutaneous, and freely movable; it felt like a fatty tumor, except in that it was not distinctly lobed, and was less firm and consistent than such tumors usually are. Both tumors had been gradually increasing for eight years, and had been painless. The patient's mother had died with hard cancer of the breast.

The tumor below the clavicle was removed. It was an oval mass in-

* Mus. Coll. Surg., No. 206.

† I believe they have been often described as such. I think, too, that some of them are included by Vogel in his group of "gelatine-tumors" (Gallertgeschwülste), of which he says gelatiniform cancers are the most frequent form.

vested by a thin fibro-cellular capsule, partitions from which intersected
it, and divided it into lobes of unequal size, distinct, but closely packed.
They all consisted of a soft, flickering, yellow, and pale ruddy substance,
widely intersected with opaque-white lines. The substance was extremely
viscid, and could be drawn out in strings, sticking to one's fingers, like
tenacious gum. Its general aspect was very like that of a colloid cancer, but it had no alveolar or cystic structure, and it was an isolated
mass, not an infiltration. Portions lightly pressed (for it needed no dis-

Fig. 70.

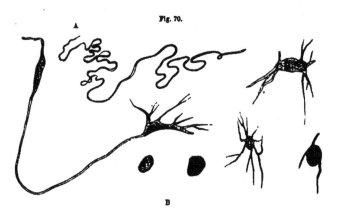

section for the microscope) showed as in the annexed figure (70), together
with a small quantity of common fibro-cellular tissue and fat, a peculiar
filamentous tissue in curving and interlacing bundles, and in separate,
very long and very tortuous, or curled filaments, or narrow flat bands
(A). The latter appeared as peculiar pale filaments, about $\frac{1}{13333}$ of an
inch in diameter ; in shape and mode of coiling resembling elastic fibres,
but not having dark edges, and extending to an extreme length. Such
fibres lay imbedded in a pellucid viscid substance, and more abundantly
scattered in the same were various corpuscles (B). Of these some were
simple, others of more complex forms. The former were, generally,
nearly round, dimly nebulous, with one or two shining particles, but
(unless in a very few instances), without nuclei. These seemed to be
free nuclei, of which many had grown to an unusual size, and measured
$\frac{1}{1000}$ of an inch in diameter. The more complex had the same texture
as these, and seemed to be also altered nuclei, and resembled most nearly
the stellate nuclei of more ordinary cartilaginous tumors. They generally had an oval, or round, or angular body or central part, from which
slender processes passed out. These followed various directions. Some
were short ; some branched once or more ; some were extremely long,
and appeared to connect adjacent corpuscles, or to be continued into
some of the tortuous bands or filaments, like which, as they extended

further, they became pale, clear, and finely edged. The chief and extreme forms are sketched, and many intermediate between these existed.

Since the operation the patient has remained well, and the tumor on the head has been stationary for four months; so that, thus far, the history has confirmed the only opinion I could form of so strange a tumor, namely, that it was composed of immature soft fibrous cartilage, not only arrested, but in a measure perverted in its development.

The softened central parts of cartilaginous masses are apt to be affected with rapid sloughing or suppuration. Such an event occurred in Sir Philip Crampton's case already quoted, and in one, presenting many features of great interest, which was under Mr. Lloyd's care, at Saint Bartholomew's Hospital.* A girl, 14 years old, was admitted with a very large tumor round the upper two-thirds of the tibia. It had been growing for 18 months, and shortly before her admission, without any evident cause (unless it were that it had been punctured), the integuments over it began to look inflamed and dusky. The limb was amputated almost immediately after her admission; and the tumor presented in its interior a large cavity with uneven broken walls, filled with brownish serous fluid of horribly offensive putrid odor. The inner surface of the walls of the cavity appeared also putrid, and gases, the products of the decomposition, were diffused in the cellular tissue as far as the middle of the thigh.

Other changes of a degenerative character may be sometimes observed in cartilaginous tumors. Parts of them may appear grumous, or pulpy, and of an ochre-yellow color.† This is probably a fatty degeneration of their tissue. And, sometimes, as I have said, their ossification is so imperfect as to be more like a fatty and calcareous degeneration, in which their substance becomes like fresh mortar, or soft chalk, and, when dry, is powdery, and white, and greasy.‡

It may serve for additional illustration of this general pathology of cartilaginous tumors if I describe now some particular forms of them.

I have said that they chiefly affect the bones. The bones of the hands are their most frequent seats; and next to these, the adjacent extremities of the femur and tibia, the parts which, for some inexplicable reason, appear to have in all the skeleton the least power of resistance of disease. After these, the humerus, the last phalanx of the great toe, the pelvis, and the ribs, appear most liable to cartilaginous growths; and after these, the number of cases is as yet too small to assign an order of frequency, but there is scarcely a bone on which they have not been seen.

* It is fully reported in the Lancet, Dec., 1850. The specimen is in the Museum of the Hospital.

† Mus. Coll. Surg., No. 200.

‡ Mus. Coll. Surg., No. 204. Rokitansky, B. i., p. 262. Mr. Humphry has particularly described this change in his Lectures, p. 143.

Of the cartilaginous tumors of the large long bones I need say little, having drawn from them the greater part of the general description. Only, the relations of the growths, according to the part of the bone in or near which they lie, may be worth notice.

When, then, the tumor grows at or about the articular end of a large long bone, it is almost wholly placed between the periosteum and the bone. Here it usually surrounds the bone, but not with a uniform thickness; and the thin wall of the bone wastes and gradually disappears as if it were eroded, or as if it changed its form, becoming cancellous, and then growing into the tumor. I have never seen such a tumor encroaching on the articular surface of a bone. But it may grow up all about the borders of the joint, and surround them. A striking

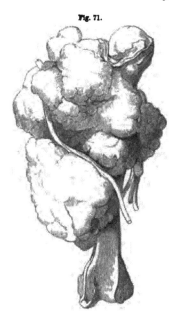

Fig. 71.

example of these relations of the cartilaginous tumor to the bone on which it grows is in one of the best and most characteristic specimens in the College Museum;[*] a cartilaginous tumor of the humerus, removed in an amputation at the shoulder-joint by Mr. Liston. His sketch of it is here copied. The patient was a naval surgeon, and the tumor had been growing for nearly forty years. The mass it now forms is nearly ten inches across; it surrounds the upper three-fourths of the shaft of the humerus, and nearly surmounts its articular surface; and it shows abundant isolated nodules, partial central ossification and central softening, and the growth of bone from the cancellous tissue of the humerus into the tumor. It shows, too, very well, how blood-vessels and nerves are imbedded in the inequalities of such tumors without being involved by them.

It is extremely rare, I think, for a cartilaginous tumor to grow within the articular end, or in the medullary tissue near it, in a large, long bone. A striking specimen, however, was presented by Mr. Langston Parker to Mr. Stanley. It was removed by amputation of the lower part of the leg, from a young gentleman in whom it had grown slowly, and had dis-

* Mus. Coll. Surg., 779. The patient recovered from the operation, but died two months afterwards with disease of the chest. The specimen is represented in Mr. Liston's Practical Surgery, p. 374, from which the sketch (fig. 71) is drawn.

tinctly pulsated. The lower end of the fibula is expanded and wasted by a growth of cartilage, mixed with a substance such as will be described in the next lecture, as the characteristic material of fibro-plastic or mye-loid tumors. The growth is rather larger than an egg, and is invested by the remains of the expanded fibula, and by the periosteum; and the relations of the chief blood-vessels make it probable that the pulsation felt during life was derived from that of the vessels within the tumor.*

When a cartilaginous tumor grows at the middle of the shaft of a large, long bone, it is, I think, usual to find coincidently both an external and an internal growth. Cartilage lies outside the shaft, beneath the peri-osteum; and another mass may fill the corresponding portion of the medullary canal. Then, in the concurrent growth of the two masses, the wall of the bone between them wastes or is broken up, and they may form one great tumor set between the portions of the shaft.† These are the cartilaginous tumors which most imitate the progress of malignant disease. They are indeed very rare; but the chance of the existence of such an one, where we might be anticipating a malignant tumor, is always to be added to the motives for amputation in cases of tumors round the shafts of these long bones.

When cartilaginous tumors grow at the attachment of tendons (and they often do so, especially about the lower part of the femur), they are peculiarly apt to acquire narrow bases of attachment. In these cases, one usually finds a layer of cartilage incrusting some cancellous and medullary bone, and the bone, as a narrow pedicle, extends into con-tinuity with the wall or the cancellous tissue of the subjacent shaft. Such tumors have then the characters of polypoid outgrowths from the bone, and may be treated accordingly; for, when cut or broken off, their stems (at least if they consist of only bone) will not grow. Indeed this stem may chance to be unwittingly broken; as in a tumor‡ removed by Mr. Lawrence. It had grown on the inner and lower part of the femur, and, when fairly exposed, was easily detached without further cutting: the narrowest part of its stem rested in a slight depression in the femur, but had no connection by tissue with it. It seemed as if the narrow pedicle of a tumor, two inches in diameter, had been by accident broken off, and the friction of the broken surfaces had smoothed and fitted them together.

* The specimen is in the Museum of St. Bartholomew's Hospital. No. 783 in the Mus. Coll. Surg. is an ossified cartilaginous tumor within the upper end of the fibula. In the Museum of St Thomas's Hospital is a most remarkable instance of cartilaginous tumors growing at once, in the scapula, the upper part of the humerus, and the lower part of the same. In the last-named part the cartilage lies within the thinned walls of the bone. The case is described by Mr. William Adams, in the Proc. of the Pathol. Soc., vol. ii.

† A specimen of this form is in the Museum of St. Bartholomew's in and upon a femur, in Ser. i. No. 111; and one of very large size, around and in the upper third of the femur, is in Guy's Hospital Museum. One also is mentioned by Mr. Hawkins as occurring in the middle of the shaft of the humerus (Medical Gazette, vol. xxv. p. 476).

‡ Mus. St. Bartholomew's, Ser. i. 183.

Such are some of the chief facts to be noted about the cartilaginous tumors on the large long bones.

On the jaws these tumors are, I believe, very rare. I know but one specimen on the upper jaw alone; a great tumor, portions of which are preserved in the Museum of Guy's Hospital, and of which the history, by Mr. Morgan, is in the Hospital Reports.

On the lower jaw, such tumors appear prone to acquire a peculiar shape, affecting the whole extent of the bone. One of the most remarkable tumors in the Museum of the College* is of this kind. The patient was a lady thirty-nine years old. The tumor had been growing eight years; it commenced as a small hard tumor just below the first right molar tooth, and gradually enlarged till it enclosed the whole jaw, except its right ascending portion. It measured two feet in circumference, and six inches in depth, and the patient died exhausted by want of food, which she was unable to swallow, and by the ulceration of parts of the tumor during the last two years of her life.

M. Lebert† has recorded a case in which a tumor like this was removed by Dieffenbach. In three successive operations he removed it by instalments, and the patient finally recovered.

The cartilaginous tumors that grow about the cranial bones and the vertebræ show, in a marked manner, that reckless mode of growth (if I may so speak) which is more generally a characteristic of malignant tumors. They grow in every direction; pressing, and displacing, and leading to the destruction of, important parts, and tracking their way along even narrow channels.

In St. Bartholomew's is a tumor,‡ composed for the most part, of cartilage, which grew in connection with the bones of the face and head of a lad sixteen years old. It involved both superior maxillary bones, extended into the left orbit, and through the left side of the base of the skull into its cavity, compressing the anterior lobes of the cerebrum; it was also united to the soft palate, and protruded the left nostril, and the integuments of the face.

The commencement of a similar growth is probably shown in a specimen in the College Museum,§ in which, together with changes effected by the growth of nasal polypi, one sees the ethmoid cells completely filled with firm semitransparent cartilage, a mass of which projects in a round tumor into the upper part of the left nasal fossa.

And here I may adduce, in proof of the tracking growth of the cartilaginous tumors, the case of one‖ originating in the heads of the ribs, which extended through the intervertebral foramina into the spinal canal, where, growing widely, and compressing the spinal cord,

---

* No. 1034 and 201. † Abhandlungen, p. 197.

‡ Mus. St. Bartholomew's Hospital. Ser. xxxv. No. 47. Drawn in Mr. Stanley's Illustrations of Diseases of the Bones, pl. xvii. fig. 4. § Mus. Coll. Surg. 2199.

‖ Mus. St. Bartholomew's Hospital, Ser. i. No. 115.

it produced complete paralysis of the pelvic organs and the lower extremities.

The cartilaginous tumors of the hands deserve a special notice.

As many, I believe, as forty cases might be collected from various records, in which the bones of one or both hands, and sometimes of the feet also, have been the seats of numerous cartilaginous tumors. Several of these cases were collected by John Bell;* many more by Müller,† who drew, indeed, from these cases the greater part of his general account of enchondroma; and many more might now be added to the list. Four admirable specimens of the disease are in the Museums of the College and of St. Bartholomew's.

The first of these,‡ from the collection of Sir Astley Cooper, consists of the amputated fingers and heads of the metacarpal bones of a girl 13½ years old. Tumors had been growing in these bones for eleven years; and now there are eleven or twelve, from half an inch to an inch and a half in diameter, and all formed of pure cartilage.

The second was presented to the Museum of St. Bartholomew's by Mr. Hodgson.§ It comprises the right hand, and the little finger of the left hand, of a lad 14 years old, in whom, without any known cause, the tumors had been growing from early childhood. In the right hand, the metacarpal bone of the thumb contains two tumors; that of the fore-finger three or four tumors, of which the smallest is an inch, and the largest is three inches in diameter: the first and second phalanges, also of the fore-finger, contain tumors; the middle finger appears normal; the third finger has one tumor in its metacarpal bone, one in its first phalanx, and two in its second phalanx; the little finger has as many, in corresponding positions. On the left hand the only tumor was that in the first phalanx of the fore-finger.

A third preparation‖ contains the fore and little fingers removed by Mr. Lawrence from a healthy lad seventeen years old. He had on his left hand four, and on his right hand six tumors; but those that were removed were alone troublesome and increasing. They varied from one inch and a half to one-third of an inch in diameter, were all covered with healthy smooth skin, and appeared to grow from the interior of the bones. No account could be given of their origin, except that they began to grow when he was five years old; and some grew more quickly than others. In both fingers a formation of cartilage has occurred in the metacarpal bones and the second phalanges, which was attended with scarcely any

* Principles of Surgery, vol. iii. p. 65.
† On Cancer. Whenever the statements made by Müller respecting the general characters of cartilaginous tumors differ from the account here given, the differences may, I think, be explained by his taking for the type the tumors of the hand. This alone could have made him regard so little the ossification of cartilaginous tumors.
‡ Mus. Coll. Surg. 775.   § Described in the Pathological Appendix to the Catalogue.
‖ Mus. St. Bartholomew's, Pathol. Appendix.

swelling: indeed, till the operation was being performed, these bones were not supposed to be the seats of disease, though their medullary cavities were quite full of cartilage.

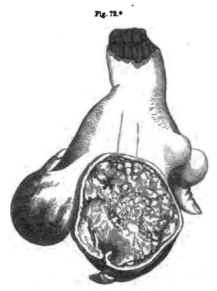

Fig. 72.*

The fourth specimen, here sketched, is, I believe, the most remarkable yet seen. I received it from Mr. Salmon, of Wedmore. It is the right hand of a laborer, fifty-six years old, from whom, when he was sixteen years old, the fore-finger of the left hand was removed with a tumor weighing 2lb. 5oz. The little finger of the same hand has a tumor about as large as a walnut: the whole length of his left tibia has irregular nodules on its anterior and inner surface, and some enlargement exists at its left second toe.

On the right hand, which Mr. Salmon amputated, there are tumors on every finger, and one spheroidal mass nearly six inches in diameter, in which the second and third fingers appear completely buried, the walls of their phalanges being only just discernible at the borders of the mass that has formed by the coalition of tumors that grew within them.

The disease which these specimens illustrate begins, I believe, exclusively in the early period of life; during childhood, or at least before puberty, and sometimes even before birth. It occurs, also, much more frequently in boys than in girls. One or more, or nearly all, of the phalanges or metacarpal bones of one or both hands may enlarge slowly, and without pain, into an oval, or round or heart-shaped swelling. When such swellings are grouped, they produce strange distortions of the hands, making them look like those of people who have accumulated gouty deposits; or, as John Bell delights to repeat, like the toes and claws of sculptured griffins. They may greatly elongate the fingers, but they more commonly press them asunder, limiting and hindering their movements.

There is no rule or symmetry observed in the affections of the hands, except that the thumb is less frequently than the fingers the seat of growths.

* Fig 72. Hand with cartilaginous tumors, described above. Reduced to one-fifth of the natural size.

In the large majority of cases, if not in all, each tumor grows within a bone, the walls of which are gradually extended and adapted to its growth. And this position within the bones is the more remarkable, because, in the cases of single cartilaginous tumors of the fingers or hands, the growth takes place not more, but rather less, often within than without the bone; these single tumors commonly growing, as those of the larger long bones do, between the periosteum and shaft.*

Thus, growing within the bones, the cartilaginous tumors may be sometimes found, even in the same hand, in all stages of growth. One phalanx or metacarpal bone may have its medullary cavity full of cartilage without any external appearance of enlargement; another may be slightly swollen-out at one part, or in its whole periphery; another so extended on one side, or uniformly, that its walls form only a thin shell around the mass of cartilage; in another the cartilage may have grown out through holes absorbed in the walls of the bone, and may then have spread out on its exterior; while from another it may have protruded through apertures even in the integuments, gradually thinned and ulcerated;† or, as the specimen sketched in fig. 72 shows, we may find not only such a protrusion through integuments, but two originally distinct tumors, growing out beyond the limits of their respective bones, and coalescing in one huge mass. In cases of this kind, the cartilaginous mass in each bone usually appears as a single tumor, with very delicate, if any, partitions. It may have a coarsely granulated aspect, but it is rarely divided into distinct nodules, or strongly intersected. Its exterior is adapted closely to the interior of the shell or bone, but is not continuous with it, except by blood-vessels. It rarely ossifies, except in a few small scattered cancellous masses in its mid-substance.‡ And it is worth observing, that the tumors often project on only one side of a bone; for when this happens in the metacarpus, it is often very hard to tell which of two adjacent metacarpal bones should be cut out in case of need.

The cases of this singular disease have shown great diversity as to the cause of the tumors, and in their modes and rates of growth; some making progress, some remaining stationary: and I believe it has often happened that at the time of manhood all have ceased to grow. But in regard to all these questions, important as they are, we are yet in need of facts.

It would be easy, and as vain as easy, to speculate on the meaning of such a disease as this. I believe no reasonable explanation of it can as yet be given, unless it may be said that these are the results of an exuberant nutrition similar to that which in the embryo may produce supernumerary limbs, but is here more disorderly and less vigorous.

* Mus. Coll. Surg. No. 772–3.

† A good case illustrating the last-mentioned fact is represented by Professor Miller, in his Principles of Surgery, p. 179. The tumor on the back of the metacarpus weighed fourteen pounds, and after protrusion bled frequently. John Bell also has recorded several such cases.

‡ Specimens of ossification are in the College Museum, No. 785–6.

The only remaining instances of cartilaginous tumors to which I shall refer are those that grow near the parotid, or, much more rarely, near the submaxillary gland.* Some of these are formed of pure cartilage, and might be taken as types of the cartilaginous tumor; but more are composed of cartilage, or fibrous cartilage, variously mixed with other tissues, and especially with what appears to be an imperfect or a perverted glandular tissue. Whichever of these forms they may have, they are commonly imbedded in the gland. They are sometimes wholly surrounded by the gland-substance, but much more commonly are more or less deeply imbedded in it, and covered with its fascia.

These tumors are generally invested with tough fibro-cellular capsules, which, though sometimes loose, are more commonly so closely attached to the surrounding parts that it is difficult to dissect them out. And the inconvenience of this is not a little increased by the frequent contact of branches of the facial nerve, which are apt to adhere very closely to the deep part of the tumor, or to be imbedded between its lobes, or may even stretch over its surface.†

The general aspect of these tumors depends much on the proportion in which the cartilage and their other component tissues are mixed. When they are of pure cartilage, or when the cartilage, or delicately fibrous cartilage, greatly predominates, they may present all the general characters that are already described. Such a case is illustrated by that to which, among all the specimens of the kind, the primacy belongs. It was removed by Mr. Hunter, and is enough to prove the skill and boldness as an operator which some have denied him. The case was that of a man, thirty-seven years old, who, sixteen years previously, fell and bruised his cheek. Shortly after the injury, the part began to swell, and the swelling regularly increased for four or five years, when he again fell and struck the swelling, which, after this, extended especially at its lower part and base. It seemed quite loose, and movable without pain. Mr. Hunter extirpated it, and with complete success. It weighed 144 ounces, and measures in its chief dimensions 9 inches by 7. It presents a striking instance of the conglomerate cartilaginous tumor, consisting of numerous round masses of pale, semi-transparent, glistening cartilage, connected by their several fibro-cellular investments; and its exterior is deeply lobed and nodulated. Its apparent composition is confirmed by the microscopic examinations of Mr. Quekett,‡ who found it composed

* These are grouped by Rokitansky as the third variety of the Gelatinous Sarcoma, with a recognition of their affinity to Enchondroma. Mr. Syme names them "Fibro-cartilaginous Sarcoma" (Principles of Surgery, vol. i. p. 89). The first good description of them was given by Mr. Lawrence (in his paper on Tumors, already often quoted). Mr. Cæsar Hawkins described them, for the most part, as "conglomerate tumors."

† The imbedding of important parts in a cartilaginous tumor need be remembered. In the Museum of St. George's Hospital is a specimen of this kind, about seven inches in diameter, which was sent to the Museum with the history, that, in removing it from the deep tissues of the thigh, the femoral artery was cut across where passing through its substance.

‡ Histological Catalogue, vol. i. p. 111. Ag. 52.

of cartilage, in which some of the intercellular substance is homogeneous, and some finely fibrous.

But when in these tumors the carti-lage is equalled or exceeded in quantity by the other tissue of which they may consist, we may find the same oval and nodular or lobed form, and the same hardness or firmness and elasticity, but they appear, on section, opaque white or cream-colored, and less glistening than cartilage.† Generally, these mixed tumors appear uniform; but, sometimes, portions of purer cartilage are imbedded in the mixed tissue, and obscurely bounded from it.‡

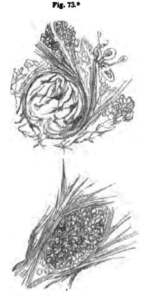

Fig. 73.*

In microscopic characters the carti-laginous parts of these tumors has, I believe, no peculiarity; different speci-mens may offer all the variety of forms to which I have already referred.

The tissue mixed with the cartila-ginous is at present, I think, of un-certain nature. In five cases I have found it, for the most part, present a lobed and clustered structure, with fibrous-looking tissue encircling spaces that are filled with nuclei and cells. These enclosed spaces look so like the acini of a conglomerate gland, that they seem to confirm the opinion one might form from its general aspect; namely, that it is an imitation of gland-tissue. And this is confirmed by the character of the cells within the seeming acini; for they have the general traits of gland-cells. They are usually small, round or oval, flattened, dimly granular, with nearly round, pellucid nuclei with nucleoli. They lie either like a thin epithelial lining of the spaces I just mentioned, or else they are clustered within them; or they may be irregularly grouped through the whole substance of the tumor; and in all cases abundant free nuclei like their own are mingled with them.

* Fig. 73. Minute structures of a mixed cartilaginous tumor over the parotid gland. In the upper sketch, a group of withered, stellate, cartilage nuclei are encircled with fibrous tissue. Others lie near the group; while, equally near, are well-formed cartilage-cells, and groups of small nuclei or nucleated cells, like those of gland structures. In the lower sketch similar corpuscles are grouped as in the acinus of a gland.

† They are among the tumors which one finds described as like turnips or like potatoes.

‡ I have often endeavored to see whence this mixture of tissues results, and especially whether the one tissue is transformed into the other; but I have not been able to discover this. It may be that these tumors are, in the first instance, composed wholly of one of the two principal tissues, and that in their further growth this primary tissue is superseded by the other. But it is, perhaps, more probable that in an apparently uniform blastema, two or more different structures should be developed, and thenceforward coincidently grow.

Such are the most general characters of these cells; but they are apt to vary from them, being more angular, or bearing processes, or being attenuated or caudate. Even if we may consider them as imitating gland-structures, yet it may be a question whether they are related to the adjacent parotid gland, or to lymphatic gland. It would be easy to discriminate between the elements of the parotid and of a lymphatic in their natural state; but a morbid imitation of either of them may deviate far enough to be as much like the other. And it is well to remember that these tumors have exactly the seats of naturally existing lymphatic glands, and are aften closely imitated by mere enlargements of these glands; so that, possibly, future researches may prove that they are cartilaginous tumors growing in and with a lymphatic gland over or within the parotid or submaxillary gland.

In general history, especially in their slow and painless growth, the absence of any morbid influence, except that produced by pressure, on the surrounding parts, the absence of proneness to foul ulceration, and of tendency to return after removal; in all these, the tumors over the parotid agree, I believe, with the other forms of cartilaginous tumors. I will therefore not delay to relate cases of them; but will draw towards conclusion by referring to some points connected with the general history and nature of the whole group of cartilaginous tumors.

First, then, concerning their origin:—They begin, in a large majority of cases, in early life; between childhood and puberty. Yet they may begin late in life. I saw one on the hand, which had been of no long duration when it was removed from a man 70 years old; another, growing in the humerus, and described by Mr. W. Adams,* had grown quickly in a man of 61; another began to grow at the same age, in a woman's thumb.† Most commonly, also, those in or near the parotid appear in or after middle age.

Then, concerning their nature: they may be regarded as, usually, completely innocent tumors, and yet there are some cases recorded, in which we must believe that, after a cartiloginous tumor has been removed, another has grown in the same place. I saw one such in a woman 30 years old, in whom, soon after the removal of one tumor from the parotid region, another grew and acquired a great size. This was an unmixed cartilaginous tumor; and I believe the first was of the same nature. Hr. Hughes Bennett‡ has related a case in which Mr. Syme removed a cartilaginous tumor of the arm by amputation at the shoulder-joint. Subsequently, the patient, a girl 14 years old, died with tumors in the stump and axilla. Mr. Liston removed a portion of the scapula, with a great tumor in its spine and acromion, which I have no doubt is a soft cartilaginous tumor.§ Three years afterwards the patient died, with

* Proceedings of the Pathological Society, ii. 344.　† Lebert; Abhandlungen, p. 191.
‡ On Cancerous and Cancroid Growths, pp. 108 and 258.　§ College Museum, No. 781.

what is described as a return of the disease. Mr. Fergusson showed at the Pathological Society a fibro-cartilaginous tumor[*] of the lower jaw, which had grown twice after the complete removal of similar tumors from the same part. In the Museum at Guy's Hospital, also, there is a cartilaginous tumor growing from the angle of the lower jaw into the mouth, which is said to have grown after complete removal of a similar tumor with the portion of lower jaw to which it was connected. Lastly, Professor Gluge[†] records two cases in which we must believe that recurrence of cartilaginous tumors ensued after complete removal. In one, a cartilaginous tumor, of 13 years' growth, and $9\frac{1}{2}$ pounds weight, over a man's scapula, clavicle, and neck, returned in the ribs, and destroyed life in a year and a half. In another, a similar tumor of the orbit returned two and a half years after removal.

We must conclude, I think, from these cases, that, although the general rule of innocence of cartilaginous tumors is established by their usual history, by numerous instances of permanent health after removal, and by cases in which, after death, no similar growths are found in lymphatics or internal organs, yet recurrence after operations may ensue. I think that when this happens it will generally be found that the recurring growths, if not the original growths also, are soft, rapid in their increase, and apt to protrude and destroy adjacent parts; as if we had, again, in these, an instance of that gradual approximation to completely malignant characters, of which I spoke in the twenty-first lecture. I think, too, that we shall find that these soft cartilaginous tumors which are apt to recur, or of which more than one exist in different parts on the same patient, affect particularly those who are members of cancerous families (see p. 431).

In connection with these points I may refer to some additional facts in the pathology of cartilaginous tumors.

First, many may exist in the same person; secondly, they are sometimes hereditary; thirdly, they are not unfrequently mingled with cancerous growths.

Multiplicity is sufficiently marked in the cases of the hands and feet, but has been observed, though more rarely, in other parts; as in a case recorded by Mr. William Adams, and already referred to, as presenting tumors at once in the scapula and parts of the humerus. The case by Mr. Bickersteth (p. 431) was probably of the same kind.

The hereditary occurrence was observed in the case of a cartilaginous tumor of the pelvis, of which I have already spoken, as examined by Mr. Donald Dalrymple. The patient's father had a large ossified enchondroma of the radius, which was removed by Mr. Martineau.[‡]

[*] Mr. Simon examined it with the microscope, and found it formed of well-marked cartilage, with a fibrous basis.

[†] Atlas der pathologischen Anatomie, Lief. iv.; and Pathologische Histologie, p. 67.

[‡] The specimens are in the Museum of the Norfolk and Norwich Hospital. In the number of the Edinburgh Monthly Journal, vol. xiii., p. 195, an abstract of the case is published by Dr. Cobbold, who relates, in addition to the facts I had learnt from Mr. Thomas Cresse,

The conjunction of cartilaginous and medullary cancerous tumors, may, perhaps, be called frequent, especially in the testicle.

A man, 88 years old, was under Mr. Lawrence's care with an apparent enlargement of one testicle, which he ascribed to a blow received eighteen months previously. Three weeks after the blow he noticed an enlargement which regularly increased, and formed an oval mass about four inches long. This, at its upper part, was moderately firm and elastic; but in the lower third it felt incompressibly hard. It was removed, and proved to be a pale, soft, grayish, medullary cancer in the testicle, having in its lower part a mass of cartilage, with scattered points of bone, and some intercellular tissue.* The patient died a fortnight after the operation; and it was interesting to observe, as illustrating the contrast between the cartilaginous and the cancerous growths, that he had soft medullary cancerous tumors in the situation of his lumbar lymphatic glands, but no cartilaginous tissue in or mingled with them.

A specimen closely resembling this, and with a very similar history, is in the Museum of the University of Cambridge. Another is in the Museum of Guy's Hospital, of which it is said that the patient died with return of the medullary disease. Müller noticed the same combination.† Virchow‡ has cited two cases and described one, all illustrating the same singular fact. In the three specimens that I have seen of conjunction of cartilaginous and medullary growths in the testicle, the cartilage appears as an isolated mass in the substance of the medullary tumor, and is enclosed in a distinct capsule. There are cases, however, in which the two morbid substances, though distinct, yet lie in so close contact that they are confused with one another. Thus, in a tumor which, as already mentioned (p. 429), was attached to the front of the lumbar vertebræ, and weighed thirteen pounds, half was formed of soft flocculent medullary cancer, and half of nodules of cartilage, some with soft, some with osseous centres.§ A tumor removed from over a woman's parotid gland by Mr. Lloyd, was invested by a single fibro-cellular capsule; but one half was cartilaginous and the other looked like medullary substance, and they were mingled, with no distinct boundary line, at their contiguous borders.║ And lastly, in a case of which preparations are in the Museum of St. Thomas's Hospital, Mr. Dodd removed a genuine and apparently unmixed cartilaginous tumor from a man's ribs; but, in three months,

---

that a brother of the man who had the tumor in the pelvis, has mollities ossium, and that "others of his kindred had been subjected to the debilitating influences of a perverted nutrition."

* The specimens and drawings are in the Museum of St. Bartholomew's.

† On Cancer.

‡ Verhandl. der phys.-med. Gesellschaft in Würzburg, i. p. 134. Baring (Ueber den Markschwamm der Hoden, Pl. ii.) has represented a similar specimen.

§ Mus. Coll. Surg. 207; Mus. St. Bartholomew's, Ser. xxxv., No. 49.

║ Mus. Coll. Surg. 207 A; Mus. St. Bartholomew's, Ser. xxxv., No. 45. The patient was alive at least seven years after the removal of the tumor.

another tumor appeared in the same part, formed of closely mingled cartilage and medullary substance. This quickly proved fatal.

I need hardly remark on the bearing which this last case may have on the question of the recurrence of cartilaginous tumors, and on that of the changes of character which may ensue in tumors generally, at their successive occasions of recurrence. It gives to all these cases a much higher interest than would attach to them if regarded only as rarities and strange things.

But it is not with the malignant diseases alone that cartilage is found in tumors. I have described it as combined with what appears like glandular tissue in the tumors over the parotid, and I have seen bone in similar combination in a tumor in the lip. Specimens are not rare in which closely grouped nodules, and irregular masses of pure white cartilage are imbedded in fibro-cystic tumors in the testicle. In speaking of the fibro-cellular tumors, I mentioned two in which cartilage was similarly mingled with their more essential constituent; and in the Museum of Guy's Hospital is a tumor removed from beneath the gastrocnemius muscle, which consists of both fibro-cellular and adipose tissue, with abundant imbedded nodules of cartilage. And lastly, similar combinations appear to exist of cartilaginous growths with those which M. Lebert named fibro-plastic, and which will be described in the next lecture as myeloid tumors. Such is, I believe, the composition of three tumors in the Museum of St. Bartholomew's—of which one surrounds the head of the tibia;* another involves the bones of the face, and extends into the cranium;† and a third occupies and expands the lower end of the fibula.‡ The compound structure of the last was ascertained with the microscope, which easily detected the two materials irregularly mingled in every part of the tumor.

In all these facts concerning its combination with other morbidly produced structures, there must be something of much importance in relation to the physiology of cartilage; but as yet, I believe, we cannot comprehend it. Such combinations are not, I believe, imitated in the cases of any other structures found in tumors; even those that are thus combined with cartilage do not, I think, combine with one another, if we except the cases of intra-uterine morbid growths. As yet, however, the interest that belongs to all these injuries is scarcely more than the interest of mystery, and of promise to future investigators. As yet, we can think scarcely more than that, as innocent tumors, generally, are remote imitations of the abnormal excesses of development which occur in embryo-life, so it might be expected that, in some of them, many of the tissues would be combined in disorder, which, orderly arranged, make up the fœtus.

* Series i. 41; and Mr. Stanley's Illustrations, Pl. 15, fig. 3.
† Ser. xxxv. 47; and the same Illustr., p. 13, fig. 4.
‡ Appendix to Pathol. Catal.

LECTURE XXVIII.

PART I.

MYELOID TUMORS.

THE Tumors for which I venture to propose the name of Myeloid (μυελωδής, marrow-like), were first distinguished as a separate kind by M. Lebert.* Before his discovery of their minute structure, they were confounded with fibrous tumors, or included among the examples of sarcoma, and especially of osteo-sarcoma. M. Lebert gave them the name of "fibro-plastic," having regard to their containing corpuscles like the elongated cells, or fibro-cells, which he has called by the same name, and to which I have so often referred as occurring in the rudimental fibro-cellular and fibrous tumors, and in developing lymph and granulations. But the more characteristic constituents of these tumors, and those which more certainly indicate their structural homology (i. e. their likeness to natural parts) are peculiar many-nucleated corpuscles, which have been recognised by Kölliker† and Robin‡ as constituents of the marrow and diploe of bones, especially in the fœtus, and in early life. It seems best, therefore, to name the tumors after this their nearest affinity. On similar grounds, they must be regarded as having a nearer relation to the cartilaginous than to the fibrous tumors; for their essential structures, both the many-nucleated corpuscles and the elongated cells, are (like those of cartilaginous tumors) identical with normal rudimental bone-textures. Moreover, as I have already said, portions of myeloid structure are sometimes mixed with those of cartilaginous tumors, and they are sometimes developed into naturally constructed cancellous and medullary bone. The structures of this group of tumors are, indeed, essentially similar to those found in granulations which grow from, and may be transformed into, bone (see page 128); and to a section of such granulations some specimens bear, even to the unaided eye, no small resemblance.

The myeloid tumors may be found in many situations; but they are far more frequent in or upon the bones than in connection with any other tissue. I have seen them in the mammary gland, and I think in the neck, near the thyroid gland; and M. Lebert mentions many other parts as occasionally containing them, especially the eyelids and conjunctivæ, the subcutaneous tissue, the cerebral membranes, and the uterus.§

* Physiologie pathologique, ii. p. 120; and Abhandlungen, p. 123.
† Mikrosk. Anatomie, B. ii. p. 264, 378.
‡ Comtes Rendus. . . de la Société de Biologie, T. i. p. 150; T. ii. p. 8, and Memoires, p. 143.
§ L. c.; and in Virchow and Reinhart's Archiv, B. iii. p. 463. But I think that in several

As usually occurring in connection with the bones, a myeloid, like a fibrous tumor, may be either enclosed in a bone whose walls are expanded round it, or, more rarely, it is closely set on the surface of a bone, confused with its periosteum. The sketches in p. 105, of fibrous tumors within and upon the lower jaw, might be repeated here for myeloid tumors; and the two kinds are about equally common in the same positions, both within and upon the upper jaw. When enclosed in bone, the myeloid tumors usually tend to the spherical or ovoid shape, and are well defined, if not invested with distinct thin capsules; seated on bone, they are, as an epulis of this structure may exemplify, much less defined, less regular in shape, and often deeply lobed. They feel like uniformly compact masses, but are, in different instances, variously consistent. The most characteristic examples are firm; and (if by the name we may imply such a character as that of the muscular substance of a mammalian heart) they may be called "fleshy." Others are softer, in several gradations to the softness of size-gelatine, or that of a section of granulations. Even the firmer are brittle, easily crushed or broken; they are not tough, or very elastic, like the fibro-cellular or fibrous tumors; neither are they grumous or pulpy; neither do they show a granular or fibrous structure on their cut or broken surfaces.

On section, the cut surfaces appear smooth, uniform, compact, shining, succulent with a yellowish, not a creamy, fluid. A peculiar appearance is commonly given to these tumors by the cut surface presenting blotches of dark or livid crimson, or of a brownish or a brighter blood-color, or of a pale pink, or of all these tints mingled, on the grayish-white or greenish basis-color.* This is the character by which, I think, they may best be recognized with the naked eye, though there are diversities in the extent, and even in the existence, of the blotching. The tumor may be all pale, or have only a few points of ruddy blotching, or the cut surface may be nearly all suffused, or even the whole substance may have a dull Modena or crimson tinge, like the ruddy color of a heart, or that of the parenchyma of a spleen.†

Many varieties of aspect may thus be observed in myeloid tumors; and, beyond these, they may be even so changed that the microscope may be essential to their diagnosis. Often, they partially ossify; well-

---

of these instances he has included in his account tumors containing only the elongated "fibro-plastic" cells; whereas I have reckoned, as belonging to this myeloid group of tumors, none but those which, together with such cells, contained also the large many-nucleated corpuscles, which alone are a peculiar constituent. A tumor containing elongated fibrocells alone, I should expect to be a rudimental fibro-cellular, or fibrous, or recurring fibroid tumor. They may, also, appear as a chief constituent in tumors containing abundant inflammatory exudation.

* Lebert says the greenish-yellow color that they may show depends on a peculiar sort of fat, which he calls Xanthose (Abhandl. 127).

† I believe that many of what have been named spleen-like tumors of the jaw have been of this kind. The color they present is not due only to blood in them; more of it is appropriate to their texture, as that of the spleen is, or that of granulations: and it may be quickly and completely bleached with alcohol.

formed, cancellous bone being developed in them. Cysts, also, filled with bloody or serous fluids, may be formed in them, occupying much of their volume, or even almost excluding the solid texture. In the last case the recognition of the disease is very difficult. I lately amputated the leg of a woman, 24 years old, for what I supposed to be a cancerous tumor growing within the head of the tibia. She had had pain in this part for eighteen months, and increasing swelling for ten months; and it was plain that the bone was expanded and wasted around some soft growth within it. On section, after removal, the head of the tibia, including its articular surface, appeared expanded into a rounded cyst or sac, about $3\frac{1}{2}$ inches in diameter, the walls of which were formed by thin flexible bone and periosteum, and by the articular cartilages above. Within, there was little more than a few bands or columns of bone, among a disorderly collection of cysts filled with blood or blood-colored serous fluids. The walls of most of the cysts were thin and pellucid; those of some were thicker, soft, and brownish-yellow, like the substance of some medullary cancers; a likeness to which was yet more marked in a small solid portion of tumor, which, though very firm, and looking fibrous, was pure white and brain-like.

None who examined this disease with the naked eye alone felt any doubt that it was an example of medullary cancer, with cysts abundantly formed in it. But, on minuter investigation, none but the elements which I shall presently describe as characteristic of the myeloid tumors could be found in it: these, copiously imbedded in a dimly granular substance, appeared to form the substance of the cyst-walls, and of whatever solid material existed between them. The white brain-like mass was, apparently, composed of similar elements in an advanced fatty degeneration; neither in it, nor in any other part, could I find a semblance of cancer-cells.

I have not seen another specimen deviating so far from the usual characters of myeloid tumors as this did; but I think that, as in this, so in any other variation of general aspect, the microscopic structures would suffice for diagnosis; for there is no other morbid growth, so far as I know, in which they are imitated. They consist essentially of cells and other corpuscles, of which the following are the chief forms:—

1. Cells of oval, lanceolate, or angular shapes, or elongated and attenuated like fibro-cells or caudate cells, having dimly dotted contents with single nuclei and nucleoli (fig. 74, A).

2. Free nuclei, such as may have escaped from the cells; and, among these, some that appear enlarged and elliptical, or variously angular, or are elongated towards the same shapes as the lanceolate and caudate cells, and seem as if they were assuming the characters of cells.

3. The most peculiar form;—large, round, oval, or flask-shaped, or irregular cells and cell-like masses, or thin disks, of clear or dimly granular substance, measuring from $\frac{1}{500}$ to $\frac{1}{1000}$ of an inch in diameter, and

containing from two to ten or more oval, clear, and nucleolated nuclei (fig. 74, B: see also fig. 76, p. 458).

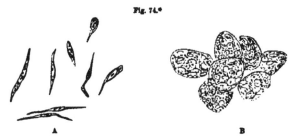

Fig. 74.*

A   B

Corpuscles such as these, irregularly and in diverse proportions imbedded in a dimly granular substance, make up the mass of a myeloid tumor. They may be mingled with molecular fatty matter; or, the mass they compose may be traversed with filaments, or with bundles of fibrocellular tissue and blood-vessels: but their essential features (and especially those of the many-nucleated corpuscles) are rarely obscured.

Respecting the general history of the myeloid tumors, the cases hitherto minutely observed are too few and too various to justify many general conclusions. Not that the disease is a rare one: for there can be little doubt that many cases recorded as examples of epulis, of fibrous tumors of the jaws, of osteo-sarcoma, and even of cancerous growths about the bones, should be referred to this group. At present, however, I can refer to no cases but those by M. Lebert, and those which I have myself been able to observe. From these, the most general facts I can collect are, that the myeloid tumors usually occur singly; that they are most frequent in youth, and very rare after middle age; that they generally grow slowly and without pain; and generally commence without any known cause, such as injury or hereditary disposition. They rarely, except in portions, become osseous; they have no proneness to ulcerate or protrude; they seem to bear even considerable injury without becoming exuberant; they may (but I suppose they very rarely) shrink, or cease to grow; they are not apt to recur after complete removal; nor have they, in general, any features of malignant disease.

I may illustrate these general statements by abstracts of some of the cases I have recorded; selecting for the purpose those which were, on any ground, the more remarkable.†

A lad, eighteen years old, was under Mr. Stanley's care, between five and six years ago, with a tumor occupying the interior of the symphysis,

* Fig. 74. Microscopic structures of myeloid tumors. A, elongated cells, or fibro-plastic cells (Lebert). B, a cluster of mani-nucleated cells. Magnified about 350 times.

† The specimens obtained from all the following cases are in the Museum of St. Bartholomew's.

and immediately adjacent parts, of his lower jaw-bone. It had been observed gradually increasing for eight months without pain, and in its growth had disparted the walls of the jaw, hollowing out a cavity for itself, and projecting into the mouth through one of the alveoli. Mr. Stanley removed the portion of the jaw, from the first left true molar to the first right premolar tooth. The tumor presented the greenish and grayish basis, blotched with crimson and various brownish tints, and the characters of firmness, succulency, and microscopic texture, which I have described as most distinctive of the myeloid tumors. It was the specimen from which some of the microscopic sketches were made, and might be considered typical. This patient is still in good health, with no appearance of return of the disease.

Mr. Lawrence had under his care a woman, twenty-one years old, with a tumor in the alveolar part of the front of the upper jaw. This was of about twelve months duration, and had sometimes been very painful. It was seated in the cancellous tissue between the walls of the alveolar and adjacent portion of the upper jaw, projecting slightly into both the mouth and the cavity of the nose, and raising their mucous membranes after passing through the wasted bone. After cutting away the front wall of the jaw, the tumor was cleared out from all the cavity in which it lay imbedded. It was in all microscopic characters like that last mentioned, and resembled it in general features, except in that it had in every part the dark ruddy color of a strong heart. The operation was performed two years ago, and there has been no reappearance of the disease, such as would have occurred in the case of a malignant tumor, if an attempt had been made to remove it without the bone in which it was growing.

A woman, 22 years old, was under Mr. Lawrence's care, in March, 1851, from the alveolar part of whose right jaw, growths which were regarded as examples of epulis had been four times removed in the previous thirteen months. In the operation in August, 1850, the growth was found to extend through the socket of the first molar tooth into the antrum, or into a cavity in the jaw. It was wholly removed (as it was thought), and the wounds healed soundly; but nine weeks afterwards a fresh growth appeared, that seemed to involve or arise from nearly the whole front surface of the right upper jaw-bone: it was firm, tense, and elastic, but not painful, projecting far on the face, as well as into the nostril, and into the cavity of the mouth at both the gum and the hard palate. This swelling, under various treatment, rapidly increased; and in December, 1850, a similar swelling appeared at the left canine fossa, and grew at the same rate with that of earlier origin. Of course the coexistence of two such swellings led to the fear, and in some minds to the conviction, that the disease was cancerous; and the more, because, at nearly the same time with the second of these, two soft tumors had appeared on the parietal bones. Still, the patient's general health was but little impaired; and when the mucous membrane of the hard palate ulcerated over the most prominent parts of the tumors, neither of them protruded, or bled, or grew more rapidly.

In April, 1851, the growth of the tumors appeared to be very much retarded, and for the next month was hardly perceptible; and the patient being very urgent that something should be done to diminish the horrible deformity of her face, Mr. Lawrence, in May, cut away the greater part of the front and of the palatine and lower nasal parts of the right upper jaw, and removed from the antrum all that appeared morbid, including, doubtless, nearly every portion of the tumor.

The excised portion of the jaw-bone was involved and imbedded in a large, irregularly spherical tumor, composed of a close-textured, shining, soft, and brittle substance, of dark grayish hue, suffused and blotched with various shades of pink and deep crimson. It was not lobed, but included portions of cancellous bone, apparently new-formed, and was very closely adherent to all the surrounding parts. To the microscope it exhibited all the characters that I have described above; and the many-nucleated corpuscles were remarkably well defined and full. They composed nine-tenths of the mass, and were arranged like clustered cells. The patient perfectly recovered from the effects of the operation; and, to every one's surprise, the tumor on the left upper jaw, which had been in all respects like that removed from the right side, gradually disappeared. It underwent no apparent change of texture, but simply subsided. The swellings on the parietal bones, also, the nature of which was not ascertained, cleared away; and when the patient was last seen, a few months ago, she appeared completely well, and no swelling could be observed.

No case could better show than this did the conformity of the myeloid tumors with the general characters of innocent growths: on the other hand, the following might well have been regarded as a malignant disease, if its structure and limitation to a single part had not been considered.

A farmer's boy, 15 years old, was under Mr. Stanley's care, in the winter of 1851, with a large tumor covering the upper part of his head, rising to a height of from one to two inches above the skull, extending nearly from ear to ear, and from the occipital spine to the coronal suture. This had been in progress of constant growth for three years, and was believed to have originated in the effects of repeated blows on the head. The head now measured 21 inches in circumference, and 16½ inches over its transverse arch. Just before his admission he had become blind in one eye, and nearly so in the other; his gait was unsteady; he had severe pains in and about the forehead, but his intellect was not affected, and he appeared in good general health. The scalp over the tumor was exceedingly tense, and, at the most prominent part, rather deeply ulcerated. The temporal and occipital arteries were very large and tortuous: the corresponding veins felt like large sinuses.

In the last two months of his life, while in the hospital, his blindness became complete; he lost nearly all power of hearing, and suffered severe paroxysms of headache. A large portion of the scalp and of the subjacent tumor sloughed, leaving a great suppurating cavity, in the still growing tumor. At length, two days before death, convulsions ensued, which were followed by coma; and in this he died.

Fig. 75.

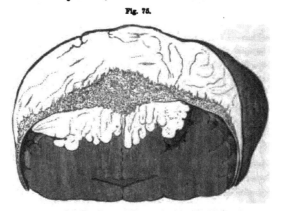

The tumor covered all the surface of the skull, in the extent above mentioned, rising gradually from its circumference to a height of two inches at and about its central parts. A similar growth of somewhat less dimensions existed within the corresponding parts of the interior of the skull, included the dura mater and longitudinal sinus, and deeply impressed the cerebrum. And, again, material similar to that forming these growths was infiltrated in and expanded the included parts of the bones of the vault of the skull. From both surfaces of these bones osseous spicula and thin lamellæ extended into the bases of the corresponding parts of the tumor. The adjacent sketch (fig. 75), from the preparation in the Museum of St. Bartholomew's, shows the relations of this singular growth to the skull and brain, as seen in a transverse section.

The extra-cranial portion of the tumor had a nearly uniform dense and elastic texture, of dull yellow color, mingled with white. Its cut surface appeared smooth, without distinct fibrous or other structure, and to the unaided eye looked like the firmest medullary cancer, involving the pericranium, and partially exposed by ulceration of the scalp. The intracranial portion was soft, easily crushed and broken into pulp, purple, streaked with pale gray and pink tints. It looked obscurely fibrous, and was intersected by shining bands derived from the dura mater and falx involved in it. To the naked eye it was like a softer medullary tumor, and was closely connected with the impressed surface of the brain, in the substance of which, just beneath it, was a large abscess.

Different, however, as the two parts of the tumor appeared, there was no corresponding difference in their microscopic elements: these were essentially the same in both parts; and though the tumor was so like cancer in its general aspect, yet its minute structures were not cancerous. They were chiefly as follows:—(1) Regular, oval, and well-defined cells, about $\frac{1}{700}$ of an inch in diameter, containing dimly-granular or dotted substance, in which many oval nucleolated nuclei were imbedded (fig. 76, A). They corresponded exactly with the corpuscles characteristic of the myeloid tumors; but they had more distinct cell-walls than I have seen in any other case, and some had even double contours, as if with very thick cell-walls.   (2) Irregular masses or fragments, of various sizes and shapes, having the same apparent substance as the contents of the cells, and containing similar numerous imbedded nuclei, but no defined cell-walls (fig. 76, B). In these also, the identity with the constituents of myeloid tumors was evident.   (3) More abundant than either of these forms were bodies like the many-nucleated cells, but having on their walls, as it were wrapped over them, one or more elongated caudate nucleated cells (c).   They seemed to be formed like the peculiar corpuscles in epithelial cancers, in which one finds cells or clusters of nuclei invested with layers of epithelial scales concentrically wrapped round them. Their borders presented two or three concentric lines, as if laminated; between these were one or more nuclei; and often the innermost of the lines was bayed inwards towards the cell-cavity, leaving a space in which a nucleus was lodged.   Sometimes, from the circumference of such bodies, one could find curved nucleated elongated cells dislodged (D).

Fig. 76.*

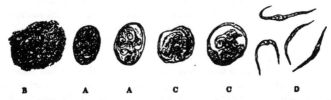

B   A   A   C   C   D

In most instances these laminated cells were filled with the dimly granular substance and the many nuclei; but in some there were clear spaces that seemed to contain only pellucid liquid. The elongated cells that could be sometimes detached from these laminated cells agreed, in general characters, with the remaining principal constituent of the growth; namely, (4) narrow, long, caudate, and fusiform cells with out-swelling nuclei, like those of developing granulations, and such as I have described as constant elements of the myeloid tumors.

All the minute structures just described were found closely compacted, and making, with free nuclei and granular matter, up the mass of both

* Fig. 76. Microscopic elements of the myeloid tumor of the skull, described in the next. Magnified 250 times.

portions of the tumor; and the only apparent difference was, that, in the intra-cranial portion, they appeared more generally to contain granules, and to be mixed with granule-cells and granule-masses, as if this part of the tumor were more degenerate than the other.

I fear that even so abbreviated a record of this case as I have ventured to print may seem very tedious; but it is not for its own rarity alone that the case is important. It would be difficult to find a tumor more imitative of cancer than this was, in its mode of growth, its infiltration of various tissues, its involving of important parts, its apparent dissimilarity from any natural structures. And yet it certainly was not cancer; the microscopic elements were like those of natural parts: not a lymphatic or any other organ was affected by similar disease, and death seemed to be due solely to the local effects of the growth.

But while these, and many other cases may be enough to prove that the myeloid tumors are generally of innocent nature, yet I suspect cases may be found in which, with the same apparent structures, a malignant course is run. Of such suspicious cases, the two following are examples:—

A woman, 50 years old, was under Mr. Stanley's care, in 1847, with an irregular, roundish, heavy tumor, between two and three inches in diameter, in her left breast. It projected in the breast, and the skin over it was red and tense, and at one part seemed to point, as if with suppuration. Some axillary glands were enlarged, but not hardened.

This tumor had existed about nine months, had been the seat of occasional pain, and was increasing. It was considered to be hard cancer; but, on the removal of the breast, was found to be a distinct growth, completely separable from the mammary gland, which was pressed aside by it. Its character was obscured by suppuration in many points of its substance; yet, after a careful examination of it in the recent state, and a repeated examination of the notes and sketches that I made of its structure, I can only conclude that it was a myeloid tumor suppurated, or, possibly mingled with cancer.

Eighteen months after the removal of her breast this patient returned to the hospital, with a large ulcerated tumor in the lower part of her left axilla, which had begun to form as a distinct tumor six months after the operation. This was like a large flat ulcerated cancer: it often bled freely. Her general health was deeply affected by it, and she died in two or three months after her readmission.

The malignant character manifested in this case was yet more decidedly marked in another. A man, 53 years old, of healthy appearance, was under Mr. Lawrence's care with an oval tumor, extending, under the mastoid muscle, from the angle of the jaw to the clavicle. Bloody serum oozed from it through three small apertures in the integuments. The anterior part of the tumor felt as if containing fluid; the posterior part felt solid, firm, and elastic. He had observed this tumor for ten months, having found one morning, when he awoke, a lump nearly as large as an egg, which regularly increased. In two months it had become very large: it was punctured, and about one-third of a pint of reddish serum was discharged from it. In the succeeding eight months it was tapped thirty-four times more, about the same quantity of similar fluid being each time evacuated. It was also six times injected with tincture of iodine, twice traversed with setons, and in various other ways severely treated. The only general result was, that it increased, and seemed to become, in proportion, more solid. When admitted under Mr. Lawrence, all the parts over the tumor were extremely tense and painful, and cerebral disturbance appeared to be produced by its pressure on the great blood-vessels of the neck. It was freely cut into, and the surface which was exposed presented well-marked characters of the myeloid tumors such as I have described. Some small portions that were removed enabled me to confirm this with the microscope. The elongated, and the many-nucleated cells, were, to all appearance, decisive. The incision of the tumor produced temporary relief; but the tumor continued to grow, and death occurred nearly twelve months from its commencement. In exami-nation after death, the solid portion of the tumor formed fifty-sixths of its bulk, the rest consisting of a suppurating cavity. The microscopic characters of the solid part were exactly like those of the portions removed during life, though the substance appeared firmer and whiter than before, and yielded, when scraped, a creamy fluid. Four small masses of similar substance were found in the lungs; and a similar material was diffused in one cervical gland.

Now, in both these cases, and especially in the last, the whole history of which seems full of anomalies, there were certainly such features of dissimilarity from the usual general characters of the myeloid tumors, that, although the microscopic characters appeared identical, yet they are not enough to prove even the occasional malignancy of the disease: they are enough to make us cautious; enough to induce us to study this dis-ease very carefully, as one of those that may, in different conditions, or in different persons, pursue very different courses; appearing in some as an innocent, in others as a malignant disease. The use of such terms as "semi-malignant," "locally malignant," "less malignant than cancer," and the like, in relation to growths of this kind, involves subjects of sin-gular interest in pathology, as well as in practical surgery. But I will not now dwell on them. The whole subject may be more appropriately discussed in the lectures on malignant tumors.

LECTURE XXVIII.

PART II.

OSSEOUS TUMORS.

MUCH of the general pathology of osseous tumors has been considered in the last two lectures, which have treated of the tumors composed of rudimental bone-textures. Ossification may ensue in either a cartilaginous or a myeloid tumor. In the latter it is rarely, if ever, more than partial, in the former it may be complete; and the cartilaginous may be transformed into an osseous tumor. The name of osseous tumor is, however, not usually applied to those in which ossification is in progress. It is reserved for such as are formed wholly of bone, and of these alone I shall now speak.

Osseous tumors, even more generally than cartilaginous, are connected with the bones, with which, moreover, though they may have the other characters of tumors, they are almost always continuous, after the manner of outgrowths. They are, however, occasionally found in soft parts, as distinct and discontinuous tumors, invested with fibro-cellular capsules. Thus in the College Museum (No. 208), is a small, completely osseous tumor, formed of soft cancellous tissue with medulla, which lies over the dorsal surface of the trapezial and scaphoid bones, completely isolated from them and all the adjacent bones. In the Museum of St. George's Hospital is a tumor formed of compact bony tissue, which lay over the palmar aspect of the first metacarpal bone, loosely imbedded in the fibro-cellular tissue, and easily separated from the flexor tendons of the finger.* It had been growing five years in a middle-aged woman. So, but rarely and imperfectly, the cartilaginous tumors over the parotid gland are ossified;† and those in the lungs‡ and testicle.

At present, these isolated osseous tumors are interesting for little more than their rarity. It is to those connected with bones that I must now particularly address myself.

I have already said that these have the character of continuous growths; that they are like outgrowths rather than tumors. And it is not easy to draw any line of distinction between what deserve to be considered as tumors, and such accumulations of bone as may ensue in consequence of superficial inflammation, or other disease, of the bone or periosteum. The exostoses and hyperostoses of nosology are not to be severally defined without artifice; but, in general, we may take this as a convenient, and per-

---

* An account of it is reported in the Medical Times, Aug. 3, 1850.
† Mus. Coll. Surg. No. 204.
‡ Museum of St. Thomas's Hospital.

haps a just, method of dividing them : namely, that those may be reckoned as osseous tumors, or outgrowths of the nature of tumors, whose base of attachment to the original bone is defined, and grows, if at all, at a less rate than their outstanding mass.* Those which are not of the nature of tumors are generally not only ill-defined, but widely spread at their bases of attachment; and the additions made to them increase their bases rather than their heights or their whole masses.

Of osseous tumors, thus roughly defined, two chief kinds may be observed: namely, the cancellous and the compact or ivory-like, which, generally speaking, may be said to resemble respectively, the medullary tissue, and the walls or compact substance, of healthy bone. In both alike, the bone is usually true and good bone. By my own observations of it I know no more than this; but Mr. Quekett, who has submitted to microscopic examination portions of all the osseous tumors in the College Museum, confirms the general statement in all particulars. In different specimens there may be varieties in the proportion and arrangement of blood-vessels, and in the size and development of the bone-corpuscles or lacunæ and their canals; but the proper characters of the bone of the species in which the tumor occurs are not far departed from.

I believe the homology of the osseous tumors is, in chemical qualities, as perfect as it is in structure; and that as with the natural bones, so with these, we may not ascribe differences of hardness or density to the different proportions of the organic, and of the saline and earthy components; but to the different manner in which the similar material that they compose is, in different specimens, compacted. Their varieties of hardness depend on mechanical rather than on chemical differences.

Of the general methods of ossification of cartilaginous tumors I spoke in my last lecture, and then noticed that in nearly all cases when the ossification of the tumors is completed, they consist of a very thin layer or wall of compact tissue, covering in a mass of cancellous and medullary substance: and thus they are composed, whether the cartilage-growth began within or upon the bone. It is probable that, in some instances, the hardest osseous tumors may be also formed by transformation of cartilage into bone. Thus, in an exceedingly hard ivory-like tumor at the angle of the lower jaw, in the Museum of the College,† has so exactly the nodular and irregularly spheroidal shape belonging to cartilaginous tumors, and to the rare cancellous bony tumors in the same part, that we can scarcely doubt it had a primeordial cartilaginous condition. So, too, Professor Goodsir tells me, there is in the Museum of the University of Edinburgh a tumor of the humerus, half of which is as hard and compact as ivory, and half is cartilaginous. In the Museum of Guy's Hospital there is a somewhat similar specimen: in which, however,

* Mr. Stanley particularly remarks this in relation to operations for removal of exostoses. (On Diseases of the Bones, p. 150.)

† No. 1035: it may be compared with a cancellous tumor of the same form, in the Museum at St. George's Hospital, removed by Mr. Tatum.

the hardness of the bone may be due to inflammatory induration of an ordinary cancellous osseous growth.

These, however, are probably exceptions to the general rule concerning the compact or ivory exostoses; for, for the majority of these, Rokitansky says truly that no preparatory cartilage is formed. As, in the natural ossification of the skull, the bone is formed, not in a matrix of cartilage but in fibrous tissue, layers of which are successively ossified, so probably are the hard bony tumors of the skull formed.

The general characters of the cancellous bony tumors are so nearly described in the account of the cartilaginous tumors from which they commonly originate, that I need only briefly refer to them. They usually affect a round shape, with projecting lobes or nodules, which answer to those of the conglomerate cartilaginous tumors, and are often pointed or angular. They may, however, be very smooth on their surface, whether they have grown within bones, whose extended walls form now their outer layer, or without them under the periosteum. When completely ossified, their respective tissues, compact and medullary, are usually continuous with those of the bone on which they are planted; and the later periods of growth seem attended with such mutual adaptation as may tend towards making one continuous, though deformed, mass of the old and the new bone.

The singularities of position in which the osseous tumors may be found, and the important hinderances that may result from their interference with adjacent parts, I need not detail; they are amply enumerated by Mr. Stanley.

Of their rates of growth little is known; but I believe that when a cartilaginous tumor is completely ossified, the growth of the bony tumor is extremely slow. However, osseous tumors may be found of an enormous size. The largest that I know is in the Museum of the College.* It nearly surrounds the upper two-thirds of a tibia, in an irregularly oval mass, with a nodulated surface, almost entirely covered in by a thin layer of compact tissue, and cancellous in all its interior. It measures exactly a yard in circumference, and the limb, which was amputated by Mr. Gay, a former surgeon of St. Bartholomew's Hospital, weighed forty-two pounds.

Another tumor of large size is in the Museum of the same Hospital.† A great nodulated mass of bone is attached to the ischium and pubes, and formed part of a tumor of which the rest was undulated cartilage.

The compact, hard, or ivory-like bony tumors occur, especially about the bones of the head, and present several diversities of form. Some

---

* No. 3220. It is engraved in Cheselden's Osteographea, Tab. 53, f. 1, 2, 3. A painting of it is in the St. Bartholomew's Museum.

† Series 1 A. No. 133; and Series 1, No. 118.

are uniform and simple; others variously lobed or nodular. The simple tumors are commonly attached to the skull by narrowed bases, over which their chief masses are prominent on one side, or all round. A good specimen of this kind is in the Museum of St. Bartholomew's Hospital,* which shows, besides, that these tumors may consist of an exterior hard, and interior cancellous, tissue, respectively resembling and continuous with the outer table and the diploe of the skull. Some of these hard tumors have the shape of biconvex lenses, resting with one convex surface on the skull; and of such as these more than one may be found on the same skull.†

A disease much more formidable than these exists in the nodulated and larger hard osseous tumors connected with the bones of the skull. These are not like outgrowths from the outer table and diploe; for they often, or I believe usually, grow first between the tables of the skull, or in the cavities of the frontal or other sinuses. Increasing in these parts, they may tend in every direction, penetrating the tables of the skull, and forming large masses, projecting as much into the interior of the skull as on its exterior.

The most frequent seat of such tumors is in the frontal bone, especially about its superciliary and orbital parts; and they are horrible by their pressure into the cavities of both the cranium and the orbit, compressing the brain, and protruding one or both eyes.

The characters of the disease, so far as the growth is concerned, are well shown in a huge mass which grew from the forehead of an ox, originating apparently in the frontal sinuses.‡ It is like a great spheroidal mass of ivory, measuring 8½ inches in diameter, and weighing upwards of sixteen pounds. Its outer surface, though knobbed and ridged, is yet compact, like an elephant's tusk: and, in similar likeness, its section shows at one part a thin investing layer, like the bone covering the ivory. It is nearly all solid, hard, close-textured, and heavy; only a few irregular cavities, and one with smooth walls, appear in its interior, and you may trace the orifices of many canals for blood-vessels. Mr. Quekett found that this tumor had a higher specific gravity than any bone, except that which is found in what are called the porcellaneous deposits, or transformations, in the heads of bones affected with chronic rheumatism. But it has in every part the structure of true bone.

Just like this, in the general characters of their tissue, are the hard bony tumors from the human frontal bone. In one, an Hunterian specimen,§ such a tumor, 2½ inches in diameter, deeply lobed and knotted, fills the frontal sinuses and the upper part of the left orbit,

---

* Series 1, 71. Series 1 A, 124, in the same Museum, and No. 3215 in the Museum of the College, are nearly similar specimens.

† Mus. Coll. Surg. 793. See also Miller's Principles of Surgery, p. 476.

‡ Mus. Coll. Surg. 3216.

§ Mus. Coll. Surg. 795. It is engraved in Baillie's Morbid Anatomy, Fasc. x. pl. 1, fig. 2; and in Home, Philosoph. Trans., vol. lxxxix. p. 239.

encroaches into the right orbit, and projects for nearly an inch on both the surfaces of the skull. It appears to have originated in the ethmoidal or frontal cells, and, in its growth, to have displaced and destroyed by pressure the adjacent parts of the tables of the skull and the wall of the orbit. It is, for the most part, as hard as ivory, but in its central and posterior portion is composed of very close cancellous tissue.

A specimen, far surpassing this in size, but resembling it in all its general characters and relations, is in the Museum of the University of Cambridge, and is represented in fig. 77. It is the largest and best specimen of the kind that I have seen, and its osseous structure is distinct; only, as Professor Clark has informed me, it is irregular: in the hardest parts there are neither Haversian canals nor lacunæ; in the less hard parts, the canals are very large, and the lacunæ are not arranged in circles around them; and everywhere the lacunæ are of irregular or distorted forms.

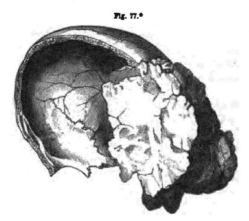

Fig. 77.*

A smaller specimen is in the Museum of St. Bartholomew's Hospital. A girl, twenty years old, was admitted with protrusion of the left eyeball, which appeared due to an osseous growth projecting at the anterior, upper, and inner part of the orbit. None but the anterior boundaries of this growth could be discerned. It had been observed protruding the eye for three years, and had regularly increased; it was still increasing, and produced severe pain in the eyeball, and about the side of the head and face. It seemed, therefore, necessary to attempt the removal of the tumor, or at least to remove some part of it, with the hope that the disturbance of its growth might lead to its necrosis and separation. A portion of it was with great difficulty sawn off; but the patient died with suppuration in the membranes of the anterior part of the cerebrum.

Now all these cases, corroborated as they are by others upon record, prove the general character and relations of these tumors. Their nodular form, and uniform hard, ivory-like texture; their growth in the diploe or sinuses, as isolated or narrowly attached masses; their tendency to extend in all directions; their raising and penetrating the bones of the skull, and growing into the cavities of the skull and orbit; all show the

---

* Fig. 77. Hard bony tumor of the skull: from the Cambridge University Museum.

exceeding difficulty and peril of operations on them. The simpler kinds, that only grow outwards, may indeed be cut off with advantage, though seldom without great difficulty; and, often, the attempt to remove them has been made in vain; but these larger and nodular tumors about the brow can very rarely be either cut off or extirpated.*

The extirpation, however, which may be impossible for art, is some-times effected by disease; these tumors are occasionally removed by sloughing. Such an event happened in a case related by Mr. Hilton;† and the great ivory-like mass, clean sloughed away, is in the Museum at Guy's. So, too, in a case by Mr. Lucas, a bony tumor at the edge of the orbit, after growing eight months, was exposed by an incision through the upper eyelid. The wound did not heal; the tumor continued to grow; and, twelve months afterwards, it became "carious," and was de-tached. The course of treatment which these cases suggest has been, I believe, the only one worth imitation; namely, exposure of the tumor, and application, if need be, of escharotics to the surface of the bone.

These hard, osseous tumors are very rarely found in connection with any bone but those of the skull. In the College Museum, however, is a well-marked specimen in the lower jaw; a nodulated mass, nearly three inches in diameter, invests the right angle of the jaw, and is, in its whole substance, as hard and heavy as ivory. I have already, also, referred to cases of similar hard tumors on the humerus: but they are extremely rare.

Osseous tumors of the lower jaw appear to be less rare in animals in-ferior to man; for the College Museum contains three specimens,‡ taken respectively from a Virginia opossum, a cat, and a kangaroo; and, which is more singular, one from a codfish. In this specimen,§ a disk-shaped mass of bone, two inches in diameter, extremely heavy and compact, is attached to the inner surface of the superior maxillary bone.

In the texture of these very hard, bony tumors connected with the bones of the skull and the lower jaw, we may observe an instance of the general rule or likeness between tumors and the parts most near to them; for their bone is like no other natural bone so much as the internal table of the skull, or the petrous bone, or inferior maxilla.

The same likeness is observable in the osseous tumors that are frequent on the last phalanx of the great toe, which, alone, now remain for me to speak of.‖

No adequate explanation, I believe, can be offered for the occurrence of these growths. They may be sometimes referred to injury; yet the effects of injury to the great toe are so inconstant, that we cannot refer

* The histories of some specimens in the Museum of St. George's Hospital illustrate these statements very well. See, also, Mr. Hawkins's Lectures (Med. Gas., vol. xxi.)
† Guy's Hospital Reports, vol. i.
‡ Nos. 1036-7-8.
§ No. 1039. A similar specimen is in the Museum of the Boston (U. S.) Medical Society.
‖ Mus. Coll. Surg., 787-8-9, 790.

to injury, as other than an indirect cause of the growth of tumors, so singularly constant as these are in all their characters, and so nearly without exception limited to the one toe of all that are exposed to injury. They grow almost always on the margin, and usually on the inner margin, of the end of the last phalanx of the great toe; in only one specimen have I seen such a tumor springing from the middle of the dorsal surface of the phalanx; and, in only two similar tumors from the last phalanx of the little toe. Growing up from the margin, they project under the edge of the nail, lifting it up, and thinning the skin that covers them, till they present an excoriated surface at the side of the nail. Their growth is usually very slow, and when they have reached a diameter of from one-third to one-half of an inch they commonly cease to grow, and become completely osseous. They are among the tumors whose independence is shown not only by abnormal growing, but by the staying of their growth when they have attained a certain natural stature.

I believe that they are not uniform in their method of development. In some specimens I have seen no cartilaginous basis; the bone appeared to form in fibrous tissue, as it were following, and at length overtaking, the fibrous growth. In another, the outer part of the tumor was formed of a thin layer of fibrous tissue, and between this and the growing bone was a layer of cartilage, which had externally the stellate nuclei, and internally the nuclei of ordinary form, among which the processes of bone were extending.

Whichever way the bone is formed, it is, like that of the phalanx itself, cancellous but very hard, and with small spaces, and comparatively thick cancelli or laminæ bounding them. The outer layer, too, is rough and ill-defined, so that the growth looks like a branch from the phalanx, and, like a branch, is apt to sprout again when cut away, unless at least the end of the bone on which it grows be removed with it.

The account of osseous tumors would be very incomplete, if there were not added to it some notice of those growths which are most like them, though they may lie beyond the range of any reasonable or convenient definition of tumors. Among these are certain growths of the bones of the face, tumor-like in their most prominent parts, and yet unlike tumors in that their bases of connection with the bones are very ill-defined, and that from their bases the morbid changes in which themselves originated extend outwards, on the same or even to other bones, gradually subsiding. In no instances can it be plainer than it is in these, that a nosological boundary of "Tumors" must be an arbitrary one.

Such growths as these are not very rare in the superior maxillary bone. Its ascending process may become enlarged and prominent, with an ill-defined hard swelling, very slowly increasing, and sometimes stopping short of any considerable deformity. But a much more formidable disease exists when a large portion of the bone, or the whole antrum, is involved: especially, because this is apt to be associated with diseases in the adjacent bones.

An extreme case is shown in a specimen in the College from the Museum of Mr. Langstaff.* Two large masses of bone, of almost exactly symmetrical form and arrangement, project from the upper jaws and orbits, and have partially coalesced in the median line. They are rounded, deeply-lobed, and nodular; nearly as hard and heavy as ivory: perforated with numerous apertures, apparently for blood-vessels. They project more than three inches in front of the face, and an inch on each side beyond the molar bones; they fill both orbits, the nasal cavities, and probably the antra, and they extend backwards to the pterygoid plates. Part of the septum of the nose, and the alveolar border of the jaw, are almost the only remaining indications of a face. The disease appears to have begun in the superior maxillary bones, and thence to have spread over the bones of the face; similar disease, in a less degree, existing in the bones adjacent to the chief outgrowths.

The patient, who was sixty years old, believed the disease had been eighteen years in progress, and ascribed it to repeated blows on the face. He suffered much pain in the face, eyes, and head. His eyes projected from the orbits: the right, after suppuration and sloughing of the cornea, shriveled; the left was accidentally burst by a blow. During the last two years of his life he occasionally showed symptoms of insanity, and at last he died with apoplexy of the cerebral membranes.

The disease very rarely attains so horrible a state as is here shown. More commonly it is almost limited to the antrum. In this case it may exist with little deformity. In the Museum of St. Bartholomew's Hospital (i. 62), is a specimen in which both the antra appear nearly filled by the thickening and ingrowing of their walls; only small cavities remain at their centres. The new bone is hard, heavy, and nearly solid; yet it is porous or finely cancellous, and is neither so compact nor so smooth on its cut surface as that of the "ivory exostosis." The same disease is manifest in a less degree upon the outer surfaces of the maxillary bones, and on the septum and side-walls of the nose.

The disease has a manifest tendency to concentrate itself in the maxillary bones; so much so, that if a case be met with where only one of these bones is diseased, it may be removed with a fair prospect that the disease will not make progress in the adjacent parts. I believe, indeed, that this has been done, with a satisfactory result, in a case where already slight increase of some of the bones near the maxillary was observable: and there was good reason to anticipate the same result in a case on which Mr. Stanley operated. The patient was a girl, 15 years old, in whom enlargement of the nasal process of the superior maxillary bone had been observed for eight years, and was still increasing. It had as yet produced no pain, and no deformity of the cheek, the orbit, or the palate: but it

* Mus. Coll. Surg. 3236, A.

was regularly increasing; and as it could be certainly expected to increase even more in width of base, than in prominence (this being the common tendency of the disease), it was thought right to remove the superior maxillary bone while yet the disease was limited to it. The patient died, ten days after the operation, with erysipelas. The specimen displays exactly the same disease as do those last described.

Now it sometimes happens that growths like these spontaneously perish, are separated with the ordinary phenomena of necrosis, and thus are naturally cured. Such an event was observed in a case under the care of Mr. Stanley.

A man, 37 years old, was admitted with a slight convex smooth prominence of the nasal process of his right superior maxillary bone, which he had observed increasing for two years, but which of late had not increased or given him any inconvenience. Indeed, he came to the hospital not for this, but for a swelling of the right gum and the mucous membrane of the hard palate, through fistulous openings in which one could feel exposed dead bone. These had existed for a month. The swelling of the nasal process was so characteristic of the disease I am describing, as to suggest, at once, the existence of such a growth; but the suppuration and necrosis threw obscurity on the case; and it was only watched and treated according to such indications as arose, till, after four months, the whole of the mass of bone with which the antrum had been filled up was separated and pulled away.

The appearance of the sequestrum, a nearly spherical mass of hard, heavy, and finely cancellous bone, an inch or more in diameter, leaves no doubt of the nature of the disease.* The great cavity which remained, opening widely into both the mouth and the nose, gradually contracted, or was filled up, and the man recovered perfectly.

A similar event, I imagine, happened in a man who exhibited himself at most of the hospitals in London, two years ago, with a great cavity where all his right upper jaw bone and his turbinated bones had once been, and through which one could see the movements of his pharynx and palate. This he said had been left after the separation of a great tumor of bone.

The growths of this kind seem to merge gradually into elevations of cancellous porous bone, which may be found on various parts of the bones of the skull, but of the exact pathology and relations of which we have, I believe, no clear knowledge. Specimens of them are in the Museum of the College, and the Museum of St. Thomas's Hospital is peculiarly rich in them. In some there are great thickenings of one or both tables of the skull, raising up bosses of new bone from half an inch to an inch in depth, one one or both the parietal bones, or on the occipital or frontal. In some, all the bones of the face are involved in similar changes. In some, similar elevations are produced by growth of bone between the

* The specimen is in the Museum of St. Bartholomew's Hospital.

tables of the skull, which themselves remain healthy. But, as yet, I believe, we can only look at these as strange and uninstructive things.

The last form of bony growths that I shall mention comprises the instances in which numerous exostoses occur in the same patient, and the examples of what has been called the ossific diathesis or dyscrasia. In the large majority of cases, both cartilaginous and osseous tumors occur singly: a few exceptions might be found among such as I have been describing, yet the rule is generally true. But in certain instances a large number of the bones bear outgrowths which, at least in external shape, are like tumors. These are commonly regarded as of constitutional origin. Some, indeed, appear to be so in that sense of constitutional disease, which implies a local manifestation of some morbid condition of the blood; but others can be so called only in that sense, by which we intend some original and inborn error of the formative tendency in certain tissues or organs.

Of these last we may especially observe that the tendency to osseous overgrowths is often hereditary, and that its result is a symmetrical deformity. A boy, six years old, was in St. Bartholomew's Hospital, five years ago, who had symmetrical tumors on the lower ends of his radii, on his humeri, his scapulæ, his fifth and sixth ribs, his fibulæ, and internal malleoli. On each of these bones, on each side, he had one tumor: and the only deviations from symmetry were that he had an unmatched tumor on the ulnar side of the first phalanx of his right forefinger and that each of the tumors on the right side was rather larger than its fellow on the left.

I saw this child's father, a healthy laboring man, 40 years old, who had as many or even more tumors of the same kind as his son; but only a few of them were in the same positions. All these tumors had existed from his earliest childhood; they were symmetrically placed, and ceased to grow when he attained his full stature: since that time they had undergone no apparent change. None of this man's direct ancestors, nor any other of his children, had similar growths; but four cousins, one female and three male, children of his mother's sisters, had as many of them as himself.

The swelling on the little boy's forefinger was an inconvenience to him, and at his parents' request Mr. Lloyd removed the finger. The swelling consisted of an outgrowth or projection of healthy-looking cancellous bone, full of medulla, and coated with a thin layer of compact tissue; its substances being regularly continuous with those of the phalanx itself.

Many similar cases of symmetrical and hereditary osseous outgrowths might, I believe, be adduced;* and all their history suggests that they are to be regarded as related not less closely to malformations, or monstrosities by excessive development, than to the osseous tumors or

* See Mr. Stanley's Treatise on Diseases of Bones, p. 152; and Mr. Hawkins's Lectures on Tumors of Bones (Medical Gazette, vol. xxv. p. 474).

outgrowths of which I have been speaking. Indeed, at this point the
pathology of tumors concurs with that of congenital excesses of development and growth.

We must distinguish from these cases the instances of multiple ossifications of tendons, muscles, and other tissues, that are occasionally met
with; for these only imperfectly imitate the forms of tumors, and are
probably connected with such a morbid condition of the blood as really
may deserve the name of ossific dyscrasia or diathesis.

Before ending, it may be proper to point out the chief distinctions
between the osseous tumors, and those growths which are connected with
other tumors springing from the bones; for, under the vague name of
osteo-sarcoma, many include together, and seem to identify, all growths
in which bone is mingled with a softer tissue.

The growths that may chiefly need distinction are those of osteoid
cancers, and the bony skeletons of certain medullary tumors of bone.
Osteoid cancers are probably examples of firm, or hard, or fibrous cancers,
ossified: and the best marked among them present an abundant formation of peculiarly hard bone. The distinctions usually to be observed
between these hard osteoid cancers and the hard osseous tumors are
mainly in these particulars :—(a) the osteoid mass, in its mid-substance,
may be compared with chalk, the osseous with ivory; the one is dull
and powdery, the other bright and wholly void of friability; (b) the
osteoid is new bone infiltrated, as it were, in some softer tissue, or in the
tissues of the original bone, which disappear as it increases; the hard
osseous tumor is a distinct growth, attached in a comparatively small
part of its extent to the bone on which it grows; (c) the outer surface of
an osteoid growth is porous and rough, and, if laminated, its laminæ have
their edges directed outwards; (d) lastly, the minute characters of bone
are far less perfect in the osteoid than the osseous growth : bone-corpuscles
existing, indeed, but small, round, irregular, with very small, if any,
canaliculi, and imbedded in a porous, chalky-looking, basis-substance.

And, 2dly, for distinction between the softer osseous skeletons of
medullary cancers, and the cancellous osseous tumors, we may chiefly
observe that, (a) the bone in cancers is more dry and friable than the
cancellous bone of the osseous tumors; and (b) the bone in cancerous
growths has no medulla, the interspaces between its laminæ being filled
with cancerous matter ; while medulla is a constant constituent, I believe,
of all the cancellous osseous tumors.

Such are the chief differences generally to be observed between the
bone of innocent and that of malignant tumors ; differences which it is
well to establish, since the fact is sufficiently confusing, that any normal
tissue should be formed in subordination to the growth of cancers. The
subject will be again adverted to in the lecture on Osteoid Cancer.

LECTURE XXIX.

PART I.

GLANDULAR TUMORS.

WE may call those tumors "glandular" which, in their structure, imitate the glands; whether the secreting glands, or those organs which we name glands, because, though having no open ducts, they are of analogous structure.

The most frequent example of these glandular tumors is the kind which imitates, and occurs in or near, the mammary gland; the chronic mammary tumor of Sir A. Cooper; the pancreatic tumor of Mr. Abernethy;* the fibrous tumor of the breast of M. Cruveilhier.† Other tumors of the same general kind are more rarely found in the lips, and in or near the prostrate and the thyroid glands. Probably, too, some other tumors, to which no name, or a wrong one, has been hitherto assigned, may yet have to be placed in this group: indeed, I think it nearly certain that there are lymphatic gland-growths, which we usually regard as enlarged glands, but which are really new growths, of the nature of tumors, even in the most limited sense of the term. At present, however, I will have in view only such gland-tumors as may be clearly recognized; namely, such as the mammary glandular tumor, the labial, the prostatic, and the thyroid.

Some of the pathology of these tumors has been already sketched in the account of the glandular proliferous cysts (p. 323 and 358). To that account I may again refer, so far as to the point at which it is believed that an intra-cystic growth has completely filled the cyst in which its growth began, and has coalesced with the walls, so as to form a solid tumor (p. 359).

Now it is perhaps probable that all glandular tumors may be formed after this plan: for, in those occurring in the breast, we find sometimes one circumscribed mass, composed, half of a proliferous cyst, and half of a solid glandular tumor;‡ sometimes two such growths lie apart, yet in the same gland (fig. 49); and often, we find such structures as we doubt whether to call proliferous cysts nearly filled, or mammary tumors (fig. 51).

However, if all the mammary and other glandular tumors are thus of intra-cystic origin, it must be admitted that many of them very early lose the cystic form, and continue to grow as solid masses; for we find

---

* The mammary tumor described by Mr. Abernethy was probably a medullary cancerous disease.

† Anatomie Pathol. liv. xxvi. pl. 1; and Bulletin de l'Académie de Médecine, to ix. p. 429.

‡ Mus. Coll. Surg., 177–8.

them solid even when they are very small; and they are traced growing from year to year, yet apparently maintaining always the same texture.

I shall speak now of the solid tumors alone; and, first, of the Mammary Glandular Tumors.

Sir Astley Cooper may be said to have had a good insight into their nature, when he called them "chronic mammary," and said they were "as if nature had formed an additional portion of the breast, composed of similar lobes."* The analogy of their structure was also recognised by Mr. Lawrence.† But I believe nothing more than this general likeness had been observed, till these tumors were examined with the microscope by M. Lebert,‡ who found in them the minute glandular structure imitative of ·the mammary gland, and recognized many of their relations to the proliferous cysts. Mr. Birkett,§ by independent and contemporary observations, made on the great collection of these tumors in Guy's Hospital, confirmed and extended the conclusions of M. Lebert, and has cleared up much of the obscurity that existed previous to his inquiries. Both these gentlemen apply such terms as "Imperfect Hypertrophy of the mammary gland" to these tumors: but, highly as I esteem their observations (and not the less, I hope, because they corrected errors of my own),‖ I would rather not adopt their nomenclature, since, if we do not call these "tumors" I hardly know to what innocent growths the term could be applied. Nearly all innocent growths are imperfect hypertrophies, in the same sense as these growths are; nay, these are, in many respects, the very types of the diseases to which the name of tumors is by general consent ascribed, and which can be distinguished, even in verbal definition, from what are more commonly regarded as hypertrophies.

The mammary glandular tumors may be found in any part of the breast; over, or beneath, or within the gland, or at its border. Their most rare seat is beneath the gland; their most common at its upper and inner part, imbedded in, or just beneath, its surface. They are usually loosely connected with the gland, except at their deepest part, where their capsules are generally fastened to it; but the connection is of so

* On Diseases of the Breast, p. 54.

† On Tumors; in Med.-Chir. Trans., vol. xvii. p. 29. It seems only just to observe that this recognition of the obvious resemblance between the structure of these tumors and that of the mammary gland was almost always sufficient, after the description by Sir A. Cooper, to enable the surgeons of this country to avoid the confusion between the "chronic mammary" tumors and the cancers of the breast, which M. Lebert describes as still prevalent in France, notwithstanding his own clear description of the points of diagnosis.

‡ Physiologie Pathologque, t. ii. p. 201.

§ On the Diseases of the Breast, p. 124.

‖ In the Catologues of the Museums of the College and of St. Bartholomew's Hospital these tumors are classed with the fibro-cellular. In most of the specimens that I had examined the fibro-cellular tissue was very abundant, and I thought too lightly of the glandular tissue which I found mingled with it.

small extent that they slide very easily under the finger, and are peculiarly movable in all directions.

The tumor is commonly of oval shape; superficially, or sometimes deeply, lobed or nodular; firm, or nearly hard, elastic, and often feeling like a cyst tensely filled with fluid. The parts around appear quite healthy. The mammary gland is pushed aside; but it undergoes no other change than that of atrophy, even when stretched over a tumor of the largest size. The skin under distension may grow slightly livid, but else is unchanged. The veins, if the growth of the tumor be rapid, may be dilated over it, as over or near a cancer of the breast. The tumor is usually invested with a complete capsule, isolating it from the surrounding mammary gland, and often adhering less to it than to the gland. This capsule may appear only as a layer of fibro-cellular tissue, like that round any other innocent tumor; but it is not unfrequently more perfectly organized in layers, and smoother on its inner surface; conditions that we may perhaps ascribe to its having been a perfect cyst within which the glandular growth originated, and which the growth has only lately filled.

On section, these tumors present a lobed construction, in which it is sometimes not difficult to discern the remains, or the imitation of the plan, of the lobed, or foliated and involuted intra-cystic growths. In some the fibro-cellular partitions among the lobes converge towards the centre of the mass, as if they were the remains of clustered cyst-walls; or, there may remain a cavity in the centre of the tumor, as if clustered cysts and growths had not quite filled up the space. In some, however, no such plan is discernible; the whole mass is disorderly lobed, and its lobes have the shapes derived from accidental mutual pressure, and are bounded by loose fibro-cellular partitions.

In structure as in construction, these tumors may present several variations; but they may be artificially arranged in three or four chief groups.

Some are really very like the normal mammary gland in an inactive state. These have a pure opaque-white, and soft, but tough and elastic tissue; they are lobed, and minutely lobulated, with undulating white fibres. Such an one is well shown in a specimen from Sir Astley Cooper's collection,* in which, moreover, his injection of the blood-vessels shows a moderate vascularity, about equal to that of the surrounding normal gland-substance.

We might take such as this as the examples of the medium form of this kind of tumor; and the other chief or extreme forms are represented by those which deviate from this in two directions. In one direction we find much softer tumors;† these, though closely textured, are soft, brittle, and easily crushed; their cut surfaces shine, or look vitreous or half

---

* Mus. Coll. Surg., No. 2772. In this specimen there is also a peculiar warty growth in the skin over the tumor.　　　　　† Such as No. 2774 in the College Museum.

translucent; they are uniformly grayish-white, or have a slight yellowish or pink hue, which deepens on exposure to the air; or they may look like masses of firm, but flickering jelly; and commonly we can press from them a thin yellowish fluid, like serum or synovia. Such as these have the usual lobed and lobular plan of construction; and I think the intersecting partitions commonly extend from a firm, fibrous-looking central or deep part, towards the circumference of the tumor.

In the other direction from the assumed average or medium form, we find firmer tumors. These have a drier and tougher texture; they are opaque, milk-white, or yellowish, like masses of dense fibro-cellular tissue, lobed, and having their lobes easily separable; as in the great specimen, weighing seven pounds, in the College Museum (No. 208).

To such as these varieties we might add many, due not merely to intermediate forms, but to the degrees in which the intra-cystic mode of growth is manifested; or to the development of cysts, which may take place as well in this new gland-tissue as in the old; or to the various contents of the cysts, whether liquids or organized growths.*

I believe we cannot at present always connect these various aspects of the tumors with any corresponding varieties in their histories. Neither, I think, have any investigations proved more of the corresponding varieties of microscopic structure, than that, as a general rule, the tougher any tumor is, and the slower its growth has been, the more it has

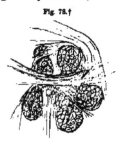

Fig. 78.†

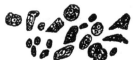

of the fibro-cellular, mingled with its glandular, tissue; while the more succulent and vitreous one is, and the more rapid its growth, the less perfectly is the glandular tissue developed.

The microscopic structures may be best described from a medium specimen: from such an one I made these illustrative sketches. The patient was 33 years old; the tumor had been noticed seven months, and was ascribed to a blow; it was painful at times and increasing; and it had the several characters that I have already described. The patient has remained well since its removal.

In such a tumor one finds in thin sections, traces of a minute lobular or acinous form; the miniature, we might say, of that which we see with the naked eye. The lobules may be merely

---

* I believe these include the chief examples of Müller's Cysto-sarcomata. One of these tumors containing simple cysts would constitute his cysto-sarcoma simplex: the cysts being proliferous with gland growths would make his cysto-sarcoma phyllodes.

† Fig. 78. Minute structures of a mammary glandular tumor, described in the text: magnified 350 times. The microscopic examinations of several specimens may be found in Lebert (Phys. Pathol. ii. 190; and Abhandlungen, p. 269): Birkett, On the Diseases of the Breast, pl. 2, 3, 4, &c.; and Bennet, On Cancerous and Cancroid Growths, p. 52.

placed side by side, with little or no intervening tissue; their form may appear to depend on the arrangement of their contents, and these may seem scarcely bounded by membrane. But, I think, more commonly, especially in the firmer specimens, the plan of lobules or acini is mapped-out by partitions of filamentous-looking tissue, fasciculi of which, curving and variously combined, appear to arch over, and to bound, each acinus or lobule. But great varieties appear in the quantity of this tissue; it may be nearly absent, or it may so predominate as to obscure the traces of the essential glandular structure.

This proper gland-structure consists of minute nucleated cells and nuclei, clustered in the lobular form, or in that of cylinders or tubes, and often, or perhaps always in their most natural state, invested with a simple, pellucid, limitary membrane.

Thus, the likeness is striking between the structure of such a tumor and that of an inactive mammary gland, such as that of a male, as Mr. Birkett has pointed out. We have here what may be compared with the round or oval cæcal terminations of the gland-tubes clustered together and often seeming grouped about one trunk-tube; and in these we have the simple membrane and the gland-cells and nuclei within; only, the main duct is wanting, and the communication with the ducts of the proper gland. It is as if the proper secreting structure of a gland were formed without connection with an excretory tube; the tumor is, in this respect, like one of the glands without ducts.

The mammary glandular tumors are singularly variable in all the particulars of their life. They sometimes grow quickly; as did the largest figured by Sir. A. Cooper, which, in two years, acquired a weight of a pound and a half. In other cases their growth is very slow: I have known one* which, in four years, had not become so much as an inch in diameter. In some instances they remain quite stationary, even for many years. One† was removed from a woman 27 years old: it was observed for 14 years, and in all that time it scarcely enlarged; yet after this it grew so rapidly, that in six months, it was thought imprudent to delay the removal. Cases of this arrest or extreme retardation of growth must have been seen by most surgeons; but there are few cases so striking as one related by M. Cruveilhier, in which a lady had, for more than 20 years, three of these tumors in one breast, and one in the other. She died in consequence of the treatment employed against them, and after death no similar disease was found in any other part.

Equal variations exist in regard to pain. Commonly these tumors are painless; but sometimes they are the seats and sources of intense suffering; even of all that suffering which is popularly ascribed to cancer, but which cancer in its early stages so very rarely presents. The irritable tumor of the breast, as Sir A. Cooper named it, was in most of his cases

* Museum of St. Bartholomew's, Ser. xxxiv. No. 23.   † Mus. Coll. Surg., 207 ʙ.

a mammary glandular tumor;* and the character of the pain, like that of the painful subcutaneous tumor (p. 394), is such as we may name neuralgic.

A tumor,† evidently glandular, was taken from the breast of a woman 25 years old, where it had been growing for two years; it had often been the seat of the most intense pain. I referred to a similar case while speaking of neuralgic tumors (p. 396), and I removed a similar tumor from the breast of a young lady, who begged for its removal only that she might be relieved from severe suffering. In all these cases the minute glandular structure was well marked.

A peculiarity of these tumors is, that they not unfrequently disappear; an event very rarely paralleled in any other tumor. They are most likely to do this in cases in which any imperfection of the uterine or ovarian functions, in which they may have seemed to have their origin, is repaired by marriage, or pregnancy, or lactation. And the fact is very suggestive: since, in many cases, it appears as if the discontinuous hypertrophy, which constitutes the tumor, were remedied by the super-vention of a continuous hypertrophy for the discharge of increased functions of the gland.

On the other side, these tumors often continue to grow indefinitely and they may thus attain an enormous size. One was removed by Mr. Stanley, which, after twelve years' progress, in a middle-aged woman, measured nearly twelve inches in length, and weighed seven pounds. It was pendulous; and, as she sat, she used to rest it on her knee, till the integuments began to slough. Mr. Stanley merely sliced it off, cutting through the pedicle of skin; and the patient remained well for at least seven years. The tumor was one of the firmest and most filamentous of the kind.‡

In the College Museum is a tumor§ of the same kind, but softer and much more succulent, which was removed by Mr. Liston from a woman 44 years old, and which weighed twelve pounds.

Respecting the origin of these tumors, little more, I believe, can be said than that, occurring most commonly in young unmarried or barren women, their beginning often seems connected with defective or dis-ordered menstruation. The law which, if we may so speak, binds to-gether in sympathy of nutrition the ovaries and the mammary glands, the law according to which they concur in their development and action, is not broken by one with impunity to the other. The imperfect office of the ovary is apt to be associated with erroneous nutrition in the mam-mary gland.

I have seen only one specimen of the mammary glandular tumor in a male. A portion of it was sent to me by Mr. Sympson, and its characters

---

* Under the same name, however, he included some that were more probably "Painful subcutaneous Tubercles:" see his pl. viii. figs. 2, 4, 5, 7.

† Mus. St. Bartholomew's Hospital, Ser. xxxiv. No. 22.

‡ Mus. Coll. Surg., No. 208.   § Mus. Coll. Surg., No, 216.

were well marked. It was removed by Mr. Hawden, from a country-man, 25 years old, in whom it had been growing irregularly, and oc-casionally diminishing or disappearing, for about five years. When re-moved, it formed a circular, flattened, and slightly lobulated tumor, $3\frac{1}{4}$ inches in diameter, and an inch in thickness, invested with a distinct fibro-cellular capsule, which loosely connected it to the adjacent tissues.

There are, I believe, no facts to suggest that the glandular tumors are, as a rule, other than innocent. More than one may grow in a breast at the same or several successive times; but I have not known of more than three either at once or in succession. Neither am I aware of any facts which prove what is commonly believed, that, after a time, these tumors may become cancerous. Such things may happen; and, on the whole, one might expect, that if a woman have a tumor of this kind in her breast, cancer would be more apt to affect it as a morbid piece of gland, than to affect the healthy gland. But, I repeat, I know no facts to support this; and some that I have met with are against it. Thus, in the Museum of St. Bartholomew's, is a portion of breast,* from a young woman 32 years old, in which there lie, far apart, a small mam-mary glandular tumor that had existed four years, and a hard cancer that had existed four months. A second specimen† shows a hard cancer and a proliferous cyst, in the breast of a patient, who died some time after its removal with recurrence of the cancer. A third case, just like the first, was under Mr. Stanley's care. In these cases, at least, the tumor was not selected as the seat for cancer; and I believe that they are not counterbalanced by any of an opposite kind.

And yet, while all the characters of innocent tumors are generally, if not always, observed in these, there are facts concerning a seeming connection between mammary glandular tumors and cancer which must not be passed by here; though they may need to be again stated in the last lectures on cancer.

It has sometimes happened that a glandular tumor has been removed from a breast, and, within a short time, the same breast has become the seat of cancer.‡ I believe that the explanation of such cases as these may be, that a woman, prone to cancer by some constitutional condition, or, especially, by hereditary disposition, had (as any other might) a glan-dular tumor in her breast; and that the operation for removing this tumor inflicted a local injury, and made the breast apt to be the seat of cancer, of which already (as one may say) the germ existed in the blood. Such events may prove only an accidental connection between the glan-dular tumors and the cancer; but they are enough to suggest great caution in operating on the breasts of those who may be suspected to be, by inheritance, peculiarly liable to cancer.

* Ser. xxxiv. No. 17.   † Mus. St Bartholomew's Hospital, Ser. xxxiv. No. 16.
‡ See such a case, by Mr. Erichsen, in the Lancet, Feb. 14, 1852; and the history of a series of preparations in the Catalogue of the Museum of St. Bartholomew's. vol. i. p. 446.

But, again, cases sometimes occur in which, I think, the mammary glandular tumors supply examples of what I have already suggested as, probably, a general truth: namely, that the children of a cancerous parent, or those in whose family cancer is prone to occur, are apt to have tumors which may be like innocent tumors in their structure, but may resemble cancers in a peculiar rapidity of growth and a proneness to ulceration and recurrence after removal. A striking instance of this occurred in Mr. Lawrence's practice. He removed the breast of a lady from one of whose sisters Mr. Ashton Key had removed a breast said to be affected with "fungoid" disease, whose mother had died with well-marked hard cancer of the breast, and in other members of whose family cases of cancer were believed to have occurred. The breast removed by Mr. Lawrence comprised a huge sloughing and ulcerating mass of yellowish, soft, flickering substance, like the softest of these mammary glandular tumors, or like the very soft pellucid growths which I have described as occurring in some of the proliferous cysts of the breast. The diseased state of the mass (in consequence of escharotics having been recklessly used) was such, that minute examination showed little more than the absence of distinct cancer-structures. During the healing of the wound, and for some months after it, fresh growths repeatedly appeared. Some of these which I examined were yellow, pellucid, soft, viscid, almost like lumps of mucus, or of half-melted gelatine, imbedded in the tissues of the integuments or scar. With the microscope I found only granules and granule-masses with elongated nuclei, themselves also granular, set in abundant pellucid substance. I found no sign of cancer-structure or gland-structure. The substance resembled that which I have mentioned (p. 362) as found in some imperfect proliferous mammary cysts.

Now, after repeated removals of such growths as these, the wounds completely healed, and the patient has remained well, and in good general health, for eighteen months.

At nearly the same time, a third sister of this family was under Mr. Lawrence's care; and he removed one of her breasts in which was a great mass, which had grown quickly, and was chiefly composed of well-marked grandular tissue, either in separate solid growths, or inclosed in proliferous cysts. But some parts also of this tumor were soft, pellucid, and gelatinous; and others were as soft, but opaque and dimly yellow. In the firmer parts, the glandular texture was as distinct with the microscope as with the naked eye: in the softer parts no such structures were seen, but abundant free cells and nuclei, of most various and apparently disorderly shapes; some elongated, like small shriveled fibro-cells; some flattened, like small epithelial cells. I would not venture on an opinion of what these were or indicated: I think they were not cancerous, that the disease has not returned. The main fact of all the cases is, and three daughters of a cancerous mother had mammary tumors; in two, at least, of them the structure was probably not cancerous; and yet the rapid growth, the recurrence in one of them, and the defective or disordered modes of growth in both, were such as marked a wide deviation from the common rules of mammary glandular or any other innocent tumors, and a deviation in the direction towards cancer.

LABIAL GLANDULAR TUMORS may be briefly described, for their general characters correspond closely with those of the foregoing kind; or, they may appear intermediate in character between the foregoing and those tumors which I described as lying over or near the parotid gland, and as consisting of mixed glandular and cartilaginous tissue. Their likeness to these tumors over the parotid was manifest to Mr. Lawrence, who has added to his account of the tumors by the parotid, the only case of labial glandular tumor that I have found on record.[*]

The most marked case of labial glandular tumor that I have seen was that of a healthy-looking man lately under the care of Mr. Lloyd. A tumor had been growing in his upper lip for twelve years. It was not painful, but the protrusion of the lip was inconvenient and ugly, the swelling being an inch in diameter. It was imbedded in the very substance of the lip, both the skin and mucous membrane being tensely stretched over it. Its form was nearly hemispherical, its posterior surface being flattened as it lay close on the gums and teeth, its anterior convex and smooth. Its whole substance was firm, tense, and elastic.

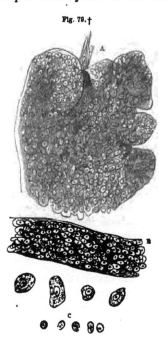

Fig. 79.[†]

Mr. Lloyd removed the tumor with the mucous membrane over it, leaving the skin entire. The tumor was firm, slightly lobed, yellowish-white, smooth. In general aspect, it resembled the mixed tumors over the parotid, but in minute structure it presented as perfect an imitation of lobulated or acinous gland-structure as any mammary glandular tumor. Its tubes and their dilated ends had distinct limitary membrane, and were filled with nuclei and nucleated cells, like those of the labial glands (fig. 79). I heard some

* Medico-Chirurgical Transactions, vol. xvii. p. 28.

† Fig. 79. A, structure like the cæcal terminations of gland-ducts in an acinus; B. a separate portion of gland-like tube; c, separate gland-cells, and free nuclei; from the labial glandular tumor described in the text. A and B, magnified 300 times; c, magnified 400 times.

months afterwards that another tumor was growing in the same lip; but
the patient was lost sight of.   Such a recurrence, even if it rarely happened, would be no sufficient evidence of malignancy.

I removed a similar tumor from the upper lip of a man about 30 years
old.   It had been regularly growing for four years without pain, and
projected far externally, reaching to the same distance as the end of his
nose.   This had a texture of glandular kind, but less distinctly marked
than that in the former case.   Moreover, in the centre of the mass was
a portion of bone; a peculiarity which existed also in Mr. Lawrence's
case, and which may add to the probability of relationship between
these tumors and the mixed glandular and cartilaginous tumors over the
parotid.

Lastly, I may again refer to a specimen in the Museum of St. George's
Hospital, in which, in one tumor, a cyst and what looks like one of these
glandular growths are combined (see p. 362).

PROSTATIC GLANDULAR TUMORS were briefly referred to in the first
lecture (p. 328), as examples of the abnormal growths by which tumors
appear to be connectd with simple hypertrophies of organs; and I can
add little to what was then said of them.

We owe to Rokitansky* the knowledge that the tumors in the prostate
gland, which were commonly, and till lately even by himself, regarded
as fibrous tumors, are composed of tissues like those of the prostate gland
itself.   In enlarged prostates they are not unfrequently found.   In cutting through the gland, one may see, amidst its generally lobed structure,
portions which are invested and isolated by fibro-cellular tissue, and may
be enucleated.   Such portions have, I believe, been sometimes removed
tumors, or as portions of prostrate gland, in operations of lithotomy.
They lie embedded in the enlarged prostate, as, sometimes, mammary
glandular tumors lie isolated in a generally enlarged breast.   They look
like the less fasciculate of the fibrous tumors of the uterus: but, to microscopic examination, they present such an imitation of the proper structure of the prostrate itself, that we cannot distinguish the gland-cell or
the smooth muscular fibres of the tumor from those of the adjacent portions of the gland.   Only their several modes of arrangement may be
distinctive.

At present the examinations of these tumors have been too few to furnish a complete history of them: neither can I add any cases or references to those which were adduced in the first lecture.

The THYROID GLANDULAR TUMORS were similarly referred in the same
lecture.   Their history is merged in that of bronchoceles, with which
they are usually associated, whether imbedded as distinct masses in the
enlarged gland, or lying close by it, but discontinuous.   Yet I suspect

* Ueber die Cyste, 1849; and, Anatomie des Kropfes.

that similar growths, of substance like thyroid gland, may occur, as tumors, further from the normal mass of the gland.

Mr. Stanley removed a tumor from the neck of a woman 62 years old. It had been observed for 50 years; for the first 30 of which it was like a little loose "kernel" under the skin, and scarcely increased. In the next ten years it grew more quickly, and in the next ten more quickly still; and now, the skin over it ulcerated, and it protruded and occasionally bled, but was never painful. It looked like an ulcerated sebaceous cyst, seated upon the subcutaneous tissue at the lower part of the neck, just in front of the trapezius. No cause could be assigned for it.

On section it appeared as a solid tumor with a thin fibro-cellular capsule, partitions entering from which divided it into distinct round lobes. Its proper substance was soft, elastic, glistening, yellowish, blotched and streaked with brownish pink and blood colors. It was, to the naked eye, like a piece of bronchocele, with such an arrangement of its parts as would exist when numerous cysts are filled with the glandular growth, and compacted. And the general impression hence derived was confirmed by microscopic examination, which showed that the tumor consisted, chiefly, of round and oval bodies, or minute sacculi, from $\frac{1}{160}$ to $\frac{1}{150}$ of an inch in diameter, filled or lined with nucleated substance, or with nuclei imbedded in a dimly molecular blastema, and not nucleolated. These bodies were closely apposed, but frequently appeared separated by thin filaments, or fibro-cellular partitions. The nuclei were very uniform, circular, about $\frac{1}{1600}$ of an inch in diameter, and in general aspect like the nuclei of vascular glands or lymph-glands. Numerous similar nuclei appeared free; and some appeared imbedded in a dimly molecular blastema, which was not enclosed in cysts or sacculi, nor divided by fibro-cellular partitions.

I have seen no other tumor like this; nor any natural texture that it resembled, except the thyroid gland. Future observations must prove whether thyroid glandular tumors can be formed so far from the normal gland, with the cervical fascia, great blood-vessels of the neck, and other adjacent parts intervening between them.

LECTURE XXIX.

PART II.

ERECTILE OR VASCULAR TUMORS.

THE ERECTILE OR VASCULAR TUMORS include most of the diseases which are described as vascular nævi, and of which the types are the subcutaneous nævi. Among them, also, are the growths to which John

Bell gave the name of aneurism by anastomosis, and those which have been called Telangeiectasis.

The name "erectile tumor" has, of late years, come into general use, as expressing a principal fact concerning these diseases, namely, that many of them resemble very closely in their texture that of erectile or cavernous tissue. Mr. Humphry[*] has, indeed, rightly objected to the use of the term, that these tumors present no imitation of the erectile tissue in the power of filling themselves with blood, as if by some internal force. But, since this occurrence in the true erectile tissue depends as much on the accessory structures of nerves and muscles as on the tissue itself, we may fairly apply the term "erectile" to the tumors: remembering only this, as for other structures occurring in tumors, that the imitation of the natural tissue is imperfect, or partial. However, if any be scrupulous in the use of these terms, they may call these tumors vascular, or cavernous, or even Telangeiectasis.

The likeness which these tumors bear to the erectile tissue, as exemplified in the corpus cavernosum penis, is sometimes, in general appearance, perfect. A well-marked specimen is in the Hunterian collection, from which the adjoining sketch was made (fig. 80). It was removed from under the lower jaw, and its cut surface displays a close network or spongy of fine, smooth, shining bands and cords, just like those of the corpus cavernosum penis, only less regular in their arrangement. The opportunities of examining such tumors in the recent state are very rare; and they are usually spoiled by the operations for removing them; but what I have seen, and the descriptions which others have recorded, leave little doubt that the imitation of erectile tissue is a frequent character among them.

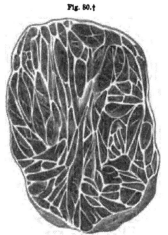

Fig. 80.[†]

John Bell's account[§] of the aneurism by anastomosis, which is by far the most vivid and exact, in relation to the history of the disease, that has yet been published, accords with this statement. Although he has chiefly in view the arterial variety of these tumors, yet of one he says,— "The substance of it was cellular, stringy, and exactly resembling the corpora cavernosa penis . . . the cells were filled with blood from the arteries, which entered the tumor in all directions." Another he exe-

pares to a sponge soaked in blood; and the descriptions of other examples, though less explicit, imply the same. The descriptions by Mr. Wardrop[*] and Mr. Cæsar Hawkins,[†] and the more minute accounts of structure by Mr. Goodsir,[‡] and Mr. Liston,[§] and Rokitansky,[||] confirm this view; and neither Mr. Birkett's[¶] nor any other that I have met with, is discordant from it.

The essential structures of the disease are, according to these descriptions, derived from such a growth of blood-vessels, or rather of blood-species, that, in imitation of erectile tissue, the whole mass seems formed of cells or spaces, opening widely into one another: and, in extreme cases, no remains exist of the walls of the vessels, except those narrow bands and cords that bound and intersect the cell-like spaces.[**]

The division, often made, of erectile or vascular tumors into such as are named, respectively, "arterial," "capillary," and "venous," is convenient, and probably well-founded. The most frequent examples of subcutaneous nævi, and the more frequent superficial nævi, which are like them in structure, though different in position, appear to consist, mainly, of closely arranged minute blood-vessels, of which some are as small and as simple as medium-sized capillaries, while others, of various size, appear as dilated capillaries, or as small arteries and veins densely clustered, but in just proportions to one another. These are such as may be called "capillary;" understanding, only, that they probably affect minute arteries and veins as well as capillaries. But, on the one hand, deviating from these specimens, we find that in some cases, the enlargement of arteries far exceeds, in proportion, that of the veins; the swellings pulsate, and are florid and over-warm, and, if injured, throw out arterial blood. These constitute the "arterial" form of the disease: the "aneurism by anastomosis." And, on the other hand, are tumors formed mainly of dilated, sacculated, and overgrowing veins; to these, arteries of comparatively small size pass, while from them proceed very large veins: and they are subject to changes of size in all the events that affect, not the arterial, but the venous, part of the circulation.

Now, I believe that, in a majority of cases, the arterial and the venous forms of the disease are constituted by a dilatation of large branches, of one or the other kind, being superadded to such a condition of the small vessels and capillaries as exists in the common, or "capillary" erectile tumors. But I have, also, no doubt that, in rarer instances, arterial

---

[*] Med.-Chir. Trans., vol. ix. p. 201, and pl. vi.

[†] Medical Gazette, vol. xxxvii. p. 1027.

[‡] Northern Journ. of Medicine.   [§] Med.-Chir. Trans., vol. xxvi. p. 125.

[||] Pathologische Anatomie, i. 276.   [¶] Med.-Chir. Trans., vol. xxx. p. 193.

[**] What tissue may remain between the blood-vessels depends on the seat of the nævus. The elements of the organ or tissue in which it has its seat will remain between its vessels, wasted or altered by compression or defective nutrition. They are seldom present in any distinct form; but a case is well described by C. O. Weber, in which abundant fibrous and fatty tissue occupied the space between the dilated vessels of an erectile tumor in a child's neck (Müller's Archiv, p. 74.)

tumors are formed by arteries alone, convoluted or anastomosing in a heap, whence, as from an arterial "rete mirabile," normal arteries proceed and lead to capillaries. And, on the other hand, there are, doubtless, venous tumors, which are formed of veins alone, and through which, since they are seated altogether beyond capillaries, the blood passes (according to Rokitansky's comparison) as it passes through a portal vein.

Since few accounts of the minute characters of the erectile tumors have been published, I will briefly describe those which I have examined, beginning with an instance of the medium form, in a capillary subcutaneous nævus.*

A child, two years old, which had a nævus of this kind on the side of the chest, died exceedingly emaciated after measles and diarrhœa. The tumor had grown from birth-time, and had appeared as one of the most ordinary subcutaneous nævi or erectile tumors; soft, compressible, dimly blue as seen through the skin, swelling in forced expiration, thinly scarred over its centre, in consequence of an ulcer which had spontaneously formed and healed. After death it had shrunk into a very thin layer of brownish tissue between the emaciated skin and the fascia covering the serratus magnus. It was well defined, and could be dissected out cleanly from the adjacent parts. Its surfaces and sections had a distinct lobular arrangement, many lobes projecting from its borders, and those within it being separated by fibro-cellular partitions derived from the tough skin and fascia between which the tumor lay. In its shrunken state, it most resembled, in its obvious characters, a piece of parotid gland; being pale brown in color, lobulated, soft, but tough, and yielding but little blood on pressure.

About six small collapsed veins proceeded, in a tortuous course, from the surfaces and borders of the tumor. Its arteries were too small to be distinct. Examined with the microscope, the whole mass appeared composed of blood-vessels interlacing in fibro-cellular and elastic tissue, which probably belonged to the natural subcutaneous structure. No parenchymal cells or abnormal forms of tissue were found; the disease seemed to be of the blood-vessels exclusively.

The vessels, which were very difficult to extricate, in any length, from the matted tissue about them, were of all sizes, from $\frac{1}{1000}$ to $\frac{1}{80}$ of an inch in diameter; but I think none were larger. Nearly all of them were cylindriform: a few were unequal, or varicose, or sacculated, with small pouches projecting from their walls (fig. 81). I could not discern their arrangement; but they did not appear to branch often; neither am I sure that they differed in structure from the normal vessels of subcutaneous tissue, except in that they were, considering their size, of less complex structure: they were as if minute vessels were enlarged without acquiring the perfect form of those which they equalled in calibre. In

* All the specimens described are in the Museum of St. Bartholomew's Hospital.

some parts, I found long cords of fibro cellular tissue, which, probably,
were obliterated blood-vessels.

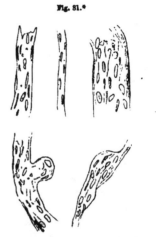

Fig. 81.*

I have examined other tumors resembling this but in less favorable
conditions. From all, however, as well
as from the descriptions of others, I believe the common structure of this form
of erectile tumor is a collection of
minute blood-vessels, dilated, and closely arranged within a limited area of
some natural texture. In the subcutaneous tissue, arteries usually appear to
pass into the vascular mass from the
under surface of the skin; and veins
radiate from it, larger than the arteries
and more numerous, but scarcely exceeding the proportion between the
normal cutaneous veins and arteries.
Within the tumor (which thus, as well
by the relation of its vessels as by their minuteness, justifies the epithet
"capillary") it is probable that some of the vessels are always sacculated
or varicose. Virchow's[†] account of this state exactly confirms what I
have described; and, with more detail, Robin[‡] describes an erectile tumor
in which, along the track of the vessels, numerous little culs-de-sac existed, which the blood might be made at will to enter and quit, by alter-
nately pressing and letting-free a piece of the tumor on the field of the
microscope. These could be seen on vessels as small as $\frac{1}{4}$ of a millime-
tre in diameter; they were generally smaller at their connection with
the vessels than at their other ends, and were commonly twice as long as
the vessels were wide.

But although the vessels within the tumor be thus dilated, yet, as a
general rule, in this form of the disease, the dilatation (if there be any
in those proceeding to and from the tumor,) extends but a short distance
from it: the arteries enlarge (if at all) only just before they enter the
tumor; the veins regain their calibre soon after they leave it: and
hence the general safety with which John Bell and many others have cut
out such tumors, when they attended to the rule he lays down with such
emphatic repetition, that in treating such a tumor we are "not to cut
into it, but to cut it out." However, this limitation of enlargement to
the vessels within and near the tumor, is not so usually observed in the
next two forms of the disease, as in this which I have just described.

* Blood-vessels of the erectile tumor described in the text. Magnified about 200 times.
† Archiv. für Pathol. Anatomie, B. iii. p. 437.
‡ In Lebert; Physiologie Pathologique, t. ii. p. 99.

31

The best example of the arterial erectile tumor, that I have been able to examine, was from a man who died under the influence of chloroform at St. Bartholomew's Hospital.   He was 23 years old, and the disease occupied the external ear, the adjacent subcutaneous tissues, and part of the scalp.   The back of the auricle, in nearly the whole extent, was puffed out by a superficially lobed, soft, easily compressed, and elastic swelling, which all pulsated fully and softly.   Two similar and continuous lobes of swelling were under the scalp above and behind the auricle; and these were well-defined above, but gradually subsided below.   The skin covering the swelling was for the most part dusky-purple, but, except where it was scarred, appeared of healthy texture; the skin of the interior of the auricle and its fibro-cartilage also appeared unaffected, except in the turgescence of the blood-vessels.   A posterior branch of the superficial temporal artery passing by the front of the swelling, and a branch of the posterior auricular artery passing behind it, felt large, and pulsated strongly: the common carotid artery, also, on this side, pulsated more fully than that on the other.   A distinct soft bruit was audible, synchronous with the pulsation in the tumor; and distinct pulsatile movement was visible.

This disease had been noticed like a very small pimple when the patient was four years old.   It had from that time regularly increased. On four occasions severe bleeding had taken place from it, through an ulcer in the skin over it, or through a prominent part over which the skin was extremely thin.   After the first of these bleedings a piece of the swelling had been tied, and had sloughed away.   A month before the patient's death, Mr. Lloyd had tied and compressed the branch of the temporal artery and two other principal arterial branches at the borders of the swelling; and by this and subsequent treatment had diminished the size of the tumor and the fulness of the pulsation in and around it.

Much of the tumor had been spoiled by this treatment, but enough remained to show that a great part of its substance was like that last described, and probably, like it, consisted of minute blood-vessels collected in a soft spongy mass.   But, while the veins proceeding from the swelling were of no considerable size, the arteries passing to it and within it were very large, convoluted, and thin-walled.   This was especially observed in the posterior auricular artery, which had not been interfered with in the operations.   A lobe of the swelling (as it seemed) had pulsated strongly below and behind the lobule of the ear; and it was for the operation of tying this that the chloroform was given to the patient.   This proved to be only a part of the posterior auricular artery which, from a short distance beyond its origin, was large, and more collapsed and flattened than the other branches of the external carotid. At the beginning of its enlarged part, this artery was from a line to a line and a half in diameter; and from this point its trunk, as well as its branches (which were not unnatural in either number or anastomosis), were tortuous and coiled up in heaps, which had felt during life like pulsating masses. The dilatation of the arteries was uniform, not sacculated, though in parts the suddenness of the curves made it appear so. The small intervals between them were filled either with the natural fibro-cellular tissue, or with the minute blood-vessels that composed the chief mass of the tumor.

I believe that this specimen presented a fair example of the ordinary structure of the arterial form of vascular or erectile tumors; and that they consist, essentially, of the minute vessels of a limited portion of tissue enlarged and closely clustered, so as to form a tumor, in the substance, as well as about the borders, of which are arteries much more enlarged, and convoluted into pulsating heaps.

The existence, and even the preponderance, of the minute vessels in such tumors was manifest in a specimen sent to me by Dr. Ormerod. A healthy woman, about 60 years old, had for many years a pendulous growth in the lower and inner part of the left axilla. Lately it had grown quickly to the size of the closed hand. It was dark, hard, and knotty, with a distinct pulsation, and hung on a pedicle in which a large artery could be felt. A ligature was tied on the pedicle, and a few hours after another was applied, and the pedicle was cut through.

The tumor was gorged with blood, ecchymosed, and too much damaged for complete examination. Its general aspect was like that of the pedicled outgrowths of skin; but nearly its whole mass consisted of minute blood-vessels confusedly arranged and of various sizes. Their walls showed nuclei, which were generally shorter than those of healthy arteries: but in many instances were placed, as in them, regularly in layers, the external lying longitudinally, others within these transversely, and, still within these, others that were obliquely or variously placed. Besides the blood-vessels, I could find in the tumor only a comparatively small quantity of fibro-cellular tissue; and Dr. Ormerod's examinations, made when the tumor was more recent, had similar results.

Some, I think, have described the arterial tumors as formed by the convolutions of a single artery; and the characters of the swelling formed by the trunk and commencing branches of the posterior auricular artery, in the first of these cases, make me ready to believe that this description may be sometimes true. But I think that, more commonly, many branches of arteries are engaged in the tumor. Such was the case in the tumor of the ear, and in an instance recorded by Mr. Coote.* Arteries of the lip, which, in their natural state, might not have had a greater diameter than a large pin, were dilated for about an inch of their course into sinuses or canals, and were equal in diameter to the adult radial artery. Similar to this was a very formidable case, cured by compression, under the care of Mr. Lloyd. The temporal, supraorbital, and occipital arteries, all exceedingly dilated and tortuous, converged to a

* Medical Gazette, vol. xlv.

large pulsating swelling over the sagittal suture, the general characters of which agreed exactly with what I have described.

In the arterial vascular tumors the veins are comparatively small; and the difficulty of transit for the abundant blood flowing into them, doubtless adds materially to the fullness of the tumors, and of the pulsations seen and felt in them. In the venous tumors the opposite condition obtains; the veins are very large, the arteries comparatively small. Of this kind of tumor the following case presented a good example.

A man, 32 years old, was under the care of Mr. Lawrence. He had a hoof-shaped tumor projecting from the middle of the outer part of his thigh. It was from six to eight inches in diameter, and looked like some strange outgrowth of skin. Its base rested on the fascia lata; it was covered with skin, which was healthy, except in one excoriated place, and adhered closely to it. It was firm, but compressible and elastic, and by long-continued pressure could be reduced to nearly half its size, as if by squeezing blood from it. Several small arteries pulsated at its base; and very large veins, like tortuous sinuses, converged from it towards the upper part of the saphena vein.

The patient was in feeble health, apparently through the effects of a life in India, where, in the army, he had received a wound by a musket-ball, to which he referred as the cause of the growth of this tumor. Before the wound, he believed the part was quite healthy. The injury appeared superficial, and he was absent from duty only two days; but, six months afterwards, he observed a small tumor, and this, growing constantly and with severe pain, had increased in ten years to the present mass. The skin had been slightly ulcerated for twelve months, and severe hemorrhages had occurred from the ulcerated part, reducing his already diminished strength.

Mr. Lawrence cut away the whole tumor. Its connections were slight, except to the skin covering it; the arteries at its base bled freely, but for a short time; the great veins bled very little.

A section through the tumor showed that, while some parts of it appeared solid and close-textured, like a mass of firm fibro-cellular tissue, the greater part was like the firmest cavernous, or erectile tissue. Sections of blood-vessels, of various sizes and in various directions, were so thick-set, that the surface looked all reticulated and grooved with them. The general color of the tumor, which seemed to have almost emptied itself of blood during the operation, was nearly white; but in some parts it had a pale ruddy tinge, and in a few was blotched with small rusty and ochry spots.

The microscopic examination was less instructive than the general aspect of the tumor. Its tissue was very hard to dissect, and displayed (as its chief constituent) matted and crooked fibres, like those of close-textured longitudinally striated membrane of blood-vessels, with shrivelled nuclei imbedded in membrane, some of these nuclei being round, some oval, and some very narrow and elongated. I think the obscurity of the microscopic appearances was due to the tenacity with which the blood-vessels were imbedded in the elastic fibrous or nucleated tissue; it seemed impossible to extricate complete vessels; and one obtained by dissection only fragments of their walls confused with the intermediate tissues.

Other cases of venous nævi, which I have been able to examine less completely, have confirmed the foregoing account, especially in regard to the small size of the arteries in comparison with the veins, the generally dilated and varicose state of the latter, and the imitation of the characters of erectile tissue, which appears always more marked in the venous than in the other forms of vascular tumors.

Such are the principal facts that I can cite regarding the structure of the vascular or erectile tumors. They are very meagre, and much is left for future inquirers; especially the manner in which the larger vessels are connected with those smaller ones which, in most cases, make up a chief part of the swelling; and the changes of structure, if any, which exist in the proper tissues of the walls of the blood-vessels. Still, from even these few facts, some general considerations may be derived.

That which is common to all the vascular or erectile tumors is an over-extension of blood-vessels or blood-spaces within a circumscribed area. Their chief varieties depend (1) on the kind of vessels affected, and (2) on the nature of the tissue in which these vessels lie. The varieties of the first class have been pointed out; but all of them alike present the singular instance of the apparent primary growth of blood-vessels. In all other tumors, as in all abnormal products, the formation of blood-vessels appears to be a consequent and subordinate process. As in the natural development of parts, so in what is morbid, organization to a certain point precedes vascularity, and the formation of blood-vessels follows on that of the growths into which they pass. But here the case appears reversed. The calibre of the blood-vessels increases and the solid tissues between them diminish; all the growth of an erectile tumor is an enlargement of blood-vessels, with diminution of the tissues in which they ramify; or, rather, it is often an enlargement, not of blood-vessels, but of blood-spaces: for though, in the first stages of the disease, the walls of the vessels may grow, and elongate, so that the vessels become tortuous, yet, after a time, the walls waste rather than grow; apertures seem to form through mutually opposed blood-vessels, and at length, while the blood within the tumor increases, the blood-vessels containing it diminish, together with the parts in which they ramified. Hence, at last, in place of branching and anastomosing tubes, there is only a net-work formed of the remains of their walls. This is an increase of blood-spaces rather than of blood-vessels; so far as solid tissue is con-cerned, we might call it a wasting, rather than a growth; no new materials seem to be added, but step by step the blood-vessels are dilated, and the intervening tissues clear away, leaving room for more and more blood.

Such a fact constitutes a great contrast between these and any other diseases named tumors. And yet perhaps we may properly regard these as being overgrowths of blood-vessels, comparable with the overgrowths of the various other tissues illustrated in the preceding chapters. And their relation to such overgrowths seem, sometimes, distinctly proved in the gradations of morbid changes that connect them with mere enlargement of blood-vessels. If we examine different specimens of these tumors, or sometimes even the condition of the vessels adjacent to one of them, we may observe a regular gradation from the erectile tumor, through clusters of dilated and tortuous vessels, to that which we regard as merely the varicose condition of the veins or arteries. Such transitions are well shown in some of Cruveilhier's plates, and in a remarkable case by Dr. Hake and Mr. Image;* as well as in two of the cases that I have related.

In relation to the tissues in which this overgrowth of blood-vessels may take place, we may hold that there are two chief classes of cases. In some the vessels of a natural part are affected; in others the vessels of a new growth. In the former class, I think, are the greater part of the common erectile tumors of the skin, and of the other parts in which they are most frequently seated; as the muscles,† the bones,‡ the orbit, and the liver. In these the remains of natural tissues may be found in the interstices of the blood-vessels, and, either in or near the tumor, well-known arteries or veins are involved. In the latter class, examples of which have been cited in the tumors on the side (p. 483) and on the thigh (p. 484), the blood-vessels of new-formed parts are affected. To this class, also, may be referred, I think, the florid and highly vascular growths that are frequent at the orifice of the female urethra,§ and perhaps many others.‖

As I have hitherto chiefly had in view the subcutaneous erectile

---

* Medico-Chirurgical Transactions, vol. xxx. p. 109.

† See especially a case by Mr. Liston, Med. Chir. Trans. xxvi. 120; and one by Mr. Coote, l. c.; and Cruveilhier, livr. xxx. pl. 5.

‡ Among these may be included, probably, some of the cases described under the name of Aneurism of Bone and Osteo-Aneurism; as by Dr. Handyside, "Probationary Surgical Essay," Breschet, and others. But I am far from convinced that, in all the cases thus entitled, the blood-vessels of the bone were primarily or chiefly diseased. My impression is that, in many of them, the disease was really medullary cancer of the bone with excessive development of vessels, and that, in some, it was such a blood-cyst as appears to be sometimes formed in the course of a myeloid or cancerous disease.

§ The specimens of these growths which I have examined have displayed a very abundant and tessellated epithelium covering a small quantity of fibro-cellular tissue, with closeset and looped blood-vessels. They might be regarded as warts with excessive formation of vessels.

‖ While this sheet was being printed I received Rokitansky's essay " Ueber die Entwickelung der Krebsgerüste," including his most recent account of the formation of the erectile or cavernous structure of tumors. I shall refer to it in the description of the filamentous tissue or skeleton of medullary cancers in the 31st lecture.

tumors or nævi, so I will now, in describing the general characters of the disease, refer to them alone for examples. Even of these, indeed, it is difficult to give a general account, since we can make only an artificial distinction between such as may bear this name, and those extended dilatations of cutaneous vessels, which with little or no swelling, form the cutaneous nævi, port-wine spots, and the like. These are, evidently, essentially the same disease; the terms, cutaneous and subcutaneous nævi, respectively applied to them, imply only their difference of seat; they have no real difference of nature, and are very often associated. But, if we include only such as are for the most part or wholly subcutaneous, then it may be said that they are generally round or oval, disk-shaped, or spheroidal, but are often ill-defined, the morbid state of the blood-vessels in which they consist gradually merging into the healthy state of those beyond them. Sometimes, and especially those of most venous character and of longest duration, the mass is circumscribed by fibro-cellular tissue, which forms a kind of capsule, is penetrated by the blood-vessels passing to and from the tumor, and is very intimately connected both with the surrounding parts and with the tumor.

The vascular tumors are remarkable by their frequent beginning before birth, and their especially quick growth in early childhood. Beyond all comparison they are the most common of congenital tumors. Hence, mother-spot is almost synonymous with nævus, and nævus with erectile tumor. But they may begin, or accelerate their growth, at any period of life. I have seen one of which no trace existed till the patient was twenty-five years old; and another in which the rapid growth began, for the first time, when the patient was past fifty. Dr. Warren mentions a case of erectile pulsating tumor about the angles of the eyes and the forehead, which began in a girl seventeen years old. Many others, no doubt, have seen similar cases.

Their origin is generally unknown; but, as one of the cases I have related shows, they may commence in the results of injury; or, rather, a tumor may originate in injury, and in this tumor an exceeding formation of blood-vessels may ensue.

Their growth is uncertain; they may seem at rest for many weeks after birth, and then grow quickly, and then again may stay their growth: and having attained a certain size, may remain therein limited, or may decrease or disappear, the vessels, in whose enlargement the growth consisted, regaining their natural calibre or becoming obliterated.

Their maintenance of life, if I may so term it, is not strong. They are much more apt than the natural tissues are to slough or ulcerate after injury; and, in general disturbances of the health, they may perish altogether. I know a case in which a large subcutaneous nævus in a child's forehead sloughed, while another on its back, of much less size, was in process of sloughing after the application of nitric acid. Similar apparently spontaneous sloughings have occurred during, or in the debility following measles or scarlatina. Such events may be connected with the extreme slowness of the movement of blood in the tumors; for though they contain abundant blood, they probably transmit it very slowly. Venous tumors not unfrequently contain clots of blood and phlebolithes; such, probably, as would form only where the circulation is most slow; and even in the arterial tumors the full pulsation seems to indicate a retarded stream.

The diseases of the vascular tumors are of much interest; especially two amongst them,—namely, the formation of cysts, and that of malignant structures in their substance.

I just referred to the formation of cysts in erectile tumors, when speaking, in the second lecture (p. 341), of serous cysts in the neck, and of sanguineous cysts. The history of the changes by which an erectile tumor becomes in part or wholly cystic is very incomplete; for the opportunities of observing them, except when they are accomplished, are rare. The principal facts are, that, next to the erectile tumors, those that are composed of clusters of serous or sanguineous cysts appear to be the most common congenital form, and that in some cases the two forms appear in one mass. I referred, in the second lecture (p. 341), to such a case as recorded by Mr. Coote. Mr. Cæsar Hawkins,* also, had before described similar cases. He says of one, "You may see, in addition to the usual vessels, that several apparent cells exist. Some of these were filled with coagulum; their structure appeared identical with the other veins, of which they constituted, as it were, aneurismal pouches . . . . There were, however, besides these, some other cysts, which contained only serous fluid, and which were, to all appearance, close-shut sacs— serous cysts—their size being about that of peas."

In other instances, no erectile or nævus structure can be found, but the communication existing between one or more among a cluster of cysts and some large blood-vessel, makes it probable that they had the same origin. Thus, Mr. Coote traced a vein, as large as a radial vein, opening into the cavity of a cyst, which formed one of a large cluster removed by Mr. Lawrence from a boy's side. The mass formed by these cysts had existed from birth; some of them contained a serous fluid, others a more bloody fluid. In another similar cluster† removed from a boy's groin, one cyst appeared to communicate with the femoral vein, or with the saphena at its junction with the femoral. In one case mentioned by Mr. Hawkins,‡ when a cyst in the neck was opened, arterial blood gushed out. In another, the patient died with repeated hemorrhages from a cyst in the neck, and this cyst was found after death to be one of several, in some of which the blood-vessels of the isthmus of the thyroid gland opened.

It is difficult to interpret the formation of such cysts in nævi, or in

* Medico-Chirurgical Transactions, vol. xxii.; and Medical Gazette, vol. xxxvii., p. 1027
† The specimen is in the Museum of St. Bartholomew's Hospital.
‡ Clinical Lectures, in the Medical Gazette, vol. xxviii., p. 838.

connection with them or with veins. It may be that, as Mr. Hawkins believes, cysts are formed in these, as they may be in many other tumors, and that gradually, by the absorption produced by mutual pressure, they are opened into communication with one or more of the veins, or of the sacs connected with the veins. Or, as Mr. Coote suggests, it may be that certain of the dilatations of the vessels are gradually shut off from the stream of blood, so as to form shut sacs; and that after this their contained blood is absorbed, and replaced by serous fluid.

Lastly, respecting the production of cancerous disease in the tissue of erectile tumors, it seems to be generally regarded as a frequent event, and these are commonly believed to afford the most frequent instances of malignant growths supervening on such as 'were previously innocent. I will not doubt that such events have happened. In one case recorded by Mr. Phillips,* the transitition appears to be very clearly traced. Yet, I think that in many of the cases which have gained for erectile tumors their ill repute, a clearer examination would have proved that they were, from the beginning, very vascular medullary cancers, or else medullary cancers in which blood-cysts were abundantly formed. Or, it may be that the erectile tumors have been presumed to be liable to cancer, through having been supposed to share in the peculiar liability of the pigmentary nævi, or moles, to be the seats of melanosis.

LECTURE XXX.

SCIRRHOUS OR HARD CANCER.

PART I.—ANATOMY.

THE foregoing lectures have comprised the histories of the INNOCENT TUMORS; and in the first of them I related the characters generally appertaining to the MALIGNANT TUMORS or CANCERS, which it now remains to describe.

For an account of this class of tumors it will, I hope, suffice if, after reference to the twenty-first lecture, I describe, in order, each of the chief forms in which cancers occur, and then gather such conclusions as may be drawn respecting the general pathology of the whole class, and the relations of the several forms to each other, and to other tumors.

The chief forms of cancer are named severally Scirrhous, Medullary, Epithelial, Colloid, Osteoid, Melanotic, Fillous, and Hematoid. These, at least, are the names most frequently applied to them. The degrees of difference between the diseases to which they are severally applied are

* On Vascular Tumors, in the Medical Gazette, vol. xii. p. 10.

not nearly equal; and, probably, under certain of them, two or more diseases are included, which are sufficiently different to justify their separation with distinct names. But these are points which, having just mentioned, I may leave to be discussed in the account of each form of cancer, or in the concluding lectures.

First, I will speak of Scirrhous or Hard Cancer.

Being both more frequent and more obvious than any other form of cancer, this was, to the beginning of the present century, the type and chief example of the disease; and so, in regard to its physiology, and many particulars of its structure, it may still remain. It has received many names,* such as scirrhus, scirrhoma, and others, expressing that hardness of texture which is its distinctive and especial characteristic; or such as Carcinoma reticulare, implying certain minute peculiarities of structure. I believe, however, that these peculiarities are too inconstant and accidental to justify the division that they suggest: I will therefore include them all under the name of Scirrhous or Hard Cancer, and will use these terms for all stages of the disease, avoiding that which seems always a confusing distinction, in which, before ulceration, the disease is called Scirrhus, and after it, Cancer.

I will describe the Scirrhous cancer first, as it occurs in the breast, because here the disease is far more frequent than in any other part, and presents, openly, most of its varities of appearance according to its successive stages, and the accidents to which it is exposed.

The scirrhous or hard cancers in the breast are very far from being so uniform that they may be briefly described. I believe that they are always primary cancers; always infiltrations; and almost always seated, in the first instance, in some part of the mammary gland; but, when we compare their other characters in any large number of specimens, we find in them many and great diversities. Probably, therefore, it will be best if I describe first and chiefly the ordinary characters of the disease; the form in which it is most frequently seen, when it has not been changed by softening, ulceration, or any other morbid process. I can then add to this description, by way of comparisons, some accounts of the principal deviations from the more usual form; and, in the next part of the lecture, can give the history of the changes that ensue in the progress of hard cancers towards destruction, or in their much rarer regress.

Most frequently, the scirrhous cancer of the breast appears as a hard mass occupying the place of the mammary gland, or of some portion of it. In the cases I have collected it has not been more frequent in one breast than in the other. It is least frequent at or near the inner margin of the mammary gland; but with this reservation, it is not more frequent in one than in another part of the gland, or in any part than in the whole.

* Enumerated by Dr. Walshe: On Cancer, p. 10.

While part of the gland is cancerous, the rest is, commonly, healthy; but, according to the age and condition of the patient, it may be more or less atrophied and withered; or excess of fat may be accumulated round it; or it may contain numerous small cysts, one or more large cysts most confusing to the diagnosis; or, more rarely, it may be the seat of mammary glandular tumor (p. 473), or of some morbid change of structure. As yet, however, I believe no connection can be traced between any of these conditions and the growth of cancer, unless it be that it is peculiarly apt to happen in breasts that are being defectively nourished.

The hardness of the cancer, as compared with that of other tumors, is in most cases extreme: it is about equal to that of a lump of fibrous cartilage, and is associated with a corresponding rigidity, weight, and inelasticity. Cases, however, are not unfrequent, especially when the cancer grows quickly, in which the mass is less hard—very firm rather than hard—about as flexible and elastic as the body of an unimpregnated uterus.

The size of a hard cancer is seldom very great, in most cases, it is rather smaller than the part of the gland which it occupies was in the healthy state; so that, e. g. if half a mammary gland become cancerous, and half remain healthy, the latter may be two or three times larger than the former; or, if the whole gland become cancerous, it may be reduced

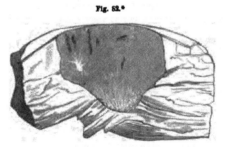

Fig. 82.*

to less than half its natural size. The exceptions to this diminution in the size of the cancerous gland, are, I believe, in cases of very rapid growth, in which the cancer-material seems to be added more rapidly than the materials of the glands can be removed.

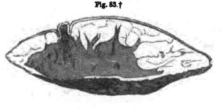

Fig. 83.†

The shape of the hard cancer, also, depends chiefly on the part of the gland that it affects. Generally, it may be said that when the cancer does not extend beyond the limits of the gland, it does not much deviate from the shape of the affected part; only, it gathers-up, as it were, the gland-

* Fig. 82. Section of a hard cancer, extending from a border-lobe of the mammary gland to the superjacent skin, and affecting both these and the intervening tissues. Natural size.
† Fig. 83. Section of a hard cancer of a whole mammary gland. Half the natural size.

lobes into an irregular lump, in which their outline is not lost, but blunted. Hence, according to their seats, we may observe different shapes of hard cancers of the breast.   At the anterior surface of the gland it is usually convex or obliquely shelving; at the posterior surface it is flat or slightly concave, resting on the pectoral muscle; in the middle, or thick substance, of the gland, it is commonly rounded and coarsely tuberous, knotted, or branched; at the borders it is often discoid, or else is peculiarly apt to extend from them in a mass reaching to the adjacent skin (fig. 82); and when the whole gland is affected, the cancer has commonly a low conical shape, or is limpet-shaped, with the nipple set on the top of the cone (fig. 83).*

From any such cancerous lump, processes, like crooked, gnarled, and knotted branches, may extend outwards, in correspondence with the out-lying lobes or processes of the gland.   But shapes like these are compa-ratively rare; and scarcely less so are the instances in which portions of the gland, after becoming cancerous, are detached from the chief mass; or those in which, in the same gland, more than one cancer forms at the same time.   Such cases do, however, happen; and I have known the smaller detached cancers nearly escape removal in operations.

As we dissect towards the surface of a hard cancer, especially of one of which the growth is not very rapid, we may observe that relation of the tissues around it which is so characteristic; I mean, their contraction towards it, and their progressive absorption.   It is as if, in its progress, the cancer were always growing more and more dense, by the contrac-tion and compacting of its substance, and by the absorption of the tissues it involves; and as if, in this concentric contraction, it drew all parts towards itself.   To this it is due, that, even from the first, and when it is yet very small, a hard cancer in the breast feels as if it could only be moved with the gland around it; it does not slide or roll under the finger as a mammary glandular tumor does.   To this, also, is due the slight dimpling of the skin over the nearest adjacent part of the cancer, even long before the two have become adherent; and to this we must ascribe the more numerous depressions, seaming and wrinkling the surface of the breast, and making it appear lobed, when, in a case of cancer occupying the whole of a large and fat breast, many parts of the skin are drawn inwards.   To the continuance of this contraction and absorption, also, are due the sinking-down of the retracted nipple, and the uplifting of the superficial fibres of the great pectoral muscle; and then, the deeper furrowing and the adhesion of the sunken skin or nipple, and the firm conjunction of the pectoral muscle with the deepest portion of the cancer.

* The terms "ramose," "tuberous," and "infiltrated," have been applied to specify the hard cancers, according to their shapes; but at present the shape appears so little con-nected with any other character of the disease,—it seems so nearly accidental,—that it cannot well be adopted for a ground of specific appellation. Moreover, there is no reason for especially calling the cancers that affect the whole gland, infiltrated; for all the hard cancers of the breast are infiltrations in less or more of its structure.

Sometimes one finds bands of tough tissue extending from the retracted parts of the skin to the surface of the cancer. These are commonly supposed to be always cancerous,—"claws," or outrunners from the cancer; but the supposition is only sometimes true; they often consist of only the cellular tissue between the lobes of the subcutaneous fat, condensed and hardened.

A scirrhous cancer in the breast has no distinct or separable capsule of cellular tissue investing it: the proper tissues of the breast, that are in contact with its surface, adhere to it very intimately; and the more so, the more slowly it has grown. The general boundary between them is, indeed, distinct to the sight; yet it is not easy to dissect out the cancer; and, at certain parts, it is evident that the tissues around the cancer are continuous with some of those within it. Especially, we can often see that the lactiferous ducts pass, from the nipple, or some healthy portion of the gland, right into the substance of the cancer.

When we cut through an ordinary hard cancer of the breast, such as I am chiefly describing, the surface of the section becomes at once, or in a few minutes, slightly concave. This is a very characteristic appearance, though not a constant one: I know no other tumor that presents it. In all others, I think, the surface of the section either rises, and becomes slightly convex, especially at its borders, or remains exactly level. In well-marked hard cancer the cut surface becomes concave, sinking in towards its centre, through the persistence, I suppose, of that tendency to contraction, to which, during life, we have to ascribe the traction of the surrounding tissues, and which is now no longer resisted by them.

The cancer seldom appears, on its cut surface, divided into lobes: it is one mass, variously marked perhaps, but not partitioned; neither has it any distinct *grain* or fibrous plan of structure; its toughness and tenacity are complete, and in every direction equal. It has, generally, a pale grayish color, and is glossy, and half-translucent; often it is slightly tinged with a dim purple hue, or, in acute cases, may be more deeply and more darkly suffused. Very often, too, its grayish basis is marked with brighter whitish lines, like interlacing bundles of short straight fibres, and with minuter ochre-yellow lines, or small yellow spots, and with various transverse and oblique sections of ducts.

The explanation of these various appearances, and of the minuter characters of the cancer, can be understood only by recollecting (what all the foregoing description will have implied), that the cancerous mass is composed not only of structures proper to the cancer, but of more or less of the tissues of the mammary gland, or other parts, among which the cancer-structures are inserted. And the differences implied in the words "more or less," may be considered as explaining many of the differences of appearances that hard cancers present.

The consideration of the influence of cancer-formations on the tissues that they occupy belongs, more properly, to the general pathology of the disease; but I must here just refer to the main facts concerning it.

As I have said, the formation of a scirrhous cancer of the breast consists in the production of peculiar structures—cancer-cells and others—in the interstices of the proper tissue of the part (see fig. 84, p. 496). Virchow* has fairly likened it, so far as the relation of the new and old materials is concerned, to the condition of pneumonia in a lobule of the lung, in which the lymph is deposited among the natural textures, so as to be thoroughly mixed up with them, and to form one mass with them.

Thus, then, we have, in any such cancer of the breast, a mixture of cancer-substance and breast-substance. But among many cancers we should find many diversities in the proportions of these two substances; which diversities are determined, first, by the original proportions in which the two substances are mingled; and, secondly, by the degrees of wasting, and other changes, that may occur in either or both of them. For example, a large quantity of cancer-substance may occupy so small a portion of the gland, that this portion, spread out as it is in the substance of the cancer, may be scarcely discernible, and the cancer may look like a completely isolated tumor; or, on the other hand, the whole of an atrophied gland may be condensed within a comparatively small cancer.

Moreover, after the original proportions of the two substances are determined, they may not remain the same; for their subsequent proportions of increase or of decrease may be different. Generally, as the cancer-substance increases, so the involved structures of the breast diminish or become degenerate, till they can hardly be recognized, and the cancer is where the natural structure was: a complete "substitution," as M. Lebert names it, is thus accomplished. But the original tissues do not thus disappear at any given rate, or all in the same rate or order. The gland-lobules, I think, waste very early: I have never found them clearly marked within a hard cancer. The larger gland-ducts remain much longer; their cut orifices may be often seen on the section of the cancer, or they may be traced right into it from the nipple, or fragments of them may be found in microscopic examinations. The small gland-ducts, with their contents, often appear, in branching buff and yellow-ochre lines, imbedded in the substance of the cancer. The fat of the breast is commonly quickly wasted: we find sometimes portions of it encircled by the cancer, and sometimes its yellow tinge is diffused through parts of the cancer, as if they were thoroughly mingled: but both these appearances are limited to the superficial and more lately formed portions of the growth: they are always lost in the central and older parts. There is the same gradual disappearance of the elements of the skin when it is involved; so that we might say that the regular process in the formation of a cancer of the breast is, that, as the cancer-substance increases, so the natural tissues involved by it degenerate and waste. I repeat, we might say this, if it were not for the fibrous tissue that inter-

* In his Archiv, B. L., p. 95.

venes among the lobes and ducts of the gland; for this seems either to waste more slowly than any other part, or to remain unchanged, or even in some cases to increase with the progress of the cancer. To these conditions of the fibrous tissue I shall again refer.

Now, if to the progressive varieties that may arise, through these changes in the involved tissues of the breast, we add that parts of the proper cancer-substance may degenerate or waste, or may vary in their method of development, while other parts are merely increasing, we may apprehend, in some measure, the meaning of those great varieties of appearance which we find in any large series of cancers. They are mainly due to the different modes and measures in which the constituents of the cancer-substance and of the original tissues are, first, mingled together, and then increased, degenerated, or absorbed.

After this necessary explanation, let me return to the description of the mingled mass. We find, as I have said, in any ordinary cancer of the breast, a grayish basis, which contains the proper elements of the cancer, but which is or may be intersected by visible fibres, ducts, and yellow lines or spots, which belong chiefly, or entirely, to the textures of the breast. One may usually press or scrape, from the cut surface of such a cancer, a pale grayish, thick, and turbid fluid, which is easily diffused through water, and is much more abundantly yielded, when the cancer has been macerated for a day or two in water. It is not creamy, but rather like thick gruel, and is usually composed of a mixture of the proper cancer-substance, and of the softened tissues of the breast, and the contents of the blood-vessels and remaining gland-ducts. It is called the " Cancer-Juice," and what is left after it is expressed, is called the " Stroma" of the cancer (see further, p. 501). I should state, however, that about the central and deeper parts, or sometimes in the whole masses of the hardest cancers, no such fluid can be obtained; they yield to pressure or scraping, only a small quantity of yellowish fluid, like turbid serum.

The remaining description of the hard cancer must be, chiefly, from its microscopic appearances.

In very thin sections it is not difficult to see the infiltration, or insertion, of the cancer-substance in the interstices of the affected tissues. It may be most clearly seen in sections of any part of the skin recently invaded by the cancer, for here, in the meshes of the reticulated fibro-cellular and elastic tissues, the cancer-particles are quite distinct, filling every interval, and not obscured by the débris of the gland-ducts and their contents. I am not aware of any more orderly plan of arrangement of the materials of the cancer than that which may be expressed by saying that they fill the interstices of whatever tissue they may lie in. They may either expand these interstices, when they accumulate quickly and abundantly; or, when they shrivel and degenerate, they may allow the tissues to collapse or contract.

The elementary structures of the cancer-substance, thus infiltrated in the breast, are chiefly two: namely (1), certain cells and other corpus-

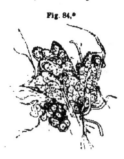

Fig. 84.*

cles; and (2), a fluid or solid blastema, or nearly homogeneous substance, in which these lie imbedded. We may study these, but, it must be admitted, in some confusion and uncertainty, in the material obtained by the pressure from the cancer.

The blastema, or intercellular substance, presents, I believe, no peculiar features.† As obtained by pressure, it is made very impure by the admixture of blood and other fluids; and it would be unsafe to describe it more minutely than as a pellu-cid or dimly granular substance, which in certain cases, yet I think rarely, assumes an appearance of fibrous texture. The corpuscles of hard cancer are chiefly nucleated cells. In ordinary cases, and where the cancer has not been deflected from its normal course, their characters are constant and peculiar, and may be described as for the types of "cancer-cells," fig. 85.

Fig. 85.‡

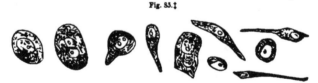

In shape they are various. Usually a large majority are broadly oval, or nearly round; in some specimens, indeed, all may have these forms; but, in other specimens, though these prevail, yet many cells have one or more angles, or outdrawn processes, and some are pyriform, some fusiform, some reniform, some nearly lanceolate.

It would be useless to describe all the shapes that may be found, for we can, at present, neither explain them, nor connect them with any corresponding differences in the general structure or history of the can-cers in which they severally occur. But we may observe, as Bruch and others have done, on this multiformity as a feature of malignant struc-tures: I know no innocent tumors, except the cartilaginous, in which it is imitated.

In size, the hard cancer-cells range from $\frac{1}{1800}$ of an inch to $\frac{1}{1?}$ of

* Fig. 84. Cancer-cells filling interstices among the bundles of the fibro-cellular tissue, in the skin of a breast. Magnified about 200 times.

† Its structures are minutely discussed by Virchow, in his Archiv, B. i. p. 110; and will be again referred to in the lecture on the general structure of cancers.

‡ Fig. 85. Cells and free nuclei of scirrhous cancer: from breasts. Magnified about 500 times.

an inch in diameter. Their medium and most frequent sizes are from $\frac{1}{1500}$ to $\frac{1}{1800}$: the smaller dimensions are usually found in the cancers of quickest growth.

In structure and general aspect they most nearly resemble, I think, the secreting gland-cells. Examined immediately after removal, and without addition of water, they appear clear and nearly pellucid; but changes quickly ensue, which water accelerates, and which bring them to the characters more generally ascribed to cancer-cells. They become nebulous, or dimly granular, or dotted, as if containing minute molecules; and they look no longer quite colorless, but very lightly grayish or yellowish. The cell-wall is, if it can be seen at all, peculiarly thin and delicate: but it is often impossible to discern any; and my belief is, that the cancer-cells are often only cell-shaped masses of some soft though tenacious substance, within which are nuclei.

The nuclei in hard cancers are more constant in their appearances than the cells, and I think, are even more characteristic. They are always comparatively large, having an average long diameter of about $\frac{1}{1700}$ of an inch, and varying from this size much less than the cells do from theirs. They are regular, oval, or nearly round, clear, well defined, scarcely altered by commencing decomposition, or by water, or any moderately diluted test substance. A single nucleous is usually contained in each cell; two nuclei in a cell are frequently found, but not in all specimens of hard cancer; more than two are rare: when more than one are found in a cell, they are generally smaller than those that are single.

Among the materials of a hard cancer, a certain number of free nuclei are usually found. It may be difficult to prove that these have not escaped from cells during the examination: but I think they are naturally free nuclei; for they are often larger than those contained in cells, and they sometimes deviate from the common shape, after methods which are more often noticed among the corpuscles of medullary cancers, and which will be more fully described in the next lecture.

Each nucleus has one, two, or rarely more, nucleoli, which, like itself, are large in comparison with the ordinary proportion between nucleoli and cells, and are peculiarly bright and well defined.

These seem to be the normal elements of hard cancer; and such as we find them in the breast, such are they, but less mingled and confused with other forms, in the hard cancers of the skin, the bones, and other organs. Indeed, these characters are so nearly constant and so peculiar, that an experienced microscopist can very rarely hesitate in forming upon them a diagnosis of the cancerous nature of any tumor in which they are observed.

But it would seem as if hard cancer seldom long maintained an undisturbed course; for we seldom find these structures, without finding also cells mingled with them, in which degeneration or disease has taken place.

32

Some of them are withered (fig. 86); some contain minute oily particles; some are completely filled with such particles, or are transformed into granule masses (fig. 87); and with these, we always find abundant molecular and granular matter, in which, as in the débris of cells, the nuclei lie loose. This débris, too, let me add, is always increased when the cancer is kept a day or two before examination, and when water acts upon it. The loss of clearness by the cancer-cell, of which I have already spoken (p. 497), is only the first of a series of changes, in the course of which the material of the cells breaks up into molecular and amorphous débris: fragments of it may hang about the nuclei; but, finally, the cells are completely disintegrated, and the nuclei, comparatively unchanged, are set free.

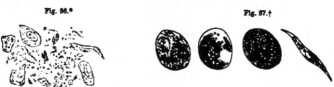

Fig. 86.*   Fig. 87.†

Among the tissues of the breast itself which are involved by the cancer, the gland-lobes, I have already said, are quickly removed; but their débris may contribute to the molecular matter which is mingled with the proper corpuscles of the cancer.

The larger gland-ducts, involved in the cancer, often appear thickened; and their contents, which are usually a thick, turbid, greasy fluid, present abundant granule-masses, withered cells, like epithelial cells of ducts, fragments of membrane, free nuclei shriveled and deformed, molecular and granular matter: all these being, I suppose, their natural contents, degenerate and disintegrated.

But the more remarkable and characteristic appearances are produced chiefly or in great part by the smaller gland-ducts, and the fibrous tissue inclosed in the cancer. The former chiefly constitute that which has been named "the reticulum" of hard cancer, and which has suggested the name of carcinoma reticulare for the specimens in which it is well seen.‡ The most usual appearances of what is now described as "reticulum" are two; and these may exist separately, or may coincide. In one, which is the most characteristic, and, indeed, the only one to which the name can apply, we see fine, branching, and variously interlacing and netted

* Fig. 86. Withered hard cancer-cells, with débris.

† Fig. 87. Hard cancer-cells, showing the progress of fatty degeneration.

‡ Under the name of Carcinoma reticulare, Müller included many cancers that could not have been scirrhous or hard cancers. On this ground, I think the name had better not be retained; for, whatever the "reticulum" be formed by, it is too accidental to be considered a specific character, and is associated with too great diversities of other characters, to be used, even arbitrarily, for the determination of a species. It is not even confined to cancers: corresponding appearances may be found in fibro-cellular, cartilaginous, fibro-nucleated, and probably several other tumors (see p. 384, 420, 433).

lines, of an opaque-white, buff or ochre-yellow hue. They appear as if formed of thickly sprinkled dots. They traverse the very substance of the cancer; and it is important to observe that when the cancer occupies but a small portion of the mammary gland, these netted lines are found only in that part of it which corresponds with the gland-substance.

In the other and rarer form of what is also called "reticulum," we find larger dots or small masses of ochre-yellow substance, such as are compared to seeds. These lie more widely scattered in the substance of the cancer, and may often be pressed from it, like the comedones, or retained white secretion from obstructed hair follicles.

I believe that these yellow "seed-like bodies," which are apt, if we examine them superficially, to be confounded with the degenerate contents of the larger ducts, are always small portions of the cancer degenerated and softened, or partially dried. We find in them abundant granule-cells and granule-masses, some entire, some in fragments; fragments, also, of granular and nebulous blastema (as it seems), and often of nucleated membrane; and these lie in molecular and granular matter diffused in liquid, with minute oil drops, and often with crystals of cholestearine. But with these products of complete degeneration, we may commonly find, also, cancer-cells, of which the great majority are either degenerate, filled with fatty matter, like granule-cells, or disintegrated; or else (when the substance is drier) shriveled and dried up, like the lymph and pus corpuscles that we may find in chronic inflamed lymphatic glands (fig. 86, 87).

Similar to these in their component structures are the larger masses of friable yellow substance, like tuberculous deposits, which are rarely found in hard cancers, but are very frequent in the medullary cancers.

Now, these appearances of yellow spots,—whether seedlike or in larger masses,—are not exclusively found in the breast, or in glandular structures: they may be seen in any hard cancer, and are yet more frequent in soft cancers in all organs. But the fine branching and netted lines that compose the more characteristic reticulum are found, especially, in cancers of glandular organs: and in those of the breast I have so often found, among the products of degeneration in them, what appeared to be portions of withered ducts and epithelium, that I feel nearly sure that the essential characters of this reticulum, in the scirrhous cancers of the breast, are to be ascribed to the minuter lactiferous tubes, which, involved in the cancerous infiltration, are now, with their contents, compressed, degenerate, and wasting.*

Lastly, respecting the fibro-cellular and elastic tissues involved in the cancer, the fate of these, I have said, appears different in different cases. We sometimes meet with a cancer of the breast, which, having just involved the skin, shows us the interlacing bundles of cutaneous fibres spread out or expanded by the insertion of the cancer structures among them (as

---

* We may compare them with a kind of black reticulum seen in cancers of the lungs or bronchial glands.

in fig. 84). The skin in such a case appears thickened, and its section is glossy, gray, and succulent, like that of hard cancer, but dimly marked with whitish fibrous bands. In other and more frequent cases the marks are absent; and the fibrous and elastic tissues of the skin are not to be found: we may presume that they have been absorbed as the cancer-structures increased. I think this removal of the fibrous and elastic tissues is the more frequent event, both in the skin and in the gland; yet in some of the hard cancers, and in the central hardest parts of others, the fibrous tissue of the gland—all that which encompasses the gland-tubes and becomes, proportionally, so abundant when the secreting structures waste—all appears to be even increased and condensed or indurated.

Such cancers as these have been regarded as examples of a special form, named Carcinoma fibrosum, and the fibrous tissue found in them has been commonly considered as a proper cancerous structure, a result of the fibrous development of the cancerous blastema. Now, I shall have to refer to certain genuine instances of fibrous hard cancer, as occurring especially in the ovaries; and I would not deny that part of the cancerous material deposited in a breast may be developed into fibrous tissue; but I am sure that, in the large majority of cases, the fibrous tissue which is found in a cancer of the breast is only that which belonged to the breast itself, and which, involved in the cancer, may now be either wasted or increased. For the fibrous tissue in hard cancers of the breast is not like morbid or new tissue, nor like that which is found in really fibrous cancers, but is like the natural fibrous or fibro-cellular tissue, either healthy or indurated and condensed. It is also generally mixed with fibres of elastic tissue, such as are intermingled with the natural fibro-cellular tissue, but never, I think, occur among the proper constituents of cancer, and are very rare in even the more highly organised of the innocent tumors. I may add, in confirmation of this view of the nature and origin of the fibrous tissue in cancers of the breast, that when hard cancer occurs in organs which have little or no fibrous tissue,—such as cancellous bone, the brain, the liver, or the lymphatic glands,—it presents as little or none of the same tissue: however hard it may be, it is formed almost entirely of corpuscles.* The difference in this respect is often, indeed, very striking between the hard cancer of the breast and that of the corresponding axillary glands. Both may be equally hard and manifestly identical in nature; yet, while the cancer of the breast may include abundant fibrous tissue, that in the glands may have scarcely a trace.†

* See, respecting the hard cancer of the brain, a case well described by Dr. Bedfern (Monthly Journ. December, 1850). I think all that Virchow, Lebert, and some others have written, is quite consistent with this view, though they seem to hesitate in accepting it.
† If it seem strange that in some hard cancers the fibrous tissue of the involved organ increases, while in others it is diminished, the strangeness may be made to seem less by the more glaring examples of difference among cancers of bones;—from the eroding secondary

I have dwelt the more on this point because the current method of describing all cancers as composed of a peculiar " stroma," the meshes of which are filled by a peculiar " cancer-juice," appears to me very deceptive, and often incorrect. The expressions, as they are commonly used, imply that the fibrous tissue or stroma, and the cells and other materials which form the juice, are alike proper and essential to the cancer. But I believe that in the large majority of cancers of the breast, the only "stroma," the only substance that would remain, after removing all that is cancerous, would be the structures of the breast itself. And so, in other cancers, my belief is, that if we except the rare examples of the really fibrous and osteoid cancers, to which I shall hereafter refer, there are few in which more than a very small quantity of fibrous tissue is formed.

In the foregoing description I have had in view, almost exclusively, the forms of hard cancer which are most frequent in the breast; instances of the ordinary or typical characters of the disease. But, as I said at the outset, the deviations from these medium forms are neither few nor inconsiderable, even though we do not count among them any of the varieties of appearance which are due to degeneration or to disease of the cancerous structure, or to varying conditions in the parts about the mammary gland.

And, first, varieties appear which may be referred to different degrees of activity or intensity of the disease. The examples which I have hitherto chiefly described might hold a middle place in a series, at the opposite ends of which would be those of what have been sometimes called the "acute" and the "chronic" cancers.*

The well-marked examples of the former kind are distinguished, not only by rapid progress, but by structure. They are scarcely to be called hard—they are, at the most, firm, tense, and elastic; and they may even, though not morbidly softened, present a deceptive feeling of fluctuation. Their cut surfaces do not become concave; they are succulent, and yield abundant fluid upon pressure; they are often suffused with vascularity, especially about their borders. The quantity of cancer-structure in them is very large, in proportion to the quantity of gland in which it has its seat. Hence the section of an acute cancer appears more homogeneous, and its growth produces a manifest enlargement or swelling, the morbid material expanding the tissues around and involved within it. The surrounding tissues, also, are less closely connected with the cancer than they usually are, and it may appear like a distinct isolated tumor, rather than an infiltration.

hard cancers, in which the osseous tissue wholly disappears, to the medullary cancers, in which the osseous tissue increases commensurately with the cancer and grows out into it as a spongy skeleton or framework.

* Most of the acute forms are such as some call *elastic* cancers : most of the chronic would be classed as *fibrous* cancers by those who adopt that term. " Hypertrophic" and " atropic' have also been applied to them as terms of contrast.

In all these conditions the acute scirrhous cancers approximate to the characters of medullary cancers; and perhaps the expression is not unjust, that they are examples of an intermediate form of the disease. And the approximation is shown in some other characters, especially in their more rapid growth; in their usually affecting those whose mean age is below that of the subjects of the harder and more chronic cancers; and in the signs of larger supply of blood.

In the chronic hard cancers the opposites of all these characters are found. The cancerous mass is comparatively small; and, as time passes, it often seems to shrink and contract, rather than increase. It is intensely hard, knotted, and dry; the adjacent tissues appear tight-drawn to it, and firmly adherent; and on its cut surface, which usually appears deeply concave, it may show more of the increased and indurated fibrous tissue of the breast than of the proper cancer substance. All the history of the chronic cancers accords with these signs of inactivity: they occur generally in those that are beyond the mean age; they are attended with no increase of vascularity; and if the skin became involved in one, it is only ruddy or palely livid at the very seat of adhesion. The tissues of the breast itself usually appear to suffer a corresponding atrophy; the gland commonly shrivels, and the skin becomes lax and wrinkled, or else is filled-out with superabundant fat accumulating round the shrinking gland.

Either of these forms of cancer may affect, in some cases, the whole gland; in others, only a portion of it. The characters of both are most marked when they occupy the whole gland, for now the enlargment attending the acute cancer, and the shrinking that accompanies the chronic, are most manifest.

In general, the respective characters of the acute and the chronic cancer are consistent throughout all their course: yet cases are not rare in which a scirrhous cancer has shown all signs of rapid progress at the beginning of its career, but, after a time, has inexplicably retarded its course, and passed into a chronic state. Nor, on the other hand, are those rare in which patients are seen dying quickly, because a cancer, which has been slowly and almost imperceptibly progressive for several years, at length assumes the rapidity and destructiveness of an acute inflammation.

A second series of hard cancers, deviating from the usual forms, consists of cases in which the nipple and the skin or other tissues of the mammary gland are peculiarly affected.

Commonly the hard cancer extends from the mammary gland to the nipple and areola, involving these as it may any other adjacent part. When seated at or near the centre of the gland, it commonly draws down the nipple, which descends as it were into a round pit sunk below the general level of the breast. As it extends, also, the cancer-structures deposited in the nipple make it hard, or very firm and elastic, inflexible, and comparatively immovable. But the changes which thus usually occur later, or in a less degree, than those in the gland, may commence or predominate in the nipple or the areola. The former may be found quite hard and rigid; or, in the place of the latter, there may be a thin layer of hard cancerous substance, with a superficial ulcer, like an irregular excoriation, while the structures of the gland itself are yet healthy.

In other cases, we find the skin over and about the mammary gland exceedingly affected. In a wide and constantly, though slowly, widening area, the integuments become hard, thick, brawny, and almost inflexible. The surface of the skin is generally florid or dusky with congestion of blood; and the orifices of its follicles appear enlarged, as if one saw it magnified,—it looks like coarse leather. The portion thus affected has an irregular outline, beyond which cord-like offshoots or isolated cancerous tubercles are sometimes seen, like those which are common as secondary formations.. The mammary gland itself, in such cases, may be the seat of any ordinary form of hard cancer; but I think that at last it generally suffers atrophy, becoming, whether cancerous or not, more and more thin and dry, while the skin contracts, and is drawn tightly on the bony walls of the chest, and then becomes firmly fixed to them.

I might add to the account of these deviations from the ordinary forms of cancer of the breast, notices of some others; but these may suffice, and if it be remembered that each of these, as well as of the more common forms, is liable to change by the various degenerations and diseases of the cancer, enough will have been said to illustrate the exceeding multiformity in which the disease presents itself in the breast. Something, however, must be added respecting the characters of scirrhous cancers in other parts of the body: and from these I will select chiefly those parts in which it has the greatest surgical interest, or has received the least attention from morbid anatomists.

In the LYMPHATIC GLANDS, the scirrhous or hard cancer appears very frequently as a secondary disease; indeed there are few cases in which cancerous patients reach their average of life without affection of the glands connected with the organ primarily diseased. But, as a primary disease, scirrhous cancer of the lymphatic glands is very rare: the cancer which most commonly appears first in them is the medullary; especially, I think, that of the firmer kind.* A specimen is in the Museum of St. Bartholomew's,† which shows well-marked scirrhous cancer in an

* The Index will, I hope, in some measure correct the disadvantage, which is here evident, of separating the accounts of the different forms of cancer in the same organ. The disadvantage is, I think, more than compensated by the avoidance of confusion in the descriptions of the different forms; and in the Index the reader will find, under the title of each chief organ or tissue (so far as they are here described), the references to all the forms of cancer occurring in it. † Series xxi. 2.

inguinal gland. The gland is increased to an inch and a half in length, and, while retaining its natural shape, nearly the whole of its proper texture appears replaced by structures exactly resembling, in hardness and all other properties, the ordinary scirrhous cancer of the breast. It was removed by Mr. Lawrence from a lady, who remained well about three years after the operation, and in whom the disease then recurred in another inguinal gland, which was also removed, and presented the same characters. They were equally marked in the progress through destructive ulceration which ensued in a primary scirrhous cancer of the axillary glands, also observed by Mr. Lawrence. I believe I saw a third instance in some inguinal glands, which formed an exceedingly hard swelling in and below the groin; but I had no opportunity for minute examination of them. There was no probability, in any of these cases, that any other part was the seat of cancer before, or at the same time with, the lymphatic glands.

Cases sometimes occur in which the disease in the glands may be so nearly coincident with that in the organ to which they are related, that we may believe the gland-cancer to be primary, though not alone. And sometimes the disease in the glands greatly preponderates over that in the organ, even though its primary seat was in the latter. A woman, 60 years old, was lately in St. Bartholomew's Hospital, in whose right breast there was a hard lump, less than a pea in size, which felt exactly like a hard cancerous tumor imbedded in the gland. This had existed unchanging for twenty years; and in the right axilla a cluster of lymphatic glands had been rapidly enlarging for twelve months, and now formed a great mass so uniformly hard, heavy, and nodular, as I have never seen formed by any glands but those affected with scirrhous cancer. The case is, however, imperfect, for the patient would submit to no operation, and there may remain some doubt as to the nature of the small tumor in the breast.

All these, however, are comparatively rare events. The ordinary course is, that after the scirrhous cancer has existed for a time (the length of which seems at present quite uncertain), in the breast or any other organ, the lymphatic glands in and near the route from that organ towards the thoracic duct become the seats of similar disease. I shall speak elsewhere of the probable method of this extension of the cancer to the glands. Its effects are shown in a process which, in all essential characters, imitates that preceding it in the organ primarily diseased. Usually the cancerous material is deposited, and its structures are formed, in the first instance, in separate portions of one or more glands. The separate formations appear as masses of very firm and hard whitish or grayish substance, of rounded shapes, imbedded in the glands, and contrasting strongly, as well in texture as in color, with their healthy remaining portions. But, as the separate portions in each gland enlarge, they gradually coalesce till the whole natural structure of the gland is overwhelmed and replaced by the cancer. Similarly, the same changes ensuing at once in many glands, they form a large and still increasing cluster, and at length coalesce in one cancerous mass, in which their several outlines can hardly be discerned.

The minute texture of the hard cancer of lymphatic glands differs, I believe, in nothing that is important from that already described in the cancer of the breast. Only, in microscopic examinations we find the proper structure of the lymphatics, in the place of those of the mammary gland, mingled with the cells and other constituents of the cancer. Neither is there any essential difference in the mode of deposit of the cancerous material; it is, in both alike, an infiltration, though circumscribed.

Occasionally, it is said (but I have never seen it), the secondary cancer of the lymphatic glands is soft and medullary, while that of the organ primarily diseased is scirrhous. Very often, before becoming cancerous, the lymphatic glands enlarge without hardening,—through "simple irritation," as the expression is. From this condition they may subside after the removal of the primary cancer, or when corresponding "irritation" in it is relieved. But the condition, whatever it may be, is probably not one of mere slight inflammation; for glands which may have thus subsided, or which have not been visibly affected, may become the sole or primary seats of recurrent cancer, even two or more years after the removal of the primary disease. There seems to be a peculiar state of liability to cancer, long retained in lymphatic glands, sometimes testified by enlargement, but often not discernible except in its results.

Scirrhous Cancer of the SKIN is another of the affections commonly occurring secondarily, yet sometimes appearing as a primary disease. Its occurrence, when the disease extends continuously from the mammary gland, is already described. In a similar manner it may be found extending from lymphatic glands, or any other subcutaneous organ; and I have described (p. 503) how it sometimes precedes and surpasses in extent the scirrhous cancer of the breast. But its most frequent appearance, in connection with cancer of the breast, and that which is imitated when it occurs as a primary disease in other parts of the skin, is in tubercles or rounded hard masses.

Such tubercles are generally grouped irregularly, but in constantly widening areas, about the primary disease in the breast; in other parts, and as primary cancers, they may be single or numerous. They are almost incompressibly hard, tough, circumscribed masses or knots; they are usually of oval, flat, or biconvex form, or, when large, are tuberous or lobed; they are imbedded, as infiltrations of cancer-structures, in the exterior compact layer of the cutis. They are generally equally prominent above, and sunken beneath, the level of the surface of the skin; and this condition is commonly acquired as well by those which commence like little prominent papulæ, as by those which at first appear like knots just subcutaneous.   The skin covering them is thin, tense, and shining; it is usually of a deep ruddy pink color, tending to purple or brownish-red, or it may seem tinged with brown, like a pigment-mark.   This change of color extends a little beyond the border of the cancerous mass, and then quickly fades into the natural hue of the skin.   Such cancers are movable with, but not in, the surrounding skin, and even with it the mobility is very limited when they are large and deep.   They may be found of various sizes; in circumscribed masses, ranging from such a size as can just be detected by the touch, to a diameter of two inches; or, when diffused in the skin, occupying it in an expansion of hardly limited extent.

The minute structures, equally with the general characters, of the scirrhous cancers of the skin, are, in everything, conformed with those already described; and the characters of cancer-cells, and their mode of disorderly insertion in the interstices of the natural tissues, are in no parts more distinct.*

In general, I think, the scirrhous cancers of the skin have a chronic course, not painful, nor soon ulcerating; but, as primary diseases, they are too infrequent for a general history of them to be written at present. I have seen only four examples of them independent of previous cancer in other parts.   In one of these the seat of disease was nearly the whole skin of the front of the left side of the chest of a woman 78 years old; in another, it was in the skin of an old woman's leg; in another, an elderly man's scalp had two large, hard, cancerous masses in it; in a fourth the disease was in the scrotum of a man 53 years old; but I believe the elementary structures of scirrhous cancer were mingled with others resembling those of the more frequent epithelial soot-cancer of the same part.†

In the MUSCLES, scirrhous cancer is commonly associated with its most frequent form in the skin: that, namely, in which it occurs in groups of tubercles about the primary disease of the breast.   We may, indeed, draw a close parallel between the secondary cancers in the skin and muscles respectively: for in both parts alike we find, in some cases,

* In the foregoing account I have not had in view that which is commonly called the "cancerous tubercle of the face," and which so often occurs as the precedent of the destructive process constituting the so-called "cancerous" or "cancroid ulcer" of the face in old persons.   I have not been able to examine minutely one of these tubercles before ulceration, but all I have seen of the materials forming the base and margins of the ulcers which follow them, and all the characters of their progress, make me believe that no cancerous structure, whether scirrhous, epithelial, or any other, exists in them.   I shall revert to this subject in the lecture on Epithelial Cancer.

† This specimen is in the Museum of St. Bartholomew's.   Cases of cancer of the skin are related by Lebert, Walshe, and others, in their appropriate chapters; but it is not clear that any of them were primary scirrhous cancers.   Those which were not epithelial cancers appear to have been either medullary, of the firmer sort, or (in Lebert's cases) melanotic. All these forms of cancer are more frequent in the skin, as primary diseases, than that which I have described: they will all be considered in the following lectures.

discrete cancerous tubercles, in others extensively diffused cancerous deposits; and in the muscles, as in the skin, the latter form occurs especially when the disease extends continuously; the former when it is multiplied contiguously to its primary seat.

I have never seen a primary scirrhous cancer in a muscle; and only once seen such a cancer forming a distinct isolated tumor in an inter-muscular space. It may be doubted, indeed, whether this tumor were the primary disease; yet, because of the exceeding rarity of scirrhous cancers in any other form than that of infiltrations of the textures of parts, it deserves mention. It was taken, after death, from a man 54 years old, in whom it had been observed for a month, and who died, exceedingly emaciated and exhausted, with similar disease in his axillary and bronchial lymphatic glands, his lungs, muscles, occipital bone, and other parts. This tumor was about four inches in length, oval, surrounded by a distinct fibro-cellular capsule, and seated between the branchialis anticus and biceps muscles, outspreading both of them. It had the same hardness, weight, and density, and the same microscopic cell-structures, as the ordinary hard cancers of the breast; it was milk-white; slightly suffused with pink and gray, and distantly spotted and streaked with ochre-tints. The other cancerous masses had for the most part the same characters; but some, which by their size and positions might certainly be considered as of latest production, were soft, and like the most frequent medullary cancers.

In the BONES, as in the muscles, the scirrhous cancer seldom, if ever, occurs except as a secondary disease: the primary cancers of bones are, I think, always either medullary, osteoid, or colloid. The structures of the scirrhous cancer may be infiltrated or diffused among those of the bone, or they may form distinct masses; but in neither case do they so increase as to form considerable tumors. In some of the cases of infiltration, the cancerous substance is diffused through the cancellous tissue of the bone, while its walls are comparatively little changed: in others all the bony structures are expanded into an irregular framework of plates and bands, the interstices of which are filled with cancerous substance, hard, elastic, gray and shining.* On the other hand, when separable cancerous masses are formed, they are usually round or oval, or adapted to the shape of the inner walls of the bone, within which they are, at least for a time, confined. They generally appear as if, while they were growing, the original bony textures around them had gradually wasted or been absorbed, making way for their further growth.†

* Nos. 822-3 in the College Museum are examples of the first form; and No. 5 (Appendix) in that of St. Bartholomew's may exemplify the second. The latter specimen was taken from a case in which a cancerous femur was broken eight months before death, and the new bone, with which it was repaired, was infiltrated with cancer as well as the original textures.

† See, respecting the occasional "preparatory rarefaction" of bones, previous to cancerous deposits in them the excellent observations of Walshe (p. 555) and Virchow (Archiv, 1. 126.)

And thus the growth of the hard cancer, with absorption (whether previous or consequent) of the bone around it, may continue till not only the medullary tissue, but the whole thickness of the wall, is removed, and the cancer may project through and expand beyond it, or may alone fill the periosteum, retaining, with very little change, the original shape and size of the bone.†

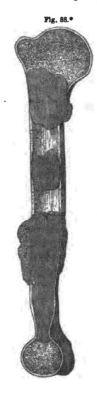

Fig. 88.*

In both these sets of cases the cancer-cells are alike, and they form, without fibrous tissue, a hard, or very firm, elastic, grayish substance, shining, and sometimes translucent, sometimes, with an obscure fibrous appearance. The likeness to the common hard cancer of the breast is complete, in both general and microscopic characters; and not less complete the contrast with the usual forms of the medullary cancer, which, as I have said, is the more frequent primary disease of the bones. Intermediate specimens may, indeed, be found; yet, on the whole, the contrast between medullary and scirrhous cancers is as well marked in the bones as in any other part.‡

The bones thus cancerous become liable to be broken with very slight forces; and to these conditions a certain number of the so-called spontaneous fractures in cancerous patients may be assigned. But some are due to the wasting and degenerative atrophy which the bones undergo during the progress of cancer, and which seems to proceed to an extreme more often than it does in any other equally emaciating and cachectic disease.

The hard cancer of the INTESTINAL CANAL, exemplified most frequently in the upper part of the rectum, in the sigmoid flexure of the colon, and, sometimes, in a very striking form, in the ileo-cæcal valve, appears, usually, as an infiltration of hard cancer-structures in the submucous tissue. Here it is usually of annular form, and occupies the whole circumference of the intestine, in a length of from half an inch to an inch. The cancer may, at the same time, or in other instances, occur

---

* Fig. 88. Section of a humerus with hard cancer, as described above. Mus. of St. Bartholemew's.

† As in Nos. 817-8-9, in the Museum of the College, and in several specimens lately added to that of St. Bartholomew's.

‡ Medullary cancer may appear as a secondary disease in the bones, as well as in other parts, after primary scirrhous cancer in the breast. The cases I have examined would make me think that the scirrhous cancer is, in these events, the more frequent: but M. Lebert (Traite des Maladies Cancereuses, p. 714) describes none but soft cancers as occurring in the bones, whether primarily or secondarily.

externally to the muscular coat, and in this case is usually not annular but in separate tubercles, which, until ulceration ensues, project with flattened and sometimes centrally depressed, round or oval surfaces, into the cavity of the intestine. Very rarely (it is said) it may affect the whole circumference of a large extent of the rectum, and may in the same extent involve many adjacent parts.

It sometimes happens that the hard cancer of the submucous tissue is associated with growths of softer medullary cancer into the cavity of the intestine, or with formations of colloid cancer. The mingling of these forms is certainly more frequent in the digestive canal than in any other part. But that which is most remarkable in the hard cancers of the rectum (as an example of those of other portions of the canal), is derived from the tendency which the cancer has here, as in other parts, to contract and condense, and adhere to the parts around it. To this it is due, that, when an annular cancer of the rectum exists in the submucous tissue; even the exterior of the bowel appears constricted; instead of swelling, the bowel is, even externally, smaller at the cancer than either above or below it: and the stricture, or narrowing of the canal, which would be trivial if it depended only on the cancerous

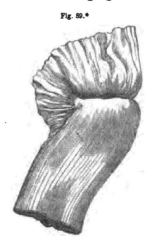

Fig. 89.*

thickening of the coats, is made extreme by the contraction of the coats around and with the cancer. The same conditions which, in hard cancer of the breast, produce retraction of the nipple and puckering of the skin over the morbid growth, here produce contraction of the muscular and peritoneal tissues around the growth, and a concentric indrawing of the growth itself.

With similar likeness to the hard cancers of the breast, those in the insestine (in the rectum, for example) give rise to close adhesion of the tissues round them to other adjacent parts. Thus the cancerous part of the rectum may be fixed to the promontory or front surface of the sacrum quite immovably; or the colon may become united to the urinary bladder, or to some other portion of the intestinal canal.

Many other important facts in the history of this affection are connected with the dilatation and hypertrophy of the intestine above the stricture; the final paralysis of the dilated part, and the phenomena of ileus chiefly due thereto, with displacement of the diseased part by the weight of

* Fig. 89. Hard cancer of the rectum, showing the constriction of the peritoneal and muscular coats around the cancer of the submucous tissue. Mus. of St. Bartholomew's.

fæces accumulated above it; the occasional variations of the degree of stricture, according to the afflux of blood swelling the diseased part, or its ulceration or sloughing decreasing it, and so, for a time, widening the canal; but these I need only enumerate, while I can refer to Rokitansky* for ample accounts of them all.

The large intestine is, probably, next to the mammary gland and the stomach, the organ in which the well-marked scirrhous cancer is most frequently found as a primary disease.   It very rarely, indeed, occurs secondarily, except when extending to the intestine continuously from some adjacent part; and in this case, as it usually affects, at first, only part of the circumference of the intestine, it may become much more extensive without producing stricture; for the unaffected part of the wall may dilate so as to compensate, for a time, for the contraction of the diseased part.   Moreover, when it is a primary disease, the cancer of the intestine is one of the forms in which the disease may exist longest without multiplication, although often, even in its early stages, it is associated with exceeding, and seemingly disproportionate, cachexia.

I have spoken of the occurrence of fibrous tissue in the scirrhous cancers of the breast, and have said (pp. 499, 500) that this appears to be no proper element of the cancer, but the natural fibro-cellular and elastic tissues of the part involved in the cancer, and often increased and condensed.   If this be always so, and if, as I have also said, little or no fibrous tissue be found in cancers affecting organs which naturally contain none, it will follow that the name *Carcinoma fibrosum* is not well applied to any examples of hard cancers described in the foregoing pages. Yet there are cancers which contain not only abundant but peculiar fibrous tissue; and these may well be called "fibrous cancers," and may be considered as a distinct form or species, unless it should appear that they are always associated, as secondary diseases, with scirrhous cancers of the more ordinary structure : so that we may suppose that the same blastema is, in one organ, developed into fibrous tissue; in others, at the same time, into cancer-cells.

The most remarkable examples of hard cancers with fibrous structures that I have yet seen, have been in the ovaries of certain patients with common hard cancer of the breast or stomach.† In these cases, the place of the ovary on either or on both sides is occupied by a nodulated mass of uniformly hard, heavy, white, and fibrous tissue.   The mass appears to be, generally, of oval form, and may be three or more inches in diameter : its toughness exceeds that of even the firmest fibrous tumors; and its component fibres, though too slender to be measured, are peculiarly hard, compact, closely and irregularly woven : they are not undulating, but, when they can be separated singly or in bundles, they appear

---

* Pathologische Anatomie, iii. 276 and 282.
† Museum of the College, No. 240, 2636; and of St. Bartholomew's, xxxi. 17, and, probably, xxxii. 14.

dark-edged, short, and irregularly netted. With these I have found only few and imperfect cancer-cells; with more numerous nuclei, elongated and slender. They are not mingled·with elastic or other "yellow element" fibres.

It may be not unfairly supposed that the same blastema, which in other organs may be developed into cancer-cells, may become fibrous in organs of so singular capacity for morbid as well as natural development, as are the ovaries. But fibrous cancers are not found in the ovaries alone. Peculiar stiff-fibred tissue is sometimes contained, together with less abundant cancer-cells, in the harder cancers connected with periosteum. So I have seen it in the pelvis, and in the unossified parts of osteoid cancers, where neither its relations nor its minute texture were such as to suggest that it was morbidly increased periosteum. However, the occasions that I have had of examining truly fibrous cancers have been two few, to justify any conclusion respecting the propriety of separating them, as a distinct form, from the scirrhous cancers. And I cannot complete my own imperfect observations with the records of other pathologists; for I think that none have endeavored sufficiently to discriminate between the two kinds of fibrous tissue that may be found in cancers; namely, that which is developed from cancerous blastema, and that which is derived from the original fibrous tissue of the affected organ, whether in its natural state, or increased, condensed, indurated, or otherwise morbidly changed. Yet the distinction is an essential one: for the former is truly cancer-structure, the latter is only the structure in the interstices of which the cancer has its seat. A similar distinction will have to be made, in a future lecture, between the osseous tissue that grows so as to form the frame-work, or interior skeleton, of certain medullary cancers of bone, and that which is the chief constituent of osteoid cancers: the one is a morbid growth of a bone affected with cancer; the other is a proper cancer-structure ossified.

LECTURE XXX.

SCIRRHOUS OR HARD CANCER.

PART II.—PATHOLOGY.

THE former part of this lecture being devoted to an account of the structures of the chief examples of hard or scirrhous cancers, I propose, in this second part, to consider their history, their mode of life, their pathology as contrasted with their anatomy. And here, even more nearly than in the former part, I will limit myself to the histories of those of the breast; for, concerning the primary hard cancers of other parts, we have too few data for any general history.

First, concerning the conditions favorable to the origin of these scirrhous cancers:—

(a.) They exist, in great preponderance, in women. Probably, of every 100 cases of scirrhous cancer of the breast, 98 occur in women; and, I believe, it is chiefly this that makes cancer, on the whole, more frequent in women than in men, for in every other organ common to both sexes, the greatest frequency is, I think, found in men.

(b.) The age of most frequent occurrence of scirrhous cancer of the breast, is between 45 and 50 years. Nearly all records I think agree in this. The disease has been seen before puberty; but it is extremely rare at any age under 25; after this age it increases to between 45 and 50; and then decreases in frequency, but at no later age becomes so infrequent as it is before 20.

The following table, drawn from the records of 158 cases, of which the diagnosis cannot be reasonably questioned, will illustrate the foregoing statement:—*

2 cases were first observed between 20 and 25 years of age.†							
4	"	"	"	25	"	30	"
9	"	"	"	30	"	35	"
26	"	"	"	35	"	40	"
33	"	"	"	40	"	45	"
40	"	"	"	45	"	50	"
17	"	"	"	50	"	55	"
11	"	"	"	55	"	60	"
9	"	"	"	60	"	70	"
6	"	"	"	70	"	80	"
1	"	"	above 80				"
158							

These numbers may represent the absolute frequencies of the occurrence of hard cancer of the breast at different ages. But it is more important to know the relative frequencies in proportion to the number of women living at each of the successive periods of life. To ascertain this I have added to the cases in the preceding table those tabulated, in a nearly similar manner, by M. Birkett‡ and M. Lebert;§ making a total of

---

* This and most of the following tables are drawn from a general table of 365 cases of cancers of all kinds. Of the whole number nearly half were observed by myself. Of the remainder, I have derived about 50 from the records of the Cancer-wards in the Middlesex Hospital, for access to which I am much indebted to the surgeons of the hospital: more than 60 were very kindly communicated to me by Mr. Humphry; others I owe to Mr. Lowe and Dr. Paget; nearly all the rest were collected from the works of Wardrop, Langstaff, Baring, Bruch, Bennett, and Sedillot.

† The ages assigned in this table are those at which, in each case, the disease was first observed *by the patient;* and no case is included which was recorded only, or chiefly because it was an example of the disease occurring at an unusual period of life.

‡ On Diseases of the Breast, p. 218.

§ Des Maladies Cancereuses, p. 354. The particulars of both these tables accord very nearly with those given above; but the numbers of cases below 20 and above 80, in Mr. Birkett's table, are very large; probably because he has included cases that were recorded on account of their rarity in respect of the patients' ages.

354 cases originating between the ages of 20 and 80 years. Then, comparing the number of cases in each decennial period of life, with the number of women alive in the same period in England and Wales (according to the Population-Returns for 1841), it appears that the comparative frequencies, relatively to the whole number of women, may be stated in the following numbers :—

Ages.	Relative frequency of the origin of hard cancer.
20 to 30	6
30 " 40	40
40 " 50	100
50 " 60	76
60 " 70	38
70 " 80	32

In other words, the proportions between these numbers may represent the degrees in which the conditions of women's lives, at the successive decennial periods, are favorable to the first growth of hard cancer in the breast.

One is naturally led to suppose that the great liability to cancer of the breast between 40 and 50 years of age, and especially the maximum between 45 and 50, are connected with some of the natural events that are then occurring in the nearly related reproductive organs; such as the cessation of the menstrual discharge, and of the maturation of ova; or else with the wasting and degeneracy of the mammary glands. And yet it is difficult to prove such a connection with any single event of the period.

The event which is generally regarded as most important is the cessation of the menstrual discharge. But I find that among 52 women with scirrhous cancer of the breast, in whose cases this point is noted, 27 were still menstruating for at least a year after their discovery of the cancer; and 16 had ceased to menstruate for a year or more previous to it; so that less than ⅓ of the whole number afforded examples of the cessation of the catamenia and the discovery of the cancer occurring within the same year.

The following table shows the ages at which menstruation ceased in 400 women,* and the ages at which hard cancer of the breast was first detected by an equal number :—

Ages.	Cessation of menstruation.	First observation of the cancer.
Below 35,	9	36
35 to 40,	51	62
40 to 45,	140	78
45 to 50,	159	101
Above 50,	41	123
	400	400

* From Dr. Guy's tables, in the Medical Times, 1845. The numbers in the third column are obtained by doubling those in a table of 200 cases, collected from those of M. Lebert and Mr. Birkett, as well as from my own.

33

All these calculations are sufficient to prove the great influence which the events of life, at and about the time of the cessation of the menstrual process, exercise in the production of cancer; but they do not prove that the defect of that process has more influence than others of the coincident events. I think we may most safely hold that the aptness of this time of life for the development of hard cancer is chiefly due to the general failure of the process of maintenance by nutrition, which usually has at this time its beginning, and of which the most obvious natural signs are in the diminution of the powers of the reproductive organs. It is in favor of this view, rather than of any special influence of the reproductive organs, or of change in the mammary gland, that, so far as we can estimate, with so small a number of cases as are yet on record, the ages of increasing frequency of hard cancer in the male breast,* and of primary hard cancer in other organs, coincide with the results of the far more numerous cases in the female breast. This would hardly be so if it were the condition of the female breast itself, or of any nearly related organ, that alone or chiefly determined the greater frequency of the cancer at particular periods of life.

(c) To these conditions of sex and age, as favoring the production of scirrhous cancer, we may add an hereditary disposition, and the effects produced by injury or previous disease. The influence of these conditions is not generally, but is often very clearly manifested. In 88 patients with hard cancer (including four men and four cases of hard cancer of other organs than the breast), 16 were aware of cancer having occurred in other members of their families. In 40 tabulated by M. Lebert only 6 could be deemed hereditary.† Probably, therefore, not more than 1 in 6 patients with hard cancer can be reckoned as having hereditary tendency thereto. And it does not appear that such a tendency, even where it exists, leads to an unusually early manifestation of the disease; for the mean age of the hereditary cases which I have collected is very nearly the same as that of the others; namely, about 48½ years. The occurrence of hard cancer in many members of a family cannot, then, be deemed frequent; yet, when it is observed, it is often too striking to leave any doubt about the reality of an hereditary tendency to the disease.

(d) So, with regard to the effects of injury and previous disease, I find that, among 91 patients, only 16, i. e. less than one-sixth, ascribed the hard cancer to injury or any such local cause. The proportion is so small (it is less even than that of the patients with other tumors, who

---

* The four men in whom I have seen hard cancer of the breast were respectively 40, 44, 48, and 52 years old at the discovery of the disease.

† The difference in the proportions of M. Lebert's cases and in mine is probably due to my having reckoned as hereditary, three cases in which members of the family had had cancers of the lip. These would be excluded as only "cancroid" by M. Lebert; and so excluded and added to the non-hereditary cases, they make the proportions very nearly equal in both our estimates.

ascribe them to the same cause*), that we might be disposed to deny the influence of injury altogether, if its consequences were not, in a few cases, so manifest and speedy.

(e) I pass by some other conditions supposed to be favorable to the occurrence of scirrhous cancers; such as mental distress, particular occupations and temperaments. Concerning all these, the numerical evidence at present gained is insufficient to justify any conclusions. But, respecting one point much discussed, namely, the general health of women at the time when hard cancer is first found in them, I would observe that a remarkable majority present the appearance of good health. I find that in 91 cases in which I have notes on this point no less than 66 patients presented the general characters of robust, or, at least, good health; 9 were of uncertain or moderately good health; and only 16 were sickly or feeble. It does not follow that all these were manifestly ill when the cancer began to form; but, granting that it may have been so, it would still appear that scarcely more than one-fourth of the subjects of hard cancer are other than apparently healthy persons. From all this it is evident, that, except in relation to the comparative liabilities of different ages, we have little knowledge of the events that are, in any sense, the predisposing causes of hard cancer. Indeed, so insignificant in their whole sum are those that are already ascertained, that, in a large majority of cases, the patient finds the cancer by some accident. She chances to touch her breast attentively, or she feels some pain in it, or her friends notice that it is smaller or larger than it used to be; and now, already, there is a cancer of, it may be, large size, of whose origin no account whatever can be rendered.

The fact last mentioned may explain why we so rarely have an opportunity of seeing what a hard cancer is like at its very beginning. I have examined only three that were less than half an inch in diameter. All these were removed within two months of their being first observed, and all had the perfect cancerous structure, such as I have described as the type. I believe they illustrated what is generally true—namely, that the cancerous structure has, from the first, its peculiar hardness. The formation of it appears to be attended with gradually increasing induration, only in the cases in which, from the beginning, it affects the whole gland, and those in which it acquires even more than usual hardness, by the gradual predominance of the increased and indurated fibrous tissue.

From the extreme of smallness the cancer grows; but at various rates, in different cases, and even in the same cases, at different times. I believe no average rate of increase can be assigned. Cases sometimes occur, especially in lean, withered women, whose mammary glands share in the generally pervading atrophy, in which two, three, or more years pass

---

* See p. 329. Of 79 tumors not cancerous 15 were ascribed to injury or previous disease, i. e. 1 in nearly 5¼.

without any apparent increase in a cancer; and the progress even of ulcerated cancer is, in such patients, sometimes scarcely perceptible, even in the lapse of years.   On the other hand, cases are found sometimes of most rapid increase.   I saw such an one last summer.   A hard cancer grew in five months from the size of the tip of a finger to a mass five inches in diameter.   This was in a woman 32 years old, in whom the disease began while she was suckling, and immediately before, even while suckling, she again became pregnant.   Extensive and speedy sloughing followed this rapid growth, and she died in seven months from the first observation of the disease.*

We may very probably connect this singular rapid progress of a hard cancer with the condition of determination of blood to the breast in which it occurred, and to the early age of the patient,—for, as a general rule, though malignant tumors may, in their plan and mode of growth, deviate never so widely from the normal tissues, yet for their rate of increase they are dependent, in a certain measure, upon the supply of blood, and the general activity of the nutritive processes.   Hence it needs to be always borne in mind, in questions of operation, that among the cancerous they that seem most robust may succomb most quickly; while the aged and withered commonly live longest and with least discomfort.

The increase of a hard cancer appears to be by gradual superaddition of new particles on the surface of the mass already existing, and in the interstices of the tissue immediately bounding it.   It is a nice question to determine how far from a mass of cancer already formed, say, in the breast, the parts to be next added to it will be formed.   Practice professes to have settled this in the rule that the whole mammary gland should be removed when only a portion of it is manifestly cancerous.   But whatever be the facts on which this rule is founded,—and I believe they are enough to justify it,—they may be explained by the advantage resulting from the removal of all the part in which the cancer would be most apt to recur: they do not prove that cancer is already present in the part of the breast that appears healthy.   It is, indeed, rare to find more than one cancerous mass in a mammary gland.   I do not remember to have seen it more than four times in about 100 cases; and in one of these the second cancer appeared to have been detached, not to have grown separately, from the principal mass.   I have looked with microscopic help at the tissues close by a hard cancer, and have found, I think, cancer-cells one or two lines distant from the apparent boundary of the chief mass, as if the disease had already begun where neither the naked eye nor the finger could have discerned it.   Beyond this little distance I have not found reason to believe that cancerous matter in any form exists in the parts of a cancerous mammary gland that appear healthy.

After an uncertain time and extent of growth of hard cancer, ULCERA-

---

* This was the same case as that related by Mr. Gray, in the Proc. of Pathol. Soc 1851-2, p. 444.

TION almost constantly follows. This may ensue in various ways; it may be accelerated or retarded by many extraneous circumstances, according to which, also, its characters may vary; but there are two modes of ulceration which are especially frequent, and are almost natural to the course of the cancer.

In one of these the ulceration begins superficially, and extends inwards; in the other the changes leading to ulceration begin in the substance of the cancer, and thus make progress outwards.

The superficial mode of ulceration is commonly observed when the cancerous growth has slowly reached and involved the skin. The best examples are those in which the hard cancer first affects a border-lobe of the gland. From this, as it grows, it extends towards the skin, occupying as it extends, the subcutaneous fat, and all the intervening tissues (fig. 82). The skin, as the cancer approaches, whether raised or depressed towards it, adheres closely to its more prominent parts, or to its whole surface. It becomes now, while cancerous matter infiltrates it, turgid with blood, thin, tense, and glossy, florid or dusky red, or livid or pale ruddy brown : the congestion does not extend far, nor very gradually fade out, as in an inflamed integument, but is rather abruptly circumscribed, just beyond the adhesion of the skin to the cancer.

In the next stage, the surface, in one or more places, appears raw, as if excoriated; or else, by some sudden stretching, it is cracked; or a thin yellow scab forms over part of it, which, being removed, exposes an excoriated surface, and is soon reproduced. After a time the excoriated or the cracked surface appears as a more certain ulcer; scabs no longer form, but a copious, acrid, thin fluid exudes. The ulcer is apt to extend very widely ; and if there have been more than one, they soon coalesce; but they very rarely extend deeply, and their surfaces rarely appear otherwise than pale, hard, dry, and inactive. The growth of the cancer continuous, as usual, after the ulceration ; and with the growth and the involving of more skin, the ulceration is generally commensurate.

Now the ulcer thus formed has, in itself, no so-called specific characters: examined by itself, it has not the features assigned to the cancerous ulcer; we recognize its nature through that of the mass beneath it. And yet there is much in the occurrence of this form of ulceration that is characteristic. For we may always notice that, though it is effected as if by the destruction of the skin, and is not unlike the ulceration that ensues over a great firm tumor that has stretched the skin to its extreme of tolerance ; yet its occurance is determined, not by the bulk of the cancer and the tension of the skin, but by the adhesion and confusion of the skin with the cancer. As the cancer approaches the skin, so the skin, without any stretching, becomes thinner and thinner ; then its residue becomes cancerous; and then, at length, it is excoriated. The cancer, exposed through the superficial ulcer, is not apt to be exuberant: it does not become or throw out "fungous growths," it manifests no peculiar tendency to further ulceration. Granulations* of ordinary aspect, or such as are only too pale and hard, may cover it, and it may often scab, or even skin over; or, if it deepen itself, it may be with no assumption of cancerous shape, but like a common chronic ulcer deepening by sloughing or accute inflammation.

Far different from this, though sometimes superadded to it is the form of ulcer of the breast which begins in the substance of the cancer. I will not now enter upon the discussions about the softening of cancers (as a normal tendency of their structure), or upon those about their interior suppuration: I will only state that, in certain cases of hard cancer, we find cavities filled and walled in with softened and disintegrated cancerous matter. In these, the dull, ochre-yellow, soft material, consists mainly of degenerate cancer-cells and their débris. It may be mingled with an ill-formed pus; and as these mingled materials increase and enlarge the cavity, so, finally, they are discharged by ulceration. Their discharge leaves in the solid mass of cancer a deep excavated ulcer, a cavity like that of a widely open abcess, except in that it is all walled in with cancerous matter, the remains of the solid mass. Then, as the walls of this cavity ulcerate on their internal surface, and at the margin of the opening into it, so their outer surface is increased by superaddition of the cancerous matter; i. e. as one part of the cancer wastes, by ejection of its ulcerating surface, so is another part increased. Hence the ulcer constantly enlarges: but the ulceration does not destroy the cancer: that increases the faster of the two, extending more and more, both widely and deeply, and involving different tissues more and more continually, to the end of life. In all its course it yields a thin, ichorous, and often irritating discharge, that smells strongly, and almost peculiarly.

In all its later course, when not disturbed, this form of cancerous ulcer has certain characteristic features, which are chiefly due to the concurrent processes of ulceration at one surface, and of predominating fresh formation at the other surface, of the cancer. Thus the edge of the ulcer is raised by the exuberant formation of cancer in and beneath the boundary of skin: the exuberance of the growth necessarily everts the margin, which is too rigid to stretch; and the margin thus raised and everted is hard, nodular, and sinuous, because the growth under it, like the primary cancer, is often formed after a knotty tuberous plan. The base of the ulcerated cavity is similarly hard and knotted, or covered with hard, coarse, cancerous granulations. Lastly, when we cut through such an ulcer, we divide a thich layer of cancer, infiltrated in the subjacent tissues, before the knife reaches any normal structures.

It would be vain to try to describe all the various and dreadful forms of ulcer that follow the accute inflammations and sloughings of scirrhous cancers, or all the aggravations of the disease by hemorrage from the

---

* These granulations are formed of cancer-structures; yet, let it be observed, they take the shape and construction of such as are formed in the healing of any common ulcer.

ulcerating surface, or by obstructions of the lymphatics or the veins. As
I passed by the effects of these accidents of the disease, in describing its
structure, so, much more, must I now. Only I would state that these
are the events which produce, in cancerous patients, the most rapid and
the most painful deaths. When inflammation is averted from it, a cancerous ulcer may exist very long, and make slow progress, without
extreme pain or disturbance of the health; it may be no worse a disease
than the "occult" cancerous growth; and ten or more years may pass
with the health scarcely more impaired than at the beginning. Sir B.
Brodie* has related two such cases; and I may add to them one which I
have lately seen in a cook, who has for eight years had hard cancer of
the breast. During five of these years it has been ulcerated, and yet
none of those with whom she lives is aware that she is diseased.

Such cases of arrest of cancer are, however, very rare; they are only
rare exceptions to the general rule of that progress towards death, the
rate of which is far less often retarded than it is accelerated by such
accidental inflammations of the cancer as I have already referred to.
Still more rare are the exceptions in which an ulcerated cancer heals.
Such cases, however, may be met with, especially among the examples
of the more superficial ulcer. The ulcers may be skinned over (as any
common ulcer usually is), and the cancerous mass beneath it may waste
and be condensed, so that the disease may be regarded as obsolete, if not
cured.

The conditions under which this healing and regress of the ulcerated
cancer may take place are, I believe, as yet quite unknown. In the
following case they seemed to be connected with the development of tuberculous disease, as if the patient's diathesis had changed, and the cancer
had wasted through want of appropriate materials in the blood.

I removed the breast of a woman 25 years old, including a large
mass of well-marked scirrhous cancer of three months' duration. She
appeared in good general health, and could assign no cause for the disease. The progress of the cancer had been very rapid; it had lately
affected the skin near the nipple; and all its characters were those of
the acute form. The axillary glands had been enlarged and hard, but
had subsided with rest and soothing treatment. Six months after the
operation, and after the patient had been for four months apparently
well, cancerous disease reappeared in the skin about the scar, and in the
axillary glands. In the skin it rapidly increased; numerous tubercles
formed, coalesced, and ulcerated; and the ulceration extended till it
occupied nearly the whole region of the scar, and often bled profusely.
Thus the disease appeared progressive for twelve months after its reappearance; but at the end of this time the ulcer began to heal, and in the
next six months a nearly complete cicatrix was formed; only a very
small unhealed surface remained, like an excoriation covered with a scab.

* Lectures on Surgery and Pathology, p. 211.

The disease in the axilla, also, nearly subsided; one hard lump alone remained of what had been a large cluster of hard glands. But even during and after the healing of the cancerous ulcer she lost strength, and became much thinner, and at length, gradually sinking, she died, nearly two years after the operation, and six months after the cancer had so nearly healed.

In the examination after death I found in the situation of the scar of the operation, a low nodular mass of the very hardest and densest cancer extending through the substance of the scar and the pectoral muscle, and nearly all covered with thin scar-like tissue. In the axilla was one hard cancerous gland, and in the liver were many masses of cancer as dense and hard as that on the chest. In all these parts the cancer-structures appeared to be condensed and contracted to their extreme limit.

The lungs contained no cancer, but were full of groups of gray succulent tubercles and grayish tuberculous infiltration in every part except their apices, where were numerous small irregular tuberculous cavities. The other organs appeared healthy.

The contrast was very striking, in this case, between the appearances of active recent progress in the tuberculous disease, and of the opposite course in the cancerous disease found after death; and I can hardly doubt that, during life, the progress of the one had been at first coincident, and then commensurate, with the regress of the other.

But leaving, for the present, the questions of the relations between cancerous and tuberculous disease, I would observe that this case illustrated the two modes of healing that may occur in cancer; namely, the formation of a scar over the ulcer, and the shriveling of the cancerous mass. The first appears to be accomplished according to the ordinary method of the healing of ulcers: the second is probably similar to the contraction and induration of deposits of inflammatory lymph. So far as I know, the process of superficial healing has not been minutely examined in relation to the changes ensuing in the elementary structures of the cancer. Only, one sees cuticle forming on the surface of apparently cancerous granulations. In the process of shriveling the cancerous mass becomes smaller, denser, drier, and harder; it contracts and draws in more tightly the adjacent parts; it yields no turbid "juice," but a thin serous-looking fluid may be scraped from it in very small quantity. One finds in such fluid, sparingly distributed, cancer-cells and nuclei, with molecular and granular débris-like matter; but (in the breast) the chief mass of the shriveled cancer seems to consist of the proper tissues of the organs, indurated and condensed. We cannot doubt that, during such a change, cancer-cells and other elemental structures are absorbed; but the changes preparatory thereto are not, I think, satisfactorily explained.*

* The whole process is minutely discussed by Virchow, in his Archiv, B. i. p. 185, et seq.

Such may serve as a general history of the progress of a scirrhous cancer in the breast. Let me add a brief notice of the pain, cachexia, and some other of its accompaniments.

Among the many inconstancies in the life of cancers, none, I think, is more striking than that which relates to the attendant pain. One sees cases, sometimes, that run through their whole career without any pain. In a case of deeply-ulcerated cancer of the breast, the patient, who had also a cluster of cancerous axillary glands, begged that the disease might be removed, but only because it was "such a terrible sight." It had never once given her the least pain. In another case a patient, from whom a cancer involving the whole mammary gland was removed, was quite unaware of any pain or other affection in her breast till, a few weeks before the operation, some of her friends observed its diminished size. The largest hard cancer of the breast that I have yet removed was equally painless. Another patient, who died with rapidly progressive and ulcerated cancer, had not a pain in its two years' duration.

On the other hand, we sometimes meet with cases that quite exemplify the agony which is commonly regarded as the constant accompaniment of hard cancer. In such a case the patient could "wish herself dead," for the sake of freedom from the fierce anguish of her pain,—pain as if a hot dart were thrust swiftly through her breast, or right through her chest,—pain, startling with a sudden pang, and then seeming to vibrate till it fades out slowly; or, sometimes, more abiding pain, likened to the burning and scalding of hot water or of molten lead. With such resemblances as these do patients strive to describe the agonies, which are indeed beyond description, and of which the peculiar intensity is perhaps best evidenced by the fact, that the sufferers almost always thus liken them to some imaginary pain, and not to anything that they have felt before. The memories of those who have suffered even the pains of child-birth supply no parallel to that which is now endured; the imagination alone can suggest the things with which it may be compared.

Now, although both these classes of cases be exceptions from the general rule concerning the painfulness of cancer of the breast, yet they are interesting, both for their own sakes, and because they illustrate the nature of the pain attending tumors; they show that it is, in great measure, independent of the merely mechanical condition of the parts; that it is due not to pressure on the nerves, or to their tension or displacement, but rather must be considered as a subjective sensation, a neuralgia due to some unknown morbid state of nerve-force. That this is so is nearly sure from the fact, that if we compare the most painful and the least painful cancers with each other, we may find their structure and relations exactly similar. Any of the forms that I have described may in one case be attended with intense pain, in another may exist without discomfort. They may present no other difference than the immense difference of painfulness.

However, as I have said, both the very painful cancers and those that are always without pain are exceptional cases. The more general rule seems to be (1), that in the early part of its course (for instance, in ordinary cases for the first year or year and a half), the hard cancer of the breast is either not painful at all, or gives only slight and occasional pain, or is only made painful by handling it; (2) that during this time, its pain has usually no peculiar character; is not generally lancinating, but more often, and especially after manipulation, is dull and heavy; (3) that after this time the cancer becomes progressively more painful, and the pain acquires more of the darting and lancinating character; (4) that the pain is generally increased when the cancer grows quickly, and more constantly when it is inflamed and ulcerating, or about to slough: (5) that the pain is yet more intense when the cancer is progressively ulcerating, and now adds to its lancinating character, or substitutes for it, the hot burning or scalding sensation.

With the advance of the local disease the signs of general disorder of the health usually increase; and the cancerous "cachexia," which may at first have been absent or obscure, is established. It would be very difficult to describe this state exactly, and much more so to analyse it. The best description of its most frequent characters is, I think, that by Sir Charles Bell :*—"The general condition of the patient is pitiable. Suffering much bodily, and everything most frightful present to the imagination, a continual hectic preys upon her, which is shown in increasing emaciation. The countenance is pale and anxious, with a slight leaden hue; the features have become pinched, the lips and nostrils slightly livid; the pulse is frequent; the pains are severe. In the hard tumors the pain is stinging or sharp; on the exposed surface it is burning and sore. Pains, like those of rheumatism, extend over the body, especially to the back and lower part of the spine; the hips and shoulders are subject to those pains. Successively, the glands of the axilla and those above the clavicle become diseased. Severe pains shoot down the arm of the affected side. It swells to an alarming degree, and lies immovable.

"At length there is nausea and weakness of digestion: a tickling cough distresses her; severe stitches strike through the side; the pulse becomes rapid and faltering; the surface cadaverous; the breathing anxious; and so she sinks."

This vivid sketch is generally true of, perhaps, a majority of the cases of hard cancer of the breast; but I doubt whether any one of the signs of cachexia here indicated is constantly present. Even emaciation is not so; for many die, exhausted by the suffering and discharge, in whom fat is still abundant, or appears even increased about the cancer itself. This want of constancy adds greatly to the difficulty of analys-

* Medico-Chirurgical Transactions, xii. 223.

ing the phenomena of the cachexia. We can see little more than that they include two mingled groups of symptoms: of which one may be called "primary," depending on the increasing morbid and peculiarly cancerous condition of the blood, and the other "secondary," depending on the local disease, and the effects produced on the blood by its pain, discharge, hemorrhage, and various accidents. In the confusion of symptoms thus arising analysis seems impossible.

The last concomitant of the scirrhous cancers of the breast, that I need now speak of, is their multiplication; but I will here only enumerate the methods in which this may happen; for its explanation belongs to the general pathology. These, then, are the methods :—

First, and most frequently, the disease extends to the lymphatic vessels and glands; or to their contents; for it seems most probable that, as Mr. Simon has suggested, its progress is along the continuity of the lymph from the breast to the glands.

(2.) Next, I think, in order of frequency, are the multiplications of the cancer in the same region; not, indeed, in the same gland, but in the skin and muscles near it, and then in areas gradually widening round it.

(3.) It is less frequent for the scirrhous cancer to appear secondarily in the similar tissue of the opposite breast. Indeed, its multiplication, if it may be so considered, is less frequent in this direction than in that of some organs of more different texture, especially the bones, the liver, and the lungs. These, among parts distant from its primary seat, are by far the most frequent seats of secondary disease; but with these, or, much more rarely, alone, nearly every tissue has been found affected.*

The structures of many examples of these secondary cancers are already described (p. 503, &c.). It is often said that the cancers which appear as secondary to the scirrhous of the breast are of the medullary kind; an error which I think must have arisen from the belief that the scirrhous cancer is always fibrous. I have already explained that it very rarely is so, and only appears to be so when it grows in parts containing fibrous tissue; and that what has been generally deemed the fibrous structure of the cancer is usually that of the organ in which it is seated. The secondary cancers are, usually, in all points conformed to the primary, and consist, like them, essentially of cells compacted into a hard mass. They may appear fibrous when growing in fibrous organs: but, inasmuch as their more usual seats are in organs that naturally contain little or no fibrous tissue, they are more commonly formed of cell structures alone. The change from hard to soft cancer is rare; it may, however, take place, especially in the latest growths; and it is the best illustration of the affinity between the two forms of the disease.

To end this history of the scirrhous cancers of the breast, I must

* M. Lebert has given a table of the relative frequencies of secondary cancers in different organs after primary disease in the breast. It is drawn from 23 autopsies. Mr. Birkett has given a similar table of 37 cases examined after death.

speak of their duration. There is a striking contrast between the certain issue, and the uncertain rate, of their progress. Cases are on record in which life has been ended in four months; and others in which it has been prolonged to twenty-five years; but I am not aware of a single clear instance of recovery : of such recovery, I mean, as that the patient should live for more than ten years free from the disease, or with the disease stationary.

The average duration of life, from the patient's first observation of the disease, is a little more than four years. In 66 cases, tabulated without selection, I find it something more than 49 months.*

Among 61 of these 7 died in between 6 and 12 months.

"	"	7	"	"	12	"	18	"
"	"	8	"	"	18	"	24	"
"	"	10	"	"	24	"	30	"
"	"	2	"	"	30	"	36	"
"	"	12	"	"	3	"	4	years.
"	"	6	"	"	4	"	6	"
"	"	3	"	"	6	"	8	"
"	"	1	"	"	8	"	10	"
"	"	5	"	"	10	"	20	"

The cases are too few to allow of many conclusions: but they suffice at least to show that the average duration of life in these cancerous patients would afford a wrong estimate of the probable duration of life in any single case; since the number who live beyond the average is far less than that of those who die within it, and the mean average is raised by the lives of those few who survive long periods.

It seems at present impossible to estimate many of the conditions which determine the duration of life; but none among them seems more weighty than the age at which the disease commences. There are, indeed, many exceptions to the rule, yet, on the whole, the earlier the disease begins the more rapid is its course. Thus, among those who lived not more than 18 months, I found that the average age at which the disease was first observed was 43 years. Among those who lived between 18 and 26 months, it was 51 years; and among those who lived between 3 and 8 years, the average at the commencement of the disease was 56·7 years.†

* I say " something more," because I have reckoned in the cases of five patients who are still living more than 49 months from the first observation of the disease. In the first table on the next page six similar cases are reckoned with those from which the general average is derived. Of the patients already dead, the average duration was, for those in this table, 49·36 months ; for those in the next table, 48·9 months. The difference is far less than I believed it to be when the lecture was delivered ; I was deceived at that time by using too small a number of cases, and a table containing some cases that were recorded only because they were examples of rarely long life.

† The average for those who lived more than 8 years was only 45 years. But this will not materially invalidate the rule as stated above, if, as I suspect, these long lives owe their unusual duration to something interfering with the more normal progress of the disease ; and if, as is also probable, the deaths from cancers, commencing in those whose average age is near 60, are often prevented or accelerated by the other diseases which destroy so large a proportion of persons living at that age.

In all the cases from which the foregoing deductions were made, the disease ran its course uninterrupted by operative treatment.

In 47 cases, in which the cancer was once or more removed by operation, the average duration of life, after the first observation of the disease, was again something more than 49 months. I believe, therefore, that the removal of the local disease makes no material difference in the *average* duration of life; but if the following table be compared with that of the preceding page, it will seem probable that the course of the more rapid cases is retarded by the operation. Among 41 of those patients who are already dead,

4	died in between	6 and	12 months.		
4	"	"	12 "	18	"
2	"	"	18 "	24	"
5	"	"	24 "	30	"
3	"	"	30 "	36	"
11	"	"	3 "	4	years.
8	"	"	4 "	6	"
2	"	"	6 "	8	"
1	"	"	8 "	10	"
1	"	"	10 "	20	"

It would seem, I repeat, as if the course of cancerous disease, that otherwise would be very rapid, were retarded by the removal of the growth; for, while in some respects the two tables closely correspond, it may yet be noticed that the proportion of those who die within two years is 36 per cent. of those in whom the disease is allowed to run its course, and only 24 per cent. of those from which the growth is once or more removed. The number of cases from which this is concluded is indeed small; but other facts might lead us to expect the same, especially that in general the most rapidly fatal cases are those in which the local disease has the greatest share in the death.

The constitutional part of the cancerous disease, little, if at all, affected by the removal of the local part, manifests itself by the recurrence of cancerous growths in or near the seat of operation, or in the lymphatics of the breast, or in some more distant part. In 74 cases, comprising 21 collected by M. Lebert and 53 by myself, the periods of recurrence after the operation were as follows :—

Between	1 and 3	months in	23 cases.		
"	3	6	"	22	"
"	6	9	"	8	"
"	9	12	"	6	"
"	12	24	"	7	"
"	2	3 years in	3	"	
"	3	4	"	1	"
"	4	6	"	2	"
"	6	8	"	2	"

Neither of us has yet met with a case in which recurrence was delayed beyond eight years.

The table confirms the view that the removal of the local has little influence on the constitutional element of the disease; for even if we believe that many of the cases, reported as recurrences between 1 and 3 months, were examples of continuous, rather than of recurrent, local disease, still the small proportion of cases in which recurrence was delayed more than twelve months after the operation might suggest the belief, that after an operation the constitutional disease continues and increases, till it manifests itself in recurrent local disease, in about the same time as it might have appeared in some secondary cancer, if the operation had not been performed.

The recurrent local disease appears generally to be less intense than the primary. This is probable, both from the fact mentioned at page 525, respecting the smaller proportion of rapidly fatal cases in those submitted to operation, and from the fact that when recurrent cancers are removed, the secondary recurrences sometimes ensue more slowly than the first did. In 12 cases in which recurrent cancers of the breast were removed I find that the period of second recurrence, *i. e.* the interval between the second operation and the reappearance of the disease, was

> Between 1 and 3 months in 4 cases.
>   "   3 " 6   "   3 "
>   "   6 " 12   "   1 "
>   "   2 " 3 years in 2 "
>   "   5 " 7   "   2 "

And, among these late-recurring cases, is one to which the first recurrence was after 24 months, the second after 60; another of first recurrence in 12 months, and second in 84; and another of first recurrence in 2 months, and second in 24.

It is believed by some that the cancer of the breast (and they would say the same of other cancers) is in the first instance a local disease; and that the constitutional disease which is manifested by recurrence after operation, or by multiplicity of cancers, or by cachexia, is the consequence of the slowly-acting influence of the local disease. If this opinion were true, we ought to find that the average interval between removal of the disease and its recurrence bears an inverse proportion to the time of duration of the cancer before removal. No such proportion, however, exists: nor does it even appear that recurrence is, on the whole, later after early, than after delayed operations. The following table shows the times of recurrence in 56 cases, in which the removal of the cancer was effected within various periods, from three months to four years, after its first appearance:—

TIME OF OPERATION.	Within 6 months.	Between 6 & 12 months.	More than 12 months.	No. of Cases.
Under 3 months,	4	2	2	8
Between 3 and 6 months,	5	2	2	9
" 6 " 12 "	5	4	5	14
" 12 " 24 "	9	1	3	13
" 24 " 48 "	7	3	2	12

The following table shows that the duration of life is not greater after early than after late operations: but this is, doubtless, because the most acute cancers are, on the whole, the most early removed:—

Time of operation.	Average duration of life after the operation.	Number of cases.
Under 3 months, ...	20 months	4
Between 3 and 6 months, ...	12 "	6
" 6 " 12 "	39 "	8
" 12 " 24 "	17 "	8
" 24 " 48 "	21 "	5

Lastly, I can find, in the cases I have collected, no confirmation of the received (and possibly true) opinion, that when some of the axillary lymphatic glands are cancerous, and are removed with the cancerous breast, the recurrence of the disease, and its fatal termination, are more speedy, than after operations in which the breast alone is removed, the glands appearing healthy. In 20 cases of removal of the breast alone, the average time of recurrence was eight months, and that of death twenty-four months, after the operation: while in 10 cases of the removal of the breast with some axillary glands, the recurrence ensued, on an average, in thirteen months, and the death in twenty-four months, after the operation.

I find as little clearly recorded evidence for the similarly unfavorable opinion generally entertained of the effects of the removal of cancers adherent to the skin, or already ulcerated. I would be far from holding that these opinions are incorrect; but their truth is not yet proved; and it is not supported by such cases as I have been able to collect. The recurrences and deaths after these "unfavorable" cases are indeed sure and speedy; but I am not yet clear that they are more so than those are which follow the operations that are undertaken in some of what are deemed the most favorable cases.

The foregoing facts, relating to the influence of the removal of cancerous breasts, on the progress of the disease, and on the duration of life, may be considered from two points of view—the pathological and the practical. Mere pathology may study these operations as so many experiments for determining the mutual influences of the local and the constitutional elements of the cancerous disease; or, the questions entertained by some respecting their priority; or, the share taken by each in destroying life. I trust that the tables I have given may be of some avail for the settlement of these and other similar questions, to which I shall again refer in the concluding lectures. But at present, few of the facts, which mere pathology can gather from inquiries such as these, are sufficiently clear or pronounced to serve for guidance in the practice of surgery, in which we have to deal with single cases, not with many at once, and in which each case presents many questions that cannot yet be solved by general statements.

In deciding for or against the removal of a cancerous breast, in any single case, we may, I think, dismiss all hope that the operation will be a final remedy for the disease. I will not say that such a thing is impossible; but it is so highly improbable, that a hope of its occurring in any single case cannot be reasonably entertained.

The question, then, is, whether the operation will add to the length, or to the happiness of life. The conclusion from the foregoing tables might be that the length of life would be the same, whether the local disease were removed or not. But such a conclusion cannot be unconditionally adduced for the decision in a single case. The tables do not include cases in which the operation was fatal by its own consequences: yet these are not few. In 235 operations for the removal of cancerous and other diseased breasts, I find 23 deaths: and probably this mortality of 10 per cent. is not too high an estimate,—at least, for the results of hospital practice. We have to ask, therefore, whether it is probable that the operation will add to the length or comfort of life, enough to justify the incurring this risk from its own consequences.

I cannot doubt that the answer may be often affirmative.—1. In cases of acute hard cancer the operation may be rightly performed: though speedy recurrence and death may be expected, its performance is justified by the probability (see p. 525) that it will, in some measure, prolong life, and will save the patient from dreadful suffering. 2. On similar grounds, the operation seems proper in all cases in which it is clear that the local disease is destroying life by pain, profuse discharge, or mental anguish, and is not accompanied by evidences of such cachexia as would make the operation extremely hazardous. 3. In all the cases in which it is not probable that the operation will shorten life, a motive for its performance is afforded by the expectation that part of the remainder of the patient's life will be spent with less suffering, and in hope, instead of despair; for when they are no longer sensible of their disease, there are few cancerous patients who will not entertain and enjoy the hope of long immunity, though it be most unreasonable and not encouraged.

On the other side, there are many cases in which the balance is clearly against the operation.—1. In well-marked chronic cancers, especially in old persons, it is so little probable that the operation will add to either the comfort or the length of life, that its risk had better not be incurred. These are, indeed, the cases in which the operation may be longest survived; but they are also those in which, without operation, life is most prolonged and least burdened. 2. In cases in which the cachexia, or evident constitutional disease, is more than proportionate to the local disease, the operation should be refused: it is too likely to be fatal by its own consequences, or possibly by accelerating the progress of cancer in organs more important than the breast. On similar grounds, and yet more certainly, it should not be performed when there is any reasonable suspicion of internal cancer. 3. If there be no weighty motives for its performance, the operation should be avoided in all patients whose general health (independently of the cancerous diathesis) makes its risk unusually great;—in all, for example, who are very feeble, very fat, over-fed, intemperate, or in any of those conditions which make persons unfavorable subjects for surgical operations.

The above rules leave unconsidered a large portion of the cases of hard cancer of the breast; and I fear that, at present, no other statement can be made concerning the cases which do not fall within such rules as these, than that each must be decided, by weighing the probability that the operation will prove fatal, or, by weakening the patient, will accelerate the progress of the constitutional disease, against the probability of its adding to the comfort, and thereby to the length of life. The first of these probabilities must be estimated by the same general principles (vague as they are) by which we reckon the dangers of all capital operations: the estimate of the second may be, I hope, assisted, though it cannot be settled, by the evidence collected in the foregoing tables. In every case we should keep in view the twofold method of destruction by this disease. It may destroy life by its consequences as a local disease; or by its primary and specific cachexia, which may be progressive independently of the local affection. Usually, indeed, its local and constitutional parts mutually affect and aggravate each other, and both contribute to the fatal issue: but, since they do not always contribute in the same proportions, our object should be to ascertain, in each case, which will contribute most,—the local disease, which the operation can remedy, or the constitutional, which, if at all affected by the operation, may be made more intense.

LECTURE XXXI.

MEDULLARY CANCER.

PART I.—ANATOMY.

FROM the long list of names which Dr. Walshe, with his usual profound research, has found assigned to this disease, I select that of MEDULLARY CANCER, because it has been sanctioned by the longest usage and by many of the best pathologists. It is true that the term "medullary" is vague and unmeaning; yet even this seeming defect may have some advantage, since, after long custom, we may now employ the word, as we do inflammation, cancer, and many others, without any reference to their original meaning, and, therefore, without any danger, of too much limiting our thoughts to the likenesses which they express. The very precision and fixity of such terms as encephaloid, cerebriform, cephaloma, and the like, are objectionable, by directing the mind to a single character

34

of diseased structures, and that an inconstant one; for the likeness to brain is observable in only a portion of the tumors to which the names of brain-like and its synonyms are applied.

The boundaries of the group of medullary cancers can be only vaguely drawn; for, although, on the whole, and as a group, they have peculiarities, both of structure and of history, which sufficiently distinguish them from the scirrhous and other cancers, yet, define them by whatever character we may, a series of specimens might be found filling every grade between them and each of the other chief forms. The term "soft cancer," often applied to them, expresses their most obvious, though not their most important distinction from the scirrhous or hard cancers, and, used comparatively, it might, for the present, suffice for the definition of the group. But, in the group thus defined, there are included many forms that appear widely different from each other; and there is, as Rokitansky has well said, no disease of which the examples present more deviations from any one cardinal character. It might be right to arrange the examples of some of these deviating forms under distinct titles; but, at present, it may be more useful to make no other division of the group, than into such as may be called, respectively, *soft* and *firm* medullary cancers. In any large series of specimens, the softer kind would constitute about two-thirds, the firmer about one-third of the whole number. The former would include such as are described as encephaloid, brain-like, milk-like, pulpy, placental, &c.; the latter would be such as have been called mastoid, solanold, nephroid, apinoid, &c.*

Certain transitional specimens would be found in the series, which might be arranged in either division, or between the two; but these, though they may prove that there is no specific distinction between the two chief divisions, do not invalidate the utility of speaking of them separately.

The medullary cancers, whether soft or firm, may grow either as separable tumors, or as infiltrations. In the former condition, they are most frequent in the intermuscular and other spaces in the limbs, in the testacle, the mammary gland, and the eye: rarely, they are thus found in the bones. In the latter condition, they most frequently occupy the substance of the uterus, the digestive canal, the serous membranes, the periosteum, and the bones.

We have, herein, the first point of contrast, in addition to that of their consistence, between the medullary and the scirrhous cancers. The latter are almost always infiltrations of natural parts: the former appear, in nearly equal frequency, as infiltrations, or as distinct growths, of cancer-substance.

The contrast is equally marked between them in regard to their

---

* I believe, also, that many examples of "albuminous sarcoma" have been firm medullary cancers.

respective seats and allocations. Of every 100 primary hard cancers, I believe that not less than 95 would be found in the breast; and there is no other organ in which they are not very rare. But, among 103 tabulated instances* of medullary cancer in external parts, the seat of primary disease was in the

Testicle, ...	in 29 cases.	
Bones, (most frequently in the femur), . . .	" 21	"
Limbs (especially in the intermuscular spaces), .	" 19	"
Eyeball or orbit, ...	" 10	"
Breast, ...	" 7	"
Walls of the chest or abdomen, ...	" 5	"
Lymphatics, ...	" 4	"
Various other parts, ...	" 8	"

———
103

Let me now, for general examples, describe such soft medullary tumors as often occur in the intermuscular spaces of the limbs or trunk.

To the touch they present a peculiar softness, or a deceptive sense of the slow fluctuation of some thick liquid; so that, even to the most experienced, their diagnosis from collections of fluid is often doubtful; and the achievement of experience in relation to them is caution rather than knowledge.

In shape, these tumors are commonly round, oval or spheroidal, fitting the adjacent parts. But they may be variously lobed; and when they are so, these following things may be noticed in them, as well as in the firmer kinds. (1) Their lobes are peculiarly apt to extend into muscular and other interspaces, far away from their chief mass. Thus (as I have seen) in the foot, they may track through the interosseous metatarsal spaces, or between bones of the tarsus; or about the hip or knee, portions may extend deep down to the immediate coverings of the joint; or, from behind the ankle-joint, they may reach with the flexor tendons, far into the sole of the foot. (2) Thus deepening as they grow, parts of these tumors may acquire unexpected deep-seated attachments. It is frequent to find them so attached in the neck, even when, in their beginning, they were easily movable tumors, or such as patients call "kernels." (3) In the same extension, they are much more apt than other tumors are to grow round, and completely inclose, important vessels and nerves. I have thus seen, in one case, the phrenic nerve, in another the pneumogastric, in another the femoral artery, in others the carotid artery and jugular vein, passing right through medullary cancer which, at first appeared freely movable and not deeply fixed, and even now had no characters of infiltration.

* It need hardly be said that this table, containing no cases of medullary cancer in the uterus or other internal organs, is not intended to prove anything concerning the relative frequency of the disease in each part of the body. I know no records by which this could be proved. Its only purposes are, to show the contrast between medullary and scirrhous cancers in relation to their usual seats in external parts, and to indicate the kind of cases from which many of the other tables in this lecture are derived.

The parts around a separable medullary cancer are generally only extended, as they might be round an innocent tumor. They are usually not contracted, or adherent, as those next to a hard cancer are. Even such a tissue as the glandular substance of the testicle may be cleanly separated from the surface of a medullary cancer, round which it has been stretched. Sometimes, however, the parts near the principal tumor contain smaller detached growths; and more rarely they are infiltrated with cancer.

When a distinct capsule exists round a medullary cancer, it is usually composed of fibro-cellular tissue, forming a very thin layer, from the interior of which partitions may pass, intersecting the substance of the tumor, or investing its several lobes. Generally, such a capsule contains numerous tortuous blood-vessels; and is tensely filled, so that, as soon as it is cut, the tumor protrudes, or, when very soft, oozes out like a thick turbid fluid. It is, usually, easy to separate the capsule, or part of it, from the surrounding tissues; but it may be closely adherent, and, I think, generally is so in the cases of medullary cancer in the breast.

In section, the soft medullary cancers usually appear lobed; and the partitions between the lobes, derived from the investing capsule, are often so complete that they may appear like separate cysts filled with endogenous growths. The lobes are of various sizes and shapes, through mutual compression; and they may even seem very differently constructed.

The material composing these cancers (when not disordered by the effects of hemorrhage, inflammation, or other disease) is a peculiar, soft, close-textured substance, having very little toughness, easily crushed and spread out by compression with the fingers. It is very often truly brain-like, most like foetal brain, or like adult brain partially decomposed and crushed. Many specimens, however, are much softer than brain; and many, though of nearly the consistence of brain, are unlike it, being grumous, pulpy, shreddy, or spongy, like a placenta, with fine soft filaments. Very few have a distinct appearance of fibrous or other regular structure.

In color, the material may be white, but most commonly, when the cancer is fresh, it is light gray (like the grayness of the retina after death). The tint is usually clear; it is in many cases suffused with pale pink or lilac, or with a deeper purple; and in nearly all, is variegated with effused blood and full blood-vessels, whose unequal abundance in different parts of the tumor produces a disorderly mottled appearance. Masses of bright yellow or ochrey substance also, like tubercle, are often found in or between the lobes, as if compressed by them, while withering and dying in the midst of their growth.

When pressed or scraped, the soft medullary cancers yield abundant "cancer-juice," a milky or cream-like, or some other turbid, material, oozing or welling up from their pressed mass. There is no better rough test for the diagnosis of medullary cancers than this is; and the substance thus yielded is generally diffusible in water, making it uniformly turbid, not floating in coarse shreds or fragments.

When the greater part of the softer and liquid substances are thus pressed out, there remains a comparatively small quantity of tissue, which appears filamentous, with abundant blood-vessels, and, to the naked eye, is spongy and flocculent, like the tissue of a placenta. This is the so-called "stroma" of the cancer; and it differs from that which, in the hard cancers, has been so named (p. 500), in that it is not part of the tissue in which the cancer has its seat, but is probably formed from the proper blastema of the cancer, and is as truly a part of the cancer as the cells and other corpuscles are.

Such are the most general or normal characters of the soft medullary cancers. It would be vain to attempt to describe all the varieties to which they are subject by the mingling of cysts within or on the surface of their mass; by hemorrhage into their substance; by inflammation; and by the various degenerations of their proper substance, of the extra-vasated blood, and of the inflammatory products. There are, I think, no other examples in which the diseases of the products of disease are so frequent, so various, or so confusing as in these.

It is in the medullary cancers alone that the blood-vessels have been minutely studied; and in these alone that it is easy to distinguish the vessels of the cancer itself from those of the organ in which it is seated. M. Lebert and his colleagues have made numerous injections, displaying arteries, capillaries, and veins, arranged in networks of various closeness, in the substance of medullary cancers of the ovary, omentum, uterus, and other parts. They have thus disproved the belief that the vascular system of these tumors is exclusively either arterial or venous. I may add, that the minute blood-vessels, though, in proportion to their size, they are thin-walled and easily torn, have the same structures as those in other new-formed parts.

In some medullary tumors we may notice a remarkable abundance of even large blood-vessels. Next to the proper cancer corpsules, they may appear to be the chief constituent. The cancer that contains them may thus appear, in many respects, like an erectile tumor, and may often vary in size, according to the fulness of its blood-vessels. (See p. 544, note.) When the blood-vessels are chiefly arterial, the whole mass of the tumor may have a soft full pulsation—a condition which seems peculiarly apt to be found when the tumor is part imbedded in, or supported by, bone, and in part held down by fibrous tissue, such as that of the periosteum.*

To the same abundant vascularity of these tumors we may ascribe not only their liability to internal apoplectic hemorrhage,† but the great

* See Mr. Stanley's paper on the "Pulsating Tumors of Bone," in the Med. Chir. Trans. vol. xxviii. 303.

† It is chiefly to the medullary tumors changed by internal, and prone to external, hemorrhage, that the name of fungus hæmatodes has been applied.

bleedings that may ensue when they protrude through ulcers, or are wounded. I have twice seen the difficulty of distinguishing a medullary cancer of the testicle from a hematocele enhanced by the fact, that when the swelling was punctured with a trocar, blood flowed in a full stream through the canula, and continued so to flow till the canula was withdrawn. The size of the swelling was not diminished, as that of an hematocele would have been, by the abstraction of the blood; and in both cases it proved to be a large medullary cancer, very vascular and very soft. So, when such tumors are cut into the limbs, the vessels that bleed are far larger and more numerous than in any other tumor, except the erectile.

The vessels, moreover, often appear defective in muscular power; for, as Mr. Hey* noticed, the bleeding from them scarcely decreases even when a tourniquet compresses the main artery of the limb. It is as if they could not contract so as to close themselves, even when the force of the blood is diminished to the amount with which it traverses the anasto-mosing channels.

Lastly, we may connect with the great vascularity and rapid growth of these soft tumors, the large size of the veins near them; though this is not peculiar to them, but is found, I think, with nearly all tumors that grow rapidly and to a large size.

Lymphatics have been injected in two specimens of medullary cancer of the stomach and of the liver, by Schroeder van der Kolk.† In both instances the vessels passed into the very substance of the cancer.

Of nerves I believe that none have been found in these or in any other cancers, except such as they have involved in their growth.

The same structures which alone form the separable medullary cancers may be infiltrated among the natural structures of parts. Thus infil-trated, the natural structures are expanded and rarefied; sometimes, indeed, they seem to be, in a measure, thus changed, even before the cancerous material is deposited among them.‡ Finally, most of them disappear, as in the infiltrations of scirrous cancer; and the can-cerous mass may now seem like a separately-growing tumor; or, when its material is very soft, it may appear as a quantity of creamy liquid, collected, like the pus of an abscess, in a defined cavity.

Exceptions to the general rules of the wasting of the infiltrated tissues are often observed in the fibrous tissues and the bones: both these may increase during soft cancerous infiltrations.

Medullary cancers may be found in the articular ends of bones, form-ing distinct tumors around which the walls of the bone are expanded in a thin or imperfect shell. But more commonly the cancer is infiltrated. In these cases, it usually occupies, at once, the cancellous tissue, the

* Observations in Surgery, p. 258.

† Lespinasse: De vasis novis pseudomembranarum, 1842, p. 41.   ‡ Walshe, l. c. p. 353.

wall of the bone, and the periosteum : and it seems probable that the disease begins simultaneously in all these parts ; or, at least, that when they are affected in succession, it is not generally by extension from one to the other.   Hence we commonly find that a tumor surrounds the bone, or, in the case of a flat bone, covers both its surfaces ; and that the portion of bone thus invested is itself infiltrated with cancer, which is collected most evidently, but not exclusively, in its cancellous tissue.   When a medullary tumor thus surrounds a long bone, it is usually of unequal thickness : when both surfaces of a flat bone are covered, the tumor is usually biconvex lens-shaped, and is, on both surfaces, of nearly equal extent.

The periosteum may seem to be continued over a medullary cancer thus placed ; but is really, with the exception of a thin outer layer, involved in it, and intersects its substance.   The intersecting portions of periosteum chiefly traverse the exterior tumor, extending from the layer which invests its surface to the wall of the bone.   They form branching and decussating shining bands, which to the microscope present a perfect fibrous tissue infiltrated with the cancerous materials.   They may, also, be much increased by growth, so as to give the section of the tumor an appearance of "grain," or of a tissue with fibres set vertically on the bone.   Or, the periosteal tissue thus growing may ossify.   In this event, it forms, in a large majority of cases, a light, spongy, and friable growth of bone, which is like an internal skeleton of the cancer.

Most of the specimens of "spongy" or "fungous" exostoses are such skeletons of cancers, examined after the maceration and removal of all the morbid structures that filled their interspaces.   The new bone is often formed in thin plates and bars or fibres, the chief of which extend outwards, at right angles to the surface of the bone on which they grow ; they may pass deeply into the substance of the cancer, but they seldom reach its outer surface : no medulla is formed with them ; and they sometimes form a denser and harder tissue, like that which belongs to the osteoid cancers (see p. 466).

In the walls, or compact substance, of the bone thus enclosed by cancer, it is common to find the laminæ separated by cancerous deposit, mingled with a ruddy, soft material, like diploe.   In other cases, the structure of the walls is rarefied, and converted into a light, soft, and porous or finely spongy tissue, whose spaces contain cancer-structures.   The Haversian canals, also, may be enlarged ; cancerous matter being formed within them.   Sometimes, a peculiar appearance is derived from an unequal separation of the laminæ of a bone's walls ; large spaces being found between them like cysts, which may be filled with blood or softened cancer.

Lastly, in the diploe or cancellous tissue, a corresponding state exists. The soft cancerous material excludes the medulla, and, commonly, its formation is attended with a disturbed growth of the bony cancelli, so that they form a finely spongy, dry and brittle structure, or more rarely a dense and hard structure, resembling the skeleton of the external mass of cancer.*

It remains that I should describe the FIRM MEDULLARY CANCER. In all their general relations,—as to seat, shape, size, and connections, —these correspond with the softer kind.   Like them, they may be separate masses, or infiltrated; may have distinct investing capsules, or may extend indefinitely in the proper substance of organs; like them, they are apt to affect a certain part or place rather than a single tissue: or may be the seats of various degeneration or disease: their only peculiarities are in their own structures.†

They are firm masses: not hard, like scirrhous cancers: but firm, elastic, tense, compact, and moderately tough ; they are as tough as the more pliant examples of fibrous cartilage, and merge into exact likeness to the less hard and more elastic scirrhous cancer.   They are not evidently fibrous, but tear or split as very firm coagulated albumen might. Their cut or torn surfaces appear peculiarly smooth, compact, shining, and sometimes translucent: in some instances, they are uniform and without plan; in some, more regularly and minutely lobed, or even imitating the appearance of any gland, such as the mammary or parotid in which they lie.   Sometimes they present a strongly marked grain, as if from fibres: but this results, I believe, from a peculiarly fasciculate and linear arrangement of elongated calls.

In color, the firm medullary cancers are hardly less various than the softer kind.   They may be pure white; but more often are white, tinted or streaked with pale pink, or yellow; or they may be in nearly every part buff-colored, or gray; or these tints may be mingled and mottled with blood-color, though not so deeply, or with such effusions of blood, as are frequent in the softer tumors.

On pressure, especially after contact with water, they generally yield a characteristic creamy or grayish fluid, which sometimes appears strangely abundant, considering their firmness of texture.   In a few instances, however, this character is wanting; the firmest tumors may give only a thin, turbid fluid.

Among the points of contrast, in the description of Medullary and scirrhous cancers, is the wider range of variety exhibited by the former in the original characters of its growths.   For the diversities which I have been describing are not to be referred to changes ensuing in different stages of the same disease; the firmer cancers do not gradually be-

---

* I have twice seen a formation of very firm fibrous substance, like the basis of the osteoid cancers, in the cancellous tissue of bones that were surrounded with very soft medullary cancer.   I have, also, seen a light brittle skeleton formed in the cancer external to a bone of which the cancellous tissue was converted into hard osteoid substance.

† Generally, I think, when they affect bones, the osseous tissue is apt to soften and waste, rather than to grow as it does in the soft medullary cancerous affections.   Certainly, the firm medullary cancers rarely have internal skeletons.

come soft, nor the soft become firmer; they are not to be connected (as the chief varieties of scirrhous cancer may be) with the acute or chronic progress of the disease, or with its different modes of growth, or with the differences of age in which it occurs: rather, the peculiar features of each specimen, and of each chief group, appear to be original and constant,—provided they are not affected by degeneration or disease. Now, equal diversities exist in the microscopic structures of medullary cancers. There are, indeed, certain characters to which nearly all are conformed: the microscopic diagnosis is, therefore, seldom difficult, very seldom doubtful; yet many varieties of appearance need to be learnt, both that the disease may be always recognized, and that we may, if possible, hereafter accurately divide the inconveniently large group into smaller ones. At present such a division is impracticable; for we can only sometimes trace a correspondence between a peculiarity of microscopic structure, and one of general aspect, in the tumors; but it should be a chief object of future inquiries.

The varieties exist in both the corpuscles and the basis, stroma, or intercellular substance of the cancers.

Among the corpuscles, the most frequent, and that which seems the normal, form, is that of nucleated cells, which, in all essential characters, are like those of hard cancer (p. 496, fig. 85). Examples of such cells may be found in nearly every specimen, although, in certain instances, other forms may predominate over them. There is, I believe, no mark by which they may be always distinguished from the cells of hard cancers. They may be softer, less exactly defined, more easily disintegrated by water, flatter than the cells of scirrhous cancer are; but there is in these things no important distinction. The only constant difference is in the modes of compacting, and in the relations of the cancer-materials to the natural structures in which they are placed. Cells such as, in scirrhous cancers, are closely placed, with a sparing, firm, intermediate substance, or are tightly packed among the contracted structures of a mammary gland, are in the medullary cancers more loosely held together, in a more abundant, and much softer or liquid intercellular substance.

The chief varieties of microscopic forms in medullary cancers may be described as affecting, severally, the nuclei, the cells, and the intercellular substance; and it may be generally understood that each peculiar form may occur in combination with a predominant quantity of the ordinary or typical cancer-structures, or may, in rarer instances, form the greater part, if not the whole, of a cancerous mass.

(a) Free nuclei, suspended in liquid or imbedded in a soft, nebulous, or molecular basis-substance, may compose the whole of a very soft medullary cancer. Appearances of cells may be seen among them, because of the adhesion of the basis-substance to them; and appearances of many-nucleated cells, when fragments of the basis are detached in which several nuclei are imbedded. But certainly, in many instances, formed cells are rare or absent: the structure is as if abundant nuclei were developed in a blastema, but had not appropriated the several portions of it, which in further development might be shaped into cells.

The nuclei (fig. 90) are like those of the typical cancer-cells (p. 496); they are oval or round-oval, having a long diameter of from $\frac{1}{1100}$ to $\frac{1}{1000}$

Fig. 90.*

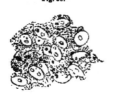

of an inch, bright, pellucid, perfectly defined, largely, and often doubly nucleolated.

It is in the structures thus formed that the minute blood-vessels of cancer may be best examined without injection; for the soft material in which they ramify may be washed away from them, so as to leave them nearly alone, and fit for examination as transparent objects.

(*b*) Free nuclei (fig. 91), which may be considered as grown or developed, are often mixed in various proportions, with other cancer-structures. Some, retaining the usual shape, are much larger than the average: others, rarer and more peculiar, are elongated, narrow, strip-like, caudate, or pyriform. Some of these are very small, slender, and apparently of simple structure: others more nearly acquire the size and other characters of cells. Their contents are not so simple and pellucid as those

Fig 91.†

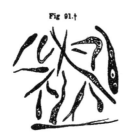

of ordinary nuclei; in the smaller they are darkly dotted or granular, but no contained particles appear larger than common nucleoli. In others, larger, oval, pellucid corpuscles, like small nuclei, are contained; and these seem to be formed by the enlargement of the nucleoli, which thus approach or attain the characters of nuclei, while the nuclei that contain them are advanced to the condition of cells. Most commonly, the cells, that thus seem formed out of nuclei, are singly nucleated; but two or three nuclei are found in a few of large size.

(*c*) In a few specimens of medullary cancer of the breast (p. 546), and of the parotid, I have found the chief constituent to be free or clustered nuclei, of round or round-oval shape (fig. 92), from $\frac{1}{1500}$ to $\frac{1}{2000}$ of an inch in diameter, well-defined, but not darkly, nebulous or molecular rather than pellucid, and appearing to contain four, five, or more shining granules, but no special or distinct nucleolus. They might have been taken for large corpuscles of inflammatory lymph, but that neither water nor acetic acid affected them. They were imbedded in a small quantity of molecular basis, and sometimes arranged in groups, imitating the shapes of

* Fig. 90. Nuclei of soft medullary cancer, imbedded in a molecular basis-substance. without cancer-cells. Magnified 500 times.

† Fig. 91. Various grown and developed nuclei of medullary cancer, as described in the text. Magnified 500 times.

acini of glands. A few of smaller size, but similar aspect, appeared to be within cells.

(d) In a remarkable case, lately at St. Bartholomew's Hospital, a

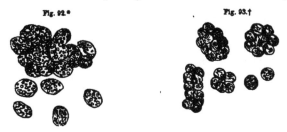

Fig. 92.*   Fig. 93.†

woman, 67 years old, had two very large and several smaller tumors connected with the skull, a tumor in the lower part of the neck, and similar small growths in the lungs. They were all very soft, close-textured, white, or variously covered with extravasated blood, enclosing large cavities filled with bloody fluid. Except that they yielded no creamy fluid till after they were partially decomposed, one could not hesitate to call them medullary cancers. But they were composed, almost exclusively, of round, shaded nuclei, with three or four minute shining particles, and in general aspect very like the dotted corpuscles of the spleen. Many of these were free; but more, I think, were arranged in regular clusters or groups, of from five to twenty or more, composing round, or oval, or cylindriform bodies (fig. 93). A few similar nuclei were enclosed singly in cells in the cancerous growths in the lungs.

Such are the chief varieties in the nuclei of medullary cancers. Scarcely less may be found in cells, mingled, let me repeat, in diverse proportions, with cells or nuclei of typical form, and rarely surpassing them in number.

(e) Besides those varieties in the shapes of cells, which were described among the microscopic characters of hard cancers (p. 496), and which are equally, or with yet more multiformity, found in these, we may note the occasional great predominance of elongated caudate cells in some examples of medullary cancers. I have hitherto observed this in none but some of the firmest specimens of the kind. Many such contain only typical cancer-cells; but in some the caudate and variously elongated cells predominate, and, by their nearly parallel and fasciculate arrangement, give a fibrous appearance to the section of the tumor. The following sketch (fig. 94) is from the cells of a very firm tumor that grew round the last phalanx of a great toe.‡ Its cancerous nature was proved

* Fig. 92. Dotted nuclei of medullary cancer, described in the text. Magnified 500 times.

† Fig. 93. Clustered nuclei of a medullary cancer, described in the text. Magnified about 400 times.

‡ Mus. Coll. Surg. 252; and of St. Bartholomew's, Series xxxv. No. 54.

not only by its structure, but by its recurrence after amputation, and by similar secondary disease of the inguinal glands. I found scarcely any cells but such as are drawn. Some were narrow, tongue-shaped, broad, and rounded or truncated at one end, and at the other elongated and tapering. Some were elóngated at both ends; some oat-shaped; some very slender, with long awn-shaped or cloven processes. All these had large, oval, well-defined clear nuclei, like those of ordinary cancer-cells, and with distinct nucleoli. Their texture, also, appeared to resemble that of common cancer-cells; they differed only in shape, being, in this, most like the cells of recurring fibroid tumors (p. 412).

(f) In the two instances I have found cancers which, by their general

Fig. 94.*   Fig. 95.†

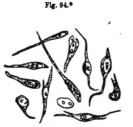 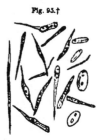

characters and history, should be called firm medullary cancer, and which were, in great part, composed of much smaller, narrower, and proportionally more elongated cells than those last described. One of these was a large deep-seated tumor behind the inner ankle and in the sole of the foot, enclosing the posterior tibial and plantar vessels and nerve, and the flexor tendons. In the other case, the primary tumor involved the gum and larger part of the front of the lower jaw; and similar secondary disease was diffused through part of the right lobe of the thyroid gland, and, in small masses, in both lungs. All the tumors were very firm and elastic; the fluid that they yielded was not creamy, but viscid and yellowish. The tumor on the foot was gray, shining, minutely lobed, intersected with opaque-white fibrous bands, and in its own tissue appeared fibrous. That on the jaw was grayish white, suffused with pink, glistening, but with no appearance of fibrous or other texture. In all there were much molecular matter and granular debris, cancer-nuclei, and a few cells of ordinary form; but their essential structures were (as in fig. 95) very small, narrow, and elongated cells and nuclei. The cells were of various shapes; some sharply caudate, some swollen in the middle, some abruptly truncated. They looked wrinkled and pellucid. They measured, generally, about $\frac{1}{1000}$ of an inch in length. Some had elon-

* Fig. 94. Caudate and variously elongated cells of a firm medullary cancer, described in the text. Magnified 450 times.

† Fig. 95. Small elongated cells and nuclei, with a nuclei of ordinary shape, from a firm medullary tumor, as described above. Magnified 500 times.

gated clear nuclei; in others no nuclei appeared. Many free nuclei had
the same shapes as these cells, and of many corpuscles it was hard to
say whether they should be called cells or nuclei.

(g) Sometimes one meets with cells, in medullary cancers, in which
nuclei are not at first discernible. They are round, large, nebulous; they
contain many minute granules; and, when water is added, it diffuses
their contents, and may display a round nucleus, smaller, and more nebulous or granular than those of the typical cancer-cells.

(h) Cells containing many nuclei are regarded by some as frequent in
certain medullary cancers. I believe that such cells may occur, and that
occasionally endogenous cells may be found within those of larger size
and probably older growth; but I am more sure that cells containing
cells, or containing more than three nuclei are very rare. What have
been described as brood-cells in medullary cancers, or as cells which, by
the multiplication of their nuclei, were effecting rapid increase of the
cancer, were, I believe, in some instances, the many-nucleated cells of
myeloid tumors, and, in more instances, detached masses or fragments of
molecular basis-substance in which nuclei were imbedded. I may add,
that I have not found in medullary cancers, any structures similar to
those of the laminated cysts or capsules which occur in epithelial cancers.

Such are the chief varieties of the corpuscles of medullary cancer:
these, at least, are what I have found them presenting in their natural
state. Much might be said respecting the changes effected in them by
the fatty and other degenerations and diseases, and about the confusion
brought into the microscopic diagnosis by the granular masses, free
granular matter, and various débris hence derived. But for these I must
refer to the general account of degenerations in previous lectures.* It
remains that I should speak of the substance with which the cells are
associated—the basis, intercellular substance, or stroma.

I need not repeat what has been said (p. 501) respecting the "stroma,"
so-called, of a cancerous infiltration,—that it is only the tissue of the
organ in which the cancer is seated. What I have now to describe is the
substance which is proper to the cancer, and in which the cancer-corpuscles are suspended or imbedded.

(a) The cells and nuclei of medullary cancers may be suspended in
liquid alone; and the two, like a collection of fluid rather than like a
tumor, may be infiltrated in tissues, or, more rarely, may be contained
in small cavities. This is not unfrequently the case in very rapid productions of cancerous matter, especially in secondary deposits. The
liquid (cancer-serum, as it has been named) is turbid; it dims transmitted
light, and has a fimely molecular appearance. With the cancer-corpuscles,
and usually with granular matter, it makes the "cancer-juice;" the peculiar thick, creamy liquid, tinted with yellow, gray, pink, or purple, and

---

* Or, with more advantage, to Lebert's admirable account of the changes of the cancer-
cells, in his "Traité pratique," p. 23.

easily diffusible in water. The quantity of corpuscles in proportion to the liquid is various; it may be so small, and the corpuscles themselves may be so lowly developed, that the liquid, like a mere blastema, may appear the chief constituent of the cancer.

(b) The same kind of liquid which, in the cases just referred to, forms the only material suspending the corpuscles, exists, also, in the solid medullary cancers: it is the liquid of the "cancer-juice." But in the more solid growths it appears to be diffused through some solid tissue, or in the interspaces of a kind of spongy texture. This, which may be more properly called a stroma of medullary cancer, is, in its simplest form, a nearly pellucid substance, having either no trace of structure, or only imbedded roundish or elongated nuclei; but sometimes it appears fibrillated.

(c) Sometimes a framework, enclosing and supporting cancer-cells, appears to be formed by elongated fibro-cells arranged in series of communicating lines. But, more commonly, a framework is constructed of delicate, pellucid or nucleated membrane, with filamentous tissue. In the last case one obtains from a medullary cancer, after expressing as much as possible of its "juice," a kind of sponge, flocculent and shreddy, constructed of membrane and filamentous tissue, with blood-vessels and still-adhering cancer-particles. One thus sees that, in even the minuter parts, the substance of the growth is intersected with such partitions as are visible with the naked eye, separating its larger lobes.

(d) Lastly, when medullary cancer is formed in bone or periosteum, these tissues may, as I have said, grow excessively, and make for it a fibrous or osseous skeleton (p. 535). Or, in other cases, new fibrous or osseous tissue may be formed in the cancer, apparently by the development by its own blastema, and may be as a stroma for the cancer-cells. Medullary cancers thus composed are the chief examples of transition-forms to the scirrhous cancers, on the one hand; and, on the other, to the osteoid cancers, in which the cancer-cells are wholly or nearly superseded by the imperfect ossification of the cancerous blastema.

Rokitansky has lately published an essay* on the development of the stroma or skeleton of cancers, an abstract of which, with copies of some of his illustrations, may find here an appropriate place. It relates, almost entirely, to that kind of stroma, in medullary cancers, which is described above (c, p. 541).

In certain examples of such a stroma or skeleton, two interlacing networks, or meshed structures, may be seen (figs. 96, 97). One of these (b) consists of slender bands, beams, or tubes (fig. 96, c) of an hyaline substance, which contains oblong nuclei, and may be in part fibrillated or transformed into filamentous tissue. The other and younger struc-

* Ueber die Entwickelung der Krebsgerüste, 1852, from the Sitzungsberichte der kais. Akademie.

ture (a) is composed of larger opaque bands or beams, which are made up of nucleated cells, with elementary granules, and variously per-
forated. These form a network interlacing with that formed by the hyaline structures. Moreover, with these opaque beams, form-ed of the same structures, and projecting from them, or from the hyaline struc-tures, there are hollow fiask-shaped or villous pro-cesses or outgrowths (fig. 97). Many of these pass through the apertures or meshes in the networks, projecting through them with free ends; and the apertures with which many of them are perforated, enlarging by absorption, give them the appearance of netted hollow bands or cords. Some of these same processes, also, ap-pear pellucid, hyaline, and nucleated at their bases or pedicles of attachment, or through more or less of their length.

These several conditions of the stroma indicate, Ro-kitansky says, that it is con-structed on that plan of "dendritic vegetation," of

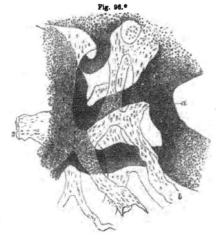

Fig. 96.*

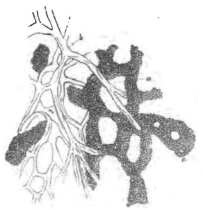

Fig. 97.*

which the type and best example is in the villous cancers. The growth of the stroma takes place, at first, in the form of hollow, flask-shaped, budding and branching processes or excrescences, which are composed of hyaline membrane, and filled with nucleated cells and granules. These processes constantly increase, throwing out fresh off-shoots of the same shape as themselves first had (comparably with the increase of the exogenous villi of the cystic chorion, described at p. 356). At the same time the cells, or part of the cells, within the processes unite or fuse their cell-walls, while their nuclei remain and are elongated. Thus the texture of the

* Figs. 96 and 97. Development of cancer-stroma, described in the text. Magnified 90 times. From Rokitansky.

growing stroma becomes hyaline, nucleated, or at last filamentous, and tubular; and, as apertures are formed in it by partial absorption of its textures, it becomes also meshed and reticulate or sponge-like. Fresh dendritic vegetations arising, on the same plan, from the network thus formed, pass with interlacements through its meshes; and, by repetition of the changes just described, increase the stroma and the complexity of its construction.

The production of cancerous elements is commensurate with the growth of the stroma, and they fill all the interstices, as well as, in some cases, the tubules of the networks.*

The foregoing descriptions, though illustrated by only a few examples, might suffice, I believe, for the medullary cancers of nearly all parts. Yet it may be useful, if, after the example of the other lectures, I describe some of the peculiarities which this form of cancer presents in certain organs,—making a selection on the same grounds as in the last lecture (p. 503).

In the TESTICLE, the medullary cancer is, usually, of the softer kind: the firmer kind is not uncommon; but examples of the scirrhous, or any other form of cancer, except the medullary, are of exceeding rarity.

The medullary cancer commonly appears as a regular oval, or pyri-form mass, which the toughness of the enclosing fibrous coat of the testicle permits to grow to a great size without protrusion. As the fibrous texture is distended by the growth, so it commonly also increases in thickness. The surfaces of the tunica vaginalis are generally partially adherent; and what remains of the cavity, usually at its upper part, is filled with serous or blood-tinged fluid. Part, or the whole, of the glandular tissue of the testicle may, I think, be always found outspread on

---

* Rokitansky holds that the same method of construction is to be traced in the formation of the layers of false membrane, which are found with reticulate or areolar surfaces, or, later, with interlacing laminæ of fibres, on the pleura and other serous membranes. He illustrates it, also, by the reticulate deposits on the interior of arteries; and lastly, by the examples of cavernous or erectile tumors, *i. e.* not of such as he admits to be formed by dilatation of blood-vessels, but of such as are entirely new-formed structures. I have supposed these (see p. 486) to be new growths, in which the blood-vessels greatly enlarging produce the character of an erectile tissue. Rokitansky says that processes spring from the bands and the cords of the cavernous tissue of such tumors, which processes end with flask-shaped swellings, and are either opaque, and formed of nucleated cells, or are formed of nucleated hyaline tissue, or of long fibro-cells, or of fibro-cellular tissue. From these likenesses he deduces for the cavernous tumors the same plan of development as for the stroma of cancer. He believes, moreover, that the blood which some of them contain is formed in them; saying that in small, lately-formed, erectile tumors, no anastomosis between their blood-spaces and the blood-vessels in the parts around them can be found.

Lastly, he says (and the statements may be added to what is mentioned at p. 489) the affinity of the cavernous blood-tumor with cancer is more than a formal one. They not unfrequently exist together in the same organ, *e. g.* in the liver; and the stroma of the cancer may be exactly like the mesh-work of the vascular tumor. Cavernous tumors, also, may be found in large numbers at once in the most different organs and tissues: for example (as in a case related by him), in the whole peritoneum, the costal pleura, the subcutaneous tissue, one of the psoas muscles, the choroid plexuses, and the fat at the base of the heart.

the surface of the tumor; the epididymis, often the seat of similar disease, is generally flattened and expanded. Separate medullary cancers may lie near; especially in the loose cellular tissue of the spermatic cord: or, the growth may perforate the tunica albuginea, and extend exuberantly about the testicle in the sac of the tunica vaginalis, or in the loose tissue of the scrotum: or, without communication, part of the cancer may be within, and part around, the tunica albuginea.*

The general characters of the cancer-structure in the testicle are usually conformed to the type already described, yet these points may be considered worthy of note: (1) Sometimes the lobes of the cancerous mass are severally so invested with fibro-cellular tissue that they may have the appearance of cysts filled with endogenous cancerous growths.† (2) Portions, or whole lobes, of the tumor, degenerate and withered into a yellow substance, like tuberculous or "scrofulous" matter, are usually seen; especially near the central parts of the cancer. (3) Large cavities full of blood may exist, and add to the difficulty of the diagnosis from hæmatocele. (4) The conjunction of medullary cancer with cartilage is more frequent in the testicle than in any other part (see p. 444). (5) The disease very rarely affects both testicles, either at once or in succession.

The medullary cancer of the EYE so rarely deviates from the general characters of the disease, and, since Mr. Wardrop's first account of it, has been described, in all works in Ophthalmic Surgery, so much more fully than would here be reasonable, that I shall advert to only two points which it illustrates. (1) It is especially apt to present, either in parts or throughout, the melanotic form; a fact which we can hardly dissociate from that of its growth near a seat of natural black pigment, and which illustrates the tendency, even of cancers, to conform themselves, in some degree, to the structures of adjacent healthy parts. (2) It shows a remarkable disregard of tissue in its election (if it may be so called) of a seat of growth. I fully agree with M. Lebert in his denial of the opinion that either the retina, or any other tissue of the eyeball, is in all or even in a large majority of cases the place of origin of the cancer. Rather, we have, here, a striking instance of what may be called the *allocation* of cancers: of their growth being determined to certain places rather than to certain tissues. Any of the tissues within or about the globe of the eye, or any two or more of them at a time, may be the primary seat of the cancer; and, probably, each of them is more liable to be so than any similar tissue elsewhere is: the locality, therefore, which they all occupy, may be assumed as that to which the can-

---

* Mr. Prescott Hewett showed me a specimen in which healthy testicle was surrounded by medullary cancer. Examples of similar cancers in the spermatic cord, the testicles being healthy, are in the College Museum, No. 2462-3: some affecting the undescended testicles are related by Mr. Arnott (Med.-Chir. Trans. xxx. p. 9).

† Mus. Coll. Surg. No. 2396.

cerous growth is directed, rather than any of the tissues themselves. And so it appears to be, when, after extirpation, the cancer returns, as if with preference, in the same locality, although the whole of the first growth, and of the tissues which it occupied, are removed.

The BREAST is among the parts which are most rarely the seats of medullary cancer. So rare, indeed, is well-marked medullary cancer of the breast, in this country, that Mr. Lawrence, in his immense experience, has met with but two examples of it; and, in our Museums, it is very rarely seen. This rarity is the more remarkable by its contrast with the occurrence of the disease abroad. In France, according to M. Lebert,* about one-fifth of the cancers of the breast are "soft and encephaloid." In America, Dr. J. B. S. Jackson has assured me that the proportion is not less than one-fifth; and I gather, from the records of German writers, that it is with them about the same.

I have never seen, in the recent state, a medullary cancer of the breast which had a brain-like or any other usual appearance:† but I have observed four cases of what must be regarded as medullary cancer, though widely deviating from the usual characters, and not resembled by any of the same kind except some of those occurring in the brain. They may be worth description, because they are with difficulty distinguished from hard cancers, on the one hand, and from mammary glandular or cystic tumors, on the other. If a general description may be drawn from these few cases, it may be to the following effect.

The tumors are separable masses, closely connected with the surrounding mammary gland or fat, but not incorporated with them, and having, in some instances, distinct thin capsules,—a character, at once distinguishing them from all the scirrhous cancers of the breast that I have yet seen. They are, generally, seated on or near the surface of the gland, "floating," as mammary glandular tumors often do. The skin over them is upraised, thin and tense; not depressed, or morbidly adherent, or itself cancerous; but when ulceration is at hand, becoming livid, then ulcerating sparingly, and then everted with the protruding and outgrowing tumor. The tumors are oval, flattened, rounded or nodular; firm, sometimes very firm, but not hard or very heavy like scirrhous cancers, and at or about their centres they feel like cysts tensely filled with fluid. They may grow quickly, and to much larger size than scirrhous cancers; are not remarkably painful; and appear prone to be associated with the formation of large serous cysts. Their general history is that of ordinary medullary cancers.

With these characters alone, the diagnosis of such medullary cancers of the breast is very difficult; all these equally belong to mammary glandular

* Des Maladies Cancereuses, p. 326.

† I do not so consider two specimens in the Museum of St. Bartholomew's, Series xxv. 28, 29, removed from the front of the chest after amputation of the breasts on account of extreme hypertrophy.

tumors or proliferous mammary cysts.   But the same disease may exist
in the axillary lymphatic glands, forming quickly-growing masses, apt to
be much larger than those in scirrhous cancer.   And, if ulceration ensue
in the tumor, it becomes exuberant, with lobed and coarsely-granulated
firm growths, discharging offensive ichor, and sometimes profusely
bleeding.

When such tumors are removed, they are found, as already stated,
separable from the mammary gland; it is pressed away by them, but is
itself healthy.   The section of the tumor is minutely lobed, with lobes or
"granulations" closely grouped, like those of a mammary glandular
tumor.   Their texture is close, more or less firm, easily crushed, shining
on the cut surface.   In color, they are grayish, varied with dots and
irregular lines of yellow (which do not follow the course of the gland-
ducts), or, in parts, suffused with livid or deeper purple tints.   Parts of
them, or even whole lobes, may be soft, shreddy, pale yellow, like tuberculous infiltration; and these seem to be portions that are degenerate and
withered, like the tuberculoid materials in other medullary cancers.
They yield, not a creamy fluid, but a turbid grayish, or viscid yellowish
one.   In some instances large cysts lie in or upon them, filled with
serous, or blood-stained, or darker fluid.

In microscopic examination traces of a glandular acinous plan may be
again observed: the corpuscles of the tumor being, at least in parts,
grouped in round or oval forms, though the groups are not inclosed in
membrane.   The corpuscles may be well-formed cancer-cells and nuclei
imbedded in molecular substance.   But I have also found in them, with
these or alone, abundant nuclei (some free and some in cells), such as are
described at page 538, fig. 92.   It was, chiefly, such nuclei as these
which being clustered, gave the minute appearance of glandular construction: and in some parts, these alone, clustered and close packed,
seemed to make up nearly the whole substance of the tumor.

In the SUBCUTANEOUS TISSUE, or deeper areolar layer of the skin, the
medullary cancers, while generally conformed to the type, exhibit these
peculiarities:

(1) They are apt to assume the melanotic state; a fact allied to that
already mentioned of the cancers of the eyeball (p. 545).

(2) While, in nearly all other external parts, the medullary cancers
appear as single growths, they are here very often multiple.   Such
numerous cancers may grow after one affecting some distant organ; or
may be first formed below the cutis.   In the latter case, many may
appear coincidently; or, when in succession, none seem to be consequences
of the growth of their predecessors; they all have the characters of
primary cancers, of "cancers d'emblé."   In some cases all the tumors
appear in a single region of the body.   In an old man, lately under Mr.
Lawrence's care, two medullary cancers were removed from the scalp,

and four remained in it. In a case which I shall presently detail a large number were seated on one arm and shoulder, but scarcely any appeared elsewhere. In some cases, on the other hand, they appear at about the same time, in many and distant parts: and in some, though limited at first to a single region, they grow successively in other parts more and more widely distant. Such was the event in a remarkable case by Dr. Walshe.*

In this aptness to be the seat of many medullary tumors, the subcutaneous tissue agrees most nearly with the serous membranes and the liver and other glands. The separable tumors are generally isolable, oval, discoid, or lens-shaped: very rarely, I believe, they are pedunculated: they do not commonly grow to a great size, or tend to ulceration or protrusion, unless after injury. But there seems no limit to their number: it is as if the force of the disease, which, in other instances, is spent in a single enormous growth, were here distributed among many.

(3) It is chiefly among these examples of multiple medullary cancers that the occasional disappearance of a cancer, as if by absorption, may be observed. The old man referred to, as under the care of Mr. Lawrence, was admitted because one of the tumors on his scalp was largely and foully ulcerated. The removal of it was deferred on account of the other tumors, and especially on account of one behind the ear; but in the course of about a month this almost wholly disappeared. The largest of those remaining was now removed; and during the healing of the wound the rest nearly disappeared, becoming gradually smaller and firmer. So, in the case of multiple tumors of the arm, before the patient died, the whole of the smaller tumors were completely removed during the sloughing and suppuration of the larger.

The LYMPHATIC GLANDS, so rarely the seat of primary scirrhous cancer, are often primarily affected with medullary cancer. They are, indeed, less frequently so affected than they seem to be; for, in some instances, when the disease seems primary in them, it is only because of its predominance over that in the organ with which they are connected. But, in more instances than these the glands are first, and, for a time, exclusively affected. The most frequent seats of such primary disease are the cervical, inguinal, lumbar, axillary, and mediastinal glands: in a few very rare instances nearly the whole lymphatic system has quickly become cancerous.

The primary cancer of the lymphatic glands usually affects, from the first, more than one gland; often, it extends through a whole group, and so many tumors form in a cluster that one may doubt whether all of them are in glands. They may present any of the various forms of medullary cancer; and these peculiarities may be noticed in their course: (1) They are rarely well marked in the first instance; they appear like

* Medical Times and Gazette, Aug. 21 and 28, 1852. In his Treatise on Cancer. Dr. Walshe gives a full analysis of all the cases previously published. See, also, the singular case recorded by Mr. Ancell (Med.-Chir. Trans. xxv., p. 227.)

merely enlarged glands; their constant and accelerating increase may alone suggest the suspicion of the nature of the disease. (2) Cyst-formation is frequent in connection with them. Especially, I think, in the neck, one may find serous cysts, in elderly persons, resting on clusters of cancerous glands, and the cysts may be often evacuated, and will fill again, while the main disease makes insidious progress deep in the neck. (3) Partial suppurations may occur in the cancerous glands, rendering the diagnosis for a time still more difficult. (4) It is especially among the cases of cancerous lymphatics that we may find those occurrences of deep connection, and of enclosing of large nerves and blood-vessels, to which I have referred (p. 531). (5) Cancerous lymphatic glands often give a fallacious support to the belief that innocent tumors are apt to become cancerous; for the glands sometimes enlarge before the cancerous disease is established in them: and since, in their simple enlargement, they are like simple tumors, there is an appearance of transmutation, when in such a state they become the seats of cancer.

In the RECTUM, and in other parts of the digestive canal, I have already said that growths of medullary cancer may coexist with scirrhous cancer. Whether in this combination or alone, the former disease may appear in at least three distinguishable forms. (1) it consists sometimes in diffuse infiltration of creamy, white, or grayish cancerous substance in the submucous tissue, the mucous membrane being, for a time, healthy, but raised into the canal with low unequal elevations. (2) Much more commonly, larger, and more tuberous circumscribed masses grow in the submucous tissue, projecting and soon involving the mucous membrane, then exuberant through ulcerated apertures in it, and often bleeding. (3) With nearly equal frequency the disease has its primary seat in the mucous membrane. Here it forms broad, circular, or annular growths, of a soft, spongy, and shreddy substance. They are but little raised above the level of the mucous membrane, unless it be at their margins, which are usually elevated and overhanging, and when ulcerated sinuous and everted. They are very vascular, justifying Rokitansky's expression that the blood-vessels of the affected part of the membrane have assumed the characters of those of an erectile tissue. They might produce little stricture of the canal, if it were not that they are, I think frequently, associated with thickening and contraction of the tissues external to them.

It hardly needs to be added that in whichever part of the intestine the disease commences it extends to the rest; and from them to the surrounding tissues exemplifying here as everywhere the coincident processes of destruction and of more abundant formation.*

* When I have omitted all description of the medullary cancers of the uterus, lungs, brain, and many other organs in which they frequently occur, it will not, I hope, be forgotten that my purpose is only to illustrate the general pathology of the disease by the best examples which I have been able to study. To have entered further on the special pathology of cancer in each organ would have been beyond my purpose, and quite superfluous while the great works of Walshe and Lebert can be consulted.

LECTURE XXXI.

MEDULLARY CANCER.

PART II.—PATHOLOGY.

THE general history of medullary cancers presents the best marked type of malignant growths. Among all tumors, they appear, in a general view, the most independent of seat and of locality; the most rapid in growth; the most reckless in the invasion of divers tissues; the most abundant in multiplication: they have the most evident constitutional diathesis; they are the most speedily fatal. All these facts will be illustrated by comparison of the following sketch with the corresponding histories of the other forms of cancer.

(a) Among the conditions favoring the production of medullary cancer, the peculiarities of the female sex, though not without influence, appear far less powerful than they appear in the history of scirrhous cancers. The peculiar liability of the uterus so much surpasses that of any of the male organs of generation, that women are certainly, on the whole, more liable than men are to this form of cancer. But when the medullary cancers of the generative organs of both sexes are left out, I cannot find, either in my own tables or in those of Dr. Walshe and M. Lebert, that either sex is notably more liable than the other to medullary cancer of any part of the body.

(b) The medullary cancer is prone to occur at an earlier age than any other form; it is, indeed, almost the only cancerous disease that we meet with before puberty. The three localities in which, according to M Lebert,[*] cancer occurs at the lowest mean age are (in the order of their liability), the eye, the testicle, and the osseous system. To these, while confirming his observation, I would add the intermuscular spaces, and other soft parts of the trunk and limbs. The mean age of the occurrence of cancer in these parts is under 40; in all other parts it is above 40, and in most of them above 50. Now the four localities named above are those in which the medullary and melanotic cancers almost alone occur as primary affections.

From a table[†] of 154 primary medullary cancers of the bones, soft parts of the trunk and limbs, the eye and orbit, the testicle, breast, and various other external parts, I find that the ages at which they occurred were as follows:—

---

[*] Traité pratique, p. 140.

[†] The table is constructed from nearly equal numbers of M. Lebert's cases and my own and it may be worthy of remark, that in the case of every part the average age is higher in his cases than in mine.

	Breast.	Soft parts of limbs and trunk.	Lymphatic glands and other parts.	Bones.	Eye and orbit.	Testicle.	Total.
Before 10 years of age	—	2	—	4	15	4	25
Between 10 and 20	—	6	—	12	1	2	21
" 20 and 30	—	3	3	11	4	12	33
" 30 and 40	2	3	2	6	2	17	32
" 40 and 50	2	6	2	11	1	8	30
" 50 and 60	3	2	3	4	5	3	20
Above 60 . . .	—	1	—	6	3	—	10
	7	23	10	54	31	46	171

The striking contrast between this table and that of the 158 cases of scirrhous cancer (p. 512) needs little comment. Of the scirrhous cancers, not one occurred before the age of 20; of the medullary cancers, more than a fourth began before that age: of the former nearly half commenced their growth between 40 and 50 years of age; of the latter, little more than a sixth: of the former, nearly three-fourths commenced after 40; of the latter, little more than one-third did so.

The following table, also, may be compared with that at p. 513. It shows, by similar calculations, the relative frequencies of medullary cancers in external parts, in proportion to the number of persons living at each of the successive decennial periods of life. The greatest frequency is between 40 and 50, and, reckoning this as 100, the following numbers may represent the frequencies of the beginning of medullary cancers at other decennial periods:—

0 to 10 years	31	40 to 50 years	100
10 to 20 "	38	50 to 60 "	99
20 to 30 "	59	Above 60 "	44
30 to 40 "	79		

The chief points which this table may illustrate are (1), that the maximum of frequency, in proportion to the number of persons living at the several ages, occurs between 40 and 50, as well for the medullary as for the scirrhous cancers of external parts; but (2) that there is a gradual ascent to this maximum from the earliest period of life, and then a more gradual descent from it.

I believe, however, that, if we could reckon the frequencies of medullary cancers of internal organs, we should find no such diminution after the age of 50. Rather, it would appear that (in consequence, chiefly, of the frequency of cancer of the stomach in advanced life) the frequency of medullary cancers, in proportion to the number of persons living, continues to increase up to the latest age. There are, I believe, no tables in which the medullary are separated from other cancers of internal organs; but from those of the cancers of the uterus and stomach given by Lebert, and of the lungs by Walshe (of which, doubtless, the majority were medullary cancers), the proportionate frequencies at successive periods appear to be as follows. (For comparison's sake, the proportion between 40 and 50 years is still counted as 100.)

0 to 10 years	. . . .	0
10 to 20 "	(cancers of the lungs alone) . .	3
20 to 30 "	. . . .	15·7
30 to 40 "	. . . .	51
40 to 50 "	. . . .	100
50 to 60 "	. . . .	204
60 to 70 "	. . . .	236
70 to 80 "	(cancers of the stomach almost alone)	250

There are no data from which we could exactly reckon the relative frequencies of medullary cancer in each part of the body, but there can, I think, be little doubt that it is a disease, which, on the whole, becomes constantly more frequent, in proportion to the number of persons living at each successive period of life, from the very earliest to the latest age.

(c) The influence of hereditary tendency is, probably, about the same in medullary as in scirrhous cancer. Among 32 patients, five were aware of cancer having occurred in other members of their families, and of these five, four reported that two members of their respective families had died cancerous.

(d) Among 57 patients with medullary cancer of external parts, 17 gave a clear history of previous injury or disease of the part affected; in 7 the history was doubtful.

Certainly it would be impossible to prove, in many of these cases, that the cancer was, in any sense, consequent on the injury after which it formed; and yet, while we find that a third of the patients with medullary cancers ascribe them to injury or previous disease, while less than a fifth of those with simple tumors, or with hard cancers, refer them to such cause (p. 514), we cannot fairly doubt that these local accidents have influence in determining the place and time in which the medullary cancerous disease shall manifest itself.

The influence of injury is very clearly shown in certain cases, in which there is no appreciable interval between its immediate ordinary consequences and the growth of a medullary cancer in the injured part. For example, a healthy boy was accidentally wounded in his eye. It had been perfectly sound to this time; but, within a few days after the injury, a medullary tumor grew from the eyeball. It was removed three weeks later; but it quickly recurred, and destroyed life.

A boy fell and struck his knee. It had been perfectly healthy; but the inflammatory swelling (as it was supposed) that followed the fall did not subside: rather, it constantly increased; and in a few weeks it became probable that a large medullary tumor was growing round the lower end of the femur. Amputation proved this to be the case.

Again, a sturdy man, at his work, slipped and strained, or perhaps broke, his fibula. Three days afterwards he had increased pain in the injured part, and at the end of the week swelling, which, though carefully treated, constantly increased. Eight weeks after the injury the swelling was found to be a large medullary growth around and within the shaft of the fibula; and the limb was amputated.

We must, I suppose, assume the previous existence of a cancerous diathesis in the persons in whom these rare consequences of accidental violence ensued: nevertheless, their cases prove, as I have said, the influence of local injury in determining the time and place in which the cancer will be manifested; and they may make us believe that, in many cases, in which a clear interval elapses between the injury and the appearance of the cancer, the effect of the violence, though less immediate, is certain.

(e) Although I know of no numerical evidence to support it, yet I think the general impression must be true that medullary cancer is peculiarly liable to occur in those who have many of the features of the fair strumous constitution: in persons of fine complexion, light hair and eyes, pale blood, quick pulse, and of generally delicate or feeble health. Scirrhous cancer appears most frequent in those who have the opposite characters of temperament. A difference also exists in relation to the general health of those in whom the two forms of the disease are severally observed. I mentioned (p. 515) that nearly three-fourths of the subjects of hard cancer appear to have good general health at and soon after its first appearance: the proportion of those in the like condition with medullary cancer is not more than two-thirds; the remaining third have presented from the very begining a loss of weight and of muscular power, accelerated action of the heart, quick breathing paleness, and general defect of health.

In the growth of medullary cancer we may chiefly observe these three things—(1) their multiplicity in certain cases; (2) their generally rapid rate of increase; (3) the occasional complete suspension of growth.

I have referred to their multiplicity in the subcutaneous tissue, but again notice it, to mention the observation of Rokitansky,* that medullary cancers are sometimes developed in great number in the course and among the phenomena of a very acute typhoid fever.

I do not know what their greatest rate of increase may be: but it has in several cases exceeded a pound per month, and, except in the instances of some of the cartilaginous tumors (p. 427, 428), it is, I believe, unequalled by any other morbid growth. In general, the more rapid the growth the less is the firmness, and the less perfect the development of nuclei and cells, in the medullary tumor. Their rapid increase commonly indicates, not a special capacity of growth or multiplication of cells in the tumor already formed, but an intense diathesis, an ample provision of appropriate material in the blood. The growth is by simple increase; the materials once formed do not normally change their cha-

* Pathologische Anatomie, i. 373.

racters; there are no stages of crudity or maturity; the disease is, in its usual and normal course, from first to last the same.

But while these things justify the expression that the medullary is, on the whole, the most acute form of cancer, yet there is, I believe, none in which arrest or complete suspension of progress is so apt to occur. These cases have occurred within my own observation. A man, 88 years old, had a slight enlargement of one testicle for 15 years, and its rate of increase was often inappreciable. At the end of this time rapid growth ensued. On removal, well-marked medullary and melanotic cancer was found, and was the only apparent source of the enlargement. He died soon after the operation with recurrence of the disease.

A man, 42 years old, had a large increasing medullary tumor of the ilium. He had also a tumor in the upper arm, which had grown slowly for seven years and had been stationary for three years. When he died, the tumor in the arm had as well-marked characters of medullary cancer as that of the ilium, or of any other of the several parts in which similar disease was found.*

A man, 35 years old, had numerous medullary tumors in his right upper arm, shoulder, and axilla, all of which had commenced their growth within three months, and were very quickly increasing. One, which appeared to be in every other respect of the same kind, had been stationary for twelve years in the groin, and another nearly as long in the neck.

Sir Astley Cooper removed a gentleman's testicle for what was believed to be medullary cancer. He remained well for twelve years, and then died with certain medullary cancer in the pelvis.

Dr. Baly had a patient who had observed for several years a tumor connected with two of his ribs. It had scarcely enlarged, till shortly before his death: then it quickly increased, and, at the same time, numerous medullary cancers appeared about it and in more distant parts.†

Cases such as these occur, so far as I know, in no cancers but those of the medullary and melanotic kinds. They seem to be quite inexplicable; and as yet no facts have been observed which would show a peculiarity of structure in the arrested cancers corresponding with the strangeness of their life.

As the medullary cancers grow, the parts about them generally yield, and some among them grow at once in strength and in extent, and for a time retard both the increase and the protrusion of the tumor. Because the skin over a medullary cancer is not often infiltrated (as that over a hard cancer usually is), we do not often see the kinds of ulcer described in the last lecture (p. 517). Neither is there, in medullary cancers gene-

---

* Museum of St. Bartholomew's, Series i. Nos. 235 to 240. Case related by Mr. Stanley in Med.-Chir. Trans., xxviii. p. 317.

† The tumor on the ribs is in the Museum of St. Bartholomew's. It appears an ordinary medullary cancer, with a hard bony skeleton.

rally, any remarkable proneness to ulceration. The usual course is, that, as the tumor grows, the skin and other parts over it become thinner and more tense; then, as the growth of the tumor is more rapid than theirs, they inflame and ulcerate, and a hole is formed over the most prominent part of the tumor. There is nothing specific or character- istic in this ulceration; it is only such as may ensue over any quickly growing tumor; but the continued rapid increase of the cancer makes it protrude and grow exuberantly; it throws out fungus, as the expression is. The exuberant growth, exposed to the injuries of the external world, inflames, and hence is prone to softening, bleeding, ulcerating, and sloughing.* These may keep down its mass; yet it may grow to a vast size, having only its surface ulcerated; lower down, it usually adheres to the borders of the apertures in the skin, and overhangs and everts them. This is usually the case with the huge outgrowths of medul- lary cancer that have protruded from the eyeball, after penetrating thrrough ulcers of the overstretched cornea or sclerotica. And similar exuberant growths are often seen when medullary cancers have pene- trated the walls of various cavities or canals: thus, e.g., they grow along the canals of veins when they have entered them by, it may be, a single small orifice.

In the cases of diffuse infiltration of an exposed superficial tissue (e. g. of the mucous membrane of the stomach or rectum), the cancer usually ulcerates widely with the tissue it affects, and herein imitates more nearly the characters of the ulceration in scirrhous and epithelial cancers.

Through the constantly deepening cachexia, with which the increase in the medullary cancers is usually commensurate, and which is augmented by the various influences of the local disease, the usual course of the medullary cancer is uniformly towards death; and rapidly thither, even when the growth does not involve parts necessary to life. And yet, as Rokitansky has observed,† there is no form of cancer in which sponta- neous natural processes of healing so often occur. Doubtless nearly all the reputed cases of the cure of cancer have been erroneously so re- garded; yet instances may be easily gathered of at least temporary cure; and these are important in relation to the general pathology of cancer, since they afford the best examples of the effects of its degenerations and diseases.

The degenerations of medullary cancer are chiefly three: withering, fatty, and calcareous degeneration. Its chief diseases are equal in num- ber—hemorrhage or apoplexy, suppuration, and sloughing.

A medullary cancer may gradually decrease, becoming harder, as if by shriveling and condensing, and at length may completely disappear. I

---

* In Series xxxv. No. 60, in the Museum of St. Bartholomew's, is a large medullary tumor which had grown in the subcutaneous tissue of the back, and, after the skin over it had ulcerated, was in one mass squeezed out through the opening, while the patient was endeavoring to raise herself in bed.   † Loc. cit. p. 375.

have mentioned such cases at p. 548; and I have seen the same happen after partial removal of cancers.

A firm medullary tumor was seated deep in the substance of a young woman's parotid gland. Its removal with the knife could not be safely completed; about a fourth part of it was left behind, and the wound was left to heal in the ordinary manner. It healed quickly, enclosing the remains of the tumor; but after some time all the appearance of swelling subsided, and no renewed growth ensued till after a lapse of three months, when it was renewed, but not more rapidly than before.

A woman's humerus was amputated with a large mass of firm medullary cancer surrounding its neck and the upper part of its shaft. The same disease existed in all the muscles about this part of the bone; and the patient was so exhausted, that the dissection necessary for the removal of the whole disease could not be completed. Large portions of it were left in the deltoid and great pectoral muscles. In two months after the operation, however, the wound had very nearly healed, and no trace could be felt of the masses of the cancer in the muscles. Nor did any perceptible recurrence take place till more than four months after the operation. At that time renewed growths appeared at the scar, and in the thyroid gland, and quickly increased.

To these cases I might add at least three in which I have known portions of cancerous growths left in the orbit after incomplete operations; in all of which complete healing ensued, and one, two, or three months elapsed before any renewed growth was evident in the portion of the disease that was left. In all these cases the disappearance of the cancer may have been due in part to the disease and rapid degeneration excited in it by the injury of the operation and its consequences; and in all, the growth was renewed within three months of the disappearance; a fallacious hope was in all excited, and bitterly disappointed. But I shall have presently to refer to a case in which the removal of cancers was independent of local injury.

It is most probable that fatty degeneration coincided with the wasting and absorption of cancer which occurred in the preceding cases; for it seems to be the most frequent change when growth is hindered. I have already referred to the fatty degeneration which, in medullary cancers, as in other tumors, may give an appearance of buff or ochre-yellow lines or minute spots scattered, as a reticulum, through their substance. I have also described (p. 527) the similar but larger degeneration which ensues in those portions or lobes of medullary cancers, that are found as tuberculoid masses (phymatoid, of Lebert), yellow and half dry, among the other portions that appear actively progressive. In both cases it is probable that the altered substances are incapable of further growth; but the change, being only partial, does not materially affect the progress of the whole mass. But, though more rarely, a whole mass (especially when many exist, as in the liver), may be found white, or yellowish-white, soft, partially dried, close-textured but friable, and greasy to the touch—in a state of what Rokitansky has called "saponification." In such cases, many of the cancer-cells and nuclei have the characters of the granular or fatty degeneration, and may appear collapsed and shriveled; and they are mingled with abundant molecular matter and oil particles of various sizes, and often with crystals of cholestearine or with coloring granules. All the analogies of such changes in other parts imply that cancers thus degenerated must be incapable of increase; they are amongst those which may well be called, as by Rokitansky, obsolete. But I am not yet sure that these gradual changes have been ever followed by absorption of the altered cancer-substance, and by healing:[*] the disease ceases but does not disappear: and usually, while one mass is thus changing, others are progressive.

The calcareous degeneration is much more rare than the two preceding. It is fully described by Dr. Bennett[†] and Rokitansky,[‡] and is in all essential characters similar to that which so often occurs in degenerating arteries, calcified inflammatory products, &c. The earthy matter, in minute granules, is commonly mingled with fatty matter, and, according to the quantity of fluid, is like more or less liquid or dry and hardened mortar: if hardened it lies in grains, or larger irregular concretions, in the substance of the tumor. Its indications are the same as those of the fatty degeneration with which it is usually mingled.[§]

Among the diseases of medullary cancers their proneness to bleeding may be mentioned. Hence their occasionally abundant hemorrhages when protruding, and the frequent large extravasations of blood in them, variously altering their aspect as it passes through its stages of decolorization, or other changes. The extreme examples of such bleeding cancers constitute the fungus hæmatodes.

Acute inflammation also is frequent, especially in such as are exposed through ulcers. It may produce not only enlargement of the blood-vessels and swelling of the tumor, but softening, suppuration, and, I believe, other of its ordinary effects. The softening may be compared with that which occurs in inflammation of any natural part, like which, also, it is, I believe, often attended with a rapid fatty degeneration or a disintegration of the cancer-structures. I am not disposed to think with Rokitansky (p. 527), that the reticulum, or other ordinary yellow deposits in cancers, are due to inflammatory exudations passing into and propagating a fatty

---

[*] These supposed cases of healing of cancer of the liver, reported as having occurred at Prague, admit of other explanations. (See Lebert, Traité Pratique, p. 72.)

[†] On Cancerous and Cancroid Growths, p. 214.　　　　　　　　[‡] Loc. cit. p. 352.

[§] I have little doubt that the melanotic cancer might be truly described as a pigmental degeneration of the medullary cancer (except in the few instances in which epithelial cancers are melanotic). But part of another lecture will be devoted to this. The same lecture will comprise the colloid or alveolar cancer; and I shall have occasion to mention in it the frequent occurrence of cysts in medullary cancers, some of which might perhaps be described as a cystic disease of the cancers.

transformation; but I think that acute inflammation in a medullary or any other cancer is likely to be attended with the same degenerative softening and transformation, as we find constituting a part of the inflammatory process in the natural tissues. Thus degenerating, and whether with or without suppuration, a medullary cancer may be completely removed.

By sloughing, also, a medullary cancer may be wholly ejected; and this event is more likely to happen than with any other kind of cancer, because no other is common in the form of an isolable mass. I might collect several cases in which it has occurred, but none is more remarkable than this.* A strong man, 46 years old, under Mr. Lawrence's care, had a large firm medullary cancer deep-seated in his thigh, of about nine months' growth, painful and increasing. In an attempt to remove it, the femoral artery was found passing right through it; its connections, also, appeared so wide and firm, and bleeding ensued from vessels of so great size, that the operation was discontinued after about half the surface of the tumor had been uncovered. The tumor sloughed, and gradually was completely separated. It came away with nearly three inches of the femoral artery and vein that ran through it. No bleeding occurred during or after the separation, and the cavity that remained in the thigh completely healed. The man regained an apparently good health for a few weeks; then the disease returning in the thigh, proved quickly fatal.

In the following strange case nearly all the methods of spontaneous temporary cure which I have been illustrating were exemplified.

A tall, healthy-looking man, 36 years old, came under my care in July, 1850. In October, 1849, he thought he strained his shoulder in some exertion, and soon after this he noticed a swelling over his right deltoid muscle. It increased slowly and without pain for nine months, and was thought to be a fatty tumor, or perhaps a chronic abscess. About the beginning of July, other tumors appeared about the shoulder; and, when I first saw him, there was not only the tumor first formed, which now covered two-thirds of the deltoid, but around its borders were numerous smaller round and oval masses; in the axilla was a mass as large as an egg; over the brachial vessels lay a series of five smaller tumors, and a similar series of larger tumors over the axillary vessels reaching under the clavicle. A small tumor of several years' date lay at the border of the sterno-mastoid muscle; and one, which had been noticed for twelve years, was in the right groin. All these tumors were soft, pliant, painless, subcutaneous, movable, more or less lobed. There could be very little doubt that they were medullary cancers, and their complete removal seemed impossible; but it was advised that, for proof's sake, one should be excised. I therefore removed one of those near the chief mass. It was composed of a soft grayish substance, with a pale purple tinge, lobed, easily reduced to

* The case is fully reported by Mr. Abernethy Kingdon, in the Medical Gazette, 1850.

pulp, and in microscopic structure consisted almost wholly of nucleated cells exactly conformed to the very type of cancer-cells. The operation was followed by no discomfort; and, in a few days after it, the patient left the hospital, still looking healthy, but, I supposed, doomed to a rapidly fatal progress of the disease.

At home, near Dover, he was under the care of Mr. Sankey. In a few days after his return, the skin over the largest tumor cracked, and a thin discharge issued from it. Four days later he was attacked with sickness, diarrhœa, and abdominal pain, and in his writhings he hurt his arm. Next day, three or four more openings had formed over the great tumor, and the scar of the operation-wound reopened: the tumor itself had rapidly enlarged. From all these apertures pus was freely discharged, and in a day or two large sloughs were discharged or drawn through them. With the sloughing, profuse hemorrhage several times occurred. All the upper part of the arm and shoulder was undermined by the sloughing, and a great cavity remained, from which, for three weeks, a thin fœtid fluid was discharged, but which then began to heal, and in twelve weeks was completely closed in.

While these changes were going on in the tumors over the deltoid and in those near it, that in the axilla was constantly enlarging. It became " as large as a hat," and early in September it burst; and through a small aperture about six pints of pus were rapidly discharged. A great cavity, like that of a collapsed abscess, remained; but it quickly ceased to discharge and healed. In the same time all the tumors over the brachial vessels disappeared; they did not inflame or seem to change their texture; only, they gradually decreased and cleared away, and with them that also disappeared which had been in the groin for twelve years.

It need hardly be said that during all this time of sloughing and suppuration the patient had been well managed, and amply supported with food and wine and medicine. About the end of October he appeared completely recovered, and returned to his work. I saw him again in January, 1851. He looked and felt well, and, but that his arm was weak, he was fully capable of work as an agricultural laborer. Over the lower half of the deltoid there was a large irregular scar; and this appeared continuous posteriorly with a small mass of hard tough substance, of which one could not say whether it were tissues indurated after the sloughing, or the remains of the tumor shriveled and hardened: whatever it was, it was painless and gradually decreasing. No trace remained of the other tumors in the arm, except a small mass like a lymphatic gland in the middle of the upper arm. In the axilla there was a small swelling like a cluster of natural lymphatic glands. The tumor also remained at the border of the sterno-mastoid muscle, and was rather larger than in July.

In February, 1851, the swelling in the axilla began to increase; its growth became more and more rapid. By the end of March the arm was greatly swollen; he suffered severe pain in and about it; his health failed; he had dyspnœa and frequent vomiting, and died with pleuro-pneumonia on the 20th of April. The tumor in the axilla (the only one found after death) was about eight inches long, oval, lobed, soft, vascular, and brain-like, and consisted, chiefly, of small apparently imperfectly formed cancer-cells.

Such a case as this needs little comment. It illustrates the spontaneous removal, and, so far, the healing, of medullary cancers by absorption, by inflammation, and abundant suppuration, and by sloughing. It shows the absorption of the cancerous matter, doubtless in an altered state, accomplished without evident injury to the economy. And it illustrates the cancerous diathesis quickly re-established after being, we must suppose, suspended or superseded, for a time, during the removal of its products. Hard, therefore, as, we may say, the struggle for recovery was, it was not successful.

It is scarcely possible to give general illustrations of the pain and other phenomena attendant on the progress of medullary cancer; for these are variously modified by the many organs in which it may have its primary seat. The history of some of the medullary cancers, which grow as distinct tumors, may teach us that the pain is not an affection of the cancer itself, but of the organ which it occupies. Such cancerous tumors, in the subcutaneous cellular tissue, are, I believe, rarely the sources of pain; often they are completely insensible: yet the same kind of tumors seated among the deeper parts of limbs, or enclosed in the testicle, or in bone, seem to be usually painful, and often severely so. The difference indicates that the varying pain is not of the cancer, but of the part it fills.

The cachexia is, in the later periods of the disease, too much varied by the disturbed functions of the organs specially affected to admit of general description. But it is chiefly in this form of cancer that, early in the disease, and even while the local affection seems trivial, and involves no important part, we often find the signs of the general health being profoundly affected; the weight and muscular power regularly diminishing, the complexion gradually fading, the features becoming sharper, the pulse and breathing quicker, the blood more pale. Such events are, indeed, inconstant, both in the time of the occurrence and in their intensity; but in many cases they are far too striking to be overlooked; the defective nutrition of the early stages of phthisis is not more marked: the evidence is complete for the proof of a distinct cancerous cachexia, which is indeed commonly indicated and may be measured by a cancerous growth, but which may exist in a degree, with which neither the bulk, nor the rate of increase, of the growth is at all commensurate.

To estimate the general duration of life in those who have medullary cancers, those cases alone should be reckoned in which parts whose functions are essential to life are affected;—such as the bones and soft parts about the trunk and limbs, the testicle, the eye, and other external organs. From a table of 50 cases of medullary cancers in these parts (including eight cases of cancer of the bones by M. Lebert), in all of which the disease pursued its course without operative interference, I find the average duration of life to be rather more than two years from the patient's first observation of the disease.*

Among 45 of these patients,—

```
 6 died within    6        months
 7  "   between  6 and 12   "
11  "      "    12 and 18   "
 4  "      "    18 and 24   "
 7  "      "    24 and 36   "
 7  "      "    36 and 48   "
 3  "   more than 48 months from the commencement of the disease.
```

A comparison of this table with that at p. 524 will show, in striking contrast with the history of scirrhous cancer, the rapidity of this form in running its fatal career; a rapidity which is certainly not to be ascribed to the earlier exhaustion produced by hemorrhage, discharge, pain, or other local accidents of the disease, but is mainly due to the augmenting cachexia. The same comparison will show how small is the proportion of those in whom the disease lasts more than four years; and there seem to be no cases parallel with those of scirrhous cancer which are slowly progressive through periods of five, ten, or more years. I have mentioned instances of the apparent suspension of the disease; but these are different from the cases of constant slow progress, the rarity of which supplies an important fact in diagnosis, in the great probability that a tumor is not a medullary cancer, if it have been increasing for more than three years without distinct manifestation of its cancerous nature.

The effect of removing medullary cancers is, on the whole, an increased average duration of life; but chiefly, I believe, because in a few cases the operation is long survived, and in some, death, which would have speedily ensued, is for a time arrested. In the majority of cases the operation, if its own effects be recovered from, seems not to affect the average duration of life. Thus in 46 cases in which external medullary cancers were removed by excision, or amputation of the affected part, the average duration of life was something more than 28 months. Among 51 cases (including 9 cases of extirpated cancer of the eye, from M. Lebert) these were the several times of death, reckoning, as before, from the first observation of the disease by the patient:—

```
Within  6      months  .    .    .    .    .   1
Between 6 and 12   "    .    .    .    .    .  13
  "    12 and 18   "    .    .    .    .    .   7
  "    18 and 24   "    .    .    .    .    .   8
  "    24 and 36   "    .    .    .    .    .  11
  "    36 and 48   "    .    .    .    .    .   3
       Above 48    "    .    .    .    .    .   8
```

* I have not reckoned in this table the exceptional cases referred to at p. 554, in which the disease appears to be suspended for some years. But I have included five cases in which the patients were still living beyond the average time. In the 45 already dead, the average duration of life was 23·8 months.

36

The comparison of this table with that at top of page 561 will show that the only notable contrast between them is in their first and last lines.

If the operation be recovered from, the regular course of events brings about the renewal of cancerous growth, either near the seat of the former growth, or in the lymphatics connected therewith, or, more rarely, in some distant part. In 38 cases of medullary cancer, affecting primarily the same external organs as afforded the cases for the former tables, I find the average period of recurrence after the operation to have been seven months. I have reckoned only those cases in which a period of apparent recovery was noted after the operation; all those cases are omitted in which the disease was not wholly removed, or in which it is most probable that the same disease existed unobserved in lymphatics or other internal organs at the time of operation. Yet the average rate of recurrence is fearfully rapid.

It was observed in between—

1 and	3	months in	18	cases
3 and	6	"	11	"
6 and	12	"	4	"
12 and	24	"	3	"
24 and	36	"	2	"

Among the 51 cases in the table at the foot of page 561, those of five patients are included, who are living, without apparent return of disease, for periods of 3, 3½, 4½, 5, and 6 years after operation; and I have referred already to one case in which a patient died with cancer in the pelvis twelve years after the removal of a testicle which was considered cancerous. Of cases more near to recovery than these I can find no instances on authentic record.

The cases I have been able to collect supply little that is conclusive respecting the different durations of life, according to the age of the patient, the seat of the cancer, and other such circumstances. In children under ten years old, the average duration of life, with medullary cancers of external parts, is, I believe, not more than eighteen months: after ten years, age seems to have little or no influence. According to the part affected the average duration of life appears to be greater in the following order:—the testicle, the eye, the bones, the soft parts of the limbs and trunk, the lymphatics; but the difference is not considerable. The average for the cancers of the testicle is about 23 months: that for the tumors in the limbs and trunk nearly 30 months. It is the same, I believe, with the results of operations; recurrence and death occur, on the whole, more tardily after amputations for medullary cancers of the bones and soft parts of the limbs, than after extirpations of the eye or testicle; but there are many obvious reasons why we cannot hence deduce more than a very unstable rule for practice. The previous duration of the disease seems, also, to have little influence on the time of recurrence after the operation: the only general rule seems to be, that the rapidity of recurrence corresponds with that of the progress of the primary disease.

Now, respecting the propriety of removing a medullary cancer in any single case, much that was said respecting the operation for scirrhous cancer of the breast might be repeated here. The hope of finally curing the disease by operation should not be entertained. Such an event may happen, but the chance of it is not greater than that of the disease being spontaneously cured or arrested; and the chance of any of these things is too slight to be weighed in the decision on any single case. The question, in each case, is whether life may be so prolonged, or its sufferings so diminished, as to justify the risk of the operation. In general I think the answer must be affirmative wherever the disease can be wholly removed, and the cachexia is not so manifest as to make it most probable that the operation will of itself prove fatal.

(1) The number of cases in which the patients survive the operation for a longer time than that in which, on the average, the disease runs its course, is sufficient to justify the hope of considerable advantage from the removal of the disease. On the other hand, the number of chronic cases of medullary cancer is so small, that no corresponding hope of a life being prolonged much beyond the average can be reasonably held, if the disease be left to run its own career.*

(2) The hope that the removal of the cancer will secure a considerable addition (two or more years, for example) to the length of life, will be more often disappointed than fulfilled. But, even when we do not entertain this hope, the operation may be justified by the belief that it will avert or postpone great suffering. The miseries attendant on the regular progress of a medullary cancer, in any external part, are hardly less than those of hard cancer of the breast; they are such, and in general so much greater than those of the recurrent disease, that unless it is very probable that the operation will materially shorten life, its performance is warranted by the probability of its rendering the rest of life less burdensome.

(3) A motive for operation in cases of supposed medullary cancers may often be drawn from the uncertainty of the diagnosis. This is especially the case with those of the large bones, for the removal of which the peril of the necessary operation might seem too great for the probability of advantage to be derived from it. I have referred to cases of cartilaginous and myeloid tumors of bone (pp. 427, 448, 450) in which during life the diagnosis from medullary cancers was, I believe, impossible. In all such cases, and I am sure they are not very rare, the observance of a rule against the removal of tumors or of bones believed to be cancerous, would lead to a lamentable loss of life. All doubts respecting diagnosis are here to be reckoned in favor of operations.

* The difference here stated may seem opposed by the tables in the foregoing pages. I must therefore state that, at page 554, I have referred to all the cases of chronic or suspended medullary cancer that I have ever seen or heard of; but that the cases of operations survived for more than three years, mentioned at the foot of page 561, were not selected on this account, but occurred in the ordinary course of observation.

LECTURE XXXII.

EPITHELIAL CANCER.

PART I.—ANATOMY.

EPITHELIAL cancer has its primary seat, with very rare exceptions, in or just beneath some portion of skin or mucous membrane. Its most frequent locality is the lower lip, at or near the junction of the skin and mucous membrane; next in order of frequency it is found in the prepuce, scrotum (of chimney-sweeps), labia, nymphæ, and tongue: more rarely it occurs in very many parts,—as at the anus, in the interior of the cheek, and upper lip, the mucous membrane of the palate, the larynx, pharynx and cardia, the neck and orifice of the uterus, the rectum and urinary bladder, the skin of the perineum, of the extremities, the face, head, and various parts of the trunk. In the rare instances of its occurrence, as a primary disease, in other than integumental parts, it has been found in the inguinal lymphatic glands (in a case which I shall relate), in bones,* and in the tissues forming the bases or walls of old ulcers.†

By extension from any of its primary seats, an epithelial cancer may occupy any tissue; thus, in its progress from the lip, tongue, or any other part, muscles, bones, fibrous tissues, are alike invaded and destroyed by it. As a secondary disease, or in its recurrence after removal by operation, it may also have its seat in any of these tissues at or near its primary seat; but it more commonly affects the lymphatic glands that are in anatomical connection therewith; and, very rarely, it has been found in internal organs, the lungs, liver, and heart.‡

The essential anatomical character of the epithelial cancer is, that it is chiefly composed of cells which bear a general resemblance to those of such tessellated or scaly epithelium as lines the interior of the lips and mouth,§ and that part of these cells are inserted or infiltrated in the interstices of the proper structures of the skin or other affected tissue.‖

---

* Virchow, in the Würzburg Verhandlungen, i. 106.

† The primary seats of cancer, in the cases from complete records of which the following descriptions are drawn, were as follows:—Lower lip, 9 cases; tongue, 9; scrotum, 6; face, 3; penis, 3; labia, 2; gum, 2; integuments of the trunk, 2; of the upper extremity, 3, lower extremity, 2; ear, eyelids, interior of the cheek, neck, perineum, arms, larynx, inguinal lymphatic glands, each 1. With very few exceptions, these are cases in which the disease was removed by operation or examined after death: in all such cases the microscopic characters of the structure was observed. I may add that the account drawn chiefly from these cases is confirmed by the recollection of a much larger number which I have observed but have not recorded.

‡ In the lungs and in the heart, in the Museum of St. Bartholomew's. In the liver once by Rokitansky (Pathol. Anat. i. 386). In the lungs and in the liver, in the Museum of Berlin and Würzburg (Virchow, l. c.; and in his Archiv, b. iii. p. 222.)

§ In very rare cases the cells, or part of them, are like those of columnar epithelium (see pp. 582, 587).

‖ In assigning these two conditions as the essential characters of epithelial cancers—

The epithelial cancers of the skin or mucous membrane from which, as types, the general characters of the disease must be drawn, present many varieties of external shape and relations, which are dependent, chiefly, on the situation in which the cancerous structures are placed. They may be either almost uniformly diffused among all the tissues of the skin or mucous membrane, predominating in only a small degree in the papillæ; or the papillæ may be their chief seat; or they may occupy only the sub-integumental tissues. As a general rule, in the first of these cases, the cancer is but little elevated above, or imbedded below the normal level of the integument, and its depth or thickness is much less than its other dimensions; in the second, it forms a prominent warty or exuberant outgrowth; in the third, a deeper-seated flat or rounded mass. These varieties are commonly well marked in the first notice of the cancers, or during the earlier stages of their growth; later they are less marked, because (especially after ulceration has commenced) an epithelial cancer, which has been superficial or exuberant, is prone to extend into deep-seated parts; or one which was at first deeply seated may grow out exuberantly. Moreover, when ulceration is in progress, a greater uniformity of external appearance is found; for, in general, while all that was superficial or exuberant is in process of destruction, the base of the cancer is constantly extending both widely and deeply into the subintegumental tissues.

I believe that it will be useful to describe separately the external characters of the two principal varieties of epithelial cancer of the integuments here indicated; and (while remembering that mingled, transitional, and intermediate specimens may be very often seen), to speak of them as the superficial or outgrowing, and the deep-seated, forms of the disease.*

Among the examples of the superficial epithelial cancers, the greater

namely, both the construction with epithelial cells and the insertion of such cells among the original, though often morbid, textures of the affected part, I make a group of diseases less comprehensive than either the "Cancroid" of Lebert and Bennett, or the "Epithelioma" of Hannover. These excellent pathologists, and many others following them, would abolish altogether the name of epithelial cancer, and place the cases which are here so designated in a group completely separate from cancers, as exemplified by the scirrhous and medullary forms. It is not without much consideration that I have decided to differ from such authorities; but I believe that the whole pathology of the diseases in which the two characters above cited are combined is, with rare exceptions, so closely conformed to that of the scirrhous and medullary cancers, that they should be included under the same generic name. The grounds of this belief, which, I think, agrees with the opinions of Rokitansky and Virchow, will appear in the present lecture; and at its end I will briefly sum them up.

* I believe that either of these forms may occur in any of the parts enumerated as the usual seats of epithelial cancer; but they are not both equally common in every such part. The superficial, and especially those which have the characters of warty and cauliflower-like outgrowths, are most frequently found on mucous surfaces, especially those of the genital organs; the deep-seated are more frequent in the tongue than elsewhere; those on the extremities and in the scrotum have usually a well-marked warty character, and are rarely deep-seated. Other particulars might, I believe, be stated, but I am unwilling to state them unsupported by counted numbers of cases.

part derive a peculiar character from the share which the papillæ of the skin or mucous membrane take in the disease. These being enlarged, and variously deformed and clustered, give a condylomatous appearance to the morbid structures, which has led to their being called papillary or warty cancers, and which renders it sometimes difficult to distinguish them from common warty growths. According to the changes in the papillæ, numerous varieties of external appearance may be presented: I shall here describe only the chief of them.

In the most ordinary examples of epithelial cancer of the lower lip, or of a labium, or of the scrotum in the soot-cancers, if they be examined previous to ulceration, one can feel an outspread swelling, and an unnatural firmness or hardness of the affected skin. The width and length of the swelling are much greater than its thickness. The diseased part is enlarged; the lip, for example, pouts and projects like one overgrown; and the swelling is slightly elevated, rising gradually or abruptly from its borders, and having a round or oval or sinuous outline. Its surface, previous to ulceration, may be nearly smooth, but more often is coarsely granulated, or tuberculated, or lowly warty, like the surface of a syphilitic condyloma, deriving this character usually from the enlarged and closely clustered papillæ. The surface is, generally, moist with ichorous discharge, or covered with a scab, or with a soft material formed of detached epidermal scales. The firmness or hardness of the diseased part is various in degree in different instances: it is very seldom extreme: the part, however firm, is usually flexible and pliant, and feels moderately tense and resilient on pressure. Commonly, it is morbidly sensitive, and the seat of increased afflux of blood. Its extent is, of course, various; but, before ulceration, the disease makes more progress in length and breadth than in depth; so that when, for example, it occupies the whole border of a lip or of a labium, it may not exceed the third of an inch in thickness.

In the form of epithelial cancer just described there may be no considerable enlargement of papillæ, or it may only appear when the growth is cut through. But, in many instances, (especially, I think, in the epithelial cancers of the prepuce, glans, and integuments of the extremities,) the changes of the papillæ are much more evident. In some, as in the adjacent sketch, one sees a great extent of surface covered with crowds and clusters of enlarged papillæ set on a level or slightly elevated portion of the cutis. Singly (when the ichor and loose scales that fill their intervals are washed away), they appear cylindriform, flask-shaped, pyriform, or conical: clustered, they make nodulated and narrow-stemmed masses. They may be in one or in many groups; or groups of them may be scattered round some large central ulcer. They appear very vascular, and their surface, thinly covered with opaque white cuticle, has a pink, or vermilion, or brightly florid hue.*

* Museum of St. Bartholomew's, Ser. i. 22, 126, 127, &c., and Ser. xi. 6. Mus. Coll. Surg. 2301, 2607, 2608, &c.

In other instances, or in other parts, a large mass is formed, the surface of which, when exposed by washing away the loose epidermoid cells which fill up its inequalities, is largely granulated or tuberculated, and is planned out into lobes by deeper clefts. Such growths are upraised,

Fig. 98.*

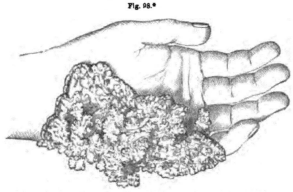

cauliflower-like; and, with this likeness, may be broken through the clefts, into narrow-stemmed masses, formed each of one or more close-packed groups of enlarged, tuberous, and clavate papillæ.† The surface of such a growth shows, usually, its full vascularity; for if it be washed, it appears bare, and, like the surface of common granulations, has no covering layer of cuticle. It may be florid, bleeding on slight contact, but, more often, it presents a dull or rusty vermilion tint, rather than the brighter crimson or pink of common granulations, or of such warts as one commonly sees on the prepuce or glans penis.

Occasionally we meet with an epithelial cancer having the shape of a sharply-bordered circular or oval disk, upraised from one to three lines above the level of the adjacent skin or mucous membrane, and imbedded in about the same depth below it. The surfaces of such disk-shaped cancers are usually flat, or slightly concave, granulated, spongy, or irregularly cleft; their margins are bordered by the healthy integuments, raised and often slightly everted by their growth. Such shapes are not unfrequent among the epithelial cancers of the tongue, of the lining of the prepuce, and of the scrotum. I removed such an one, also, from the perineum, and have seen one in the vagina.

Sometimes, again, an epithelial cancer grows out in the form of a cone. I examined such an one removed from the lower lip, which was half an inch high, and nearly as much in diameter at its base. Its base

* The papillary character is well shown in the specimen of soot-cancer of the hand, in the Museum of St. Bartholomew's (Ser. xi. 6), which is represented in fig. 98. The history of the case is in Pott's Works, by Earle, iii. 182. The patient was a gardener, who had been employed in strewing soot for several mornings: the disease was of five years' duration.

† Museum of St. Bartholomew's Ser. xxx. 35. Mus. Coll. Surg. 2609.

was a cancerous portion of cutis; its substance was firm, gray, composed of the usual elements of epithelial cancers imbedded among the fibro-cellular and elastic tissue outgrown from the skin: the subcutaneous tissue was healthy. In another instance an exactly similar cancer grew on a chimney-sweep's neck;* and in both these cases, the growth, being covered with a thick laminated black and brown scab, was, at first, not easy to distinguish from syphilitic rupia: that in the neck might even have been confounded (as some, I believe, have been) with one of the *horns* that grow from diseased hair follicles. Mr. Curling† describes a similar growth, three quarters of an inch long, on the scrotum of a chimney-sweep; and has copied, from one of Mr. Wadd's sketches, a representation of a horn 2½ inches long similarly formed.

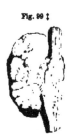

Fig. 99 ‡

Lastly, we may find epithelial cancers as narrow-stemmed or even pendulous growths from the cutis. I have seen such on the lower lip, and at the anus, like masses of very firm exuberant granulations, two inches iu diameter, springing from narrow bases in the cutis or deeper tissues, and far overhanging the adjacent healthy skin. And I lately examined one of this kind, which was removed from the skin over the lower border of the great pectoral muscle. It was exactly like the specimen sketched in fig. 99. It was spheroidal, about an inch in diameter, rising from the skin with a base about half as wide; it was lobed, deeply fissured, and subdivided like a wart, with its component portions pyriform and mutually compressed. Its surface was pinkish, covered with a thin opaque-white cuticle, which extended into and seemed to cease gradually in the fissures. Its substance, composed almost wholly of epithelial cancer-cells, was moderately firm and elastic. It was but little painful. A thin, strong-smelling fluid oozed from it. The patient had noticed a small unchanging wart in the place of this growth for ten or twelve years. Without evident cause it had begun to grow rapidly, and had become redder and discharged fluid, six weeks before its removal.§

It is almost needless to say that a much greater variety of shapes than I have here described may be derived from the different methods and

* Mus. of St. Bartholomew's. In the next year the same patient was in the hospital with a cancerous wart of the scrotum.

† Treatise on Diseases of the Testicle, p. 522. The specimen is in the Mus. Coll. Surg., 2469. In the Museum of St. Bartholomew's is an instance of a very large soot-cancer, in which, at the borders of the ulcer, there are spur-shaped sharp-pointed processes, doubtless cancerous papillæ, some of which are from ¼ to ½ an inch in length.

‡ Fig. 99. Section of a narrow-based, outgrowing epithelial cancer. It was extremely vascular, and had grown in the place of a dark mole, or pigmentary nævus, on the wall of the abdomen. Two growths had been previously removed from the same part.

§ The cauliflower excrescence of the uterus may be most nearly compared with the extremely exuberant epithelial cancers, such as are described above (see p. 557).

degrees in which the papillæ are deformed, enlarged, and involved in the cancerous disease. All, and more than all, the shapes of common warty and condylomatous growths may be produced. But the same general plan of construction exists in all; namely, a certain portion of the skin or mucous membrane is infiltrated with epithelial cancer-structure: on this, as on a base more or less elevated and imbedded, the papillæ, variously changed in shape, size, and grouping, are also cancerous; their natural structures, if we except their blood-vessels, which appear enlarged, are replaced by epithelial cancer-cells. And herein is the essential distinction between a simple or common warty or papillary growth, and a cancerous one or warty cancer. In the former the papillæ retain their natural structures; however much they may be multiplied, or changed in shape and size, they are either merely hypertrophied, or are infiltrated with organized inflammatory products; however abundant the epidermis or epithelium may be, it only covers and ensheathes them. But in the warty cancer the papillæ are themselves cancerous; more or less of their natural shape, or of the manner of their increase, may be traced; but their natural structures are replaced by cancer structures; the cells like those of epithelium lie not only over, but within, them.*

To describe the interior structure of the superficial cancerous growths, we may take as types the most common examples of cancers of the lower lip—those in which the papillæ are indeed involved, enlarged, and cancerous, but not so as to form distinct or very prominent outgrowths.

The surface of a vertical section through such a cancer commonly presents, at its upper border, either a crust or scab, formed of ichor, detached scales, and blood; or else a layer of detached epidermoid scales, forming a white, crumbling, pasty substance. This layer may be imperceptible, or extremely thin; but it may be a line or more in thickness, and it enters all the inequalities of the surface on which it lies. Its cells or scales are not regularly tessellated or imbricated, like those of the epidermis on a common wart, but are placed without order, loosely connected both with one another, and with the subjacent vascular structures, and may be easily washed away.

Such a layer must be regarded, I presume, as formed of epithelial

---

* I described the papillary origin and construction of these cancers in 1838 (Medical Gazette, xxiii. 284), but was not then aware of their minute structure. Later examinations have made me sure that the true distinction between them and other papillary growths is as above stated. But it is to be observed that cancerous growths may appear papillary or warty, though no original papillæ are engaged in their formation. Thus when papillary cancers are deeply ulcerated at their centres, the base of the ulcer, where all the original papillæ are destroyed, may be warty, like its borders where the cancerous papillæ are evident. Some of the most warty-looking epithelial cancers are those which grow from the deep tissues of the leg after old injuries. This may be only an example of cancerous growths imitating the construction of adjacent parts; but in some instances (as in cysts, and on the mucous membrane of the gall-bladder and stomach), the warty cancers are probably examples of the dendritic mode of growth. It must also be a question, at present, whether some of the most exuberant cancers of the skin are not to be ascribed to this mode of growth. It is, to say the least, extremely difficult to trace their origin from once-natural papillæ.

cancer-cells, detached or desquamated from the subjacent vascular and more perfectly organized substance of the cancer. This substance presents, in most cases or in most parts, a grayish or grayish-white color, and shines without being translucent. It is firm and resilient, close-textured, and usually void of any appearance of regularly-lobed, granular, or fibrous construction, except such as may exist near its surface, where close set and uniformly elongated vertical papillæ may make it look striped. The grayness and firmness are, I think the more uniform and decided the slower the growth of the cancer has been. In the acute cases, especially of secondary formations, or when the cancer has been inflamed or ulceration is in quick progress, the cut surface may be opaque white, or of some dull yellow or ochre tint, streaked and blotched with blood; or it may, in similar cases, be soft and shreddy, or nearly brain-like; but these appearances are very rare.

The gray substance of epithelial cancers commonly yields to pressure only a small quantity of turbid yellowish or grayish fluid: but with rare exceptions, one may squeeze or scrape from certain parts of the small cavities or canals, a peculiar opaque-white or yellowish material. It is like the comedones, or accumulated epithelial and sebaceous contents of hair-follicles; or even more like what one may scrape from the epidermis of the palm or sole after long maceration or putrefaction. This material, which is composed of structures essentially similar to those of the firmer substance of the cancer, but differently aggregated, supplies one of the best characteristics of the disease. It may be thickly liquid, but more often is like a soft, half-dry, crumbling, curdy substance: pressed on a smooth surface, it does not become pulpy or creamy, but smears the surface, as if it were greasy; mixed with water, it does not at once diffuse itself, so as to make the water uniformly turbid, but divides into minute visible particles.*

The quantity of this softer material is extremely various in different instances of epithelial cancer. According to its abundance and arrangement, the gray basis-substance may appear differently variegated; and the more abundant it is the more does the cancer lose firmness, and acquire a soft, friable, and crumbling texture. In many cases the soft substance appears, on the cut surface, like imbedded scattered dots, or small grains, these being sections of portions contained in small cavities. But, as the quantity increases, and the cavities containing it augment and coalesce, so the firmer substance becomes, as it were, cribriform; or when the softer substance is washed away, it may appear reticulated or sponge-like, or as if it had a radiated or plaited structure. Or, lastly, the soft substance may alone compose the whole of the cancer; but this, I think,

---

* In these are its distinctions from the "juice of either scirrhous or medullary cancers. But it must be remembered that, in the rare instances in which epithelial cancers are very soft, they may yield a creamy or turbid grayish fluid. It can hardly be necessary to give a caution against confounding the peculiar material described above with that which may be pressed from milk-ducts involved in scirrhous cancers (compare p. 498).

is very rarely the case, except in secondary formations and in the lymphatic glands.

Vertical sections of the more exuberant and the more distinctly papillary epithelial cancers present essentially the same appearance as I have described. The upper border, corresponding with the exposed part of the growth, may be overlaid with a thin scab or crust, or epidermoid scales, detached and disorderly, or may be bare, like that of a section of common granulations. The cut surface is generally gray, succulent, and shining, with distinct appearances of vascularity. Portions of it may yield the peculiar soft crumbling substance like macerated epidermis; but this is, I think, generally less abundant than in the less exuberant and deeper-set specimens, and is more often arranged in a radiated or plaited manner.

The vertical sections of the superficial epithelial cancers of the integuments display many important differences, in relation to the depth to which the cancer-structures occupy the proper tissues of the skin or mucous membrane.

In some, only the papillæ, or the papillæ and the very surface of the tissue on which they rest, appear to be involved. The enlarged papillæ, in such cases, usually retaining their direction and their cylindrical or slenderly-conical shape, appear like fine gray stripes or processes vertically raised on the healthy white tissue of the integument, or on its surface rendered similarly gray by cancerous infiltration. And the outlines of the papillæ are commonly the more marked because of their contrast with the opaque-white substance formed by the epidermoid scales which cover them and fill up all the interstices between them. In such cases, the cancerous material may be more abundant on the surface than in the substance of the papillæ or corium; and often the whole morbid substance is brittle, and may be separated from the corium which bears the papillæ.

But more frequently, and almost always in such cases of epithelial cancer when they are removed in operations, the cancerous structures are more deeply set. They occupy the whole thickness of the integument, or reach to a level deeper than it. The base or lower border of the diseased mass rests on, or is mingled with, the subcutaneous or submucous tissues, whatever these may be,—fat, muscular fibres, or any other. The lateral borders usually extend outwards for some distance, on each side, beneath the healthy integuments which bounds the upraised part of the diseased growth, and which is usually raised and everted so as to overhang the adjacent surface. In nearly all these, also, while the surface and central parts of the cancer are being destroyed by ulceration, its base and borders are, at a greater rate, extending more deeply and widely in the subcutaneous or submucous tissues.

The bases of the most exuberant and most distinctly papillary cancers are rarely, in the early periods of their growth, either deeply or widely set in the integument. They rarely, I believe, occupy more than the thickness of the portion of the skin or mucous membrane from which the growths spring: they sometimes occupy less. But, in their later growth, and especially when ulceration is progressive, the same deeper and wider extension of the base of the cancer ensues as I mentioned in the last paragraph.

All the foregoing description will have implied that the proper structures of the diseased parts are mixed up with the cancer-structures inserted among them: the condition of parts is here exactly comparable with that of other cancerous infiltrations. (Compare p. 498 and 500). The boundaries of the cancer, as seen in sections, usually appear to the naked eye well-defined; yet it is often easy to see portions of the natural tissues extending into it, these being continuous with those portions among which the cancer-structures are infiltrated. This is especially evident when, as in the lip or tongue, the superficial muscular fibres are involved. Pale red bands may then be traced into or within the cancer; and the microscope will prove, if need be, their muscular structure. Or, when these cannot be traced, yet we may find the fibro-cellular and elastic fibres of the involved skin of the mucous membrane.

Concerning the changes that ensue in the tissues thus involved in the deeper parts of epithelial cancers, I believe that what was said of those in cancerous breasts (p. 493 and 500) might be here nearly repeated, regard being had to the original differences of the tissues in the respective cases. In general, the natural structures in these cases appear not to grow; gradually, but not all at the same rate, they degenerate and are removed, till their place is completely occupied by the increasing cancer-structures, and an entire substitution is accomplished. So, too, what was said of the stroma of scirrhous cancers of the breast might be repeated. These epithelial cancers have no stroma of their own; their proper structures are sustained by the remains of the original textures of the affected part. And, as in the scirrhous cancers, so in these when they grow very quickly, they occupy a comparatively small area of the original tissues, and may appear like nearly distinct tumors.

In the most exuberant epithelial cancers, and in those that are prominent, like warts, or condylomata, there is more growth of the natural tissues; those, not of the papillæ alone, but of the basis of the skin or mucous membrane, may be traced into the outgrowth, forming a stroma for the cancer-structures, and surmounted by the cancerous papillæ. Such a stroma may be well traced in many soot-cancer-warts: the fibro-cellular and elastic tissues extend from the level of the cutis, in vertical or radiating and connected processes among which the cancer-cells lie; and one may compare them with the osseous outgrowths that form an internal skeleton of a cancer on a bone (see p. 534).

The tissues bordering on the superficial epithelial cancers appear generally healthy, but they are often increased in vascularity, and succulent. The adjacent corium also may appear thickened, with its papillæ enlarged, and an unusual quantity of moist opaque-white cuticle may cover them.* This condition is, however, not frequent; neither is it peculiar to the environs of cancer; changes essentially similar are often observed around chronic simple ulcers of the integuments.†

The deep-seated epithelial cancers remain to be described. In the progress of all the preceding varieties of the superficial form of the disease, especially when their surfaces are ulcerating, we may trace a constant subintegumental extension of their basis, in both width and depth; an extension which is more than commensurate with the destruction at the surface, and in the course of which no tissue is spared. Now, the same cancerous infiltration of the subcutaneous or submucous tissue, which is thus the common result of the extension of the disease from the surface, may also occur primarily: that is, the first formation of epithelial cancers may be in masses of circumscribed infiltration of·the tissues beneath healthy skin or mucous membrane. The same condition is more frequent in the epithelial cancers that form, as recurrences of the disease, near the seats of former operations, or, as secondary deposits, about the borders of primary superficial growths.

In comparison with the superficial form, the primary deep-seated epithelial cancer is a very rare disease; yet it is frequent enough for me to have seen, within the last year, three cases, which I will describe; for they were all well-marked examples.

A chimney-sweep, 32 years old, died suddenly, suffocated, in the night after his admission into St. Bartholomew's.

He had had cough for six months, and aphonia and dyspnœa for two months. A scrotal soot-cancer had been removed from his brother in the previous year.

I found a wide-spread layer of firm substance, exactly like that of the majority of epithelial cancers, under the mucous membrane of the larynx, involving the left border of the epiglottis, the left arytenoid cartilage, the intervening aryteno-epiglottidean fold, part of the right arytenoid cartilage, and the upper and posterior third of the left ala of the thyroid cartilage. In all this extent, the diseased substance lay beneath the mucous membrane, which, though very thinly stretched over some parts of it, appeared healthy, was covered with ciliary epithelium wherever I examined it, and could everywhere be separated in a distinct layer.‡ All the submucous tissues were involved; the cartilages, as it

* M. Lebert (Traité Pratique, p. 618) quotes from M. Follin, that the tissues around the disease are often "infiltrated with epidermis in a diffuse manner."

† On some of the diseases of the papillæ of the cutis (Medical Gazette, vol. xxiii., p. 285). The multiform appearances of epithelial cancers which I have described may be still more varied by the consequences of degeneration and disease. But it would be too tedious to describe them minutely, while, as I believe, they are essentially similar to the consequences of the same affections in the scirrhous and medullary cancers, of which I have already given some account.

‡ The specimen, and those referred to in the two following cases, are in the Museum of St. Bartholomew's.

were buried in the growth, appeared less changed than the softer parts. The surface of the growth, as covered with the mucous membrane, was lowly-lobed, or tuberculated, raised from one to two lines above the natural level; its border was in many parts sinuous. The cancerous substance was firm, elastic, compact, grayish and white, shining, variously marked on its section with opaque-white lines. It appeared wholly composed of the usual minute structures of epithelial cancers, including abundant laminated epithelial capsules. All the epithelial structures were of the scale-like form, though collected in the tissues under a membrane covered with ciliary epithelium.

A man was admitted into the Hospital, in a dying state, with a large

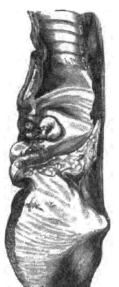

Fig. 100.

firm swelling between the lower jaw and the hyoid bone, the increase of which had produced great difficulty of breathing and swallowing. After his death, the greater part of the swelling was found to be due to cancer of the deep tissues of the tongue, and of the fauces and lymphatic glands. A section of the parts (as in fig. 100) showed that the muscular and other structures of the posterior two-thirds of the tongue were completely occupied by a firm cancerous infiltration: but the mucous membrane of the tongue was entire; its various papillary structures only were healthy and distinct; it was tight-stretched and adherent on the surface of the cancer. From the base of the tongue the cancer extended backwards and downwards on both sides of the fauces, and as far as the vocal cords, preserving in its whole extent the characters of a massive infiltration of all the submucous tissues. It was covered with healthy-looking mucous membrane in every part, except just above the right vocal cord, where it protruded slightly through a circular ulcer less than half an inch in diameter. The substance of the disease presented, to the assisted as well as to the unaided sight, and touch, the well-marked characters of epithelial cancers. The lymphatic glands were similarly diseased.

A gentleman, 64 years old, had, on the upper part and right side of his nose, a flat, lowly-lobed or tuberculated growth, an inch in diameter, gradually rising above the level of the adjacent skin, to a height of 1½ or 2 lines. It was covered with skin, which was very thin and adherent, and florid with small dilated blood-vessels, like those in the skin of his cheek. The base of the growth rested on the bones; it felt like an infiltration of all the thickness of the deeper part of the skin and subcutaneous tissue, and moved as one broad and thick layer of morbid substance inserted in the skin. In its middle and most prominent part was a fissure nearly a line in depth, with black, dry borders, from which a very slight discharge issued. It was very painful, and, beginning from no evident cause, had been ten weeks in regular progress.

I removed this disease, and found in its centre a small, roundish mass of soft, dark, grumous substance, like the contents of a sebaceous cyst.* Around the cavity in which this was contained, all the rest of the disease appeared as an outspread infiltration of firm yellowish and white cancerous substance in the tissues under the stretched and adherent but entire skin. It extended as deep as the periosteum of the nasal bones. Soft, crumbling, and grumous substance could be scraped from it; and it yielded well-marked elements of epithelial cancer, with numerous laminated capsules. During the healing of the operation-wound, a similar small growth appeared in the adjacent tissue. It was destroyed with caustic by Mr. Hester, and the patient has remained well: but only a few months have yet elapsed.

Besides such cases as these, which may suffice for a general description of the disease, many might be cited, of what may be regarded as an intermediate form, in which both the skin or mucous membrane and the subjacent tissues are simultaneously affected, but the latter to a much larger extent than the former. Such cases are far from rare in the lower lip and tongue. They are characterized by the existence of a roundish, firm, or hard and elastic lump, deep-set in the part, well-defined to the touch, with its surface little, if at all, raised, and having at some part of its surface either a portion of cancerous integument, or a small ulcer or fissure.

Now these cases of deep-seated epithelial cancers have much interest, as well in practice as in their bearing on the pathology of the disease. They are instances of the disease of which it is impossible to speak as of mere augmentations of the natural structures; there is in them no trace at all of the assumed homology of epithelial growths; there is in them no progressive formation of epithelial cells gradually penetrating from the surface into the substance of the cutis; their progress, or a part of it, is from the deeper parts towards the surface.

The epithelial cancers in or near the integuments are so prone to ulceration, that the occasions of seeing them as mere growths are comparatively rare. The state in which they are usually shown to us is that of progressive ulceration of the central and superficial parts, with more than equal growth of the bordering and deeper parts. In this state,

---

* Mr. Hester and Mr. Rye, who saw this case some weeks before I did, told me that it presented, at first, all the characters of a common sebaceous cyst; and I think it quite probable that it was an example of epithelial cancer formed in and around such a cyst.

indeed, they present the type of that which is commonly described as the cancerous ulcer; a type which is observed, also, in some examples of the scirrhous cancer (p. 518), and more rarely in the medullary.

In the superficial first-described form of the disease, the ulceration usually begins either as a diffuse excoriation of the surface of the cancer, the borders of which are alone left entire, or else as a shallow ulcer extending from some fissure or loss of substance at which the disease commenced. The discharge from the excoriated or ulcerated surface usually concretes into a scab, or a thicker dark crust, beneath which, as well as beyond its edges, ulceration gradually extends in width and depth.

A nearly similar method is observed, I believe, in the earliest ulceration of the papillary and other more exuberant epithelial cancers. The central parts ulcerate first, and the ulcer from this beginning deepens and widens, destroying more and more of the cancer-structures; but its rate of destruction is never so quick as that of the increase of the borders and base of the cancer.

In the deep-seated epithelial cancers, other methods are observed in the first ulceration. Sometimes the skin or mucous membrane over them, becoming adherent and very thin, cracks, as it may when adherent over a scirrhous cancer (p. 517). Such a crack may remain long with little or no increase, dry and dark, and scarcely discharging; but it is usually the beginning of ulceration, which extends into the mass of the cancer. In other cases, with inflammation of the cancer, its central parts may soften and perhaps suppurate; and then its liquid contents being discharged (sometimes with sloughs), through an ulcerated opening or a long fissure, a central cavity remains from the uneven walls of which ulceration may extend in every direction. And again, in other cases, especially, I think, in secondary formations, and in those under the scars of old injuries, the cancer protrudes through a sharply-bounded ulcer in the sound integument or scar, and grows exuberantly, with a soft shreddy surface, like the medullary cancer, or with a firmer, warty or fungous mass of granulations.

But though the beginnings of the ulcers be thus, in different instances, various, yet in their progress they tend to uniformity. The complete ulcer is excavated more or less deeply, and usually of round, or oval, or elongated shape. Its base and borders are hard, or very firm, because, as one may see in a section through it, they are formed by cancerous substance infiltrated in the tissues bounding it. The thickness of this infiltration is, commonly, in direct proportion to the extent of the ulcer, from a line to half an inch or more: we may feel it as a distinct and well-defined indurated boundary of the whole ulcer, hindering its movement on the deeper tissue. The surface of the base of the ulcer is usually concave, unequal, coarsely granulated, nodular, or warty: it is florid, or often of a dull vermilion, or rusty-red color; it bleeds readily, but not profusely; and yields a thin inchorous fluid, which is apt to form scabs, and has a peculiarly strong, offensive odor, something like that of the most offensive cutaneous exhalations. The borders of the ulcer, or some parts of them, are, generally, elevated, sinuous, tuberous, or nodulated; frequently, they are everted, and, to a less extent, undermined. They derive these characters, chiefly, from the cancerous formations beneath the skin or mucous membrane that surrounds·the ulcer. These formations may be in a nearly regular layer, making the border of the ulcer like a smoothly rounded embankment; but oftener, though continuous all round the ulcer, they are unequal or nodular, and then corresponding nodules or bosses, from a line to nearly an inch high, may be raised up round the ulcer or some part of it. Moreover, these upraised borders may so project as to overhang both the base of the ulcer and the adjacent healthy surface of the skin or mucous membrane: they thus appear, at once, undermined and everted. When they are everted, healthy skin is usually reflected under them, and continued beneath them to their extreme boundary. When the papillary character of the primary growth was well-marked, the borders of the ulcer often present, instead of the characters just described, a corresponding papillary or warty structure: for in these cases, the cancer continues apt to affect especially the papillæ, and widening areas of them become its seat as it extends. And, even at the base of the very deep ulcers, the cancerous granulations, though rising from the tissues far deeper than papillæ, may have a similarly warty construction.

The characters of the ulcer here described, are generally retained, however deep, and into whatever tissues the cancer may extend. For the proper tissues of the successively invaded parts, at first infiltrated with cancer-structures, seem to be quickly disparted and then removed: even the bones rarely produce any outgrowths corresponding with those that are found in medullary cancers; they become soft, are broken up, and at length utterly destroyed. Epithelial cancers thus extending produced the changes described, as characteristic of malignant ulceration. in p. 327; and by similar extension (especially in the affections of the lymphatic glands), they lay open great blood-vessels more often than any other ulcers do. I have seen three cases in which the femoral artery was thus opened by ulceration extending from the epithelial-cancerous inguinal glands.

The minute component structures of the epithelial cancers are alike among all the varieties of construction and external shape that I have now described; and, if we omit the proper textures of the part affected, they may be thus enumerated: (a) epithelial cancer-cells; (b) nuclei, either free, or imbedded in blastema; (c) endogenous or brood-cells; (d) laminated epithelial capsules, or epithelial globes. From each of these, by degeneration or other change, several apparently different forms may be derived. The proportions, also, in which they are combined are various in different specimens; but I believe that diversities of appearances to the naked eye are not so connected with these propor-

37

tions, as with the methods of arrangement, the degrees of degeneration of the component structures, and the mingling of the products of inflammation in the cancer.

(*a*) The most frequent cells (fig. 101, A), and those which may be regarded as types, are nucleated, flattened, thin, and scale-like. They are, generally, round or round-oval; but they seldom have a regular shape: their outline is, usually, at some part, linear, or angular, or extended in a process. Their average chief diameter is about $\frac{1}{700}$ of an inch; but they range from $\frac{1}{300}$ to $\frac{1}{1500}$, or perhaps beyond these limits. In the clear, or very palely nebulous cell-contents, a few minute granules usually appear, either uniformly scattered, or clustered, as in an areola, round the nucleus.

The nucleus is usually single, central, and very small in comparison with the cell, rarely measuring more than $\frac{1}{3500}$ of an inch in its longest diameter: it is round or oval, well defined, subject to no such varieties of shape and size as the cell. It is usually clear and bright, and is often surrounded by a narrow, clear area; it may contain two or more minute granules, but rarely has a bright, distinct nucleolus.

But many of the cells may deviate widely from these characters; the most various and (if the term may be used) fantastic shapes may be found

Fig. 101.*

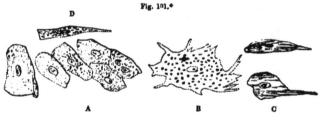

A   B   C

mingled together. The younger cells are generally smaller, rounder, more regular, less flattened to the scale-like form, clearer, and with comparatively larger nuclei. The older (as I suppose) appear drier and more filmy; they are often void of nuclei, and like bits of membrane in the shape of epithelial scales (B): they are flimsy, too, so that they are often wrinkled or folded and rolled up, so as to look fibrous (C). Independently of differences of age, some cells are prolonged in one, two, or more slender or branching processes; some are very elongated (as D); some are void of nuclei; some, within their pale borders, present one or two dimly-marked concentric rings, as if they had laminated walls.

To these varieties may be added such as depend on the progressive degeneration of the cells. The most frequent (besides the withering, which, I suppose, is shown in the shriveled, flimsy scales, without nuclei, just mentioned) is the change like fatty degeneration in other cancer-structures. One of the most frequent effects of such degeneration is, that the place of the nucleus is occupied by a circular or oval group of

* Various epithelial cancer-cells or scales. Magnified 350 times: referred to in the text.

minute oily-looking molecules, some with bright black borders, some dark (fig. 102). Others, like these, or larger, are generally scattered through the cell. With the progress of the degeneration, all trace of the nucleus is lost; the molecules increase in number and in size, till the whole cell or scale appears filled with them, or is transformed into an irregular mass of oily-looking particles, differing in shape alone from the common granule masses of fatty degenerations.

Fig 102 *

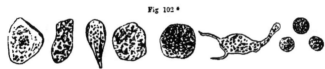

(*b*) Nuclei either free or imbedded in a dimly-molecular or granular basis, are commonly found mingled with the cells. I believe they occur in the greatest abundance in the most acute cases. They may be just like the nuclei of the cells; but usually, among those that are free, many are larger than those in the cells; and these, reaching a diameter of more than $_r\frac{1}{\overline{6\overline{0}}}$ of an inch, at the same time that they appear more vesicular and have larger and brighter nucleoli, approximate very closely to the characters of the nuclei of scirrhous and medullary cancer-cells. Indeed, I have seen many nuclei in soot-cancers, which, if they had been alone, I could not have distinguished from such as are described at page 497; yet all the other structures of these specimens were those usual in epithelial cancers, and between the different characters of nuclei there were all possible gradations. The free nuclei, like the cells, may be found in all stages of degeneration (fig. 102).

(*c*) Those which are named brood-cells, or endogenous cells, present many varieties of appearance, which may be regarded as the results of one or more nuclei, enclosed within cells assuming, or tending to assume, the characters of nucleated cells (fig. 103).† In some cells a nucleus appears very large, clear, pellucid, spherical: it loses, at the same time, its sharply-defined outline, its boundary becames shadowed, and it looks like a hole or vacant space in the cell (▲). Thus enlarging, the nucleus may nearly fill the cell, and appear as a pellucid vesicle. I think, however, that such nuclei rarely grow to be cysts, like those whose history is described in the twenty-second lecture (p. 336); for cysts containing serous or other fluids are very rarely found in epithelial cancers. Neither have I seen instances of free nuclei changed, as those in the cells are.‡

* Cells and free nuclei of epithelial cancer, in states of fatty degeneration. Magnified 350 times.

† We owe the ability to interpret these appearances, which illustrate many things interesting in the general physiology of cells, almost entirely to Virchow (in his Archiv, iii. 197), and Rokitansky, l. c. Other facts, derived from the examination of solid tumors, and illustrating the capacity of the nucleus for development, are in pages 426, 453, 538 : all these may deserve study in physiology, together with the doctrine of cyst-formation explained at p. 336, &c.

‡ Virchow, however (Würzburg Verhandl. i. 100), mentions having found, in a cauli-

The enlarged nucleus may remain completely pellucid or barren; but aften granular matter appears to fill it, and, as often, one or two corpuscles appear to form in it, which now appear as its nuclei, and make it assume the character of a cell, endogenous within the first or parent-cell (B). The sketches show many of the appearances that may be hence derived; and others may be thus explained. When a cell contains two

Fig. 103.*

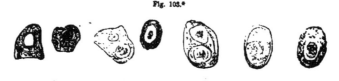

A　　　　　　B　　　　　　C　　　　　D

nuclei, one only of these may enlarge or become inflated (if I may use such a term for that which fills with liquid, not with air); the other may be then pressed against the wall of the cell. Or both nuclei may alike proceed to the grade of cells, and two cells, flattened at their place of mutual compression, appear within the parent-cell (c): or a secondary nucleus, *i. e.* one formed within an enlarged nucleus, may enlarge like its predecessor, and become like a pellucid cavity, or may become a secondary cell, and contain its tertiary nucleus: hence, possibly the concentric appearance above mentioned may be referred to the series of successively enclosed cell-walls (D). And changes such as these may equally occur with more than two nuclei: a cell of any grade, primary, secondary, or later, may be filled with a numerous "brood" of nuclei, in which all the above-described changes (but not the same in all) may be repeated.

(*d*) The laminated capsules, as I have called them ("globes épidermiques" of Lebert), are the most singular and characteristic structures of the epithelial cancers (fig. 104). They are not, indeed, peculiar to this disease; for I have found exactly corresponding structures in the contents of an epidermal and sebaceous cyst; and so has V. Barensprung;[†] and I have illustrated a corresponding mode of formation in some of the many-nucleated cells of myeloid tumors (fig. 76, p. 453.) However, they are nowhere so frequent or so well-marked as they are in nearly every epithelial cancer.

Their great size at once attracts the eye: they are visible even to

flower excrescences of the uterus, alveoli which, after the plan of the proliferous cysts, contained secondary papillary growths. The analogy of other proliferous cysts may indicate that these, also, originated in nuclei.

* Epithelial cancer-cells, with endogenous development of nuclei, as described in the text. Magnified 350 times.

† As quoted by Virchow (Archiv. iii. 200). I have said (p. 453) that I have never seen such structures in medullary cancers. Rokitansky delineates some (Ueber die Cyste, figs. 9, 10, 11), but with less perfect structures than are common in epithelial cancers. I would add, that what was said in p. 453 respecting the rarity of endogenous cells in medullary cancers relates only to such as occur in external parts; I must believe from the reports of others, that they are more frequent in cancers of internal organs.

the unaided sight, especially when the softer curdy material of the cancer, in which they are generally most abundant, is pressed out on glass. They appear, at first sight, like spherical or oval cysts, from $\frac{1}{70}$ to $\frac{1}{750}$ of an inch in diameter, walled in by irregular fibrous tissue, and containing granular matter, nuclei, or cells, obscurely seen within them (fig. 104, C). They may be clustered together in a mass or a long cylinder (D); but, by breaking them up, or looking more closely, it becomes evident that the appearance of fibrous tissue is due to one's seeing the edges of epithelial scales, which, in successive layers, are wrapped round the central space. Such scales may be broken off, in groups of two, three, or more, retaining the curved form in which they have lain (fig. 104, A). When detached, they generally appear like the driest and most filmy of the epithelial scales composing the rest of the cancer (B): often they are folded, and look fibrous, even when separated; their nuclei are shriveled or not visible; their contents are often granular. As they lie superposed, they appear closely compacted; but not unfrequently gra-

Fig. 104.*

B   C

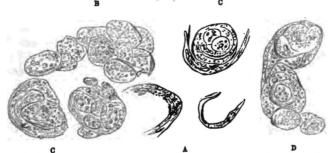

C   A   D

nules are distinct in the outer laminar spaces, or on the inner surface of detached pieces.

The contents filling the central spaces in these laminated capsules are extremely various; sometimes, or partly, granular and oily particles diffused in some nebulous material; more often, or with these, cells or nuclei (C, D). Sometimes one cell is thus enclosed, sometimes two or more: and these not scale-like, but oval or round and plump, having distinct and generally large nuclei; or a crowd of nuclei may be enclosed: and briefly, these nuclei may appear in any of those various states which I described just now in the account of the endogenous epithelial cells. Indeed it is probable that the last sentence of that description (p. 579) might begin the history of the development of these capsules; for I know no method of explaining them, except that taught by Rokitansky, and illustrated by the diagrams copied here (fig. 105).†

In one of the simplest cases, we may suppose a nucleus largely *inflated*

* Fig. 104. Laminated epithelial capsules, described in the text, magnified about 250 times.
† From his Essay, Ueber die Cyste: fig. 8.

and filled with a brood of (say four) secondary nuclei, which proceed to the formation of secondary cells (fig. 105, A). If now, only one of the

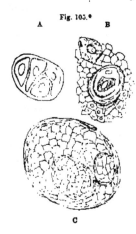

Fig. 105.*

A   B

nuclei of these secondary cells becomes enlarged, it will not only extend its own cell's wall into contact with that of the cell containing it, but it will at the same time press the three other cells into similar contact, and thus appear invested with laminated epithelial scales. Such a state, with the nuclei of the investing scales, is shown in B. A greater complexity of similar events is shown in C, in which, among a very large number of secondary endogenous nuclei, many are persistent as nuclei, while others developed to nucleated cells, are laminated around them. But among the nuclei, two are represented as enlarged and containing tertiary "broods" of nuclei, among which the same changes have ensued as in the preceding generation. And it is evident that if any in the group *a* had now singly enlarged, the rest, with all the cells and nuclei around them, must have arranged themselves or been compressed into imbricated scales, so as to form a large laminated capsule.

The component structures now described appear to be disorderly placed in the mass of epithelial cancer, in the interstices of the natural structures, or of their remains. I have never seen any of them within a natural structure, *e. g.* within a muscular fibre. The laminated capsules are, I believe, most abundant in the softer substance, but they are not confined to it. The texture of the mass is such as makes it very difficult to obtain a sufficiently thin section with the structures undisturbed; but in sections of scrotal cancers I have seen the laminated capsules imbedded at distant intervals among the simpler epithelial structures, and the turgid large capillaries ascending towards the surface and forming near it simple or undulating loops. The epithelial structures appeared to be in contact with the walls of the blood-vessels, supported by a wide sparing meshwork of fibro-cellular tissue growing up from the adjacent tissue of the scrotum.

In whatever part or organ they may be found, there is a remarkable uniformity in the characters of the epithelial cancer-structures. Deviations, however, from such as I have described as the normal structures are sometimes found. I have once seen a melanotic epithelial cancer: it grew in the deeper part of the cutis and in the subcutaneous tissue, under a dark pigmentary nævus or mole, in a woman who had many similar moles on various parts of her body: a thin layer of the cutis, with

* Fig. 105. Diagrams of the production of the laminated epithelial capsules; from Rokitansky.

its covering of dark epidermis, extended over the cancer and was slightly raised by it. The epithelial shape and texture of the cancer-cells were well marked, but most of them contained melanotic matter; in some, a quantity of brownish molecular matter was either diffused or collected about the nucleus or its place; in some, with similar molecular matter, there were two, three, or more brown corpuscles, from the size of mere molecules to that of blood-cells. Materials like those within the epithelial cells existed, also more abundantly as an intercellular substance.

Cells like cylindriform epithelium-cells may also be mingled with the more usual form. I have seen this in a case of large "cauliflower-excrescence" of the uterus, in the very substance of which the cylindriform cells were found.

Bidder describes a similar occurrence in a cancer of the stomach* and duodenum; and Rokitansky,† in the same parts.

I believe, also, that cases may be found in which the cancer-cells, or part of them, have characters intermediate, or transitional, between those of the epithelial and of the scirrhous or medullary diseases. I have mentioned the existence of the large free nuclei (p. 579), and the full plump cells in the capsules (p. 581) in epithelial cancers; and I believe that I have seen cancers with all their cells of intermediate shape. But the point is very difficult to determine. Young epithelial-cells are less flattened and scale-like, and have larger and clearer nuclei, than those of completed formation: in these characters they approach to the appearance of the other cancer-cells; and if, in a quickly-growing mass, they occur alone, they may produce a fallacious appearance of an intermediate form of cancer. Moreover, two kinds of cancer may be mingled in one mass. Lebert and Hannover have satisfied themselves of this; and such a specimen as they describe may have deceived me. As yet, therefore, I can have only a belief in the existence of such intermediate forms.

The foregoing description has been drawn, almost exclusively, from cases of epithelial cancer in integumental parts, and the varieties which it may present in different localities are so slight and inconstant that such references as I have already made to them may suffice. but certain examples of the disease, in other than integumental parts, need separate description.

The LYMPHATIC GLANDS, in anatomical relation with the primary seat of an epithelial cancer, usually become similarly cancerous in the progress of the disease; and, I think, sooner or later in that progress, in direct proportion to its own rapidity; following in this, the same rate as in other cancers. From the glands nearest to the primary seat, the disease gradually extends towards the trunk, yet seldom reaches far. I have known the whole line of cervical glands affected in epithelial cancer of the

* Müller's Archiv, 1852. p. 178.   † Ueber den Zottenkrebs, pp. 11, 18.

tongue; and the lumbar glands may become diseased with the penis or
scrotum; but much more often, the proximate cluster of glands alone
becomes cancerous, and those more distant are swollen and succulent, but
contain no cancerous matter. This, however, must not be taken to imply
a continuous extension of the disease from the primary seat to the glands;
for large intervals of apparently healthy tissues often intervene. I have
seen, with epithelial cancer of the back of the hand, the lymphatic gland
near the bend of the elbow similarly cancerous throughout; but the whole
forearm was healthy.

Last summer I amputated an old man's hand with a similar cancer;
and I have lately seen him with all his axillary glands diseased, but with
no sign of cancerous lymphatics or other disease in the arm.*

In some cases the diseased glands appear in a large cluster, forming
one lobed mass; in others, a chain of small glands is felt, such as one
might not suppose to be cancerous, except for their hardness. The cancerous elements in the glands resemble those in the primary disease;
indeed, I have found even slight modifications of general character in the
one, exactly repeated in the other.† They are inserted among the natural structures of the gland. At first, I think, they usually appear in
circumscribed masses, occupying only a certain part of the gland; but
these, gradually increasing, at length exclude, or lead to the removal of,
the whole of the original tissues.

The diseased glands are enlarged, hardened, smooth-surfaced, and usually retain their natural connection with the surrounding tissues. On
section, part or the whole of the gland presents the same appearance as
a section of primary epithelial cancer; and, generally, the opaque-white
crumbling substance, like scrapings from macerated epidermis, is abundant. One can remove masses of it, and leave only the capsule of the
gland, or some remains of gland-substance that bounded the spaces that
it filled.

Glands thus diseased are not unfrequently the seats of acute inflammation, in which, with fatty degeneration of the cancer-cells, suppuration
may ensue: they may discharge the pus, as from a common bubo, and
may continue many days thus suppurating. But the end of this is, that
large and deep cancerous ulcers, such as are already described, form in

* Such cases do not prove—they only make it very probable—that there was no cancerous
affection of the lymphatic vessels between the primary disease and the glands. Such continuous disease has been traced from scirrhous cancers of the breast to the axillary glands; and
I once found epithelial cancer-cells in the dental canal, when primary disease existed in the
gum and alveolar part of the jaw, and secondary disease in a submaxillary lymphatic gland.

† In one case of epithelial cancer of the tongue, and in another of the larynx, I found
the lymphatic glands affected with what, according to both general and microscopic characters, could only be regarded as firm medullary cancer. It is possible that, in these cases,
the primary disease was of mixed kinds—medullary and epithelial: just as there are examples of mixed cartilaginous and medullary tumors, in which only the medullary disease is
repeated in the lymphatic glands (see p. 444). But I found no evidence of this mixture of
diseases in the primary growth; and I think it equally possible that the cases may be compared
with the rare instances of secondary medullary, associated with primary scirrhous, cancer

them and the adjacent tissues, and the progress of these is often more serious than that of the primary disease.

I have seen one example of primary epithelial cancer in lymphatic glands, which I will relate, both for its own interest, and because it illustrated many of the foregoing statements. The patient, who was in St. Bartholomew's Hospital last summer, was a sweep, 48 years old: his skin was dusky and dry, and many hair-follicles were enlarged by their accumulated contents; but he had no appearance of cancer, or wart of any kind, on the scrotum or penis: yet his inguinal glands were diseased just as they commonly are in the latter stages of scrotal soot-cancer. On the right side, over the saphenous opening, a cluster of glands formed a round tuberous mass, more than an inch in diameter. It felt very firm, heavy, ill-defined, and as if deep-set. Over its most prominent part the skin was adherent, and ulcerated, and a soft dark growth protruded through it. Above this mass were three glands, enlarged, but not hardened. On the left side, below the crural arch, one gland was enlarged to a diameter of half an inch, and hard; and four others felt similarly but less diseased. All these were movable under the skin.

This disease had been observed in progress for fifteen weeks, having begun in the right groin as a hard lump under the skin, like those which were now in the left groin, and which had commenced to enlarge somewhat later. The ulceration in the right groin had existed for a week.

I removed all the glands that seemed diseased. The chief mass, from the right side, appeared, on section, lobed, soft, grayish, mottled with pink and livid tints. The same changes, but with increased firmness, were seen in the largest gland from the left side; and the material pressed from both these (a turbid, grumous, and not creamy, substance) contained abundant epithelial cancer-cells. The other glands were not evidently cancerous; but, during the healing of the operation on the right side, a gland, which I had thought it unnecessary to remove, enlarged and became hard; it was destroyed with chloride of zinc, and then the wounds healed soundly.

The Epithelial Cancer of the LUNGS, which I referred to (p. 564) as having once seen, occurred in an old man whose penis was amputated eighteen months before death. The disease soon returned in the inguinal glands and I received these and the lungs for examination. The other organs were reported healthy.

A cluster of three or four glands were compressed in a large mass, of which a part protruded through an ulcerated opening in the skin. On section, nearly the whole of the gland-substance appeared replaced by the peculiar and oft-mentioned whitish, half-dry, friable substance, with grayish mottlings and streaked with blood-vessels. In this substance all the structures of epithelial cancer, with abundant laminated capsules, were perfectly distinct; they might have been taken as types.

In the lungs there were about twenty masses of similar cancerous substance: and of one large mass, at the root of the right lung, I could not
be sure whether it were in the lung itself or in a cluster of bronchial
glands.   They were nearly all spherical, or flattened under and in the
pleura, and measured from ¼ of an inch to nearly 8 inches in diameter.
Their substance was opaque-white, marbled with pale yellow and pink,
intersected by lines of gray and black (belonging apparently to the involved
interlobular tissue of the lungs,) and marked with blood-vessels.   They
were compact, but brittle and crumbling under pressure: several of the
largest were softer and more friable at their centres than elsewhere, and
the largest three had great central cavities, filled with softened cancerous
matter and pus: they might have been called "cancerous vomicæ;" but
they were completely bounded by layers of cancer, rough and knotted
on their inner surfaces, and had no communication with air-tubes.   From
one mass an outgrowth projected into, and had grown within, a bronchial
tube; from another a similar growth extended into a pulmonary artery.

The crumbling, brittle texture of these masses, and the absence of
creamy "juice" in even the softest parts, might have sufficed, I believe,
to declare that these were not masses of scirrhous or medullary cancer:
but the microscopic examination left no doubt.   Their minute structures
accorded exactly with those in the inguinal glands: not a character of
the epithelial cancers was wanting.*

Epithelial Cancer in the HEART is illustrated in the Museum of St.
Bartholomew's.†   A man, 58 years old, had a granulated and warty
epithelial cancer, which covered the anterior and inferior third of his eye,
and was firmly combined with the conjunctiva and parts of the sclerotica
and cornea.   Mr. Wormald removed the eyeball with all the disease.
Two years afterwards, the man died with a large tumor over the parotid
gland; and a mass of cancer, about an inch and a half in diameter, was
imbedded in the substance of the apex of the right ventricle and septum
of the heart.   The mass is soft and broken at its centre, and has the microscopic structures of epithelial cancer.

In the UTERUS, and the adjacent part of the VAGINA, the epithelial
cancer may be found with ordinary characters, such as were described at
the beginning of the lecture; but its more remarkable appearance is in
the form of the "Cauliflower-Excrescence."   Only a part, however, of
the cases to which this name has been ascribed have been epithelial cancers: of the rest, some were medullary cancers, and some, perhaps,
simple non-cancerous, warty, or papillary growths.

My own observations of this disease have only sufficed to confirm

* Portions of the lungs and of the inguinal glands, in this and in the last-described case,
are in the Museum of St. Bartholomew's.

† Series xii. 60.   In the Catalogue the disease is described as medullary cancer; but I
have recently examined microscopically both it and the primary growth (Series ix. No. 11),
and they are certainly epithelial cancers.

(wherever I could test them) those far more completely made by Virchow,[*] whose results, approved by Lebert, and consistent with the best earlier records, I shall therefore quote:—" One must distinguish three different papillary tumors at the os uteri—the simple, such as Frerichs[†] and Lebert[‡] have seen; the cancroid; and the cancerous,"—[*i. e.* the epithelial cancerous and the medullary cancerous]:—the first two forms together constitute the cauliflower growth. This begins as a simple papillary tumor, and at a later period passes into cancroid [epithelial cancer]. At first one sees only on the surface papillary or villous growths, which consist of very thick layers of peripheral flat, and interior cylindrical, epithelial cells, and a very fine interior cylinder formed of an extremely little connective tissue with large vessels. The outer layer contains cells of all sizes and stages of development; some of them forming great parent-structures with endogenous corpuscles. The vessels are, for the most part, colossal very thin-walled capillaries, which form either simple loops at the apices of the villi, between the epithelial layers, or towards the surface develope new loops in constantly increasing number, or, lastly, present a reticulate branching. At the beginning of the disease, the villi are simple and close pressed, so that the surface appears only granulated, as Clarke describes it: it becomes cauliflower-like by the branching of the papillæ, which at last grow out to fringes an inch long, and may present almost the appearance of an hydatid mole.

"After the process has existed for some time on the surface, the cancroid alveoli begin to form deep between the layers of the muscular and the connective tissues of the organ. In the early cases I saw only cavities simply filled with epithelial structures; but in Kiwisch's case there were alveoli, on whose walls new, papillary, branching growths were seated—a kind of proliferous arborescent formation."

It will be evident, from this description, that the cauliflower excrescence, in the two conditions distinguished by Virchow, illustrates the usual history of the most exuberant epithelial cancers (p. 567): it might be taken as the principal example of the group. That which he calls the "simple papillary tumor" is an excessive papillary outgrowth of epithelial cancer; the later stage of the same, when it " passes into cancroid," is the usual extension of such a cancer into deeper parts,—a continuous growth of the same thing in a new direction. For the papillary structures, *composed*, as Virchow says, of epithelial cells with blood-vessels and a very little connective tissue, are the essential characters of the epithelial cancerous outgrowths; and I believe that the same composition has never been seen in any papillary or warty growths, that did not, if time were allowed, proceed to the formation of epithelial structures in the deeper parts, and thence through the usual progress of malignant disease.

* Würzburg Verhandl. 1850, B. i. 109. They were chiefly made in the cases described by Mayer in the Verhandl. der Gesellsch. fur Geburtshülfe in Berlin, 1851, p. 111.
† Jenaische Annalen, p. 7. ‡ Abhandlungen, p. 57, 150.

Before entering on the pathology of epithelial cancers it will be useful to refer briefly to the morbid anatomy of the diseases with which they have most affinity, and from which it is most necessary to distinguish them,—at least, as clearly as we can. These are, on the one side, the scirrhous and medullary cancers; and, on the other, certain rodent ulcers and warty growths of scars.*

The descriptions in former lectures of the scirrhous and medullary cancers of the skin and subcutaneous tissue may suffice for the distinction from them (compare pp. 503, 504, 547).

The RODENT ULCER is the disease which has been described under various names; such as cancerous ulcer of the face, cancroid ulcer, ulcère rongeant, ulcère chancreux du visage, der flache Krebs, moosartige Parasit, ulcus exedens, noli me tangere. In its earliest appearance, on its most frequent seat, it has been called cancerous tubercle of the face. It has been confounded by many with different forms of cancer; yet it is distinct from them in structure as well as in history, and had better be described by some name which may not add to the yearly increasing confusion that arises from the use of terms expressing likeness to cancer.

Sir B. C. Brodie thus describes the most frequent characters of the disease:—"A man has a soft tubercle upon the face, covered by a smooth skin. He may call it a wart, but it is quite a different thing. On cutting into it you find it consists of a brown solid substance, not very highly organized. A tumor of this kind may remain on the face unaltered for years, and then, when the patient gets old, it may begin to ulcerate. The ulcer spreads, slowly but constantly, and if it be left alone, it may destroy the whole of the cheek, the bones of the face, and ultimately the patient's life; but it may take some years to run this course. So far these tumors in the face, and these ulcers, are to be considered as malignant. Nevertheless, they are not like fungus hæmatodes or cancer; and for this reason, that the disease is entirely local. It does not affect the lymphatic glands, nor do similar tumors appear in other parts of the body."

The constantly progressive ulceration is a character in which this disease resembles cancer, especially epithelial cancer. The likeness in this respect may indicate some important affinity between them; but the differences between them are greater; for not only is the rodent ulcer usually unlike that of any cancer in its aspect, rate, and mode of progress, but the tissues bounding it, and forming its base and walls, never

---

* The whole of this subject is admirably illustrated by Mr. Cæsar Hawkins, in paper in the Medico-Chir. Trans. vols. xix. and xxi., and in the Medical Gazette, vols. xxvi. xxix. Indeed, I can add nothing to his account, except such conclusions as are derived from microscopic examinations of the diseases. One of Mr. Hawkins's lectures relate to cheloid growths; but to these it seems unnecessary to refer; if they could be confounded with any form of cancer, it would be with scirrhous cancer of the skin.

† In his Lectures on Pathology and Surgery, p. 333.

contain any epithelial or other cancerous structure; they are infiltrated with only such structures as may be found in the walls of common chronic ulcers.

The most usual characters of the rodent ulcer, whether on the cheek, the eyelids, upper lip, nose, scalp, vulva, or any other part, are as follows:*—It is of irregular shape, but generally tends towards oval or circular. The base, however deeply and unequally excavated, is usually, in most parts, not warty or nodular, or even plainly granulated; in contrast with cancerous ulcers, one may especially observe this absence, or less amount of up-growth. It is, also, comparatively dry and glossy, yielding, for its extent, very little ichor or other discharge, and has commonly a dull reddish-yellow tint. Its border is slightly, if at all elevated, it is not commonly or much either everted or undermined, but is smoothly rounded or lowly tuberculated. The immediately adjacent skin appears quite healthy. The base and border alike feel tough and hard, as if bounded by a layer of indurated tissue about a line in thickness. This layer does not much increase in thickness as the ulcer extends; and herein is another chief contrast with cancerous ulceration: in the progress of the rodent ulcer we see mere destruction, in the cancerous we see destruction with coincident, and usually more than commensurate, growth.

The indurated substance at the base and border of the ulcer appears, on section, very firm, pale, grayish, uniform or obscurely fibrous; little fluid of any kind can be pressed from it. It is composed of the same elementary structures as common granulations are, and these, in the deeper layers, are inserted among the tissues on which the ulcer rests. I have examined very carefully six of these ulcers, removed by excision, and have never seen in or near them a structure resembling those of epithelial or any other form of cancer. Lebert's observations, I believe, fully coincide with mine; though he classes the disease with epithelial cancers, under the general name of Cancroid. Mr. Joseph Hutchinson, also, has made several examinations of pieces cut, during life, from the margins of rodent ulcers, and always with the same result; they never contained structures resembling those of epithelial or any other cancer.

Thus the anatomical distinctions between this disease and cancer is evident, and they are equally different in pathology; the rodent ulcer, so far as it has yet been observed, is never attended by similar disease in the lymphatics or other part; and if completely removed or destroyed it does not recur.

The WARTY GROWTHS ON SCARS (Cancers of Cicatrices) are usually well-marked papillary epithelial cancers, which grow in the place of scars, re-

---

* The parts enumerated were the seats of disease in the cases from which I have drawn my description, and in which it is, I believe, most frequent; but it is not confined to them. Lebert refers to cases of it, in his account of the cancroid of the uterus, and suggests (what is highly probable) that the simple chronic, or perforating, ulcer of the stomach is a disease of the same nature.

maining after injuries or common ulcers. Mr. Hawkins,* who has given a very full account of their general characters and progress, describes cases in the scars of burns, gunshot wounds, floggings, and ulcers. All that I have seen were on the lower extremities, and connected with scars after repeated injuries.†

The description already given of the warty epithelial cancers may suffice for these. They usually exemplify very well the wide-spread growth and cancerous change in the papillæ; the enlargement, at first probably simple, and afterwards with cancerous formation, in the papillæ of the adjacent skin; the deep extension of the disease to the periosteum, and thence onwards, even to the complete penetration of the bones and other adjacent tissues; and, at a late period, the cancerous disease of the lymphatic glands. But it is important to be aware that this disease may be closely imitated by warty growths and ulcers, in and about which no cancerous matter can be found. I examined very carefully such an ulcer with prominent growths on the front of a man's leg. It was seated in the middle third of the leg, in the place of a large old scar after a scald, and the greater part of the ulcer presented high, lobed, and nodulated hard granulations. No one doubted, before the amputation, that the disease was the usual form of cancer ensuing in these conditions; yet no cancer structure could be found; in whichever part I examined, I could find only inflammatory products, and such corpuscles as compose ill-developed or degenerate granulations upon common ulcers.

I think some of the diversities of opinion respecting the nature of these warty growths and ulcers may be due to the want of distinction between those which are, and those which are not, epithelial cancers. To the naked eye and during life the two diseases may be very much alike: but the difference in their respective minute structures would indicate essential difference of nature; certainly, in the pathology of epithelial cancer, caution is necessary in reckoning any of these cases that are without microscopic examination.

I would add, that I have no doubt the epithelial growth, in some cases, proceeds from the periosteum or other subcutaneous tissues, and thence extends into and through the skin. I have seen the growth protruding through an ulcerated aperture in the scar, just as any deep-seated tumor might. Such cases justify Mr. Stanley's description of the disease as one, primarily, of the periosteum.

---

* Medical Gazette, vol. xxviii. 872; and Med.-Chir. Trans., xix. See, also, the Dub. Quarterly Journal 1850–51.

† They are amply illustrated in the Museum of St. Bartholomew's, Ser. i. and Ser. xxii. Several cases are described by Mr. Stanley (Treatise on Diseases of the Bones, p. ...

LECTURE XXXII.

EPITHELIAL CANCER.

PART II.—PATHOLOGY.

AMONG all the cancers, the epithelial present the general or constitutional features of malignant disease in the least intense form. They commence at the latest average period of life; they appear to be most dependent upon local conditions; they are least prone to multiplication in internal organs: they are associated with the least evident diathesis or cachexia. An yet I believe that, in a large survey of them, none of the features of malignant disease, as exemplified in the scirrhous and medullary cancers, will be found wanting: the difference is one of degree, not of kind.

(*a*) A large majority of the cases of epithelial cancers occur in males. In 105 cases, affecting parts common to both sexes, 86 were in men and 19 in women. In the cases affecting the sexual organs themselves, I think the proportion is nearly equal; unless we reckon the scrotal soot-cancers, which, for obvious reasons, we should more properly exclude.

(*b*) A few cases are on record, transmitted from book to book, in which what were probably epithelial cancers occurred before adult life. Sir James Earle saw a scrotal soot-cancer in a child eight years old;* so did Mr. Wadd;† and M. Lebert‡ examined a "cancroid" growth at the vulva in a child 3½ years old, in whom it was almost congenital. But cases such as these cannot be taken into our estimate of the influence of age in determining the access of the disease. In the following table, I have included no cases that were recorded merely or chiefly on account of the patients' ages.§

Age.							No. of cases.
20 to 30	.	.	.	.	.	.	9
30 to 40	.	.	.	.	.	.	22
40 to 50	.	.	.	.	.	.	40
50 to 60	.	.	.	.	.	.	32
60 to 70	.	.	.	.	.	.	30
70 to 80	.	.	.	.	.	.	10
							143

* Pott's Works, by Earle, iii. p. 178.   † Curling on the Diseases of the Testis, p. 528.

‡ Traité Pratique, p. 676. Hannover (Das Epithelioma, p. 104) quotes from Frerichs a case in which the disease extended from the ear through the petrous bone in a male 19 years old.

§ The table includes cases from Lebert, Hannover, and others. But I have omitted, both from it and from the preceding one, Lebert's cases of "cancroid" of the face. They were examples of rodent ulcers, and their contrast with epithelial cancers (of the lip, for example) is well shown, in that the average age for their coming under operation is 17 years later, and the proportionate frequencies in the two sexes is reversed. The ages assigned in the above table are, with few exceptions, those at which the disease was first observed *by the patients.*

If now, as in the two last lectures (pages 513, 551), we calculate, from this table, the frequency of epithelial cancer in proportion to the number of persons living at each of the successive periods, it may be represented by the following numbers (100 being, as before, taken to express the frequency between 40 and 50):—

20 to 30 years	12
30 to 40 "	41
40 to 50 "	100
50 to 60 "	119
60 to 70 "	163
70 to 80 "	111

We may probably deduce from this calculation, that the conditions favorable to the production of epithelial cancers regularly increase with the increase of age; for, the apparent diminution after 70 may be reasonably ascribed to the comparatively small proportion of persons beyond that age who are received into hospitals, or who are under such surgical treatment as to have their cases recorded.

The proportions expressed by the foregoing general tables are nearly true for the epithelial cancers of each part most liable to be affected: the only notable peculiarities, I believe, are, that the mean age of its occurrence is lowest in the sexual organs, and highest in the integuments of the head, face, eyelids, and upper extremities.

(c) An hereditary disposition to soot-cancer has been several times observed: as, by Mr. Earle,* in a grandfather, father, and two sons; by Mr. Hawkins,† in a father and son; by Mr. Cusack,‡ in a mother and son; by myself (twice) in two brothers. But all the persons here referred to were engaged in 'the same trade, and their exposure to the same exciting or predisposing cause of the disease diminishes the value of the facts as indications of hereditary predisposition. I have no certain record of other epithelial cancers occurring in many members of the same family; but I have found some significant facts indicating a disposition to epithelial cancer, in members of those families in which other members have had scirrhous or medullary cancers.

Among 160 instances of cancer, in most of which the point was inquired into, though none were collected for the sake of it, these cases were found :—(1) A man had medullary cancer of a toe; his father had a cancer of the lip. (2) A woman had repeated epithelial cancers of the labia: her sister, her father's sister, and her mother's brother's daughter, had cancer of the breast. (3) A man had epithelial cancer of the lip, whose grandmother had cancer of the breast. (4) A gentleman had epithelial cancer of the interior of the cheek: his aunt died with cancer of the breast. (5) A woman had medullary cancer of the breast: her mother had cancer of the uterus, and her uncle had cancer of the face. (6) A woman had scirrhous cancer of the breast, whose mother's uncle had cancer of

* Med. Chir. Trans., xii. 305.   † Medical Gazette, xxi. 842.
‡ Quoted by Mr. Curling (On Diseases of the Testis, p. 528).

the lip. (7) Of another woman with similar cancer, one cousin had cancer of the lip, another cousin cancer of the uterus. (8) A third woman had scirrhous cancer of the breast, whose grandfather had cancer of the lip.*

The proportion of these cases (only $\frac{1}{10}$ of the whole number) may seem too small to be even suggestive; yet it is too large to be referred to chance. Let it be contrasted with these facts:—(1) I have found that among 116 patients† with cancer, only one was aware of any member of the same family having had a simple tumor. This was a woman with scirrhous cancer of the breast, from whose sister a myeloid tumor of the breast had been removed. (2) Among 77 patients with non-cancerous tumors, 10 were aware of near relations having had similar diseases: but among the same 77, the only cases of family connection with cancers were the following:—(a) The cases of recurring and disorderly-growing mammary tumor related at page 474; (b) the case of anomalous cartilaginous tumors at page 531; (c) that of the same woman whose case was just mentioned as one of myeloid tumor of the breast: five years after its removal, she and her sister were at the same time in St. Bartholomew's with scirrhous breasts; (d) that of a lad with mixed cartilaginous and glandular tumor over his parotid gland, whose grandmother had cancer of the breast. Now of these cases the two first must be regarded, I believe, as instances of a cancerous disposition, modified and gradually ceasing in its transmission from parent to offspring (see page 474, &c.); the third is a very anomalous one, exemplifying the formation of a most rare tumor in the breast, not long before it became cancerous; the fourth alone is an instance of an ordinary simple or innocent tumor growing in one who had a cancerous relation.

I have referred to these cases, not to suggest that when cancer has occurred in one or more members of a family, the rest are peculiarly unlikely to have innocent tumors, but to show, by contrast, that the proportion of cases in which epithelial and other cancers occur in the same family is relatively, considerable. For if that proportion were the result of chance-coincidences or errors in observation, an equal, or nearly equal, proportion of coincidences should have appeared in the opposite set of cases. But the contrast between the two sets of cases is remarkable; and I believe the facts may be justly regarded as evidence for the close affinity between epithelial and other cancers, and as an illustration of the

* Dr. Warren mentions this:—A grandfather died with a cancer of the lip. His son and two daughters died with cancer of the breast. One of his grandsons and one of his grand-daughters had also cancer of the breast (On Tumors, p. 281). It may be objected, by some, that the cancers of the lip here referred to were not epithelial. I assume that they were, because of the exceeding rarity of any other kind in the lip: indeed, I have not yet seen one, or a complete record of one, in which the microscope did not find the epithelial structures.

† These were part of the 160 mentioned above; but I have here reckoned only the cases recorded by myself, because it is probable that, even if, among the others, any instances had occurred of innocent and malignant tumors in the same family, they would not have been mentioned.

38

modification which the cancerous and other diathesis may undergo in their hereditary transmission.

(d) Among 84 patients with epithelial cancers, 19 were aware of injury or previous morbid condition in the affected part;—a much larger proportion than is found among patients laboring under tumors of any other kind, except melanoid cancers of the skin.

In certain cases, injury by violence appears as the exciting cause. But the histories of epithelial cancers differ from those of others in that the kind of injury which is most effective in their production is such as is often inflicted—frequent blows or slight wounds on the same part; hurts of scars and other seats of old injury. It is as if it were necessary that the part should be considerably changed in structure, before it is appropriate for a cancerous growth.

It agrees with this that, in the majority of cases, patients assign, as the cause of the disease, not injury, or not it alone, but some former disease, especially such as arises from long-continued irritation of a part. Thus epithelial cancers arise sometimes in old ulcers, as on the legs, or, as I have known, in perineal urinary fistulæ; sometimes, in those of more rapid progress, as I once saw in a case of necrosis of the hard palate, and once in a case of necrosis of the angle of the lower jaw, and, as Frerichs describes, in an ulceration of the internal ear following scarlet fever. The majority of the epithelial cancers of the prepuce and glans occur in those who are the subjects of congenital phymosis, and in whom we may assume the frequent irritation of the part by decomposed secretions. In some rare cases, a mole or pigmentary nævus becomes the seat of the disease. But, among all the things referred to by patients, none are so frequently named as "warts."

The affections thus named are not usually such as are commonly called warts. They are not usually like the warts (Verrucæ, or Condylomata elevata) that grow on the genital organs during gonorrhœal or other similar irritation; nor like such warts (Verrucæ vulgares) as are common on the hands of young people before puberty; nor like the condylomata (C. lata) of syphilis. Such papillary growths as these may, I believe, precede epithelial cancer; but I think they rarely do so. The general condition of the "wart" is, I think, that a small portion of the cutis is slightly indurated; its papillæ are, generally, in some measure enlarged; and it is covered with a darkish dry crust, or with a scab, or, if the part be very moist, with a soft layer of detached scales.* The induration of the cutis, and the predominance of the crust or other covering (which apparently constitutes more of the disease than either the induration or the papillæ), mark the chief differences between this disease and any of the "warts" just referred to. The induration, which patients often describe as "a little hard knot," is usually attended with

---

* Such as these are well described by Schuh (Pseudoplasmen, p. 46), under the title "barky warts." With the same intimation of likeness, Dr. Warren (On Tumors, p. ?) called the disease "Lepoides."

elevation, but sometimes with contraction and depression of the piece of cutis. The crust consists, for the most part, of epidermal scales held together by dried secretion, or, in its deepest layers, forming whitish friable substance, and fitting between the papillæ. It is easily detached and quickly removed; and, when it is removed, the subjacent cutis does not usually appear raw or bleeding, but is tender, florid, and as if covered with a very thin glossy layer of epidermis. When a moister yellow scab covers the induration, the surface beneath it is usually more inflamed and excoriated, and the papillæ are more enlarged.

Such incrusted warts as these are very common, especially on the faces of old persons: the large majority of them lead to no further trouble; yet some become the seats of epithelial cancers, and some of rodent ulcers. A similar affection often precedes the epithelial cancer of the lower lip. Some slight violence often applied, such as that of a short pipe habitually supported by the lip, or the frequent slight rending of the surface of a dry scaly lip, or one much exposed to weather, leads to a "little crack:" this scabs over, and after repeated removals and renewals of the scab, there is a "little hard lump" or "a sort of wart," with a head or crust. And such a wart might be as often innocuous on the lip as on the face, if it were not that the lip is in the unhappy singularity of being within easy reach, at once, of the fingers, the teeth, the tongue, and the other lip; so that when it is as yet but slightly diseased, it is never left at rest.

A similarly drily scaled or incrusted warty change of the cutis often, I believe, precedes the chimney-sweep's cancer; and I suspect that the true influence of the soot in this disease is not that its continued contact determines the growth of cancers, but (at least in part) that it produces a state of skin which provides an apt locality for epithelial cancer in persons of cancerous diathesis. How it does this I cannot imagine: but this is only one of many things unexplained in this strange disease; for the whole of the peculiarities of the chimney-sweep's cancer,—its dependence on soot, while coal-dust is wholly inoperative (for the disease is unknown among colliers); its comparative frequency in England, especially in the large towns, while in other countries where soot is abundant it is hardly seen; its selection of the scrotum for its most frequent seat, —all these, and many like facts in its history, appear completely inexplicable. Still, it is certain that scaly or incrusted small warts, such as I have been describing, are very common in chimney-sweeps. In many of them, even when they are thoroughly cleaned, the whole skin is dry, harsh, and dusky; and before operation for the removal of scrotal cancers in them, it is a common question whether one or more warts or scaly patches near the chief disease should be removed with it. Nor are such warts confined to the scrotum; they may exist on every part of the trunk and limbs; and I have seen sweeps so thick-set with them, that a hundred or more might have been counted.

Such are some of the numerous morbid states, one or other of which may, in the majority of cases, be assigned as predisposing a part to become the seat of epithelial cancer. Expressions are sometimes used, implying that the part does not become the seat of a new morbid structure, but that its mode of action is changed, or that the change is only due to the extension and deepening of a common epidermoid or warty growth. The truer view, however, may be expressed by saying that the part, whatever were its previous state, becomes the seat of epithelial cancer, the structures of which, as of a new disease, are inserted among the original or previous morbid textures of the part. This evidently happens when the cancer appears in parts previously healthy, or in the deep-seated tissues, or in the walls of ulcers, or in a pigmentary nævus; for, in these cases, no morbid structures of the epithelial cancer existed previous to its access. There is more appearance of similarity and continuity of disease between the epithelial cancers and the warty growths by which they are sometimes preceded: for here both the earlier and the later disease may have, in common, an accumulation of epidermoid cells and an enlargement of papillæ. Yet the warts, whether incrusted or others, in which the epidermoid structures are only superficial, should also, I think, be regarded as only predisposing conditions of epithelial cancer; as diseased parts, not cancerous, though peculiarly apt to become the seats of this form of cancer. For the great majority of these are stationary affections, or may disappear, or be cured even in cancerous persons; they are comparatively few in which, after a certain duration as simple warts, the cancerous disease is manifested. And the time of this change in them is often well marked. Nearly all patients,—even those who can assign no date to the beginning of the wart or hardness, or other previous disease,—can refer exactly to some time of change in it, when it began to "grow up," or "be sore," or "get bad," discharge or bleed. They thus mark the time when the cancerous mode of progress was commenced; and from this time the history of all such cases is nearly uniform—even remarkably uniform if it be compared with the variety of the histories of the previous states.

Now, I believe that this change in the life of the warty or other diseased part is always associated with a change in its structure; and that whatever were its previous state, its proper tissue, whether papillæ or any others, now become the seat of the formation of epithelial cancer-cells. It is hardly possible to prove such a change of structure in any single case, but it is rendered highly probable by this,—that in those warty structures which we remove because experience makes us believe that they are in progress as epithelial cancers, we find the tissues infiltrated with the specific cancer-cells: while in those which have been long stationary, without extension or outgrowth, without ulceration or ichorous discharge, no such infiltration is found. Certain cases must be excepted from this statement because of error in diagnosis. I have known rodent ulcers excised, in the belief that they were epithelial cancers; but I never saw any growth removed as an epithelial cancer, in which the epidermoidal cells were placed only on the surface of the vascular tissues; and on the other hand, I have never seen such cells *in* the cutis or papillæ of any incrusted or other wart, in which the cancerous mode of progress was not yet manifested. The opportunities of examining such warts as observation shows to be most apt to be precursors of epithelial cancer are rare: but I have examined some on the scrotum, and one on a lower lip. The last may deserve description.

A healthy-looking farmer, 66 years old, came to me with an induration, about two lines wide and half a line thick, at the middle of the florid margin of his lower lip. The indurated part was slightly sunken, and covered with a thin yellow scab. This disease had existed two years, frequently scabbing thickly, then desquamating, never soundly healing; yet it had made no progress. I removed it, chiefly because the patient's father, when 85 years old, had had cancer of the lower lip; and because, if not already cancerous, this could not but be thought a place very likely to become so. I found, in the indurated tissue, inflammatory products infiltrated among the natural structures of the skin; but no appearance of epithelial cancer-cells. The cutis was slightly thickened; but there was no evidence of enlargement of papillæ, or of accumulated epidermis: the scab seemed formed chiefly of dried secretion.

I believe that such a description as this would apply to most of the warts that precede epithelial cancers of the lower lip, and that we may justly say of them that they are not cancerous, but are such parts as, in certain persons, are peculiarly apt to be the seats of cancer. Why only some among them should become cancerous we can no more explain than we can why, among so many injuries inflicted, so few should be followed by erysipelas or tetanus; or why, among so many pigmentary moles or nævi as may be found, only few should become the seats of melanoid cancer; or, in a yet nearer parallel, why, when a person has many such moles, the melanoid cancer should appear in only one. In these varieties of fate, there is nothing unusual in warts, if we regard them as only predisposed to become cancerous; but, if we regard them as the first stage of a cancroid or cancerous disease, such varieties of progress as they manifest would be without parallel.

(e) The general health of patients with epithelial cancer is usually good, till it is affected by the consequences of the local disease. No primary cachexia can be observed preceding the appearance of the growth; nor does a secondary cachexia ensue earlier than it probably would in any disease of equal duration and severity.

When the formation of an epithelial cancer has once commenced, its natural course is as regularly progressive to the destruction of life, as that of either a scirrhous or a medullary cancer. Only, the rate, and some parts of the method, of progress are different.

The average rate of increase of epithelial cancers is less than of either of the other kinds. It is not apt to be arrested altogether; yet it is sometimes so slow that, in a year, the cancer may gain only a line or two in any of its dimensions. In other cases, however, and especially when such a cancer has been violently injured, the progress is much more rapid. I have known three-fourths of the scrotum covered with ulcerating soot-cancer, and part of the urethra surrounded by it, in three months after a laceration received while in apparent health: in another case, a spheroidal mass of soft epithelial cancer, an inch in diameter, formed in the substance of the cheek in two months; in another, a growth more than an inch in diameter formed in ten weeks; in another, the whole depth of the lower lip, and two-thirds of its width, were occupied with epithelial cancer in three months after a blow on a little cancer at its margin; in another, within twelve months, the eyelids and a large part of the contents of the orbit were destroyed by ulceration, and tuberous masses, from one to three-quarters of an inch in diameter, were formed under the integuments of the brow, the temple, and the other boundaries of the orbit.

Cases such as these, and they are not rare, may prove the error of regarding epithelial cancer as a trivial or an inactive disease in comparison with the other forms. Its rate of progress is, like that of scirrhous cancer, widely various in different cases; it has its acute and its chronic instances. Of its modes of growth, and of ulceration, and of the usual coincidence of these processes, I have spoken fully in the former part of the lecture (p. 575); I will here only add that the ulceration, at whatever rate, seems constantly progressive. Some portions of the ulcer may appear, for a time, as if skinning over, or, portions of the disease may slough away, and the surfaces they leave may partially heal; but I do not remember to have seen any process of healing or wasting so nearly accomplished in an epithelial cancer, as I have described in some cases of both scirrhous and medullary cancer, in the former lectures (pp. 519, 558).

The progress of the ulceration, and the coincident deepening of the growth, are usually attended with great pain,—hot, scalding, and widely diffusing pain; or with pain like that of neuralgia darting in the course of nerves. With this, and the constant ichorous discharge from the ulcer, and the occasional bleedings from ulcerated blood-vessels, the patient becomes cachectic; yet probably not sooner than in other diseases of equal extent, nor in any very characteristic manner.

Primary epithelial cancers are usually single. Two growths may sometimes appear at once in the same region, as, e. g. on the prepuce and glans, or on the scrotum; but even this is rare. In the later progress of the disease, separate masses of epithelial cancer may be sometimes found in the tissues, or cancerous warty growths on the surface, around the primary growth or ulcer. Healthy tissue appears to intervene between these secondary cancers and the primary one: and they may be compared with the tubercles so often grouped around a scirrhous mammary gland.

The lymphatic glands, sooner or later in the progress of the disease, usually become cancerous. I have already (p. 584) described the manner of their infection. I feel almost disposed to think that epithelial cancer is a much worse disease in this country than in France or Denmark, when I see how far my observations on the affection of the lymphatics differ from those of Lebert and Hannover. Lebert* says that he has found the lymphatic glands affected with "cancroid" three times in 81 cases; and of these 81, 60 were certainly cases of epithelial cancer. Hannover† has even less frequently seen them diseased. Now, in 42 cases of epithelial cancer collected in the ordinary course of hospital and private practice, and including many in the early as well as in the latest stages of the disease, I have observed the lymphatics cancerous twenty times. In the greater part of these cases, the characteristic cancer-structures were found in the glands removed during life or after death: in the rest, their existence was concluded, with scarcely less certainty, from the enlargement, with induration, rapid growth, clustering, and destructive ulceration of the glands. It need not be suspected that in any of these cases the glands were enlarged merely through "irritation;" such a state does, indeed, occur with epithelial as with scirrhous cancer, but the diagnosis of this from the cancerous enlargement is seldom, in either case, difficult.

I do not suppose that the proportion cited above expresses the greatest frequency of epithelial cancer in the lymphatic glands. I believe rather, that very few cases reach their natural end without infection of the glands. Even after the primary disease has been wholly removed, and when the glands at the time of the operation appeared healthy, they are frequently, and often alone, the seats of recurrences of the disease (p. 602). Sometimes, also, with scirrhous cancers (p. 504), we find the disease in the lymphatics greatly preponderating over that in the primary seat.

My observations are scarcely less different from those of Lebert, in relation to the occurrence of secondary epithelial cancers in internal organs. In 18 autopsies (some of which, however, were made in fatal cases of rodent ulcer) he has not once found "cancroid growths" in any internal part. In 7 autopsies,‡ I have found epithelial cancer once in the heart, and once in the lungs; [its appearance in these parts is described at p. 586.] Doubtless, the internal organs are more rarely infected than in any other form of cancer; but they do not enjoy an

* Traité Pratique, p. 619.   † Das Epithelioma, p. 24.

‡ In two of these the disease had not reached its natural end; for the patients died in consequence of amputation. In another case I found epithelial cancer of the tongue, with medullary cancer of the cervical glands, and of the lungs; but as I have already said (p. 584), though no medullary cancer-structures were found in the primary disease, it was impossible to prove that they had never existed, for a large portion of the tongue had sloughed before death.

absolute immunity; the difference between the epithelial and the other cancers is, in this point again, one of degree, not of kind.

It is a peculiarity of epithelial cancers, that in nearly all the characteristics of malignant disease—whether the propagation to the lymphatics or other organs, the extension to deep-seated parts, the recurrence after removal, or the rate of progress towards death—greater differences are noted according to the seat of disease than among the medullary cancers of different parts. The anatomical characters of the disease are in all parts essentially the same, but their history, in all the particulars noted above, differs, so as to justify the expression that the disease is less malignant in some parts than in others. It is, generally, most malignant in the tongue, the interior of the mouth, and the penis; least in the lower extremities and the scrotum; in general, also, the epithelial cancers that are deep-seated are more malignant than the superficial.

These diversities make it very difficult to assign the average duration of life in persons with epithelial cancer; and the difficulty is greatly increased by the recorded cases being often mixed or confounded with those of other cancers and of rodent ulcers. I have not been able to collect more than 30 cases, traced to the end of life. Of these, 12 were not submitted to operation; in the remaining 18, the diseased parts were once or more removed, and the operation was in none of these cases fatal. The average duration of life in the former was 38.6 months; in the latter 39-3 months; the general average of the whole was 39 months. But, with these cases, I have also those of 8 patients, still living beyond 39 months; and if these be reckoned with the other 30, they raise the average to 44 months.

I believe the true average duration of life with epithelial cancer is higher than 44 months; for the cases I have collected, being chiefly those of hospital and other patients, who when first seen, were in a state to be remedied by treatment, probably contain too small a proportion of those of longest standing. Probably four years is about the true average.

The following table will show the duration of life in the 38 cases, and may be compared with those in p. 524 and 561: the total difference produced by operations appeared too slight to make separate tables necessary :—

Duration of Life.	Number of Cases.
Less than 6 months	1
Between 6 and 12 months	1
" 12 " 18 "	7
" 18 " 24 "	4
" 24 " 36 "	5
" 3 " 4 years	3
" 4 " 6 "	3 dead 6 living
" 6 " 8 "	4 dead 1 living
More than 8 years	2 dead 1 living

The chief point which this table shows, in contrast with those of other cancers, is in the proportions of patients living more than four years. The proportion is here nearly half; while in the cases of scirrhous cancers it is only $\frac{1}{3}$, and in those of medullary cancers only $\frac{1}{17}$ (or, after operations, $\frac{1}{37}$ and $\frac{1}{57}$ respectively). An equal contrast is in the proportions of those dying within twelve months of the access of the disease: the proportions being, in the cases of epithelial cancers, less than $\frac{1}{15}$; of scirrhous cancers, nearly $\frac{1}{6}$; of medullary cancers, nearly $\frac{1}{3}$. In both these respects, however, differences may be noted among the epithelial cancers of different organs. I have not yet found a case of one in the tongue surviving more than four years; nor of one in the trunk or limbs destroying life in less than three years: a majority of those in the lower lip are fatal within four years, but some few survive that period. The age at which the disease commences has no great influence on its duration. The average duration among 14 patients, in whom it commenced at or below 45 years of age, was 39 months; that among 17, in whom it commenced later, was $45\frac{1}{2}$ months; and the general average duration was not exceeded in the first list more often than in the second. There is, therefore, no well-marked correspondence, in this respect, between the epithelial and the scirrhous cancers. [Compare p. 524.]

A very trivial prolongation of life would appear, by the cases I have collected, to be obtained by the removal of epithelial cancers. But I would not use this result for more than general guidance in practice; for though I have no doubt that the common opinion of the epithelial cancers being trivial diseases, in comparison with the scirrhous and medullary, is very incorrect, yet I cannot doubt that, in some cases, permanent recovery, and, in some, a long period of health, follows their removal. I have seen a man whose leg was amputated twenty years previously for epithelial cancer commencing in or beneath a scar, and he was still well. A sweep was lately in St. Bartholomew's with a small scrotal cancer, from whom one of the same kind was excised thirty years ago. Of another, Mr. Curling* gives a history extending over twenty-two years, and including five operations. A man from whom Mr. Lawrence removed a cancer of the lip remained well for nine years, and then the disease appeared in the lymphatic glands.

Cases such as these must, I believe, be considered very rare. Too much regard to them, and the confusion of the rodent ulcers with the epithelial cancers, have led to a common belief that recovery or long life may be promised as the consequence of operations. Such a promise, if generally made, will very seldom prove true; and yet, as a general rule, the operation is to be advised, whenever the whole of the disease can be removed without great risk of life, or of producing worse deformity than already exists.

For (1) though the instances of operation followed by complete reco-

* On Diseases of the Testis, p. 535.

very, or by long immunity from the disease, are very rare, yet, in certain cases, these results may be hoped for. This is especially the case, I think, with the epithelial cancers of the lower extremity, which follow injury, and for which amputation is performed; with the soot-cancers which are not making quick progress; with the more superficial cancers of the lip. On the other side, according to present experience, such lengthening of life cannot reasonably be hoped for after operations for the epithelial cancers of the tongue, the gums, or other parts in the interior of the mouth.

(2.) In the majority of cases, and even when very little increase of life can be hoped for, the removal of the disease may give great comfort for a time. In general, also, the greater part of the time that intervenes between the recovery from the operation and the recurrence of the disease may be reckoned as so much added to life; for although we cannot deny a diathesis, or specific constitutional affection, in epithelial cancers, yet it is by the progress and consequences of the local disease that, in the majority of cases, the time of death is determined; so that, while local disease is absent, life may be shortening at scarcely more than the ordinary rate. Of course, in applying such a rule as this may suggest in practice, we must except from it certain cases in which the general health is already very deeply affected, or in which the operation would be perilously extensive.

(3.) The extension of the epithelial cancer to the lymphatic glands is not an insuperable objection to operations. The disease usually remains long limited to the glands which are nearest to its primary seat (p. 584); its complete removal can therefore be usually accomplished; and, although I can cite no instance of very long survival after operation including cancerous glands, yet, on the other side, I can cite none which would prove that the recurrent disease is quicker or more severe after such operations, than it is after those of equal extent in which the glands are not yet diseased.

(4.) The general rule concerning operations in cases of recurrent epithelial cancer may be the same, I think, as for the primary disease. A second operation is, in general, less hopeful than a first, yet not always so; for although the epithelial, like other cancers, usually make progress at an accelerating rate, yet cases are not wanting in which the intervals between successive operations have progressively increased.

I have tabulated 60 cases in which epithelial cancers were removed with the knife. In 3 the operation (amputation at the thigh) was fatal, or accelerated death; in 27 the disease recurred; the remaining 30 are lost sight of, or are still living, and among these are 3 of those 8 patients whom I mentioned (p. 600) as living beyond the average period: in these 3 the disease has not reappeared; but in 2 of the 8 the recurrent disease is still in progress.

Among the 27 cases of recurrence, the secondary disease was in or near the same place eleven times; in the lymphatic glands, eight times; in both, eight times. The periods of recurrence ranged from one to twelve months, and were, on the average, six months after the operation.

In 20 of the 27 cases, the disease after recurrence was allowed to run its course. In the remaining 7 the recurrent cancer was removed, and with these results :—(1.) Cancer of a labium removed after eight months' duration, recurred in two months; it was removed a second time, together with cancerous glands, and the patient remained well for fourteen months; then fatal recurrence ensued. (2.) Cancer of a labium was removed after thirty-six months' duration; thrice after this the disease reappeared in or near the same part, and was removed after intervals of twelve, three, and twenty-four months; the patient has already survived the last operation twenty-eight months; and, though the disease has again recurred, it makes slow progress. (3.) Cancer of the lip, of forty-eight months' duration, recurred in the cheek after three operations, with intervals of six, three, and four months; and the patient is now dying at a distance of eight months from the last operation. (4.) A cancer of three months' duration was removed from the nose; a new growth appeared near the scar a month after the operation; it was removed with *potassa fusa*, and the patient has remained well for six months. (5.) A cancer of the lip of four months' duration was removed; in a month disease reappeared; this also was removed, and the patient had no recurrence in the following six years. (6.) In a similar case recurrence ensued in two months; but the patient remained well for at least twelve months after the second operation. (7.) A cancer of the scalp was removed after eighteen months' duration; it recurred in six months, and was again removed, and there was no reappearance of it in the next eighteen months.

These, and similar cases referred to by M. Lebert, are enough to show that repeated operations may be, in certain instances of epithelial cancer, fully justified. And perhaps we may gather from them an additional motive for very free excision of the cancers; for the excision of a recurrent disease, undertaken as a nearly desperate measure, is generally more free than the first operation was; and thence, it may be, its occasionally greater success.

Let me now collect from the facts of this lecture the grounds which seem to justify the inclusion of this disease under the name of cancer. It is not unimportant to do so; for we may be certain that, in this case, the name of the disease will often guide the further study and the treatment of it.

I have excluded from the group of epithelial cancers the rodent ulcers, which M. Lebert includes with them under the name of "cancroid." The two diseases are so constantly unlike, in both structure and history (see p. 588), that their separation under different titles seems consistent with the most usual rules of nosology. I have also excluded those papillary and other affections of the skin, in which epidermoid structures are accumulated only on the surface of the affected part. For, although these may sometimes appear like the first stages of certain epithelial cancers (see pp. 569 and 596), yet the distinction between the two is commonly well-marked in the history of each case: and, in their respective anatomical relations, the distinction between a superficial and an interstitial epidermoid structure is very significant; since the former has its nearest homologue in natural epithelia, the latter in cancerous infiltrations.

Thus limiting the diseases to be included under it, the name of epithelial cancers seems justified by their conformity with the scirrhous and medullary cancers in these following respects:—

(1.) The interstitial formation of structures like those of epithelium is not an imitation of any natural tissue; it constitutes an heterologous structure; for the superficial position is more essential to the type of epithelial structures, than any shape of elemental cells or scales is.

(2.) Even that delusive appearance of homology, which exists when the structures like those of epithelium are formed in the dermal tissues, and therefore near the surface, is lost in nearly all the cases of deep-seated epithelial cancers, and in all the similar affections of the lymphatic glands and internal organs.

(3.) The interstitial formation of cells in epithelial cancer is conformed with the characteristic plan of all cancerous infiltrations, and leads to a similar substitution of new structures in the place of the original tissues of the affected part.

(4.) The interstitially-formed cells often deviate very widely from the type of any natural epithelial cell, in shape, in general aspect, in method of arrangement, and in endogenous formation (p. 579, e. s.). The difference between them and any natural elemental structures is, indeed, much greater than that between many medullary and scirrhous cancer-cells and the cells of the organ in which they grow: e. g. it is sometimes difficult to distinguish the cells of a medullary cancer in the liver from those of the liver itself.

(5.) The pathology of epithelial cancers is scarcely less conformed than is their anatomy to the type represented by the scirrhous and medullary cancers; for, not only are they prone to incurable ulceration, and to repeated recurrence after removal, but (which is much more characteristic) they usually lead to the formation of structures like themselves in the lymphatic glands connected with their primary seat, and they lead sometimes to similar formations in more distant organs (p. 583, e. s.).

(6.) In their growth, and in their recurrence, there is no tissue which the epithelial cancers do not invade and destroy (pp. 571 and 577).

(7.) A peculiar liability to them seems to exist in certain members of those families in which scirrhous or medullary cancers also occur (p. 592).

Such are the affinities between the epithelial and (as I would say) the other cancers. They are so numerous and so close, that I cannot but think we should be guided in the choice of a name by them, rather than by any other consideration. They are surely more significant of affinity with the other cancers, than the contrast between the shapes of the elemental cells is indicative of such difference as should be expressed by a different generic name.

LECTURE XXXIII.

MELANOID, HÆMATOID, OSTEOID, VILLOUS, AND COLLOID CANCERS.

OF the three chief forms of cancer which I have now described, we may observe, I think, that though two of them may be mixed in one mass, or may occur at different times in the same person, or in different members of the same family, and though there are forms intermediate and transitional between them, yet a mass of one of them does not, by any transformation, assume the characters of another. A scirrhous cancer, I think, never itself becomes medullary or epithelial; neither does the converse happen; nor do we see any indication that interference with the development of a cancer of either of these forms would lead it into the assumption of the characters of another. Combination, coincidence, succession, or interchange of these three forms may be found; but, I believe, no transformation of a growth completed or in progress.

If this be true, it indicates that the degree of difference between each two of these three forms is greater than that which exists between them and the cancers to which I shall devote this lecture. For there seems sufficient reason to believe that, by certain generally recognized processes of degeneration or disease, a medullary or epithelial cancer may become melanoid or hæmatoid; that a scirrhous or firm medullary cancer may become osteoid; that the colloid character may be, in some measure, assumed by either of the three chief forms; and that either of them may observe the villous or dendritic mode of growth. It need not always be supposed that, in the transformations here implied, the cancer-structures already perfected change their characters. It is probable, indeed, that such changes do occur in some of the instances we have to consider; but, in others, we may rather believe that the peculiarities of structure are due to something which induces degeneration or disease in the cancer-elements in their most rudimental state.

The belief that the five forms of cancer, whose names head this lecture, are modifications or varieties of one or more of the three already described, may justify my describing them more briefly, and, in many parts, by terms of comparison with the chief forms. Or, if this belief be not a good reason for such a course, it must be sufficient, that the examples of all these five forms are so rare, that complete and independent histories of them cannot, at present, be written.

It is, I think, probable that other groups of cancers besides these might be conveniently described as varieties of the principal kinds ;[*] but, at present, it seems better to defer the introduction of new names till we have attained more accurate knowledge.

MELANOID CANCER.

The Melanotic or Melanoid Cancers are, with very rare exceptions, medullary cancers modified by the formation of black pigment in their elemental structures. On this long-disputed point there can, I think, be no reasonable doubt. I have referred to a case of melanotic epithelial cancer (page 582): but with this exception, I have not seen or read of any example of melanosis or melanotic tumor in the human subject, which might not be regarded as a medullary cancer with black pigment. In the horse and dog, I believe, black tumors occur which have no cancerous character ; but none such are recorded in human pathology. The conditions, which some have classed under the name "spurious melanosis," are blackenings of various structures, whose only common character is that they are not tumors.

Melanotic cancers may have the general characters of any of the varieties of the medullary cancer; but the primary growths are rarely either very firm or very soft. They may appear as infiltrations; but are more often, I think, separable masses. Their characteristic pigment marks them with various shades of iron-gray or brown, deepening into deepest blackness. The pigment is variously arranged in them. Sometimes, we see, on the cut surface, a generally diffused brownish tint, derived from thickly sprinkled minute dots: sometimes, a whole mass is uniformly black: sometimes, one or more deep black spots appear in the midst of a pure white brain-like mass: sometimes (as in the specimen here figured), in half a tumor there are various shades of brown and black, in the other half the same texture uncolored: sometimes a whole mass is, as it were, delicately painted or mapped as with Chinese ink. There are thus to be found, in melanoid cancers, all plans and all degrees of blackening; and these diversities may be seen even in different parts of the same tumor, or in different tumors in the same person.[†] Nay, even in cancers that look colorless to the naked eye, I have found, with the microscope, single cells or nuclei having the true melanotic characters. And both the general and the microscopic aspect of the disease may yet be farther diversified by the coincidence of degenerations or hemorrhages, producing, in the

---

[*] This may be the case with what Müller named Carcinoma fasciculatum seu hyalinum. But, judging from his description and Schuh's, I cannot tell whether it is a disease which I have not yet seen, or whether (as I am more inclined to believe) the name has not been applied to some specimens of the soft, flickering, mammary or parotid glandular tumors, or to the mammary proliferous cysts that are prone to recur (see pp. 364, 470).

[†] All these varieties are illustrated in the Museums of the College and St. Bartholomew's by specimens referred to in the Indices of the Catalogues, vol. i. p. 133, and vol. i. p. xiv.

unblackened parts of the tumors, various shades of yellow, or of blood-color.

In the dark turbid creamy or pasty fluid that may be pressed from melanotic cancers, the greater part of the microscopic structures are such as might belong to an uncolored medullary cancer. It is often remarkable by how small a proportion of pigment the deepest black color may be given to the mass: a hundredth part of the constituent structures may suffice. The pigment is generally in granules or molecules: but it is sometimes in nuclei or in corpuscles like them.

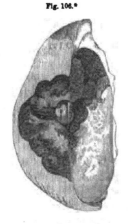

Fig. 106.*

The majority of the pigment-granules are minute particles, not much unlike those of the pigment-cells of the choroid membrane. When out of focus, they appear black or deep brown; but, when in focus, they have pellucid centres, with broad black borders. They appear spherical; and usually the majority of them are free, i. e., not enclosed in cells, and vibrate with molecular movement in the fluid that suspends them.

The greater part of the color depends on these free granules (fig. 107); but others like them are enclosed in the cancer-cells, or, more rarely, in nuclei. Sometimes those in the cells are clustered round the nucleus; sometimes they are irregularly scattered; in either case they appear as if gradually increasing till they fill the cell, and change it into a granule-mass, which, but for its color, we might exactly compare with the granule-masses of fatty degeneration. While the pigment granules are thus collecting, the nucleus remains clear; but at last, when the cell appears like a granule-mass, it is lost sight of. After this, moreover, the masses

Fig. 107.†

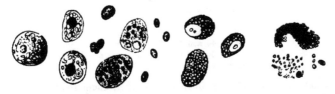

formed of pigment-granules may break up, and add their granules to those which we may suppose to have been free from their first formation.

* Fig. 106. Section of a variously shaded melanoid cancer formed beneath a mole or pigmentary nævus. Museum of St. Bartholomew's. Natural size.

† Fig. 107. Elemental structures of melanoid cancer, referred to in the text. Magnified 350 times.

The completely melanotic cells and their corpuscles, seen singly in the microscope, look not black, but rusty brown or pale umber-brown: like blood-cells, it is only when amassed that they give the full tint of color.

With the melanotic granules, there is sometimes a much smaller number of particles of the same color, and the same apparently simple structure, but of larger size: from $\frac{1}{6000}$ to $\frac{1}{4000}$ of an inch in diameter. These may be both free and in cells; in the latter case, lying mingled with melanotic granules in the contents of the cell. More rarely, corpuscles like the nuclei of cancer-cells, preserving their shape, size, and apparent texture, present the characteristic brown tint. Such corpuscles may be free; but they may also occupy the place of nuclei in cells, whose other contents are either uncolored or mixed with pigment-granules: and more rarely, a single corpuscle of the same kind may be seen in a cell containing an ordinary colorless nucleus.

In all the main facts of their pathological history, the melanotic cancers are in close conformity with the medullary; and this may be reckoned among the evidences that there is much less difference between these two forms than there is between the medullary cancers and either the scirrhous or the epithelial.

In the tables of 365 cases of cancer from which those in the foregoing lectures were derived, there are 25 cases of melanoid cancer. Seventeen of the patients were females, 8 were males. In 14 cases, the primary seat of the disease was in the skin or subcutaneous tissue; in 9, in the eye or orbit; in 1, in the testicle; in 1, in the vagina.* In this limitation to a few primary seats, and in its proneness to affect certain abnormal parts of the skin, are the chief peculiarities of this variety of cancer; but on the other points which may be settled by counting, I might have added the 25 cases to those of ordinary medullary cancer, without disturbing the results stated in Lecture XXXI.

Thus, the ages of the patients at the access of the cancer were as follows:—

Under	10	years	. .	2
Between	10 and 20	"	. .	1
"	20 and 30	"	. .	7
"	30 and 40	"	. .	4
"	40 and 50	"	. .	5
"	50 and 60	"	. .	4
Above 60		"	. .	2

The only notable difference in this table, when compared with that at page 561, is in the inferior proportion of cases before 20 years of age; a difference mainly determined by the large number of cases of uncolored medullary cancer of the eye in children.

Among 10 patients with melanoid cancer, one had had a relative who

* I once saw primary melanotic cancer of the liver; but I have no complete record of the case.

died with cancer of the breast; another had many relatives with pigmentary nævi like that in which her own cancer originated.

In 20 of the cases, the previous history of the affected part is recorded. In 3 of those in which the eye was affected it had been morbidly changed by previous inflammatory disease; in 2 it had appeared healthy. Among the 14 cases affecting the skin or subcutaneous tissue, one patient assigned no local cause; 2 referred to injury, and were uncertain of the previous condition of the skin; in 10 the disease commenced beneath a congenital pigmentary nævus, or dark mole; and in 1, what the patient called a wart of several years' standing. I shall presently revert to these facts.

In regard to their rate and method of growth, their ulceration, and their multiplying in parts near and distant from their primary seat, I believe the general history of the melanotic cancers is parallel with that of the medullary, given in a former lecture (p. 553, c. s.) But they present even a greater tendency to multiply in the subcutaneous tissue, growing here in vast numbers of small soft tubercles.

In like manner, the duration of life in melanotic nearly corresponds with that in medullary cancers. In 18 cases, in all of which the primary disease was removed (but in two only partially), the durations of life from the first notice of the cancer were as follows (and the table may be compared with that in p. 561):—

Between   6 and 12 months in 3 cases.
    "   12 and 18   "   4 "
    "   24 and 36   "   5 "
    "   36 and 48   "   1 "
    Above 48   "   5 "

Among 18 cases, whose history is known for some time after the removal of the primary disease, one has survived for three years, another for ten months, without recurrence of the disease. In the rest the disease recurred at the following periods (compare p. 562):—

Between   1 and   3 months in 7 cases.
    "   3 and   6   "   4 "
    "   6 and 12   "   2 "
    "   12 and 24   "   2 "
    "   24 and 36   "   1 "

Seeing this close correspondence in their general pathology, the rules respecting operations for melanoid cancers must be the same as for the medullary. (See p. 563.)

I have reserved for separate consideration some of the peculiarities of melanoid cancers. Three things in them especially deserve reflection, namely—(1) their color; (2) their proneness to take their first seat in or near cutaneous moles; (3) their profuse multiplication.

1. The color of the melanoid cancers is due to a pigment-formation, corresponding with that which we find, in the normal state, in the pig-

39

ment-cells on the choroid membrane, and in the rete mucosum of colored skins. Their usual primary occurrence near these seats of natural pigments may, therefore, be regarded as an illustration of the tendency of cancers to conformity, at least sometimes and in some respects, with the characters of the adjacent natural textures.

But another meaning of the pigment in melanotic cancers is suggested by its likeness to that which accumulates in the lungs and bronchial glands in advancing years, and in the darkening cuticle of many old persons. The coloring particles are probably different in these cases; they produce different shades or tinges of blackness; but their plans of formation and arrangement are in all similar. And the analogy of their formation in the aged, and in some other instances (page 75), may warrant us in regarding melanosis as a pigmental degeneration of medullary cancer. The chief characters of its minute structures agree with this, especially the gathering of pigment molecules about the nucleus, their gradually filling the cell-cavity, till, both the nucleus and the cell-wall disappearing, the nucleated cell is transformed into a dark-colored granule-mass. In all these characters there is an exact parallel between the transformations of the cells in melanoid cancers and the usual changes of the fatty degeneration. (Compare p. 498 and p. 579.)

2. The proneness of melanoid cancers to grow first in or beneath pigmentary moles is very evident: and I am not aware that such moles are peculiarly apt to determine the locality of any other tumors; for, except a case (p. 568) in which an epithelial cancer grew from one, I have met with no instance of other than melanoid cancers connected with them.

The fact is, I suppose, quite inexplicable; but it may be usefully suggestive. It seems a striking illustration of the weakness in resisting disease which belongs to parts congenitally abnormal. It seems, also, to be an evidence that a part may very long remain apt for the growth of cancer, and not become the seat of such a growth, till the cancerous diathesis, the constitutional element of the disease, is established. And this event may be very long delayed: as in a woman 80 years old, whom I saw with a large melanotic tumor, which had lately grown rapidly under a mole that had been unchanging through her long previous life. But again, this peculiar affinity (if it may be so called) of moles for melanoid cancers, may make us suspect that there may be other, though invisible, defects of first formation in our organs, which may render them, or even small portions of them, peculiarly apt for the seats of malignant and other specific diseases. It is often only the color that makes us aware of the peculiarity of that piece of a man's skin in which cancer, if it ever occur in him, will be most likely to grow: and yet color is so unessential a condition of texture, that we may well believe that all the more real conditions of such liability to cancer may be present without peculiarity of color, though, being without it, the part in which they exist may not be discernible.

I have spoken of the pigmentary moles as becoming the seats of melanotic cancers. It might seem as if the mole were, in some sort, the first stage of the cancer; but it is not so: the structures and the life of the mole are those of natural skin and epidermis, abnormal in quantity and color, but in no more essential properties: there are no structures in moles like those of cancer, till, at a certain and usually notable time, cancer begins to be formed in them. And here let it be observed, how close is the correspondence in these respects between the pigmentary moles, and the warts that are apt to become the seats of epithelial cancers (p. 595). The patient is usually aware of a time at which a mole, observed as an unchanging mark from birth or infancy, began to grow. In some instances the growth is superficial, and the dark spot acquires a larger area and appears slightly raised by some growth beneath it: in other cases, the mole rises and becomes very prominent or nearly pendulous. I believe that when the mole becomes thus prominent, the chief seat of the cancerous formation is in the superficial layer of the cutis and in the place of the rete mucosum; and that when it only extends itself, the cancerous growth is chiefly in the skin and subcutaneous tissue. In the former case, the cancer-structures are usually infiltrated among the natural structures of the affected part; in the latter, they generally form a distinct tumor, which may be dissected from, though it is closely connected with, the surrounding tissues and the thinned layer of cutis and dark cuticle that covers it. (Fig. 106, p. 606.)

The general characters of the growths thus forming correspond, I believe, in every respect with the medullary cancers of the skin and subcutaneous tissue (p. 547): color alone distinguishes them; they are equally prone to multiplicity. Often, in removing a deep-set melanotic mass, smaller masses are found imbedded in the adjacent fat or other tissue; and sometimes the formation of one or more subcutaneous growths almost exactly coincides with the outgrowth of the mole and its occupation by the cancer-structures.

3. The multiplicity of secondary melanoid formations is often very striking. I have, indeed, seen one case in which, to the last, only the lymphatic glands connected with the primary growth were diseased; and another in which only the liver and some lymphatics were affected; but the more frequent issue of the cases almost literally justifies the expression that the disease is everywhere. Are we to conclude from this that the multiplication of melanoid cancers is more abundant than that of the medullary cancers, which, in other respects they so closely resemble? I think not. We can easily see all the secondary melanoid formations, even the smallest and least aggregated; and it is often the color alone that draws attention to many which, but for it, we should not have noticed. I suspect that equally numerous formations exist in many cases of medullary cancers, but are unseen, being uncolored.

HÆMATOID CANCER.

This name may perhaps be retained to express a form of cancer which Mr. Hey had chiefly in view when he proposed the name of Fungus Hæmatodes.* It is most probable that all the cases to which he gave this name were soft medullary cancers; and his attention was especially directed to the fact, that when the morbid growth protrudes through the skin, the protruding portion may have such a shape as, in the conventional language of surgery, is called fungous, and often bleeds largely, and is so vascular, or so infiltrated with blood, that it looks like a clot.

The identity of the fungus hæmatodes of Hey with the medullary cancers was fully recognized by Mr. Wardrop and others; but unfortunately, certain foreign writers, regarding the hemorrhage as the distinctive character of the disease, included under the same term nearly all severely bleeding tumors of whatever kind.† It was an unhappy misuse of Hey's name, by which he meant to express, not a bleeding growth, but one like a clot of blood: and it led to a confusion which is still prevalent.

Leaving the term fungus hæmatodes, we may employ that of hæmatoid cancer, for such as are like clots of blood through the quantity of blood that they contain. The likeness is, indeed, I believe, only an accidental one, due to hemorrhage into the substance of the cancer, from rupture of some of its thin-walled blood-vessels. It seldom exists in the whole mass of a cancer; but, usually, while some parts have the ordinary aspect of medullary or some other form of cancer, other parts are blood-like. The best illustration of the disease that I have seen is in a large tumor,‡ of which one-half might be taken as a good type of the brain-like medullary cancer, and the other half as an equally good type of the hæmatoid. This half had been deeply punctured during life; it had bled very freely, and the simultaneous bleeding into its own substance had, doubtless, changed it from brain-like to blood-like.

Probably any cancer may thus be made hæmatoid; but the change is peculiarly apt to happen in those which are of the softest texture and most rapid growth, and which are situated where they are least supported by adjacent parts.

* Observations on Surgery, p. 239.
† Among the cases thus confused are some strange ones of profuse bleedings from supposed growths, of which little or nothing could be found after death. Such a case is related by Mr. Abernethy (On Tumors, p. 127–note); and a specimen from Mr. Liston's Museum is in the Museum of the College, 302 A. It is perhaps impossible at present to say what these diseases were; but I suspect they were medullary cancers with blood-vessels excessively developed, like those of erectile tumor.
‡ Mus. of St. Bartholomew's, Ser. xxxv. No. 28.

OSTEOID CANCER.

Müller assigned the name of osteoid tumor, or ossifying fungous growth,[*] to a form of disease of which, with admirable acumen, he collected several cases, illustrating these as its distinctive characters;—that the primary tumor consists chiefly of bone, but has, on its surface and in the interstices of its osseous parts, an unossified fibrous constituent as firm as fibrous cartilage; and that, after a time, similar growths ensue in parts distant from the seat of the first formed, and not on bones alone, but in the cellular tissue, serous membranes, lungs, lymphatics, &c. Mr. Stanley[†] has described the same disease under the name of Malignant Osseous Tumor; and single examples of it may be found under the names of periosteal exostosis, fibrous osteo-sarcoma, foliated exostosis, &c. Müller was disposed to call it osteoid cancer; and certainly this name is best suited to it, its intimate affinity with the other forms of cancer being evident in these things—(1) its correspondence, in nearly every particular of structure and of history, with the characters of cancerous disease, as exemplified in the scirrhous and medullary forms; (2) its not unfrequent coexistence with medullary cancer of the ordinary kind, either in a single mass of tumor, or in different tumors in the same person; (3) the uninterrupted gradations between it and the scirrhous and medullary cancers; (4) its mutations with the same, in hereditary transmission or in secondary productions. I cannot doubt the propriety of calling a disease cancer, in which these facts can be demonstrated; and I believe that the most probable view of the nature of osteoid cancers would be expressed by calling them ossified fibrous or medullary cancers, and by regarding them as illustrating a calcareous or osseous degeneration. (See pp. 510–11, and compare p. 77.)

The primary seat of osteoid cancer is usually some bone; but it is not limited to bones. In a case by Pott,[‡] quoted by Müller, the primary tumor lay "loose between the sartorius and vastus internus muscles." In the Museum of St. Thomas' Hospital, there is a tumor like an osteoid cancer, which was removed from near a humerus, and another from a popliteal space. In all these cases, the removal of the tumor was followed by the growth of medullary cancers with little or no bone in them.

Among the bones, the lower part of the femur is, with remarkable predominance, the most frequent seat of osteoid cancer. Among 25 cases, of which I have seen histories or specimens, 13 had this part for their seat; the skull, tibia, humerus, ilium, and fibula, were each affected in two cases, and the ulna and metacarpus each in one case.

---

[*] Ueber ossificirende Schwämme oder Osteoid-Geschwülste: (Müller's Archiv, 1843, p. 396.) [†] On Diseases of the Bones, p. 163.

[‡] Works, by Earle, iii. 313. I think that No. 2429 A in the College Museum may be regarded as an osteoid cancer of the testicle, though the bone-like substance has not the characters of perfect bone.

In most cases the osteoid growth occurs coincidently within and on the exterior of the bone, following herein the usual rule of medullary cancers; but it may exist on the exterior alone: and I have twice seen its fibrous basis in the cancellous tissue of a bone, of which the exterior was surrounded with soft medullary cancer.

In the best examples of osteoid cancer, *i. e.* in those in which its peculiar characters are most marked, it presents, if seated on a long bone. such as the femur, an elongated oval form; if on a flat bone, a biconvex form. Its elongated shape on the femur, the swelling gradually rising as we trace down the shaft, and then rather less gradually subsiding at the borders of the condyles, is almost enough for a diagnosis of the osteoid cancer from other hard tumors. It is like the enlargement produced by simple thickening of the bone or periosteum: a likeness which is increased by the smoothness of surface, the nearly incompressible hardness, and the considerable pain, which, in general, all these swellings alike present.

When we dissect down to an osteoid cancer (taking one on the femur

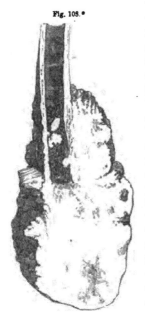

Fig. 108.*

for a type) we usually find the adjacent tissues healthy, except in being stretched round the swelling. Small masses of firm cancer may, however, be imbedded in them, distinct from, but clustered around, the chief mass. The periosteum is usually continued over the cancer, but scarcely separable from it. The surface is smooth, or very lowly and broadly tuberous. A section generally shows that the exterior of the growth is composed of a very firm, but not osseous, substance; while its interior part, *i. e.* that which lies nearest to the shaft, and that which is in the place of the cancellous tissue, are partially or wholly osseous. The two substances are closely interblended where they meet; and their relative proportions differ much in different specimens, according to the progress already made by ossification.

The unossified part of the tumor is usually exceedingly dense, firm, and tough, and may be incompressibly hard; its cut surface uprises like that of an intervertebral fibrous cartilage, or that of one of the toughest

* Fig. 108. Section of the osseous part of an osteoid cancer of the femur. Museum of St. Bartholomew's, Ser. i. 109.

fibrous tumors of the uterus. It is pale, grayish, or with a slight yellow or pink tint, marked with irregular short bars of a clearer white; rarely intersected as if lobed, but sometimes appearing banded with fibres set vertically on the bone.

The bony part of the tumor, when cleared by maceration, has characters altogether peculiar (fig. 108). In the central parts it is (in the best-marked specimens) extremely compact, scarcely showing even any pores, white, and dry. To cut, it is nearly as hard as ivory, yet, like hard chalk, it may be rubbed or scraped into fine dry powder. At its periphery it is arranged in a knobbed and tuberous form, the knobs being often formed of close, thin, gray or white lamellæ, whose presenting edges give them a fibrous look, exactly like that of pumice-stone. In this part, also, the bone is very brittle, flaky, and pulverulent.

In some specimens the whole of the bone has this delicate lamellar and brittle texture; but more generally, as I have said, the central part is very hard, and this, occupying the walls and cancellous tissue of the shaft, equally with the surrounding part of the tumor, makes of the whole such a compact white chalky mass as the sketch represents (fig. 108).

In the osteoid cancers of the lymphatic glands (fig. 109) and other soft parts, the bone is finely porous, spongy, or reticulated; or it may be finely lamellar, and look fibrous on its surface. It is always soft and brittle, and, often, it has in these parts no regular plan, but is placed in small close-set grains or spicules, which fall apart in maceration. In whatever plan or part the bone is found, it has no medulla; its interstices are filled with cancer-substance.

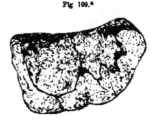

Fig 109.*

When the salts of lime are removed from the bone with acid, an organic basis-substance remains, which presents the same general aspect as the unossified part of the cancer, while retaining the lamellar and fibrous arrangement of the bone.† This basis yields gelatine; and the saline constituents are similar to those of ordinary bone, but with a disproportionate preponderance of phosphate of lime (Müller, l. c. p. 412).

With the microscope, the unossified part of an osteoid cancer appears fasciculated or banded, and is always very difficult to dissect. In some specimens, or in some parts, it has only a fibrous appearance, due to markings and wrinkles of a nearly homogeneous substance, in which abundant nuclei appear when acetic acid is added. In others, it is distinctly fibrous, but not in all parts with the same plan. The fibres are sometimes moderately broad, about $\frac{1}{3000}$ of an inch wide, have uneven, thorny edges, and, arranged in bundles, look like faggots (fig. 110, A).

* Fig. 109. Section of an inguinal lymphatic gland, with osteoid cancer, after maceration. Nat. size. Mus. of St. Bartholomew's, Ser. i., No. 109. † Mus. Coll. Surg. No. 809.

In other parts they are finer, like sharp-edged, crisp, and stiff filaments. Such as these may present a nearly regular reticular arrangement, with

Fig. 110.*

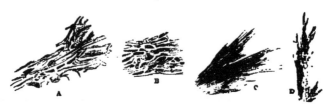

well-formed meshes (B); or they may be nearly parallel, and construct a more distinctly fibrous texture (C); or they may be closely matted, and except in their exceeding toughness, may be like the short, crooked filaments of a fibrine clot (D). I never saw them presenting the undulating glistening aspect of the filaments of an ordinary fibrous tumor, or of natural fibrous tissue.

Fibrous tissue, in one or other of the forms just mentioned, makes up the main mass of the unossified part of the cancer. But other elemental forms usually exist with it. Sometimes cancer-cells are mingled with it, as if imbedded in the interstices of the fibres. They are of ordinary form, not differing from those of common scirrhous cancers in anything, unless it be in that they are smaller and less plump. Sometimes granule-masses and minute oil-molecules are scattered among the fibres. Both these and the cancer-cells appear foreign to the fibrous tissue, as mingled with it, not part of it; but, if acetic acid be freely added, the fibrous tissue becomes clearer, and we find (what may before have been very obscurely seen) abundant nuclei imbedded in it. They are generally oval, smooth, well-defined, from $\frac{1}{1000}$ to $\frac{1}{1500}$ of an inch in length; but, I think, as the fibrous tissue becomes more perfect, they shrivel and become crooked, or like little stellate cracks in the basis-substance; or else that, as it ossifies, they are imbedded in the accumulating lime-salts, and become the lacunæ of the bone.†

Structures such as these exist in the osteoid cancers of all parts; and when a series of those occurring in the lymphatics and other organs can be compared with the primary disease on the bone (for example), I believe no other difference will be found, than that the secondary cancers are less definitely fibrous, and have a larger proportion of cancer-cells or granule-masses, than the primary disease. These, however, are no greater differences than may be found in comparing the less with the more firm parts of a single primary mass of the disease.

The microscopic characters of the ossified part of the cancer are those

* Fig. 110. Fibrous tissue of an osteoid cancer, in different forms, as described in the text. Magnified 400 times.

† Gerlach also describes this in his Essay, Der Zottenkrebs und das Osteoid, p. 52.

of true bone, but rarely of well-formed bone. In some parts—especially in the secondary cancers—that which appears to be bone is only an amorphous granular deposit of lime-salts, like those in ordinary calcareous degenerations. In other parts the lacunæ of true bone are distinct, but they are small, and their canalicules are few and short, and without order. Haversian canals also exist with these, but they have not a large series of concentric lamellæ like those in normal bone. In other instances, but these are rare, the lacunæ are more nearly perfect; their canalicules communicate with one another, and with the cavities of the Haversian canals. The bone with distinct lacunæ and canalicules is not found exclusively in the primary cancer, or near the natural bone on which it is seated: here, indeed, the complete bone is most frequent; but it may be found, also, in the secondary growths in the glands and elsewhere. These differences between the bone of the primary and that of the secondary osteoid cancers, like the similar differences of their unossified parts, are only differences of degree, such as may be found in separate parts of the same mass; they are, probably, to be ascribed only to more recent or more rapid growth.

The foregoing description of the osteoid cancers may suffice to show that their nearest affinities, judging by the structure of their unossified part, are to the fibrous cancers, of which I spoke at p. 514, and to the firmest of the medullary cancers (p. 536). When abundant cancer-cells are present they most nearly resemble the latter form; when they are almost wholly fibrous, the former. Their peculiarity, as cancers, is in their ossification. In this they may seem to approximate to the non-cancerous tumors; but, really, they remain, even when ossified, very distinct from any of them. I have enumerated (p. 466) the characters by which they are distinguished from both the hard and the cancellous osseous tumors; and the difference is as complete, and, I believe, as constant, as that of their fibrous basis is from the structure of any non-cancerous fibrous tumor.

If we consider only their osseous part, the osteoid cancers most nearly resemble those soft medullary cancers which have the most abundant internal skeletons. There is, indeed, no absolute line of distinction to be drawn between the two. It may be very evident, in the typical specimens of each, that the skeleton of the soft medullary cancer is formed by ossification of the intersecting and overgrown infiltrated periosteum (p. 535); and that the bone of the osteoid cancer is formed by ossification of the proper cancerous substance; but, between these extremes or types, there are numerous instances in which the two conditions are mingled, or through which the one condition merges into the other. And this is no more than we might expect, seeing the frequency with which the osteoid and the medullary disease appear together, or in succession.

The materials for a general pathology of osteoid cancers are very scanty; yet one may be written; for if we collect only well-marked examples of the disease, their histories will be found consistent with one another, and distinct from those of the other groups of cancers.

Among 20 cases, 15 occurred in men, and 5 in women: a preponderance on the male side approximating that observed in epithelial cancers, and (if we may trust to a result from so few cases) contrasting, in a striking manner, with the distribution of medullary and scirrhous cancers.

Among 19 of these patients, 5 were between 10 and 20 years old; 9 between 20 and 30; 4 between 30 and 40; 1 between 40 and 50:— proportions which again do not correspond with those in any other form of cancer.

Among 13 of the patients, 5 distinctly referred to injury as the origin of the cancer, and 2 to previous disease in the part: the others assigned no cause.

The growth of osteoid cancers is generally rapid, and accompanied with severe pain in and about their seat; their multiplication in the lymphatics and in distant parts takes place with proportionate rapidity; and intense cachexia occurs early in their course. There are exceptions to these things; but in all these respects the majority of the osteoid cancers appear as malignant as the medullary, and are as quickly fatal.

Among 14 cases, of which the ends are recorded, 3 died in consequence of amputations. Of the other 11, 4 underwent no operation, and all died in or within six months from the first notice of the disease. Of the remaining 7, in all of whom the disease was once or more removed, and in all of whom it recurred before death, 2 died in the first year of its existence, 1 in the second, 1 in the third; but one lived for $7\frac{1}{2}$ years, another for 24, and another for 25 years.

In all the instances of speedy death, secondary osteoid cancers existed, and the result was probably to be assigned to these and to the coincident cancerous cachexia; for the primary growths have little tendency to ulcerate or protrude, and they seem to contribute directly to death by their pain alone. In the instances of life extended beyond twenty years, the disease appeared to recur only near its primary seat.

The most frequent seats of the secondary, or recurrent, osteoid cancers are the lymphatic glands, in the line from the primary seat to the thoracic duct, the lungs, and the serous membranes: but it is not limited to these; it may be found even in the blood-vessels, as in a case which I shall relate, and has been traced in the thoracic duct.* Its condition in these secondary seats need not be described: in structure it resembles in them the primary disease, with only such differences as are already mentioned; in plan it is like the growths or infiltrations of secondary medullary cancers in the same parts. But it is to be observed that, sometimes, the secondary cancer is medullary, without osseous matter. I

* Cheston, in Philos. Trans. 1780, vol. lxx.

have mentioned three instances of this (p. 613), and Professor Langen-
beck told me that he once removed an upper jaw with a bony growth,
and the patient died soon after with well-marked medullary cancer in the
lungs. The reverse may occur: for the same distinguished surgeon told
me that he once removed a humerus with a medullary cancer, and the
patient died with osseous tumors in the lungs.

The ordinary course of osteoid cancers may be known by the foregoing
account of them, and by the cases recorded by Müller and Mr. Stanley.*
But deviations from this course are sometimes observed, which it may be
well to illustrate by cases that displayed the disease in an unusually acute,
and an equally unusual inactive, form.

A girl, 15 years old, was admitted into St. Bartholomew's Hospital,
with general feebleness and pains in her limbs, which had existed for two
or three weeks. They had been ascribed to delayed menstruation, till
the pain, becoming more severe, seemed to be concentrated about the
lower part of the back and the left hip. A hard deep-seated tumor was
now felt, connected with the ala of the left ilium. This gradually increased, with constant and more wearing pain; it extended towards the
pelvic and abdominal cavities; the patient became rapidly weaker and
thinner; the left leg swelled; sloughing ensued over the right hip; and
thus she died cachetic and exhausted, only 3½ months from her first
notice of the swelling.

A hard lobulated mass was found completely filling the cavity of the
pelvis, and extending across the lower part of the abdominal cavity. It
was firmly connected with the sacrum, both ischia, and the left ilium; it
held, as in one mass, all the pelvic organs; and the uterus was so imbedded in it, and so infiltrated with a similar material, that it could
scarcely be recognized.

The general surface of this growth was unequal and nodular. It was
composed of a pearly-white and exceedingly hard structure, in which
points of yellow bony substance were imbedded, and which had the characters of osteoid cancer perfectly marked. The ilium, where the tumor
was connected with it, had the same half fibrous and half bony structure
as the tumor itself.

The common iliac veins, their main divisions, and others leading into
them, passed through the tumor, and were all distended with hard substance like the mass around them. From the common iliac veins a continuous growth of the same substance extended into the inferior cava, which,
for nearly five inches, was distended and completely obstructed by a cylindriform mass of similar fibrous and osseous substance, 1¼ inches in diameter. At its upper part this mass tapering came to an end near the liver.

The lower lobe of the right lung was hollowed-out into a large sac, containing greenish pus and traversed by hard coral-like bands, which proved

* L. c. See also Garlach's two cases (l. c.) and that by Hunter, in the Catalogue of the
College Museum, vol. ii. p. 176.

to be branches of the pulmonary artery plugged with firm white substance intermingled with softer cancerous matter, and resembling the
great mass of disease in the pelvis. The rest of the lung was healthy,
with the exception of some scattered grayish tubercles; and so was the
left lung, except in that there were a few small abscesses near its surface,
with hard, bone-like masses in their centres, like those in the branches of
the right pulmonary artery. The skull, brain, pericardium, heart, and
all the abdominal organs, were healthy.*

I suppose that few cases of osteoid cancer can be found equal with this
in the acuteness of their progress. The opposite extreme is illustrated
by a case communicated to me by Mr. Thomas Sympson, and exactly
corresponding with one of which the specimens are in the Museum of the
College.† A swelling appeared in the upper arm of a woman 32 years
old. After ten years growth, when it had increased to seven pounds
weight, it was removed by Mr. Hewson. It had the characters of osteoid
cancer. The patient completely recovered from the operation; but,
about a year after it, a new tumor appeared about the humerus, and at
the end of four years had acquired a huge size, and a weight of 15½ pounds.
For this, which proved to be a similar osteoid growth, the arm was amputated at the shoulder-joint. She recovered from this operation also; but
the disease returned in the scapula, and, in about 10 years after the
amputation, and 24 years from the beginning of the disease, she died.

VILLOUS CANCER.

VILLOUS CANCERS (Kottenkrebs of Rokitansky),‡ are varieties of
Medullary, and, perhaps, in some instances, of Epithelial Cancers; but
they demand a separate description, not for their own sake alone, but
because they illustrate a remarkable mode of growth, which probably
prevails in a much wider range of morbid structures than is yet clearly
traced in.

Among the best examples of the villous cancer are those which occur
on the mucous membrane of the urinary bladder, and of which an excellent specimen, in the Museum of the College, is represented in the opposite sketch. Here the cancer appears of oval or spheroidal shape, attached to the mucous membrane by a narrow base, and pendulous in the
cavity of the bladder. Its base and central part may be solid, either
moderately firm, or soft, like an ordinary medullary cancer, yielding
abundant creamy fluid; but all its unattached and peripheral part is
very soft, tufted, shreddy, and flocculent, like the surface of a chorion.
It is covered with fine villous processes that float out in water, and are
usually bright or dark red, with the full blood-vessels which they con-

* The specimens from this case are in the Museum of St. Bartholomew's.
† No. 3244-5.5 A.
‡ Ueber den Zottenkrebs, in the Sitzungsberichte der kais. Akademie; April, 1852.

tain, and from which, during life, profuse hemorrhages are apt to occur. Two or more such cancerous growths may stand near together; or there may be, according to Rokitansky, a collection of delicate, spongy, and branched villous excrescences, rising from a circumscribed base; or a diffuse growth of numerous single tufts scattered over a wider extent. Commonly, the surrounding mucous membrane appears reticulated with a fine-meshed trellis-work, from the bars of which very delicate excrescences rise, in the form of fine vesicles or villi.†

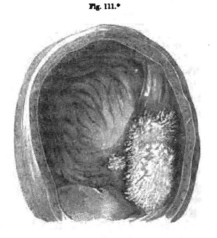

Fig. 111.*

Growths, such as these are on the mucous membrane of the bladder (their most frequent seat), may occur in many other parts. Rokitansky describes them in the stomach, the rectum, the gall-bladder,‡ the interior of ovarian cysts, on the peritoneum,§ and the dura mater. In all these positions the cancer projects into cavities, and finds, probably, the most favorable conditions for its characteristic method of growth; but Rokitansky has also observed similar growths in the brain, the liver, and the uterus; in the last-named organ growing first in its very substance, and thence protruding into its cavity.

I have had no opportunity for many years past of minutely examining well-marked villous cancers. I will therefore describe their construction in an abstract of Rokitansky's Essay.

The excrescence consists, in its stem, of a fibroid membranous structure, on which the branches and villous flocculi are borne, as larger and smaller pouch-like and flask-shaped buddings, or sproutings of a structureless hollow tissue.

The "dendritic vegetation," of which these sproutings are an example, has been already often referred to, especially in the account of the stroma

* Villous cancer of the urinary bladder, half the natural size. The specimen is No. 2005 in the College Museum: the figure, 111, is copied from that by Clift in Sir E. Home's "Observations on the Prostrate Gland," vol. ii. p. 49, pl. x. No. 2006 in the College Museum, and Nos. 2, 7, and 25, in Ser. xxvii. in the Museum of St. Bartholomew's, are similar specimens.

† So in the mucous membrane of a cancerous stomach in the Museum of St. Bartholomew's, xv. 5. Gerlach rightly dwells on this state, and the smaller tufts that surround the main disease, as constituting a preparatory villous or papillary, but not yet cancerous, state. The case is parallel with that of the warty growths that may precede and become the seats of epithelial cancer. ‡ Museum of St. Bartholomew's, xix. 3.

§ An exquisite specimen of this is in the Museum of St. Bartholomew's, xvi. 60.

of medullary cancers* (p. 542), which stroma is, indeed, only another modification of the same plan of growth as the villous cancers exemplify in a clear form. Other examples are in the endogenous growths of cysts; in the Lipoma arborescens of Müller (*i. e.* the tufted and villous growths on synovial membranes); and in the intracystic growths of thyroid and other gland-substance illustrated in the twenty-third lecture, (p. 357, e. s.).

The "dendritic vegetation" appears originally as a hollow club-shaped or flask-shaped body, consisting of an hyaline structureless membrane. It is either clear and transparent, or opaque, *i. e.* filled with granules, nuclei, and nucleated cells (fig. 97, p. 543): externally, it is either bare or covered with epithelium. The vegetation does not usually develope itself into villous growths directly on the mucous or other surface on which it rests, but on the bars of some previously formed meshed-work, such as is described at pp. 543 and 621. The further development of the vegetation is commonly in one of two chief plans. Either the membranous flask grows uniformly into a sac, which contains a serous fluid, or is filled with a delicately fibrous meshed-work; or else it grows and

Fig. 112.†

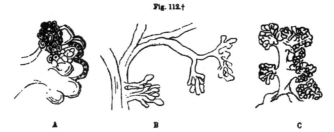

A   B   C

sprouts in various degrees and methods. Of this sprouting growth, which alone is illustrated in villous cancer, there are three types. They are represented in the adjoining copy of Rokitansky's sketches.

In the first (fig 112, A), the flask grows out in low, nearly hemispherical sprouts. These may contain serous fluid, as in the cystic disease of the choroid plexuses; or they may be filled with gland-structures, as in the thyroid and mammary intracystic growths; or they may contain and be covered with cancerous structures, as in the instance of the small excrescences within a cyst in a cancerous kidney, from which fig. 112, A, was drawn.

* The following pages contain the fuller truth of what is said in a note at p. 357, which was printed before I received the two essays by Rokitansky that are cited here and at p. 542. The same views which these essays expound were stated by him in those published in 1849, on Cysts and on Bronchocele, but so much less clearly, that I did not fully see their bearing on the pathology of the endogenous growths in proliferous cysts. The reader may not fail to observe how much of the truth concerning these cancerous growths was expressed by Dr. Hodgkin.

† Fig. 112. Methods of growth of the "dendritic vegetation," from Rokitansky. Magnified 30 times: explained in the text.

In the second type (fig. 112, B), the flask grows lengthwise into a tube, and shoots out new ones, which grow to secondary tubes, and again shoot out others, which grow to tertiary tubes, and so on. On these outgrowths abundant broader sprouts and buds appear. Thus a multiformly ramified dendritic-structure is produced. Its sprouts may be filled with fibro-cellular tissue, or fat (as in Lipoma arborescens), or with cartilage and bone (as in the pendulous growths of these tissues within joints); or they may contain and be covered with the elements of the cancer, as in the villous cancer of the urinary bladder, of which part is sketched in fig. 112, B.

In the third type, illustrated by fig. 112, c, from another villous cancer of the bladder, the flask grows with considerable dilatation into a stem, which gives off branches that do not ramify further, but break up at once into a great number of flask-shaped sprouts.

The usual arrangement of the blood-vessels of the dendritic vegetations is that (as in the synovial fringes and the villi of the chorion) a vessel runs along the contour of the vegetation, forming frequent loops, and supplying to the stem, as well as to each of the sprouts and branches, an ascending and a descending vessel. There are, however, pouches in the vegetation in which only a single vessel exists, and terminates with a rounded end. The vessels are generally large, examples of the so-called colossal capillaries, thin-walled with longitudinal, and sometimes also transverse, oval nuclei in pellucid membrane.*

In structure, the vegetation in villous cancers is often hyaline; that is, it contains, besides a clear fluid, no tissue-elements; but it often contains, together with its blood-vessels, a quantity of elementary granules, nuclei, and cells, and, especially at the ends of its sprouts, structureless simple and laminated vesicles. On its exterior, the elements of a medullary or melanotic cancer-juice adhere to it, consisting of nucleated cells of various shapes, which form a soft, or a more consistent, deposit, and are often present in such quantity that they make up the greater part of the morbid mass, into which then the vegetations seem to grow.

In other cases, a fibrous texture developes itself in the interior of the vegetation, and with it cancerous elements form, like those of the exogenous formation just mentioned. In this state the villous cancer, in consequence of the accumulation of the fibrous and cancerous structures, appears as a collection of excrescences which, in their stems as well as in their branches and sprouts, and especially towards their free ends, are swollen thick and big. They are here filled with a delicately fibrillated meshed-work, turgid with medullary cancer-juice; and, as their swollen ends are often mutually compressed, the whole appears like foliage growing on shorter or longer stems.

When the villous cancer is cut through to its base, one finds a tolera-

* Gerlach's account of the blood-vessels nearly corresponds with this (Der Zottenkrebs und das Osteoid, Taf. i. fig. 3).

bly abundant porous fibrous texture, which, on nearer examination, presents a compressed meshed-work traversed by fissure-like apertures. Its bars consist of a hyaline substance, beset with oblong nuclei and nucleus-fibres, and here and there dividing into filaments of connective-tissue. The tissue (e. g. of the mucous membrane) around the base of the cancer is traversed by a whitish fine-meshed trellis-work, the bars of which consist of nucleated cells, and often develope delicate prominences and vesicles, the beginnings of the kind of vegetation from which the cancer sprang.

The fissured and perforated meshwork in the interior of the base of the villous cancer corresponds with the stroma of ordinary medullary cancers (p. 543). Both are constructed on the plan of the dendritic vegetation. In the construction of the stroma, the sprouting growths become a meshed-work by partial absorption: in the villi of the villous cancer they lengthen into branching tubes. And these tubes have, on the one hand, the import of a stroma, in that the cancerous elementary structures cover them and fill up the spaces between them, as they do those between the bars of the more ordinary stroma. But, on the other hand, the tubes have a nearer and distinctive relation to the cancerous elements, in that they produce those elements in their interior; so that there is an endogenous as well as an exogenous production of cancer-structures.

In all the instances that have been fully examined, these structures have been like those of medullary or melanotic cancer. But I believe Rokitansky is right in the anticipation that certain epithelial cancers will be found to grow on the same plan as the villous. I have referred (p. 569) to instances of warty epithelial cancers growing where they could not have had origin in natural papillæ; Virchow also describes arborescent epithelial cancers growing in cavities where no papillæ could well be; and I have seen the same in cysts within what I believe to be an epithelial cancer of the clitoris.* The shapes of the most exuberant epithelial cancers so imitate those of the villous cancers, that it seems highly probable that some of them are produced by the dendritic mode of growth, rather than by the enlargement and deformity of papillæ.

The correspondence of the stromal structures, and the exact similarity of the cancer-elements, found in the medullary and melanoid cancers on the one hand, and in the villous cancers on the other, are enough to warrant us in regarding these as varieties of the more general form. This view is confirmed by numerous cases in which the central and basal parts of the growth are like common medullary cancer, its surface being villous; and by some in which villous cancers appear as secondary growths with primary medullary cancers of the more common kind: thus, e. g. the former occur on the peritoneum, with the latter in the ovaries. It may be anticipated that the histories of the villous cancers will equally coincide with those of the medullary and melanotic; but, as yet, the cases recorded are too few for the deduction of any general rules.

* Museum of St. Bartholomew's, xxxii. 39.

COLLOID CANCER.

Many names have been given to this form of cancer—Colloid, Alveo-lar, Gelatiniform, Cystic, and Gum-Cancer. I have adopted the first, because it seems to be now most frequently used, and expresses very well the most obvious peculiarity of the diseased structure, the greater part of which is, usually, a clear flickering or viscid substance like soft gela-tine.

The most frequent primary seats of colloid cancer are the stomach, the intestinal canal, uterus, mammary gland, and peritoneum: as a secondary disease, it affects most frequently the lymphatic glands and lungs, and may occur in many other parts.

To the naked eye, a colloid cancer presents two chief constituents; an opaque-white, tough, fibrous-looking tissue, which intersects, parti-tions, and encloses its mass; and a clear, soft, or nearly liquid material, the proper "colloid" substance. According to the proportions in which these are combined, the general aspect of the disease varies. When the fibrous texture is predominant (as I have twice seen it in the central parts of colloid cancers of the breast) it forms a very tough, white, fascia-like mass, in which are small separate cysts or cavities filled with the colloid substance. In the opposite extreme, large masses of the colloid sub-stance appear only intersected by fibrous white cords or thin membranes, arranged as in the areolar tissue, or in a wide-meshed network. These extremes often exist in different parts of the same mass, and with them are various intermediate forms, in which, probably, the essential characters of the disease may be best learned. In these, the cancerous substance appears constructed of small thin-walled cysts, cells, or alveoli, arranged without apparent order, and filled with the transparent colloid substance. The cysts or alveoli are, typically, of round or oval form, but are changed from this, as if by mutual pressure; some may appear closed, but the great majority communicate with those around them, through apertures like imperfections in their walls. They vary from an inch in diameter to a size as small as the naked eye can discern. The largest cysts, and the least abundant fibrous tissue, are usually at or near the surface of the mass; and in these large cysts, when the colloid substance is emptied from them, we can generally see intersecting bands, or incomplete parti-tions, as if they were formed by the fusion of many cysts of smaller size. The walls of the cysts appear formed of delicate white fibrous tissue, but cannot be separated from the surrounding substance, and are continuous with the coarser bands or layers of fibrous tissue by which the cancerous mass is intersected.

The colloid matter is, in different parts or in different instances, various in consistence; resembling a thin mucilage, starch-paste, the vitreous humor, size-gelatine, or a tenacious mucus. In its most normal state, it

40

is glistening, translucent, and pale-yellowish; but it may be colorless, or may have a light green, gray, pink, or sanguineous tint; and may become opaque, whitish, or buff-colored, by (apparently) a fatty or calcareous degeneration; or, in the extreme of this degeneration, may look like tuberculous matter. In water, or in spirit, it oozes from the alveoli and floats in light cloudy flocculi; and when the surface of the cancer is exposed by ulceration or by rupture, it is discharged from the opened alveoli and lies on them like a layer of mucus.

The colloid cancers have, usually, in the first instance, the shape of the part that they affect; for they are always, I believe, infiltrations of the affected part, whose tissues are gradually removed and superseded by their growth. But the growth of the colloid cancer enlarges and surpasses the part in which it is seated, and produces, in such an organ as the breast or the lymphatic glands, a considerable rounded and tuberous firm swelling, or, in such an one as the stomach or the peritoneum, a flattened expanded mass with more or less of nodular or tuberous projection.

The extent of growth is sometimes enormous, especially in the peritoneum, in which, as in a case related by Dr. Ballard,* the greater part of the parietal and much of the visceral portion may be infiltrated with the morbid structure, either in a nearly uniform layer, or in nodulated swellings formed of groups of cysts, and sometimes projecting far into the peritoneal cavity. The cavity itself may, in these cases, contain free colloid matter, discharged, I suppose, from the open superficial alveoli, and the abdominal walls may be thus distended with a fluctuating vibrating swelling like that of ascites.†

It is not unfrequent to find one or more large and thick-walled cysts near or attached to masses of colloid cancer, and imitating the characters of such proliferous multilocular cysts as are found in the ovaries. They are usually filled with colloid matter, and their likeness to the ovarian cysts may confirm the belief that many of the latter are really colloid cancers of the ovaries.

Moreover, colloid cancer is sometimes found mingled in the same mass with medullary cancer. This is, indeed, frequent in the digestive canal. Villous and melanotic cancers have been similarly combined with it; and, more frequently, in different parts of the same person, the medullary and the colloid are found in distinct masses.

Microscopic examination of fragments of colloid cancer brings into view an arrangement of delicately fibrous and lamellar structures, imitating, in miniature, the larger appearances visible to the naked eye. Fine

* Méd. Chir. Trans., xxxi. 119.

† In Dr. Ballard's case, six quarts of free colloid matter were removed from the peritoneal cavity after death. I remember an exactly similar case in which, I think, the quantity removed must have been greater, and in which it certainly appeared to be derived from the dehiscence and constant discharge of the alveoli. In the Museum of the College No. 294, is a mass of peritoneal colloid cancer, from eight to ten inches in its diameter, which was removed from the lower surface of a liver.

tough fibres, or fibred membranes, are arranged in curved bundles and
lamellæ, which, by their divergences and interlacements, encircle or
enclose oval or spherical spaces,
containing the colloid substance.

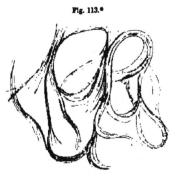

Fig. 113.*

The enclosed spaces are seldom
complete cavities; they communicate freely with one another; and
both in their plan, and in the general aspect of the tissue, remind one,
as Lebert says, of the structure of
a lung, with its communicating air-
cells. The fibres are very fine, but
appear stiff and tough, not undulating or easily parting; they are but
little and slowly changed by acetic
acid. Elongated nuclei are often seated on these fibres, and sometimes,
Lebert says, elastic fibres are mingled with them. The colloid substance
fills all their interspaces, not merely the cavities which they circumscribe,
but, as it were, mere crevices between the fibres, and spaces in the walls
of the larger cavities.

The colloid substance generally appears, however magnified, clear and
structureless; it might be invisible but for the seeming filamentous texture produced, as it often is in spread out masses, by its folds and creas-
ings. Sometimes, the colloid material is sprinkled with minute dots, like,
oily or fatty molecules,† which to the naked eye may give it a peculiarly
milky or ochrey aspect; and sometimes it is beset with clusters of such
molecules, resulting apparently from the degeneration of imbedded nuclei
or imperfect cells. With these, also, crystals of the triple phosphate,
cholestearine, and some peculiar fatty matter,‡ may be mingled.

Lebert§ has published an exact analysis of this colloid matter by
Wurtz. The main results are, that it is quite unlike any variety of gelatine, being insoluble in water, and containing only 7 per cent. of nitrogen,
a peculiarity which distinguishes it as well from all protein compounds,
and from the materials of which (imperfectly and impurely as they have
been examined) the essential structures of other cancers are composed.

Imbedded in the colloid substance, but in very uncertain quantity, are
corpuscles of peculiar form. According to Lebert (of whose description
and sketches I again gladly avail myself), they are chiefly these:—

(1) Nucleated cells lie free in the colloid substance, or enclosed within
large blood-cells, or grouped like an epithelium on the boundaries of the
alveoli or cysts. These, the so-called colloid corpuscles, are small, granular, moderately transparent cells, of irregular shape, from $\frac{1}{5000}$ to $\frac{1}{3000}$

* Fig. 113. Fibrous tissue of a colloid cancer of the breast. Magnified 70 times.
† But the observations of Dr. Jenner (Proc. of Pathol. Sec., 1851-52, p. 323) make it
probable that these are granules of phosphate of lime.
‡ Luschka, in Virchow's Archiv, iv. 411.　　§ In Virchow's Archiv, iv. 203.

of an inch in diameter, with small nuclei or none. These are, probably, cancer-cells hindered and modified in their development by the peculiar

Fig. 114.*

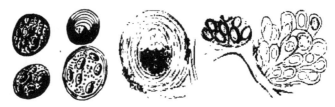

circumstances of their formation; for, with such as these, more perfect cancer-cells are sometimes found.

(2) Large compouud cells, mother-cells or brood-cells, which, in typical specimens (fig. 114 A), are from $\frac{1}{310}$ to $\frac{1}{160}$ of an inch in diameter, are in some instances very numerous. They are very pale, oval, round, or tubular, and lie in clusters: some of them display a lamillar surface, indicated by concentric boundary-lines; and they enclose one large granular nucleus, or several of smaller size imbedded in their general granular contents, or, together with such nuclei, complete nucleated cells like cancer-cells.

(3) Large laminated spaces (fig. 114 B) are also found of nearly crystaline clearness, from $\frac{1}{70}$ to $\frac{1}{160}$ of an inch in diameter. These are usually oval and grouped, so as to form a soft parenchyma. Between the lamellæ of their walls elongated nuclei are scattered; in the interspaces between them are clusters of small nucleated cells and nuclei; and they enclose brood-cells in the cavities surrounded by their concentric lamillæ.

Whether we consider the larger, or the minuter, characters of this colloid cancer, it seems difficult to believe that such a structure can have any close affinity with the cancers I have already described; they appear, at first sight, to have scarcely anything in common. Hence, some have denied altogether the cancerous nature of this disease. But if we look, not to its structure alone, but as well to its clinical history (so far as it is illustrated by the great majority of the recorded cases), we shall find in it all the distinctive features of the cancers. Thus (1), its seats of election are, remarkably, those in which the medullary cancers are, at the same time of life, most apt to occur; (2) like the typical cancers, the colloid infiltrates, and at length supersedes and replaces, by substitution, the natural tissues of the affected part; (3) like them, also, it is prone to extend and repeat itself in lymphatic glands, the lungs, and other parts near to or distant from its primary seat;† (4) the colloid is

* Fig. 114. Structures of colloid cancer described in the text. From Lebert (Virchow's Archiv, B. iv. Taf. v.) and Rokitansky (Ueber die Cyste, Taf. vi.)

† Colloid cancer was thus multiplied in ten out of eleven cases recorded by Lebert. In

often associated with other forms of cancer in the same mass, or in different tumors in the same person; (5) it appears as apt as any other form to recur after removal; (6) it may be derived, hereditarily, from a parent having scirrhous cancer, or a parent with colloid may have offspring with medullary cancer.

These facts seem enough to prove the right of including the colloid with the generally received forms of cancer; certainly they are enough, if we can explain the peculiarities of the colloid cancer as the result of any known morbid process in such elemental structures as, in other conditions, might have been conformed to the ordinary types of cancer. And such an explanation is not impossible, for, as Rokitansky shows, the colloid cancer has a near parallel in many cyst-formations in the normal structures, and especially in those forms of bronchocele in which abundant cysts, full of viscid fluid, are formed in the growing thyroid gland. It seems, therefore, a reasonable hypothesis that the peculiarities of the colloid or alveolar cancer are to be ascribed to cystic disease occurring in elemental cancer-structures. Such a cystic disease may ensue in a medullary or other cancer already formed; but in the well-marked and uniformly constructed colloid cancer, it is probable that the deviation to the cystic form ensues in the very earliest period of the cancer-structures, while each element is yet in the nascent or rudimental state.

Such may be the explanation of the structures of those cancers in which the formation of cysts is carried to its maximum; and I have reserved for this place an account of the various combinations of cysts with cancers of all kinds,—combinations giving rise to many singularities of appearance, of which I omitted the description in earlier Lectures, that I might once for all endeavor to explain them.

And first, we may divide these cases into those in which the cysts are formed independently of the cancer-structures, and those in which they are, or appear to be, derived from them.

In the first class we may enumerate many cases in which cysts and cancers are in only accidental proximity. For example, a scirrhous cancer may occupy part of a mammary gland, in the rest of which are many cysts that are in no sense cancerous, or of which the chief lactiferous tubes are dilated into pouches or cysts (see page 490). And such a cancer, in its progress, may enclose those cysts, and they may, I believe, remain for a time imbedded in it. In like manner, the ovary, or any other organ, being already the seat of common cysts, may become the seat of cancer; and the too morbid structures may become connected though not related.

a case by Dr. Warren (Med.-Chir. Trans., vol. xxvii.), the multiplication was to an amount scarcely surpassed by any medullary cancers. It is true that it is not unfrequently limited to the stomach, or rectum, and the adjacent lymphatic glands; but it is equally observable in the cases of villous and other medullary cancers, and I suspect is only an example of a general rule, that cancers (of whatever kind) on exposed surfaces are, on the whole, more apt to remain single than those growing in other parts.

In this class, also, may be reckoned the cases in which cancers grow from the walls of common cysts; *i. e.* of cysts which did not originate in cancer-structures. Thus medullary cancers may grow, especially in the villous form, from the walls of ovarian cysts, which have themselves no cancerous appearance.*

There may be other methods in which, as by a sort of accident, cysts and cancers may thus become connected; but these are the chief examples. In the second class, including those in which the cysts appear to be derived from cancer-structures, we find numerous varieties, which may be studied as a series parallel with those of the simple and the proliferous cyst-formations in the natural structures, or in innocent tumors. (Compare Lectures XXII., XXIII., and page 367.)

(*a*) Cysts filled with fluid, like serum variously tinted, and in their general aspect resembling the common serous cysts (page 339), are often connected with cancers, especially with those of the medullary form that grow quickly or to a great size. There may be one or many of such cysts, lying at the surface, or imbedded in the substance, of the cancer. Sometimes, a single cyst of the kind enlarges so as to surpass the bulk of the cancer, exceedingly confusing the diagnosis.† In other cases so many cysts are formed, that the tumor appears almost wholly composed of them, the cancerous structure only filling the interstices between their close-packed walls.‡ Such cases might justly be grouped as a "cystic variety" of medullary cancer.

(*b*) Sanguineous cysts are found, as often as the serous, in connection with the medullary and other cancers; and the changes which the blood undergoes in them add not a little to the multiformity of appearances that the cancerous masses may present.

(*c*) The colloid cysts here find their type (page 349); not only as constructing the peculiar variety of cancer just described, but as being mingled with ordinary cancerous growths; for it is common to find, with such growths, especially in the abdomen and pelvis, cysts filled with thickly viscid material, like mucus, or half-liquid jelly, in all the varieties of tint that we see in the cystic disease of the kidney or of the thyroid gland.

(*d*) While thus the principal varieties of simple or barren cysts are found in cancerous growths, as in the original tissues or in simple tumors, so may we also trace in them the production of proliferous cysts; *i. e.* of cysts from whose inner surfaces cancerous growths arise, corresponding with the glandular growths that may fill the cysts in the mammary or thyroid gland (page 358). I have already often referred to this (pp. 367, 532, 587, &c.); and, now, need only add that such endogenous growths are often to be found in the alveoli of the colloid cancer. Clusters of

---

* Museum of St. Bartholomew's, xxxi. 20.

† Bruch (Die Diagnose der bösartigen Geschwülste, p. 1); Mus. Coll. Surg., 281.

‡ Mus. Coll. Surg., 277, 279, 280, &c.; Mus. St. Bartholomew's, xxxv. 14, and others.

clavate, or flask-shaped, villous processes, like those formed in the early stages of the dendritic vegetation of villous cancer (page 622), spring from the wall of the alveolus With laminated walls, and cancer-structures, or new cysts in their cavities, such villous growths crowded together probably constitute the structures which I have described after Lebert (page 658, fig. 113, c).* To less perfect endogenous growth we must, I suppose, ascribe the cancer-structures which are found disorderly mingled with the colloid contents of the alveoli.

Thus is the general anatomy of the autogenous cysts, which I described in Lectures XXII. and XXIII., paralleled in the cysts connected with cancers. It may suffice to add that Rokitansky has traced a similar correspondence in their origin and modes of development. The account of the formation of cysts (page 336-338) might therefore be again read here; with the understanding that the nucleus, or smaller corpuscle, by whose enormous growth a cyst is formed, is here a cancerous element, while, in the cases there cited, it was supposed to be an element of some natural tissue. A part of the process is, moreover, already exemplified in the instance of epithelial cancers (page 581, fig. 104–5); but in these, the cysts, produced in the shape of laminated capsules, are very rarely barren, or filled with colloid substance.

Respecting the history of colloid cancer, the number of well-recorded cases, especially of those in which external parts were its primary seat, is too small to authorize many general statements.

Lebert has shown, by his collection of cases, that it generally corresponds with the history of scirrhous and medullary cancers; that the cases are about equal in the two sexes; that the greatest absolute frequency is at the middle period of life; that the disease is very rare in childhood;† that it is probably of somewhat slower average progress than the medullary cancers; that it more slowly affects the lymphatics and the organs distant from its primary seat; that, in general, its symptoms in each part correspond with those of other cancers affecting the same part: and this summary, I believe, includes all that can be prudently said upon the matter.

* Compare Lebert's figures with those of Rokitansky (Uber die Cyste, pl. iv. fig. xvi.)

† He adduces two cases of children, in which one was two, the other one and a half years old. Mr. Edward Bickersteth has observed two cases of colloid cancer of the kidney in children, one of whom was 3½, the other 11, years old.

LECTURE XXXIV.

GENERAL PATHOLOGY OF CANCER.

PART I.

CONDITIONS PRECEDING THE CANCEROUS GROWTH.

I PROPOSE, in this and the next Lecture, to consider the general pathology of all the forms of cancer which have now been particularly described; to gather a general history of them from the statements made concerning each; and to trace how the laws observed by them correspond with the more comprehensive laws of all specific diseases.

In the twenty-first Lecture (page 329) I stated the hypothesis which I think we must hold concerning cancers: namely, that they are local manifestations of certain specific morbid states of the blood; and that in them are incorporated peculiar morbid materials which accumulate in the blood, and which their growth may tend to increase.

In the terms which are more usual in discussions respecting the nature of cancers, I would say that a cancer is, from the first, both a constitutional and a specific disease. I believe it to be constitutional, in the sense of having its origin and chief support in the blood, by which the constitution of the whole body is maintained; and I believe it to be specific, 1st, in the sense of its being dependent on some specific material which is different from all the natural constituents of the body, and different from all the materials formed in other processes of disease; and 2dly, in the sense of its presenting, in the large majority of cases, structures which are specific or peculiar both in their form and in their mode of life.

The evidences for this hypothesis appear in the conformity of cancer to the other specific diseases, for which a similar hypothesis is nearly proved (Lect. XX.), and in the fitness of the terms which it supplies for the general pathology of cancer.

I will speak in this lecture of the conditions that precede the formation of a cancerous growth, and in the next of the growth itself.

The general history of cancers, and their analogy with other diseases that are, in the same senses, specific and constitutional, imply that, before the formation of a cancerous growth, two things at least must co-exist: namely, a certain morbid material in the blood, and some part appropriate to be the seat of growth incorporating that material, some place in which the morbid material may assume, or enter into, organic structure.

The existence of the morbid material in the blood, whether in the rudimental or in the effective state, constitutes the general predisposition to cancer; it is that which is, by some, called the predisposing cause of cancer. The morbid material is the essential constituent of the "cancerous diathesis, or constitution:" and when its existence produces some manifest impairment of the general health, independently of the cancerous growth, it makes the "primary cancerous cachexia" (see page 522).

That which evidently makes some part of the body appropriate for the growth of a cancerous tumor is a so-called exciting cause of cancer; but it is a cause of cancer only in so far as it fits some part for the local manifestation of a disease which already, in its essential material, exists in the blood.

It seems very important to keep constantly in view that these two conditions must coincide before the appearance of a cancerous growth; important not only to recognize their existence, but, if we can, to measure the several degrees in which, in each case, they are present; because, upon our recognition of the shares in which they respectively contribute to the production of the cancerous tumor, must depend the chief principles of practice in relation to the removal of such tumors. The larger the share taken by the constitutional element of the disease,—that is, by the cancerous condition of the blood,—in the production of a cancerous growth, the less is the probability of advantage to be derived from the removal of that growth; while, on the other hand, the more largely the local state enters into the conditions upon which the cancerous growth is founded, the more benefit may we anticipate from the removal of the cancer and of the locality with it.

So, too, in our considerations of the mere pathology of cancerous diseases, it seems essential to have a just regard of both these previous conditions. If we look at only a certain class of cases, we may easily find enough to persuade ourselves that cancers are, from the first, and throughout their course, wholly constitutional diseases; or, if we look exclusively at another class, which are as truly cancerous as the first (according to any natural definition of the term), we may find equal evidence for believing that they are, at least in the first instance, entirely local diseases, and that the constitutional affection which may attend them is only something consequent upon their growth.

When, for example, we see that certain organs are much more liable than others to the growth of cancer, and that, in those organs, the growth sometimes follows the infliction of a local injury, or some previous disease; and much more when we see, as in the case of the scrotal epithelial cancers, that the repeated application of a stimulus, such as soot, to a part of the body, will lead to the formation of cancer in even a large number of persons, we might assume that the growth has its origin wholly in the local state, and that whatever may follow of disease in other parts is only the consequence of the growth. On the other hand, when we consider the numerous analogies between cancers and the admitted specific blood-diseases; when we see the rapidity of outbreak with which cancerous disease sometimes manifests itself in multiple growths, apparently irrespective of the locality in which they are produced, and how, sometimes, a distinct affection of the general health, intense and destructive, exists even while the cancerous structure is yet trivial or unobserved; and when we see the insufficiency of all local causes to excite the growth of cancer in some persons, we might suppose that the cancerous disease is one wholly constitutional, wholly dependent on some morbid condition of the blood, and that the formation of the tumor is but as an accident of the disease, and is independent of the state of the part in which it occurs.

It is in correspondence with these classes of cases, too partially examined, that two distinct opinions are commonly entertained respecting the nature of cancer; some holding that it is from the beginning, and throughout, a constitutional disease; and others, that it is, in the first instance, if not through its whole course, a local one.   The reconciliation, not only of the two conflicting opinions, but of the seemingly conflicting facts upon which they chiefly rest, is to be found in this,—that the complete manifestation of cancer—the formation of a cancerous growth—is suspended till such a time as finds both the constitutional and the local conditions co-existent,—till the blood and the part are at once appropriate.

I might show how consistent the belief of the necessity of this coincidence is with what is known of other specific diseases (as illustrated in preceding lectures).   But let me illustrate it by two cases, such as may frequently be met with.   Bruch* records the following :—A woman had a child at eighteen years of age.   The child died when it was a month old, and her breasts were left to the disturbance which usually ensues in prematurely arrested lactation.   At the age of thirty-four she received a blow on the right breast.   This was followed by no manifest change of structure, but, for some days, by severe pains, and then, for a much longer time, by feelings of swelling and tension at the menstrual periods. At thirty-nine she received another blow upon the same breast, which was followed by an increase of pain.   Soon afterwards she was exposed to cold, and then there ensued erysipelatous inflammation of the breast, followed by induration of a part of the mammary gland.   This, however, continued without change for four years; but then, after menorrhagia, a tumor appeared in the breast.   When this was removed, or partially removed, it was found to be not a cancerous, but a cystic tumor, with growths from the interior surfaces of the cysts.   She remained well after this, the wound having perfectly healed, for twelve years more, and in this interval she ceased to menstruate; but now, when she was fifty-five years old, after having a whitlow and inflamed lymphatics of the right

* Die Diagnose der bösartigen Geschwülste, p. 94.

arm, another tumor formed in the breast, which had every appearance of being cancerous, It was removed; but it recurred, and ended fatally.

Now, surely, in such a case as this, we may say that all the local conditions necessary for the production of a cancer of the breast had been amply provided. They had existed, or had been reproduced from time to time, for a period of upwards of twenty years; yet, being alone, they had been insufficient; and no cancer appeared till the time when, at a more favorable condition of age, the cancerous condition of the blood was manifested, and filled up the measure of the necessary precedents of the disease.

Contrast with the cases of this kind those to which I had occasion to refer in a former lecture (page 552), and of which I may here repeat one. A boy received a cut in his eye, which had been previously sound. Within three weeks of the injury a fungus protruded from the eye. It was removed with the whole eyeball and the contents of the orbit. The wound had scarcely healed before a fresh growth appeared; and shortly afterwards the boy died with medullary disease extending from the orbit to the brain. We can scarcely express such cases as this in any other terms than that the cancerous condition of the blood existed at the time of the injury, but was insufficient for the production of a cancerous growth, and remained latent, for want of an appropriate locality for the growth, till the injury, disturbing or causing the suspension of the natural course of nutrition in the part, supplied the appropriate local condition. As one might say, the seed had been long present in the blood, but the soil was wanting, and the injury, hindering or diverting the eye from its ordinary nutrition, supplied the want, and prepared the soil for the growth of the cancer.

These cases, I repeat, are but examples of classes. In the one class, we seem to meet with all the constitutional or blood-conditions of cancerous disease complete, waiting only for the existence of some part in which the cancerous growth may be manifested; in the other class, the local conditions are abundantly present, but the disease does not appear till the cancerous condition of the blood is complete (compare p. 313).

It may, further, be deduced from these cases, in which the extremes illustrate the ordinary mean, that if either of the two conditions be present in an extreme degree, its intensity may compensate for a comparative defect of the other. Among the cases to which I have been referring, we find certain in which the cancerous disease makes its appearance in such a multiplicity of growths and of parts, that it seems indifferent to local conditions; and these are the very cases in which all the other constitutional characters of cancer are most strongly marked; in which cachexia often precedes the growth, and in which the removal of the cancer interferes in no way with the progress of the constitutional disease, unless it be to accelerate it. On the other side, we meet with cases in which the long-continued irritations, or frequent injuries of certain parts of the body, seem almost sure to be followed by cancer; and these are the cases in which the constitutional characteristics of the disease are least marked, and in which, as in epithelial cancer of the scrotum and of scars, we may hope that the recurrence of the disease may be long deferred, if that which has first appeared be removed with its seat. In this class of cases it may be said, the cancerous blood-condition is so slowly developed, that the cancerous growth can ensue in none but a peculiarly appropriated part, which part being removed, the growth is for a time, or for life, impossible; while, in the former class, the blood-condition is so highly developed, or so intense, that almost any part suffices for the seat of growth.

Let me now proceed to consider what each of these conditions, necessary as precedents of the growth of a cancer, consists in. What is the cancerous condition of the blood? and what is the state of a locality apt for the formation of a cancerous growth?

I. Concerning the state of the blood, our positive knowledge is very trivial and obscure; perhaps it would be safest to say that we have at present none. We may be sure, on grounds to which I have already referred, that there is a peculiar material in the blood which is separated from it, and constantly renewed, in the formation of a cancer; but we can say what this material is not, rather than what it is.

We may reasonably hold that, in cancerous persons, the whole constitution of the blood is not perverted; for we see that all the tissues may for a long time be perfectly nourished, even while the cancer is making progress; that injuries may be repaired with the ordinary quickness and perfection; that the products of inflammation may be like those in non-cancerous persons, and may pass through their ordinary developments; and that some other specific diseases may have their usual course. It would therefore be unreasonable to regard the whole of the blood of a cancerous person as perverted from its normal condition. The cancerous state is not a total change of the blood, but depends, probably, on some definite material mingled with the natural constituents: and this material, we may believe, is derived from a morbid transformation of one or more of the natural constituents of the blood, and is maintained, as morbid structures are, by the persistence of the same method of transformation, or by its own assimilative force.

But now, as to what this material is; or, again, is not. I believe it is not anything visible to the sight. There is not, so far as I know, anything in the blood of a cancerous person which we can recognise as a cancer-structure. There are no cancer-cells, nor, in any form, visible germs of cancer, existing in the blood, and only needing to be separated from it to make up or grow into the cancerous structure. In advanced cases of cancer, and especially in those in which the cancerous substance is very softened and broken, we may meet with portions of it in the blood.

which appear as if they had been detached or absorbed from some growth, and carried on with the stream. In similar cases we may find cancerous formations in the blood itself. Such seem to be some of the cancerous growths in the veins and the right side of the heart. For, although, among the former, there are many in which the growth has only extended into the veins, through their walls involved in cancerous tumors, yet there are others in which, as in the endocardial cancers, the internal growth takes place far from any other tumor. In these we may believe that cancerous structures have been conveyed in the blood to the part of the vein, or of the right side of the heart, at which they have been arrested, and to which adhering (either alone or with blood-clot), they have subsisted and grown on materials derived from the passing blood. But none of these cases afford any support to a belief that, previous to the existence of a cancerous tumor, any visible germs of cancer exist in the blood.

Other means for investigating the very nature of the cancerous material in the blood seem as impotent as the sight. Minute chemistry has, up to this time, done nothing; neither can we yet accept, I think, that which is in part a chemical theory, and has been especially held by the pathologists of the Vienna school,—namely, that particular diatheses or dyscrases of the blood, appropriate to such diseases as cancer and tubercle, may be recognized by a superabundance of albumen or of fibrine. The facts adduced as bearing directly on these doctrines are, at present, few and incomplete; and although the course of investigation, in which they have been observed, is the most hopeful yet entered upon, I think they are not sufficient either to establish the theories based on them, or to outweigh the general improbability, that diseases so complex as cancer and tubercle should depend, chiefly, on quantitative variations in any of the larger constituents of the blood. Neither can it, I think, in the present state of organic chemistry, and with so few analysis as we yet possess of the blood of cancerous and other diseased persons, be more than a guess, that either cancer or any other such specific disease, depends, in any sense, on qualitative modifications of the albumen, or the fibrine, or any other single constituent of the blood.

At present, I believe, the best part of the facts established, or made probably, by these investigations, relate to the antagonism or incompatibility of cancer and certain other specific diseases. I think we cannot doubt that, as a general rule, cancerous and tuberculous diseases do not make active progress at the same time; and that, in this sense, they exclude one another, and are incompatible. I mentioned in a former Lecture (p. 337), a striking case bearing on this point, in which, as it seemed, the rare event of arrest and almost complete recovery from scirrhous cancer was connected with the evolution of tuberculous disease. I believe, also, that I have seen at least one instance in which active tuberculous disease of the lungs was arrested immediately before the appearance of a scirrhous cancer in the breast; and we find, in so many of those who die with cancer, the remnants of tuberculous disease from which they have suffered in earlier life, that we may believe that the recovery from the one has been in some manner connected with the supervention of the other. So, on the other side, the rarity of progressive tuberculous disease in those that are cancerous may be because, except in such extremely rare cases as that to which I have referred, the cancerous diathesis excludes that condition of the blood in which the tuberculous disease has its rise.

To the same class of facts, as illustrating the exclusion of one morbid condition of the blood (or, as Hunter would have said, of one morbid action), by another, we may perhaps refer the occasional withering of a cancer under the influence of some fever, and the more rarely occurring complete death of one, so that during an attack of acute fever the whole mass may slough off; and this whether the feverish condition of the blood be produced by some miasma, or by medicinal means. Such, I fear, is all that can be, at present, safely regarded as matter of fact in relation to the nature of the peculiarity of cancerous blood; and it must be admitted that these facts are scarcely more than indications of the direction in which inquiry should be made. Let us next see if we can, in any measure, trace the method of its production;—whence the specific material is derived from without, and the conditions most favorable to its generation within, the body.

First, it is evident that a disposition to cancer may be derived by inheritance; that something may be transmitted from the parent to the offspring, which shall ultimately produce both the cancerous condition of the blood and the locality apt for the cancerous growth.

The proportion of cases in which this hereditary transmission is manifested is, it is true, but small. In 160 cancerous patients, there were 26, or very nearly one-sixth, who were aware of cancer in other members of their families (see pages 514, 552). The proportion may seem too trivial to reason upon, yet it is larger than could be due to chance (page 598); and its import is corroborated by the fact of so many members of the same family being in some instances affected.

That which is transmitted from parent to offspring is not, strictly speaking, cancer or cancerous material, but a tendency to the production of those conditions which will, finally, manifest themselves in a cancerous growth. There are here some facts worth dwelling upon, both for their own sake, and because they are clear instances of the manner in which the hereditary transmission of the properties of the parent body takes place.

I repeat, that which is transmitted from parent to offspring is not cancer itself, but a tendency to the production of cancer at some time far future from the birth. We have no reason to believe that a cancerous material passes with the germ. To suppose such a thing, where the cancerous parent is the male, would be almost absurd. Moreover, no reason to believe that cancerous material passes from either parent is furnished by any frequency of congenital cancer, or (so far as I know) by cancer being earlier developed in the offspring of cancerous parents than in other persons.

But while, on the one hand, we cannot assume that a cancerous material passes with the germ or impregnating fluid; on the other, we cannot understand the transmission of a tendency or disposition to any event, independently of all material conditions. The germ from the cancerous parent must be already, in some condition, different from one from a parent who is not cancerous, if, in the course of any number of years, cancers are to be formed out of the substance which the germ, in its development, or subsequent changes, will appropriate. Our expression, then, may be, that in the impregnated germ from a cancerous parent, one or more of the materials, normal as they may seem, are already so far from the perfectly normal state, that after the lapse of years, by their development or degeneration, they will engender or constitute the cancerous material in the blood, and, it may be, the locality apt for a cancerous growth.

But now, let it be observed, this tendency to cancerous disease is most commonly derived from a parent who is not yet manifestly cancerous; for, most commonly, the children are born before cancer is evident in the parent; so that, as we may say, that which is still future to the parent is transmitted potentially to the offspring. Nay, more: the tendency which exists in the parent may never become in him or her effective, although it may become effective in the offspring : for there are cases in which a grandparent has been cancerous, and although his or her children have not been so, the grandchildren have been. How admirable a discovery it would be if we could find the means by which the tendency, conveyed from the grandparent to the child, was yet diverted from its course, even after it had been transmitted to the germ of the grandchild !

Let me repeat, the cases of hereditary cancer only illustrate the common rule of the transmission of hereditary properties, whether natural or morbid. Just as the parent, in the perfection of maturity, transmits to the offspring those conditions, in germ and rudimental substance, which shall be changed into the exact imitation of the parent's self, not only in the fulness of health, but in all the infirmities of yet future age; so, also, even in seeming health, the same parent may communicate to the materials of the offspring the rudiments of yet future diseases; and these rudiments must, in the case before us, be such modifications of natural compositions as, in the course of many years, shall be developed or degenerate into materials that will manifest themselves in the production of cancer.

There is, surely, in all science, no fact so strange as this : and it need not be a barren fact, fit merely for wonder and vain speculation ; for we may deduce from it that the cancer-substance in the blood, whatever it may be, and whencesoever derived, is a result of long-continued elaboration; needing, as the normal materials of the body do, to pass through a life of continual change before it attains its complete efficiency. The period required for this completion of the cancer-material, is the time, often of long delay, during which the disease, according to various expressions, is "latent," or only "in predisposition." But such expressions are deceptive. As with other specific blood diseases, so with cancer, the predisposition to it is a substantial thing; and we should hold that, in all the time of latency, there is that thing in the blood, which will become, or generate by combination, the effective cancer-material, unless (as in the healthy generation between the cancerous grandparent and the cancerous grandchild) it be destroyed or retained in the course of natural nutrition.

In hereditary transmission, the cancer-material may be so modified, so that the form of the disease in the offspring may be different from that in the parent. The change from scirrhous to medullary cancer, and *vice versâ*, is, I believe, not rare. I have mentioned cases of alternation between these and the epithelial cancers (page 592); and a case of melanoid cancer in a patient descended from one with a scirrhous breast (page 608). Mr. Simon has told me that he removed a colloid cancer from the cheek of a woman whose child, seven years old, was dying with medullary cancer of the eye; and M. Lebert, with two cases like these, relates that the celebrated Broussais died with medullary cancer of the rectum, and his son, Casimir, with colloid cancer of the same part. With so many cases supporting it, this kind of transmission of cancer can hardly be doubted. But, I believe, we may trace further changes in the transmission; and that the material may be so altered that, as we may say, the cancerous disposition may gradually cease, or fade out in the production of tumors, whose characters are intermediate or transitional between cancers and simple growths. I have referred (pages 431, 474) to cases illustrating this opinion; and I feel sure that many more will be found; for we may observe corresponding changes, in both form and degree, in the hereditary transmission of many other diseases. Thus the syphilis of the infant is seldom exactly like that of the mother; the same family may include cases of insanity, epilepsy, palsy, chorea, stammering, and other diseases allied to these in that all are affections of the nervous centres, but differing from them in form and degree.*

The rule of hereditary transmission (a rule which, like many in pathology, has more seeming exceptions than examples)† holds for only a sixth of the cases of cancer. Can we, for the remaining five-sixths, trace any external source of the morbid condition of the blood? Inocu-

---

* Hereditary malformations display similar mutations *in transitu;* as in instances in the Museum of St. Bartholomew's, Casts A 21 to 27. The whole of this subject of the change of diathesis on hereditary transmission will repay, I believe, the deepest study.

† Page 307.

lation and contagion are the only probable sources of the kind; but concerning these the presumed facts are, at present, very few and uncertain. There are cases in which, by the inoculation of cancerous material into the bodies, or by the injection of such material into the blood, of dogs, cancer has seemed to be produced. I think that, in a large number of experiments, that result has been three times obtained; but it is quite possible that the dogs used for these three experiments were cancerous before the human cancerous matter was injected into them; for cancer is indeed a frequent disease among dogs. The instances are certainly too few for proof of inoculation.

There are, also, certain cases in which it seems possible that cancer may have been transmitted from the wife to the husband during the act of copulation. Such cases are recorded by Dr. Watson and Dr. Copland:* wives having cancer of the uterus had husbands with cancer of the penis. Of course, it must be questionable whether there were in these cases more than the accidental coincidence of persons having married, in both of whom an ordinary and independent generation of cancer ensued; and we cannot conclude that inoculation of cancer may thus occur, unless it should appear that persons thus related become cancerous in larger proportions than they do who, being otherwise in similar conditions, are not thus exposed to the possibility of inoculation.

Again, I have heard that cancerous matter having been inoculated under the skin of frogs, cancerous growths have been produced in them. I have repeated this experiment, but without effect; for all the frogs in whom I inserted the cancerous matter died soon after. But the facts, so far as I have yet heard them, have not much meaning in relation to the general pathology of cancer; for I believe it is not yet proved that the local growths of cancer, which are the consequence of the inoculation, are followed by general cancerous disease, or by the production of cancer of distant parts, as well as in that in which the matter was deposited. Unless this occurs, the experiments only prove the fact (and a very strange one it is) that materials of disease from human bodies, being inserted in the bodies of cold-blooded animals, will live and grow, even upon the materials of the cold-blooded creature. In like manner, if any one could establish the supposed cases of husbands inoculated by their wives, he might only prove that cancerous elements may subsist and increase upon other materials than those of the body in which themselves were generated. Unless the cancers thus generated, in the first instance locally, are found to multiply themselves in distant organs, these cases of isolation will prove no more than that cancer, like a parasitic growth, may be transplanted, and grow on common or indifferent nutritive material; they will have no bearing on the questions concerning the nature and origin of cancerous blood.

At the most, then, we may assume that a transference of cancer by

* Dict. of Pract. Med.; Art. Scirrhous and other Tumors.

41

inoculation is possible. But such an assumption will not materially diminish the number of cases in which we look in vain for any external source for the disease, and in which all that we can study are the conditions most favorable for its production within the body. Of these conditions I have already spoken, in relation to each of the principal forms of cancer. I need, therefore, do little more than sum up the general conclusions concerning them.

First, respecting the influence of sexual peculiarities. Women are, on the whole, more liable to cancer than men are; but in what proportion they are so cannot be exactly stated; Lebert assigns about 37 per cent. as the proportion of cancers in males: Dr. Walshe finds it scarcely more than 26 per cent. This is just one of the points on which the truth will not be known till statistics are collected by practitioners under whose charge the two sexes, and all the organs of each, fall in just proportions, and by whom the existence of internal cancers is so constantly ascertained by autopsy as that of external cancers. The frequency of cancer of the breast and uterus gives an apparently large preponderance of cases in women; but, on the other side, the cancers of the skin, bones, and digestive organs, greatly predominate in men. The liability of the breast makes scirrhous cancer by far most frequent in women; but this, in a general estimate, may be nearly balanced by the preponderance of epithelial, osteoid, and villous cancers in men.*

The influence of age may be more definitely stated. Dr. Walshe has clearly shown that "the mortality from cancer" [i. e. the number of deaths in proportion to the number of persons living] "goes on steadily increasing with each succeeding decade until the eightieth year." His result is obtained from records of deaths; but it is almost exactly confirmed by the tables I have collected, showing the ages at which the cancers were first observed by the patients, or ascertained by their attendants. In 772 cases, including cancers of all kinds, the ages at which they appeared were as follows:—

Under	10	years	.	.	.	.	.	27
Between 10 and 20	"	.	.	.	.	.	.	30
" 20 and 30	"	.	.	.	.	.	.	78
" 30 and 40	"	.	.	.	.	.	. *	130
" 40 and 50	"	.	.	.	.	.	.	200
" 50 and 60	"	.	.	.	.	.	.	152
" 60 and 70	"	.	.	.	.	.	.	98
" 70 and 80	"	.	.	.	.	.	.	57

The proportions between these numbers and the numbers of persons living at the corresponding ages (calculated in the same manner as in the previous Lectures, pp. 513, 551, 592), will show the proportionate frequency of cancer at each period of life, and may be represented by the following numbers:—

* The particular influences of sexual difference may be collected from pp. 512, 550, 591, 608, 618. On all the questions capable of being solved by statistics, the largest information is collected by Dr. Walshe.

Under 10 years							5
Between 10 and 20 years							6.9
" 20 " 30							21
" 30 " 40							48.5
" 40 " 50							100
" 50 " 60							113
" 60 " 70							107
" 70 " 80							126

Thus the liability to cancer seems always increasing from childhood to eighty years of age. A single exception to the rule (between 60 and 70) appears to exist; but this would very probably not appear in estimates from a larger number of cases. The general fact, and that of the immense increase of cancer after 40 years of age, are of exceeding value in proving that it is a disease of degeneracy.

Within this larger rule, others may be collected from the foregoing Lectures. Of the three chief forms of cancer, the medullary alone exemplifies the rule of frequency constantly increasing from earliest to latest life; but the rate of increase is, of course, different from that shown in the general table (p. 551-2). The epithelial cancers exemplify the rule after the age of 20; before that age they are scarcely found (p. 592). The scirrhous have their maximum proportionate frequency between 40 and 50* (p. 513). The melanoid cancers are nearly conformed to the rule of the medullary. The osteoid and colloid probably have rules of frequency peculiar to themselves, and depending upon local conditions; but we need more cases to calculate them.

The increase of frequency of cancer with increasing years, its great prevalence after middle age, and the conformity to this rule shown by medullary cancers which are least of all dependent upon locality for their development,—these facts may prove, as a rule, that cancer is a disease of general or constitutional degeneracy. But, as in every other part of the pathology of cancer, so, in estimating the influence of age in its production, we must consider the effect of time in making certain parts apt to be the seat of cancer. Such an effect is shown in the different liabilities which each organ manifests at different periods of life. These cannot be exactly stated; but, beyond doubt, the eye and orbit are earliest apt to become cancerous; then the bones, testicles, and the cellular tissue of the limbs and trunk. These are its chief seats before 30 years of age; from 30 to 50 it predominates in the penis, uterus, external sexual organs, and the breasts; after 50, in the integuments and digestive organs.† I fear nothing can be said of the real nature of the changes ensuing in each organ, which thus make it, at different times of life, more or less appro-

* It is probably due to this great frequency of scirrhous cancer in the female breast that (as Dr. Walshe found) the increase of mortality from cancer between 40 to 50 is so much greater in women than in men.

† More rules of this kind may perhaps be gathered from the statistics of Walshe and Lebert; but with caution, for want of such records as I have said are necessary to estimate the liability of the sexes.

priate for the seat of cancer. In some parts, as the testicles and limbs, the chief liability seems to coincide with the first attainment or mainte- nance, of full functional power; in others, it falls in with the beginning of the loss of power, as in the uterus and breast.

Two other conditions seem to have influence in producing or promoting the cancerous constitution: namely, climate, and mental distress. Dr. Walshe has collected evidence that "the maximum amount of cancerous disease occurs in Europe," and that it is very rare among the patients of the hospitals at Hobart Town and Calcutta, and among the natives of Egypt, Algiers, Senegal, Arabia, and the tropical parts of America. We cannot, indeed, be sure that this difference depends on climate; it may be due to the national differences in habits of life; possibly, as Dr. Walshe suggests (p. 415), the greater prevalence of cancer may be due to the more wasting influence of the higher state of civilization. More records are necessary to decide such questions; and it may be well if they in- clude accounts of the apparent varieties of cancer among nations whose climate and habits of life are not materially different. (See pp. 545, 598.)

It is only on a general impression, not by counted facts, that we can reckon deep mental distress among the conditions favorable to the pro- duction of cancer. I do not at all suppose that it could of itself generate a cancerous condition of the blood; or that a joyous temper and pros- perity are a safeguard against cancer; but the cases are so frequent in which deep anxiety, deferred hope, and disappointment, are quickly fol- lowed by the growth or increase of cancer, that we can hardly doubt that mental depression is a weighty addition to the other influences that favor the development of the cancerous constitution. Nor is it strange that it should be so; it is consistent with the many other facts showing the affinity between cancer and depressed nutrition.

But, after all, when we have assigned to these conditions their full weight in producing the cancerous constitution or state of the blood, that which may strike us most of all is the comparatively small influence which any known internal or external conditions possess. We are, as yet, wholly unaware of any great difference, in the frequency of cancer, among those of our own nation who are most widely apart from each other in all the ordinary conditions of life. The richest and the poorest alike seem to be subject to it; so do the worst and the best fed; those that are living in the best conditions of atmosphere, and those that are immured in the worst; those that are cleanly, and those that are foul; those of all temperaments, and of all occupations (except such as have peculiar local influences); those that appear healthy, and those that are diseased, ex- cept those with some few specific diseases. We can hardly lay our hand upon any one of the various circumstances of life, in the various orders of society in this country, to which we can refer as rendering one more or less liable than another to the acquirement of the cancerous constitution.

Dr. Walshe's evidence amply shows the want of foundation of all the general impressions opposed to this conclusion.

From this confession of ignorance respecting the production of the cancerous constitution, or, as I would say, of the cancer-material in the blood, when it is generated within the body, I will proceed to speak of some of the changes which, being once generated, it may undergo.

In all ordinary events the normal course of cancerous disease is that of steady increase, steady progress towards death. The increase is indicated by two different, but usually commensurate, series of phenomena: those, namely, of increasing formation of cancer-structures, and of increasing cachexia.

We may commmonly observe, that, from the beginning of a cancerous formation, there is a constant increase in its mass, and in the rate at which it is added to. Even the cancers that are, in part, ulcerating, are usually growing, at a greater rate at the border or surface opposite to that in which ulceration is destroying them; or else, while ulceration is going on in one cancer, there is a greater rate of increase in others; or, the number of growing masses is constantly increasing. In one or more of these methods most cases exemplify the general rule, that the quantity of cancer which is formed, within any given length of time, regularly increases from the beginning to the end of the case.

In most cases the increasing formation of cancer is accompanied by manifest indications of increasing cachexia. But it is not always thus; and, on the other hand, we find cases in which the cachexia increases without proportionately increasing cancerous formations: cases in which we may say that the cancerous condition of the blood manifests itself less plainly in the production of growths, than in its inteference with the ordinary phenomena of life. Such cases are not unfrequent among those of cancer of the rectum: we see the patient intensely ill, and dying with cachexia, to which the extent or rate of growth of the cancerous tumor bears no proportion. So, sometimes, with cancer of the liver; the cachexia is quite disproportionate to the amount of cancerous formation, and to the degree in which it interferes with the functions of the organ. In these cases, the cancerous disease exemplifies a frequent event in the history of specific diseases; namely, that when the morbid material is most intense and acute in its action, when it most manifestly affects the constitution, it may produce the least indications of local morbid influence.

In both these sets of cases, the increase of cancerous disease, and its accelerating rate, are illustrated as the rule of its career. The phenomena, in the first set of cases, may be explained by assuming that the quantity of cancer-material in the blood regularly increases; those in the second, that, with its increase, it undergoes some transformation, rendering it less appropriate for growths, but more injurious to the other offices of the blood.

(*b.*) The cancerous constitution may apparently cease; a growth already formed may maintain itself, subsisting, probably, on the normal constituents of the blood,* but its progressive increase may be, for a time suspended. I have exemplified this by cases of medullary cancer (p. 553), of which the general history was, that, after a certain period of increase, the tumors ceased to enlarge, were for a time stationary (the general health also remaining the same), and then resumed the cancerous mode of progress.

(*c*) The cancerous constitution may be in some measure changed or modified. It may manifest iself for a time in a certain form of cancer, and then in some other form. Thus scirrhous cancer may be succeeded, in secondary growths, by medullary cancer; osteoid by medullary, and *vice versâ*; and I think, epithelial by medullary. We must, I believe, in these cases assume a transformation of the specific cancerous material in the blood—a change corresponding with that which may be more regularly traced in the materials of other specific diseases (*e. g.* of syphilis) in their successive stages or periods of life (pp. 308, 315).

Lastly, the cancerous diathesis, even after it has been manifested by growths, may be superseded. Thus we may express the cessation, or retrocession, of cancer, when tuberculous disease ensues in its course.

In the last three events the rule of progress in cancer is departed from. But if we could reckon all the cases in which any of these events happen, they would make but a few exceptions to the general rule, that the cancerous constitution regularly increases at an accelerating rate, and with little change in its methods of manifesting itself.

I pass now to the consideration of the second necessary precedent of a cancerous growth, namely, the existence of some part fitted to be its seat, some apt locality. Such fittness may be natural or acquired; and in parts in which it is in some measure natural, it may be increased by accident or disease.

Certain parts of the body are evidently, and independently of external influences, far more liable than others are to become the seat of cancer. They are, thus, naturally, apt localities; not equally so throughout life, but usually becoming so at certain periods.

We have no such full and impartial statistical evidence as might enable us to state clearly the proportions in which the several organs are primarily or secondarily affected with cancer. There are at present, I believe, no large statistics on which we can place reliance for accurately determining this point : bills of mortality, founded upon diagnoses not confirmed by autopsy, and the records of those whose practice is chiefly medical or chiefly surgical, supply only unsafe or partial evidence.

* I shall revert to this point in the next lecture. The maintenance, or even the increase of a cancerous growth, does not necessarily imply that a cancerous condition of the blood is maintained : once formed, a cancer, like any other tumor, may live and grow by its assimilative power over cancerous materials.

It cannot be doubted that the uterus, stomach, and female breast hold the first place in aptness for primary cancerous growths; and the lymphatics, lungs, and liver, for secondary growths; and that among the parts least liable to either affection are, the spinal cord, tendons, tonsils, pharynx, and prostate gland. But beyond these general statements, none, I think, can be safely made. Neither does any explanation yet offered of the different liabilities of parts seem well founded. As Dr. Walshe observes, all that has been said to explain the liability of the breast and uterus may be equally well said of the ovaries, which are comparatively rarely cancerous. So, too, what has been said about the brain and stomach, and testicle, is just as applicable to the spinal cord, the duodenum, and the epididymis; yet these parts of similar systems are, severally, in complete contrast in their aptness to be the seat of cancer.

It seems impossible, at present, to discover what it is that makes one part more than another naturally fit to be the seat of cancerous growth; or any part more fit at one time of life than at another. We are, of course, disposed to look for explanation to peculiarities of tissue, and to their changes with age; and we can hardly doubt that these are chiefly influential: and yet, as the medullary cancers of the eyeball and orbit share (p. 545), we must ascribe something to locality as well as to tissue. The *allocation* of cancers is certainly not wholly determined by aptness of structures. An osteoid cancer, for example, affects at once cancellous and compact osseous tissue, medulla, periosteum, and surrounding muscles; a medullary cancer may occupy, from the first, many tissues both within and around the eyeball: when a cancerous breast is cut away, the recurrent growths appear very commonly in the scar, *i. e.* in the same locality, though all the tissues affected by the primary growth are gone. Very numerous cases such as these might be cited; they cannot, I presume, be explained, but they suggest the need of considering always that morbid products may be determined to certain *places* as well as to certain *structures*. As each natural organ has its appropriate place as well as structure, so, but with almost infinitely less regularity, morbid growth may have laws of allocation.

A question of much interest is connected with the liability of other tumors to become cancerous; it is of interest not only as a subject of pathological inquiry, but in relation to an opinion which is often made a reason for operations: namely, that if a tumor of any kind is left to its own course, it is not unlikely to become cancerous. I have looked carefully into this question, and I believe there are no facts sufficient to justify the opinion that an innocent tumor is more likely to become the seat of cancer than any other parts of the body in which it is growing. The only case supporting such an opinion is that of cystic disease of the ovary. I think there is no doubt that it is not unfrequent for cysts of the ovary to exist, for a time, as an innocent disease, and then become the seat of cancerous growths. But, then, the case of cystic disease of the ovary is so peculiar in all respects, that we cannot deduce from it any rule to be applied to instances of other tumors.

With regard to the supposed transformation of any other tumors into cancers, the facts are very few.

M. Lebert states that he has twice met with tumors which were at first of an innocent kind, but afterwards became cancerous; but he does not state whether they were in persons who had cancer in some other part: *i. e.* whether the cancer in the tumor were secondary or primary.

Sir Benjamin Brodie mentions a case in which he removed a tumor, the general mass of which appeared to be fatty substance, somewhat more condensed than usual, but "here and there was another kind of morbid growth, apparently belonging to the class of medullary or fungoid disease."* A few other cases of the same kind are related; and some would assume that in all the cases of mixed cartilaginous and cancerous tumors (mentioned at p. 444) the cartilaginous growth was being transformed into, or superseded by, the cancerous one. I see no good evidence for such an assumption: the contrary might very well be maintained in argument; or the two growths might be regarded as simultaneous in their origin.

It need not be denied that cancerous growths may occur in tumors that were previously of an innocent kind, but I feel quite sure that these may be regarded as events of the greatest rarity. My own experience has (perhaps by chance) been such as would indicate that innocent tumors are less liable to cancer than the structures they resemble; for, as I have elsewhere mentioned (p. 473), I have seen three cases in which cancer affected the natural structure of the mammary gland, while, close by, mammary glandular tumors remained unaffected.

It may be asked, whence is derived the impression that so commonly exists, that a tumor of an innocent kind is peculiarly apt to become cancerous? I believe it has arisen from several different kinds of deceptive cases.

First, there are the cases of what I have referred to as the suspension, for a time, of cancerous progress; in these the cancer seems for a time to be an innocent tumor; it is judged to be so because it remains so long quiet; and when it assumes the ordinary progress of cancer, it is said to be a tumor once innocent, but now become cancerous. This might have happened in the first and fourth of the cases mentioned at p. 554: yet, without doubt, in these cases, the tumors that made little or no progress had all along the cancerous structure.

Another class of deceptive cases have a history of this kind:—a tumor is removed which is apparently of an innocent sort: but, some time after, a cancer appears at the same part. The explanation of some of these cases is (as I suggested in p. 473), that a simple tumor has grown in a person having an hereditary or other constitutional tendency to cancer;

* Lectures on Pathology and Surgery, p. 282.

and that, in the removal of this tumor, the surgeon has unwittingly supplied, by the local injury, what was needed for the production of a cancerous growth; he has made some locality apt for the manifestation of a constitutional disease already existing.

In the third class of cases, we may find in the same person a succession of tumors, of which the first may have few or no characters of cancer, and the last, as if by gradual change, may be evidently cancerous. I have referred to this in connection with the recurring fibroid tumors (p. 418); but the facts have little bearing on the question whether an innocent tumor can become cancerous: for here the transition is effected, not in one tumor, but in a succession of tumors.

By cases such as these we may, I believe, explain away the grounds for the assumption that simple or innocent tumors are parts peculiarly apt to become cancerous. Cancers may grow in such tumors, but the event is so rare, that it cannot, in any given case, be reasonably anticipated.

It remains to consider how parts may acquire an aptness for cancerous growth in them, or, in most instances, how that aptness which they naturally posses may be increased: for it is very observable that the "exciting causes" of cancer act with far greatest effect on the parts which are, without their help, most liable to it.

Three chief conditions may be here enumerated: namely, the results of certain diseases in intrauterine life, indicated by congenital defect; the results of certain diseases after birth; the consequences of injury.

The aptness for cancer due to congenital defect is exemplified in the peculiar liability of moles or pigmentary nævi to become the primary seats of melanosis. I have already enlarged on this (p. 610), and have suggested that these defects, which we can easily see, may be only examples of a larger group, which, though invisible, are not less efficient in rendering certain parts peculiarly liable to cancer.

The aptness due to diseases after birth may be illustrated by the liability of the incrusted warts and scars, and other morbidly changed parts, to become the primary seats of epithelial cancers. For other than epithelial cancers the effect of disease in disposing parts to cancer is slight. We find no remarkable liability in parts that have been changed by inflammation, whether of common or specific kind. Few theories, I think, have been less founded than those which have regarded scirrhous or medullary cancer as, in any sense, the result or sequence of inflammation. Parts that have been the seats of inflammation may become the seats of cancer; but I doubt whether the proportion in which they do so be much greater than that in which they become cancerous when apparently healthy.

The influence of injuries is more evident. About a fifth of those who have cancer ascribe it to injury; and although, doubtless, some of these are wrong in their belief, yet, among the rest, there are some in whom the consequence of injury is too evident to admit of doubt. But here a distinction must be made as to the manner in which injury promotes the production of cancers.

In certain cases, the cancerous growth appears immediately after the common effects of the injury. A person receives (suppose) a blow, and when its direct effects are passing away, a cancer appears in the injured part. I have cited cases of this kind in the history of medullary cancers (p. 552); among which, indeed, the event seems more frequent than among those of other forms.

In other and more usual cases, a much longer interval passes between the injury and the appearance of the cancer. The injured part seems to recover, without change of structure. In most cases, indeed, such as those of ordinary blows on the breast, the direct effects of the injury are not such as we might expect to be followed by structural change; yet, doubtless, the part remains different from what it was.

In a third class of cases, which are most frequently exemplified in the epithelial cancers, the injuries appear to be ineffective unless they are repeated time after time, so as to produce, we may suppose, a real change of structure in the part that at length becomes the seat of cancer (p. 594).

It is important to remember these different relations between injuries and the growth of cancers, not only for pathology's sake, but for practice.

It is often stated, as a rule, that those cancers are least likely to return (it should be said, to return quickly), after removal, which have followed the receipt of injury, or some previous disease in the part. Now, this is only partially true; it is, probably, often true of the epithelial cancers that have grown in the seats of repeated injury, of frequent ulceration, and the like; but I know no facts relating to scirrhous and medullary cancers that will support it; and I believe that the cases in which cancers follow quickly after accidental injury are just those in which a speedy return may be anticipated after operations. The growth of a cancer immediately after an injury implies the existence of an intense cancerous diathesis, which no removal of the cancer is likely to affect; but when a part has been repeatedly injured, and only at length becomes the seat of cancer, it implies such a low degree or stage of cancerous diathesis, as we may expect to remain long "latent," if the slowly-prepared locality, with all that has grown in it, be cleanly removed. Of the intermediate cases, in which some clear time intervenes between the injury and the growth of the cancer, we must hold, I think, that the abiding effects of the injury keep the part in a state peculiarly apt for the growth, till the constitutional condition is established. This being complete, the removal of the growth cannot change it; and the injury done by the operation would be enough to prepare a place, if none elsewhere were appropriate, for a recurrent cancer.

LECTURE XXXIV.

GENERAL PATHOLOGY OF CANCER.

PART II.

STRUCTURE AND LIFE OF CANCEROUS GROWTHS.

I ENDEAVORED to illustrate, in the last lecture, those two conditions which, judging from the general history of cancers, and the analogy of other specific diseases, we must assume as necessary precedents of a cancerous growth: namely, the cancerous diathesis, constitution, or morbid condition of the blood, and the condition of some part appropriate for the growth. Now, according to the same analogy, the assumed cancer-material in the blood, if it cannot be removed by any natural excretory organ, will determine the formation of some abnormal organism in which itself may be incorporated; and this organism will have a specific structure and mode of life significant of its origin. It is of these—the general structure, composition, and life of cancerous growths—that I shall now speak.

It may be generally held that the characteristic structures of a cancer are altogether of new formation. But questions are often raised whether natural structures may not be transformed into cancerous; or, whether cancerous materials may not be simply transferred from the blood into the natural textures; or, whether natural structures can assume cancerous properties. I believe such questions may be thus answered:—

(1.) It is not probable that any structure, once completely formed, can be transformed into any other. Structures may change by degeneration; but in this their changes are as limited and as normal as in development. The instances in which natural or other structures are supposed to become cancerous are, chiefly, those in which new-formed cancer-structures are inserted or infiltrated among, or, sometimes, within, those of the affected part. Of such cases we may say that the part becomes the seat of cancer; not that it becomes cancerous.

(2.) It is possible that, in the mutation of structures effected in the nutrition of certain parts, the elemental structures successively formed may gradually assume the appearance and properties of those of cancer. It has often been observed, in cases of cancer of the liver, that every gradation of structure appears, from the natural to the cancerous; and that, among the microscopic structures, are many of which it is hard to say whether they be hepatic cells or cancer-cells. It may be that this only exemplifies the tendency of cancer-structures to be conformed, in some measure, to those of the adjacent natural parts; but it may also be, that both the fact and this well-known tendency are evidences that cancerous properties may be gradually imparted to the undeveloped blastema in a part, so that the elementary structures successively formed from it may gradually assume more of the characters of cancer. In other words. as in inflammations we observe the wider deviations from the normal methods of nutrition or secretion, the larger the proportions are in which the inflammatory exudation is mingled with the normal products of the part (page 223); so, it may be, increasing quantities of cancerous material, added to natural blastema, may be represented by successive gradations of structure. I cannot doubt that transformation into cancer is, in this sense, possible; but its occurrence is not to be assumed as frequent, and is, probably, limited to such organs as the liver, whose elementary structures are of the same general type as those of cancer, and are, in the ordinary process of secretion or nutrition, quickly changed.

(3.) It is possible that undeveloped cancer-material may be separated from the blood, with the materials of natural excretory organs, and may be for a time incorporated with the transient structures of such organs. We may assume this from the analogy of the cases in which we believe that other specific morbid materials are thus eliminated from the blood, as well as of the cases in which certain materials, which should be separated from the blood by appropriate organs, are, when the office of those organs is hindered, vicariously eliminated by others. In both these cases we believe that alien materials are, for a time, incorporated in the structures of the eliminating glands, and then discharged; and it is, in like manner, possible that cancer-materials, though their ordinary tendency is to determine the formation of peculiar structures for their incorporation, may be incorporated in those of natural glands.

So far, then, as the gradual change accomplished in a succession of structures, or the introduction of cancer-materials into the clemental structures of excretory organs, can be called a transformation, the term is not chargeable with the absurdity which some impute to it. And the belief of the possible transference of cancer-material into some gland-structure is worth holding, for it encourages one of the few hopes of curing cancer that at present seem reasonable—the hope, namely, that means may be found by which the morbid substance, transformed or combined, may be constantly eliminated from the blood through the transient structures of some gland.

But these things are only possible: the unhappy rule is, that the natural consequence of the cancerous condition of the blood is, sooner or later, the formation of a cancer with specific structures and mode of life. Concerning these, it may suffice if I collect and comment upon the principal facts detailed in the foregoing lectures.

In general construction, cancers may be either infiltrations or separate masses: i. e. their elementary structures may be either commingled, and form one mass, with those of a certain portion of a natural part, or they may be collected unmixed in a mass round which the natural tissues are extended. In any case, the mass they form is a growing part; and herein is the ground for classing them with tumors, and for separating them from those results of disease, such as inflammatory products and tubercle, which may be increased, but probably not by their own power of growth. (See p. 319, &c.)

In both their likeness and their unlikeness to other tumors, cancers exemplify what is common among specific diseases, namely, that they take certain general characters of common diseases, and, as it were, stamp them with some specific mark. Syphilitic eruptions are known by some specific character, added to those which are common to other eruptions of the same group: each specific form of ulcer has its own, together with common, characters; so, cancers have many characters in common with other tumors, but specific characters are superadded. (See page 305.)

When, as in infiltrations, the cancer-structures are mingled with those of a natural part, the most frequent event is, that the growth of the cancer preponderates, and at length excludes that of the natural structures; so that, finally, the latter disappear, and a substitution (to use M. Lebert's term) of cancer, in the place of the natural tissues, is effected. But the reverse of this sometimes happens; instead of atrophy, hypertrophy ensues in the natural structures of the affected part; and within the same area both normal and abnormal structures grow excessively. Thus it is with the growths of bone that form skeletons of the medullary cancers, and with those of fibro-cellular and elastic tissues that extend into the exuberant epithelial cancers.

The cancerous substance may be found in a rudimental state, as an undeveloped blastema. Vogel, whom Virchow generally conforms,[*] describes it as a firm, compact, amorphous substance, like coagulated fibrine, which is rendered transparent by acetic acid, ammonia, and other caustic alkalies, and sometimes includes molecular granules, which consist of modified proteine or fat.

The developed cancer-structures, if we except the few cases in which they are fibrous or osseous (pp. 510, 615), may be generally described as formed of nucleated cells, or of such corpuscles as are rudimental of, or degenerate from, the nucleated cell. Herein, and in the fact that the corpuscles are neither imbedded in formed intercellular substance, nor orderly arranged, lies one of the characters by which cancers are distinguished from all other tumors, and from all natural parts. Their chief heterology, in respect of construction, is in this disorderly crowding of their elements; and I believe it is constant, unless when they imitate the plan of some adjacent natural gland-structure (pp. 538, 547).

We observe, in the large majority of cancers, two primary or founda-

* In his Archiv, B. i. p. 111.

tion-forms of cells, of which the respective types may be found in gland-cells, and in epithelial or epidermal cells. Of the former, we have examples in the ordinary cells of scirrhous and medullary cancers (pp. 496, 589); of the latter, in the ordinary epithelial cancer-cells (p. 578); and it is, perhaps, very significant of the meaning of cancer, that the forms which its structures are most prone to assume are after the pattern of those belonging to the natural structures, whose office is to separate whatever is refuse or abnormal from the blood.

I say, the cancer-cells are formed on the types of excretory gland-cells and epidermal-cells; yet, without deviating from the general type, they have special characters by which it is seldom difficult to distinguish them. The question is often asked,—What are the characters of the true cancer-cell? or, Has the microscope discovered any structure which is decisive of cancer, wherever it is found? The answers may be,—(1.) Where cells, such as are described at pp. 496 and 578, are found alone, or chiefly composing a tumor, we may be certain that the tumor is a cancer: we may, therefore, regard these as especially cancer-cells. (2.) When a tumor is composed, chiefly or alone, of corpuscles, such as the nuclei described at p. 538, or any others which we can trace as rudiments or degenerations of the cancer-cells, the diagnosis of cancer is not less certain: structures such as these are found composing none but cancerous tumors. But if the question be changed to,—Are there any cancers which are not formed of structures such as these?—the answer must be affirmative: for there are rare tumors which present the whole clinical history of cancers, and which should therefore be called by the same name, though they have not these peculiar cancer-structures, or have them in very subordinate quantity. I do not refer here to cancers of which all the structures are imperfect, or degenerate, or diseased; but to such as the fibrous cancers (p. 510), the osteoid (p. 615), and certain varieties of the medullary (p. 588 to 540).* These all deviate from the assumed specific cancer-structures; and two of these, the fibrous and osteoid, approximate to the characters of natural tissues.

Together with the disorderly construction, and the peculiar cell-forms, we may often observe, as characteristic of cancers, the multiformity of the structures composing their mass. It is not equalled, I think, by any tumors, unless they be the cartilaginous or the mixed glandular and cartilaginous (pp. 423, 440). The variety of forms appears due, in part, to the mingling of the perfect structures with such as are in various stages of development and degeneration; and, in part, to what seems like a disorderly overgrowth and endogenous increase in cells and their

* Some pathologists would exclude from the name of cancer all these tumors, and all which are not composed of the "specific" cancer-structures; but I feel sure that we shall do right if (when a choice must be made) we choose modes of life, rather than structures, for determining the affinities of morbid products, and for arranging them under generic names. As of all tumors, so, especially, of cancers, the true nature is to be apprehended only by studying them as living things. (Compare p. 320.)

contents. All these forms have been already described; but they may be thus enumerated and arranged :—(1.) The chief of those to be referred to incomplete development are the free nuclei, and abundant undeveloped liquid or other blastema (pp. 497, 537, 579.) (2.) The chief forms due to the degeneration are the transitions from cancer-cells or nuclei to granule-masses (p. 498, 578); the withering corpuscles with fatty degeneration found in the material like tubercle in cancers (pp. 498, 499, 556;) the calcareous deposits (p. 557); the abundant granular matter; and the occasionally mingled melanoid cells (p. 607). (3.) Overgrown or abnormally developed corpuscles are seen in the various extensions of cell-walls into angles and processes (pp. 497, 540, 578); and in the enlargement of free nuclei and their assumption of the characters of nucleated cells (pp. 497, 588, 579). (4.) The endogenous increase in cells is exemplified in all that is described of the brood-cells and laminated corpuscles of the epithelial and colloid cancers (pp. 579, 628).

It would be too tedious even to enumerate more forms than these of the component cancer-structures, and I need not again describe them. It is not their multiformity, so much as the existence of many of them in a single mass, that is generally characteristic of cancer.

Various as are these corpuscles of cancers, it is yet to be observed, that there is none so entirely different from those of normal structures, that we cannot point out among them its type or parallel. No observation since Müller's time has invalidated his demonstration of this principle. The experienced microscopist will, indeed, very rarely fail in the diagnosis of a cancer by its minute structures; but he only discriminates them as specific modifications of the nucleus, nucleated cell, endogenous cells and other forms of which the types are in natural parts; he finds among them no new type-forms.*

In like manner, the elemental cancer-structures show no method of growth or development which is without parallel in natural structures; they are formed and increased according to the same general laws as are observed in the normal rudimental structures; their peculiarities, in this regard, are chiefly in the seeming disorder that often prevails among them,—in the absence of an apparent singleness of design.

The abundance of cell-structures in cancers has suggested that they are lowly organized, and many consequences have been hence deduced. The terms "high" and "low" in relation to structures, are derived from very arbitrary estimates, and are too fallacious for any important deduction in pathology; still it may be observed, that among morbid products, cancers should stand high rather than low; for their elemental forms are on a level with those of natural excretory organs, and more developed than any but the best inflammatory lymph. If there were any corre-

* This is now sufficiently evident for all the simple cells and nuclei of cancer; and the more complex endogenous cells and developing nuclei find their parallels especially in cartilage, the preparatory structure of medulla, and the thyroid and similar glands. (See especialy, Rokitansky "Die Kropf," and "Ueber die Cyste;" and Virchow, in his Archiv, B. iii.)

spondence, such as has been assumed, between lowness of organization and malignancy, the ordinary croupous or corpuscular lymph should be a much worse material than cancer; but malignant properties, like malignant spirits, are not confined to the vilest forms.

The proper structures of cancer are supported and held together by fibrous, membranous, or other connective tissue, forming their "stroma." This stroma, as I have elsewhere described, is formed, in the case of cancerous infiltrations, by the natural fibrous or other tissues of the infiltrated part, which, in different cases, are either gradually reduced in quantity or increased. In these cases the stroma is no proper cancer-structure, and varies with the nature of the affected part (pp. 500, 535, 572). But in distinct, isolable, cancerous tumors, a stroma is formed appropriate to the cancer, and in many cases, with a different mode of growth—the dendritic mode (pp. 542, 622). Generally, however, it is only in its plan or construction that the stroma is peculiar; its tissues are simply membranous, or nucleated, or filamentous, or it may be osseous: they are not cancerous.* We see, therefore, in cancers thus formed, as well as in the cancerous infiltrations with overgrowth of the natural structures, the coincident growth of morbid and of normal tissues within the same area, and out of the same mixed materials.

With the stroma of cancers are their blood-vessels, among which we must again distinguish, as in the preceding paragraph, that some are the vessels of the affected part now involved in the cancerous infiltration, others are new formed. Concerning the changes which the first named may undergo in the growth of the cancer, we have, I believe, at present, no knowledge. They are not, as in tuberculous infiltrations, gradually destroyed or removed: rather, they seem to be increased; so that an injected scirrhous cancer of the breast (for example) often appears more vascular than the adjacent substance of the mammary gland, though, in the first instance, it had only the blood-vessels of the part of the gland which it occupies. No direct, observations, however, have shown the method of this increase.

The new-formed blood-vessels of the isolable cancers and the cancerous outgrowths extend from those of the adjacent parts. It is by some thought that they are formed as an isolated system of tubes in the cancer: I know no satisfactory evidence of this; and the associated theory of blood being formed in the substance of a cancer, and out of cancer-materials, seems to me wholly untenable. The method in which the new vessels extend into cancers has not yet been traced, but is probably not

* Exceptions to this statement must be made for certain fibrous and osteoid cancers, in which the fibrous and osseous tissue, if regarded as a stroma for the mingled cancer-cells, must be admitted as a proper cancer-structure: and for some cases of medullary cancer, in which a kind of stroma is described as formed of series of elongated cancer-cells.

It must be observed, also, that the line between infiltrations and isolable tumors is here, as elsewhere, somewhat artificially drawn. It is not to be denied that the latter may involve small portions of natural tissues, which may remain intersecting or partitioning their masses, and supplying a framework upon which their peculiar stroma may be constructed.

different from that observed in other new formations (pages 145, and 237). Neither has anything specific in their structure or method of arrangement been yet observed. The descriptions already given of them (pp. 533 and 623) will show that the blood-vessels of cancers do not differ from those of other abnormal growths, except in that, generally, their calibre is more than proportionate to the thickness or complexity of structure of their walls. Hence the term "colossal capillaries;" and hence, when the blood-vessels are abundant, the likeness to the simple vascular erectile tumors: but in neither of these respects are the vessels of cancer without parallel in those of natural parts; those of the placenta and of the cavernous erectile tissue might be their types.

Such are the component structures of cancers. We might hope that chemistry, carrying its analysis far beyond the reach of sight, would find in them something as different from natural compositions, as their mode of life is from that of any natural member of the body. But it has failed to do this; and the numerous analysis made since those of Müller have not materially added to his results.* In a general comparison, the cancers are distinguished by the predominance or exclusive existence of albuminous compounds, while in the non-cancerous tumors gelatinous compounds (or in the adipose tumors, the fatty) are the chief constituents. But there are large exceptions on both sides. The fibrous and osteoid cancers yield abundant gelatine; the albuminous sarcomata of Müller (including probably, many of the least developed proliferous cystic tumors, and the recurring fibroid tumors) are as albuminous as the typical cancers. It is probable, moreover, that the broad general difference between albuminous and gelatinous growths is not directly related to their respective properties, as malignant and innocent, but to their retaining or passing beyond the cell-form.

The want of a more definite result from chemical analysis is not to be ascribed to the absence of difference between cancerous and normal materials,—we may be nearly sure that they are chemically essentially distinct,—but, rather, to the fact that an exact analysis of cancer-structures is nearly impossible. That which would be given to a chemist for examination is not a pure cancer-material, but a mixture of it with the materials of blood, blood-vessels, connective tissue, and, in many cases, of the natural or degenerate structures of the part in which the cancer has been growing. Add to this, that, in every sample, the cancer-structures themselves are probably in all stages of development and degeneration; and the search for the essential chemical properties of cancer will surely seem as difficult as it would be to find those of muscle, or of bone, in the analysis of the whole of a foetal, or of a paralytic, limb.†

* The best of these analysis may be found in Lebert's Traité Pratique, p. 44, e. s.

† The case of the colloid material may seem not open to this objection; but the colloid is, probably, not a true cancer substance, but the product of disease in cancer.

42

In studying the life of a cancerous growth, we have always to consider it as adding to the conditions of disease which already existed, and which usually still continue; it is a new factor in an already complex morbid process. The formation of cancerous material in the blood does not cease because some is incorporated in a growth; the transformations of parts, making them apt for the allocation of cancer, do not cease because one part is occupied. In all the history of cancers, therefore, we have to study the continuation of those processes which I described, in the last lecture, as preceding the growth of the cancer, and which now (with rare exceptions) are concurrent with it, and increase with it.

Before the formation of a cancerous growth, we trace two distinct, though usually concurrent, processes : namely, that which leads to the cancerous condition of the blood, and that which makes certain parts fit to be seats of cancerous growths. When once a growth is formed, it introduces a third element of disease, without necessarily removing or diminishing either of those that preceded it. As a living part, the cancer, like any other tumor, has the power of self-maintenance and of growth, which power, though favored by the continued or increasing cancerous condition of the blood, is, probably, not dependent thereon. Also, in the results of its nutrition, the cancer reacts upon the blood, and through it influences the whole economy : and these influences are added to the cancerous diathesis or cachexia which is usually, at the same time and of itself, increasing.

The manifestations of life in a cancer may be divided (but it is too artificial a division to be followed far) into those which are progressive, and those which are retrogressive. The latter are traced in the various degenerations and diseases of its structures ; the former in its growth, extension and multiplication.

The chief characteristics of the growth of cancers are seen, in those that are infiltrated, in their invasion of all tissues, as if indifferently. Thus the scirrhous cancer of the breast, though limited for a time to the mammary gland, at length extends beyond it, and gradually occupies every surrounding part alike : thus the epithelial cancer extends from the integument of the lip to its muscles, glands and all deeper tissues, and thence to the gum and jaw : and thus the medullary cancer grows into and through the walls of blood-vessels and other canals, and extends, among their contents, along their cavities. Such reckless growth (if it may be so called) is scarcely known except in cancers. They supply, also, the instances of most rapid increase; but although they do this frequently enough to make rapid growth one of the diagnostic signs of cancers, yet the cases are far from rare in which the growth is very slow. Few diseases are more variable than cancers are in this respect. (Compare p. 502, 553, 598, 427.)

It has been assumed that the appearances of endogenous increase in certain cancer-cells are indicative of a peculiar inherent capacity of growth. But this is far from certain and is made improbable by the fact that the endogenous productions are most abundant in epithelial cancers, whose average rate of increase is least; and that those medullary cancers which have only free nuclei, or imperfect nucleated cells, are among those of most rapid growth. The rule is more nearly true, which these instances exemplify, that the rapidity of growth among cancers is inversely proportionate to the development of their elemental textures. But this finds exceptions in the very quickly increasing and multiplying fibrous and osteoid cancers.

Two things administer to the growth of a cancer; namely, (1) the continued formation of the specific material in the blood; and (2) the inherent power in the cancer, as a living part, to assimilate to itself the common or indifferent materials of the blood. The first of these maintains and augments, as it originated, the growth; the second effects an independent increase, like that of a non-cancerous tumor. The effect of the first is shown in the fact, that the rate of increase in cancers is, usually, proportionate to the indications of constitutional affection; the effect of the second is shown in the increase being accelerated by whatever augments the supply of blood to the seat of cancer (p. 516) and (if the facts be as I have stated them at p. 543), in the growth of cancers after inoculation.

In ordinary cases, both these conditions are engaged in the growth of cancer; but if the first fail, the second may suffice. The cancerous diathesis may cease, or be exhausted for a time, or sometimes even permanently; cancer material we may suppose, is no longer formed in the blood; yet the cancer may subsist and increase by its own power. It does so like any other tumor; especially like those which I mentioned (p. 329) as beginning during or after some general disease, but continuing to grow when that disease has ceased.

Now, in this state, the cancer is essentially a local disease, living upon the materials of blood restored to health, though capable, probably, of infecting that blood, and inducing secondary phenomena of extension and multiplication. It illustrates, in this state, a principle which we are too apt to forget: namely, that diseases of constitutional origin may become wholly local. The origin of local diseases in constitutional conditions has been well studied, and the necessity of constitutional treatment, in chronic as well as in acute diseases, has been rightly referred to the local affections being maintained by the continued morbid condition of the blood; but it has been less considered that, after the constitutional disease has ceased, the local one may, of itself, continue, and need local treatment. Such cases are very frequent. One often sees syphilitic ulcers, which, doubtless, had a constitutional origin, and were maintained by specific material in the blood, and would have needed specific treatment of the blood for their cure; but now, while retaining their specific forms, they are curable by local treatment alone. Just so it may be, though very rarely, with cancers. While the cancerous diathesis is suspended, they may subsist by their own powers of assimilation; and I believe the few credible cases of recovery after operation are to be referred to the chances which have led to the occasional removal of such as were thus localized.

The extension of cancers (so far as it may be distinguished from their growth) is that which takes place through lymphatic vessels to their glands. The number of cases in which lymphatics, filled with cancer, have been traced from the primary growth to the nearest glands, is sufficient to make it probable that the disease often thus extends continuously from the one to the other; and that it is thus, as Mr. Simon expresses it, transferred by " continuity of blastema." But, even when such tracts of cancer cannot be traced from the primary disease to that in the lymphatic glands, I think Mr. Simon's suggestion is very probably true— that the disease is one of the lymph, not of the parenchyma or vessels of the glands. We do not, indeed, yet know exactly the derivation of the lymph, nor what is its relation to the materials of the part from which it comes; but what we do know of it is consistent with the belief, that lymph, from a seat of specific disease, is likely to contain such of the materials of the disease as may either be carried to the blood, or may be organized in the lymph after the same plan as in their primary seat.

The characters of the secondary cancers thus formed in lymphatic glands are already described (pp. 503, 548, 583, &c.); and these general principles may be gathered concerning them.

(1.) The disease in the lymphatic glands usually repeats exactly that in the primary seat; the apparent differences between them depend only on the structures among which the cancerous elements are placed. But this rule is not without exceptions (p. 505, &c., as cited above).

(2.) The cancer in the glands seldom appears before that in the primary seat has made considerable progress. At a general rough estimate, it appears about midway in the course of the disease towards death. The delay is, perhaps, not to be explained, seeing that lymph is carried from the primary disease as well in its earlier as in its later stages.

(3.) While the disease in the glands makes progress, the primary disease usually keeps the lead which its earlier origin gives it. Occasionally, however, that in the glands so far surpasses it that we are in danger of overlooking the primary disease (page 504, &c.) I do not know how the fact can be explained; but it has its parallel in the occurrence of primary cancer in the glands that are usually secondarily diseased, and in the recurrence of cancers after operations in the glands, rather than in or near its primary seat.

(4.) The lymphatic glands usually become cancerous in direct succession from the primary disease to the thoracic duct. The extension is, generally, made slowly; in scirrhous and epithelial cancers the disease often remains long limited to the glands nearest to its primary seat; in nearly all cases, also, it is prone to increase in these proximate glands much more than in those more distant. Rarely, the secondary cancer appears in distant, rather than in proximate, glands; but in these cases it illustrates the multiplication, not the extension, of disease.

The multiplication or discontinuous increase of cancer may take place in the following ways:

(1.) The cancer-growth may multiply itself, from its primary seat, to a part not directly continuous, but in contact therewith. Thus Dr. Hodgkin and Dr. Budd relate cases of cancer in abdominal and pelvic viscera, with corresponding formations on the portion of parietal peritoneum, or other parts in contact with them; and thus there may be correspondence and contact of cancers on the two layers of pleura, or on the glans and prepuce.

(2.) The multiplication may take place on a surface not in contact, but continuous, with the primary seat; as in cases by Mr. Simon (l. c.), in which cancerous growths were found scattered along the tract of mucous membrane leading from primary cancers in the kidney and lung.

In both these cases, the multiplication of the cancers seems to be the result of simple transference of the materials from the primary to the secondary seat of growth: it is effected by a kind of inoculation. The materials of a cancer, whether in formed germs or liquid blastema, pass from its mass, and develope themselves, and grow, where they rest.

(3.) Cancers are multiplied in parts neither directly continuous, nor in contact with the primary seat. In some instances the parts are near, in others remote from, the primary disease.

When cancers are thus multiplied near their primary seat by "irradiation," we find them, as it were, springing up in an area which gradually widens, and of which the primary cancer is the centre. Thus it is with the tubercles in the skin and muscles near a scirrhous breast (p. 505); and with the secondary medullary, osteoid, and melanoid growths scattered round the main disease, but separated from it by intervals of healthy tissue (p. 611, 614).

I do not know that we can explain this mode of increase of cancers otherwise than by reference to the seeming tendency of specific diseases to be allocated, not only in certain tissues or organs, but in certain places or regions (see p. 545). Certainly, peculiarities of tissue have little to do with this grouping of the cancers around the primary formation; for they may be found, promiscuously, in all the surrounding tissues within a certain area. Neither does the course of lymphatic or other vessels seem to determine their places.

In the increase of cancers by multiplications distant from the primary growth, there is scarcely an organ that may not be affected. We see this most easily in the cases of melanoid cancers; yet their multiplicity is probably not greater than that of other medullary cancers (see p. 611). The cancers that thus least frequently multiply are the epithelial and colloid, and those, of whatever kind, in the rectum, urinary organs, uterus, and brain. The organs in which the secondary cancers formed by multiplication are most frequently found are the lungs and liver; the latter, especially, in cases of cancer of the abdominal viscera; the former, especially, in those of the breast, limbs, and other parts whose blood passes to the venæ cavæ. After the lungs and liver, the most frequent seats of such secondary cancers are, I believe, the pleura, bones, lymphatic glands, and subcutaneous tissue; after these, no rule or proportion can be stated, except that many of the organs in which primary cancers are most frequent, are very rarely the seat of secondary cancer; e. g. the breast, uterus, testicle, and stomach.*

At present, probably, none but a very general explanation of this multiplication of cancers can be given: we can scarcely venture to guess what determines the above-mentioned peculiarities. The general explanation may refer the multiplication to two sources, which are independent, though concurrent and mutually influential; namely, the increasing cancerous diathesis or morbid condition of the blood, and the conveyance and transplantation of cancerous matter by the circulating blood.

The constant increase of the morbid condition of the blood was shown, in the last lecture, to be a general fact in the history of cancers. And, although it may sometimes be represented only by the accelerating growth of the primary tumor, yet we might well expect that it would often produce a numerical increase of cancers. The common indication of the most intensely constitutional cancerous disease is the simultaneous or rapid formation of numerous primary growths in different parts. This is sometimes witnessed at the very onset of the disease (pp. 548, 553); and it is, probably, also exemplified in the later period of ordinary cases. Certain cases scarcely admit of explanation, on the supposition that the first-formed cancer is, in any sense, the source of all that grow after it; such, for example, as those in which a sudden rapid multiplication of cancers takes place (p. 554), and those in which they appear some long time after the removal of the first-formed growth.

The second method of remote multiplication of cancers, that of conveyance by the blood, is sometimes visibly demonstrated, and may almost always be assumed. I have spoken of cases (p. 637) in which cancers so grow into veins, that we cannot doubt fragments may be washed from them by the blood, and may grow wherever they come to rest: and I related one instance of osteoid cancer in which this almost certainly occurred (p. 619). But, even where no such intra-vascular growths appear, similar events may occur. In a case of primary cancer of the liver, in which the growths were all tinted with bright yellow by the bile, I found numerous small cancerous masses of the same color infiltrated in the lungs; and the small branches of the pulmonary arteries leading to these were filled with bright-yellow substance, as if they had been minutely injected with chromate of lead. The accidental color of the cancer-materials, in this

* Lebert gives the best statistics on all these points (p. 81).

case, made their transference from the liver to the lungs very evident; but the same event is often, though less plainly, traceable.

The transference of cancer-materials, with the blood, from a cancer already formed, need not be always seen to be believed. Its frequent occurrence is made very probable by the many points of correspondence, which Dr. Walshe* has shown, between the dissemination of cancers, and that of secondary abscesses after the entry of pus or other degenerate inflammatory products into the veins. The peculiar liability of the liver and the lungs to be the seats of both these secondary diseases, and the evidence that they are the organs in which foreign matters, introduced into the circulation, are most commonly arrested, may nearly prove that they are, in all these cases alike, affected by materials brought to them in the blood.

We need not assume that corpuscles of pus or cancer, or any kind of germs already formed, must be thus carried for the multiplication or dissemination of disease. A rudimental liquid, an unformed cancerous blastema, mingled with the blood, may be as effectual as any germs; and must almost necessarily be assumed, in the explanation of cases in which the dissemination takes place, not in the lungs or liver, but in organs beyond them in the course of the circulation.

The materials conveyed with the blood from the primary cancer must be such as are capable of development, in order to the multiplication of the disease. In the ordinary absorptions occurring in the process of natural nutrition, and probably, also, in those that take place in the nutrition of cancers, the venous blood carries away only degenerate or refuse materials, such as we may assume would be incapable of development. I have mentioned cases (pp. 548, 558) in which masses of cancer, probably thus degenerate, were absorbed, without any appearance of consequent dissemination or other damage. We do not know what leads to the removal of such cancerous matter as can be developed; but the necessity of some change in the ordinary process of absorption is evident, and is the more worth studying, because there are corresponding similar differences in the effects of the absorption of pus and other morbid products.

Such are the various means of numerical increase of cancers—by local inoculation of parts continuous, or in contact with the primary disease; by extension, through a continuity of lymph, or of blastema, to the lymphatic glands; by transportation of potent cancer-materials with the venous blood; by the cancerous condition of the blood becoming, of itself, more intense. In certain cases the increase may be accomplished by all these means at once; the secondary cancers, also, as soon as formed, become like centres, from which a tertiary formation may be derived, as they were themselves derived from the primary; and to all this it may be added, that, with lapse of time and failing general health, all

* Nature and Treatment of Cancer, p. 106.

parts of the body are constantly becoming less resistant of disease, and more appropriate for the residence of morbid growths.

I have now to trace a general history of the retrogressive life of cancers; of that which, as I said (p. 658), is signified in their various degenerations and diseases.

The degenerations of cancer-structures are like those of natural parts, and of other products of disease. Examples may be cited of every form corresponding with those enumerated in pages (74 and 241). (1) The withering, or wasting and drying, of the structures is exemplified in many scirrhous and epithelial cancers (pp. 502, 578); (2) the fatty degeneration is so common that it might be hard to find a cancer, in some of whose corpuscles it does not exist. The granule-masses ("the mulberry-cells") of cancers are hence derived, as they are from many more morbid products. Hence, too, the "saponification" of cancers (p. 557); while to the fatty degeneration, combined with more or less of withering, we may ascribe the masses of substance, like tubercle, so often imbedded in medullary cancers (p. 532), and the minuter spots and lines of soft ochre or yellow substance traversing scirrhous and medullary cancers, like a "reticulum" (pp. 499, 556). (3) A calcareous degeneration is observed in medullary cancers, and in osteoid (pp. 557, 613, 617); and, probably, exists in many instances mingled with the fatty degeneration. (4) Pigmental degeneration is probably the essential character of melanoid cancers (p. 610). (5) Thickening of primary membrane is, perhaps, indicated in some of the cancer-cells whose walls appear simply laminated (p. 580, fig. 103 D). A liquefactive degeneration may occur in some of the softenings of cancers; but, so far as I know, it ensues only in connection with disease. (Compare pages 105, 266.)

In the interpretation of degeneracy in cancers, we must again refer to the two conditions of their life; namely, the maintenance of the morbid condition of the blood, and their inherent power of self-maintenance. The supervention of another diathesis may lead to the degeneration or death of a cancer (pp. 519, 558); but this is extremely rare. A transformation of diathesis may, I am disposed to believe, lead to the degeneration of one cancer, while it promotes the growth of one or more others; for there are cases of apparent metastasis of cancer, in which the primary disease has withered, while secondary growths appear to have increased.[*] But these cases, again, are too rare to be reasoned from; and the usual course of events indicates that degeneration of cancer is, in the great majority of cases, an essentially local thing. For, commonly, part of a cancer, or one mass in a group, degenerates, while growth continues in the rest; and extensive degeneration is often found, in cases in which the rapid progress of the disease has testified to the full maintenance of the morbid blood. Hence the unhappy rarity of the recovery from cancer. One that is degenerate or absorbed may be as ineffective for

* Cases cited by Walshe, pp. 110, 134.

harm as one that has been cut away; but the constitutional element and progress of the disease are as little affected by the natural as by the surgical process of removal.

We cannot tell what are the local events that lead to this degeneration; but I suspect that the chief of them is the local obstruction of blood-vessels by growths of cancer into them.

The diseases of cancers, like the degenerations, are essentially local processes; they are most apt, indeed, to occur in the enfeebled general health, but they do not certainly indicate a decreased diathesis. It may suffice to refer, for examples of most of the diseases, to those already cited (pp. 517, 557, &c.); but two require more consideration; namely, softening and ulceration.

Some have believed that softening is almost a natural event in cancers, a change parallel with that in tuberculous deposits, and a necessary precedent of ulceration; while others, recoiling from the error of this belief, have written of the softening of cancers as a rare and unimportant accident. The truth is about midway between these extremes. There is no probability that (as some have supposed) the hard scirrhous cancers ever become medullary by any process of softening; a softened cancer is very different from a soft one. There is no natural tendency in cancers to become soft in their later stages: those of the oldest date commonly retain, if they do not increase, their original consistence. Neither is softening a necessary precursor of the ulceration of cancers. But any scirrhous or other cancer may be softened by degeneration, or, more effectually and extensively, by inflammation of its substance. The fatty degenerations of which I have just been speaking are usually attended with a softening; but the altered substance becomes drier and more greasy than before; it does not appear, in any degree, liquefied (p. 499). That which is generally understood as softening of cancer is, so far as I have seen, a more acute process, and the result of inflammation of its substance. One may see it very well in the exposed protruding growths of medullary cancers (p. 557); or in those parts of them which lie just beneath inflamed portions of the integuments. Sometimes, also, within scirrhous cancers that have rapidly enlarged, with heat and pain, and redness of the superjacent skin, one finds large portions liquid, or else very soft, as it were rotten, shreddy, and infiltrated with pale, yellow, serous, or puriform fluid. Sometimes such softening has distinct appearance of suppuration in the centre of the cancer; but these cases (which have suggested the terms cancerous suppuration or abscess) are, I think, most frequent in the secondary epithelial and medullary cancerous affections of lymphatic glands (pp. 559, 584).

If, as I believe, these softenings of cancer are the results of inflammation, they correspond with the softenings produced by the same disease in natural parts (page 258); they are the results of such defective nutrition as always ensues in the proper textures of an inflamed part; and when pus is diffused in the softened cancer-substance, the process may be compared with ordinary purulent infiltration, which is always attended with loss of consistence in the affected part. With this view the microscopic characters of the softened cancers agree.

Such softening as this, taking place within a cancer, generally leads to ulceration, and to the discharge of liquefied and degenerate materials, with whatever of serum, or pus, or blood may have been mingled with them. This discharge is essentially similar to the opening of an abscess; but it is less regular, and the ulceration is quickly more destructive, and exposes widely the cancerous walls of the evacuated cavity.

I have already described both this and the other forms of ulceration that may ensue in cancers (pp. 517, 555, 575). They are all, like the degenerations, essentially local processes, and not indicative of any peculiar advance or transformation of the cancerous diathesis. Ulceration is, indeed, a feature of the later progress of cancer, and it is most likely to occur in those whose health is most enfeebled; it is, therefore, often coincident with an exceeding intensity of constitutional disease; but it is not the consequence of such intensity. The amount of constitutional disease is indicated by the growth, or by the multiplication, of cancers rather than by anything which, like ulceration, implies imperfect maintenance of their structures; and so we commonly see one part of a cancer growing rapidly, while another is being destroyed by ulceration, or many growing while one is ulcerating. Now the growth is, generally, the measure of the force of the constitutional disease; the ulceration is the measure of the local defect of nutrition: and in these instances we may watch, at once, both the progressive and the retrogressive phenomena of the life of the cancer.

While dwelling on the constitutional origin of cancerous growths, I must not forget their constitutional effects—the changes in the blood and other parts, which are their consequences.

I said that a cancer adds a new element of disease to those that were already in progress. And this may be said of it in consideration both of its own life, and of the influence which its growth and changes have upon the whole economy. If we assume a constant process of nutrition in cancers, it cannot but be that the blood will be affected both by what they take from it, and by what it derives from them in the process of nutritive absorption. This latter source of change of the blood has been too little considered,—the former, perhaps, too much; for the quantity of good nutrient material abstracted from the blood, in the growth of a cancer, is probably very trivial, whereas what returns to the blood is almost necessarily a morbid substance. It may be incapable of development into cancer, but, unless it can be at once eliminated, it must injuriously affect the blood. What change it works we cannot tell; nor can we tell more of the later changes produced when complete cancerous material is absorbed into the blood, or when secondary cancers multiply in important organs, hindering their functions; or when ulceration ensues with pain, hemorrhage, discharge, hectic, and all the various signs of ruined health. When these things are added to the still increasing cancerous condition of the blood, and when all, with mutual influence, are in progress, they make a state so complex that analysis seems impossible, and so various that no single or general description can be true. The general result is what is commonly called the cancerous cachexia ; but (as I have said before) it should be called the secondary cachexia, to distinguish it from the primary, which may precede the formation of a cancerous growth, or, in its independent increase, may far exceed the probable consequences of the local disease (pp. 523, 560).

The constituents of the secondary cancerous cachexia, I say, are too numerous and complicated for analysis ; still we must always recognize, in the later stages of the disease, the double source of the morbid phenomena ; namely, the progressive constitutional disease, and the effects, direct or indirect, of the local disease. How nearly independent the former is of the latter is proved by the results of removing the local disease. The secondary cachexia and many of its components may be, for a time, decreased ; pain and discharge, and all the local accidents of the disease, may cease ; but the average lengthening of life is very trivial (pp. 525, 561, 600). The fact proves, not only that the progress of the peculiar constitutional part of the disease is nearly independent of the local part, but, also, that the constitutional part generally contributes most to the fatal issue. However, in this, as well as in the times and manners of dying, and the times of recurrence after removal of the first growths, the differences in the several forms of cancer are such as should not be put out of sight by a general or summary description : death is the common, and almost constant end of all, but its circumstances should be studied separately in each.

In conclusion, let me add a few words respecting the nosological relations of the several forms of cancer to one another and to other diseases.

Here, as everywhere in pathology, it is difficult to keep the just mean of classification ; to avoid, on the one side, confusion ; on the other, too rigid circumscription. The many features of resemblance in all the forms of cancer, and the large general history which may be truly written of them, might lead us to merge all minor distinctions, and speak as of a single and uniform disease ; but it would be easy to show that, if in this view we write of the general symptoms, progress, and diagnosis of cancer, or of the history of cancers in any single organ, we write vaguely, and are obliged to omit many points of importance, for fear of contradictions. If, on the other hand, we look at contrasts rather than likenesses, we might be induced to separate some forms, as the epithelial and colloid, from the name of cancer, and to believe that the remaining forms have no affinity with any other disease.

I suspect that the errors of such extremes as these (in all nosology, as well as in that of cancers) come from our attaching too much meaning to the terms that imply specific distinctions among diseases ; from our proneness to think of them as if they meant the same as they do in zoology. Now, there is no real correspondence between the two sets of terms. A specific name, in zoology, usually implies that all to whom it is given have origin from a common stock; certain characters fixed, and not changeable, beyond certain narrow limits, by variety of external circumstances; and circumscription, *i. e.* intervals of difference between them and other species, which intervals are not filled up by varieties or intermediate forms. Now in all pathology there are, probably, no such species as these; and the terms implying the existence of genera, species and varieties of disease, mean only that the products of diseases may be arranged, and the diseases themselves considered, in larger and smaller groups, according to the number and importance of the characters which they have in common. Such terms do not mean that the borders of each group of diseases are naturally circumscribed; they allow that the borders of each are confused with those of every adjacent group.

With this meaning, I have adopted the words used in the foregoing lectures. The whole group of diseases included under the name (used like a generic name) of Cancer or Carcinoma are sufficiently distinguished by the concurrence in them of all the characters of malignant tumors enumerated in the twenty-first lecture (p. 324–329). But this group is not circumscribed; its borders are everywhere overlapped by those of diseases to which other names are given: there are no one or two characters pathognomonic of cancer, and found in it exclusively. The foregoing lectures have repeatedly illustrated this, especially in the accounts of the recurring proliferous cysts (p. 364), the malignant fibrous tumors (p. 409), the recurring fibroid and fibro-nucleated (p. 412), certain cartilaginous tumors (pp. 432, 443), some of the myeloid (p. 451) and mammary glandular (p. 474), and the rodent ulcers (p. 588). At the same time, this want of definition in the assumed genus of Cancers has been exemplified. it will be observed, chiefly by rare and exceptional cases; all the general facts collected in the lectures have illustrated the sufficiency of the concurrent signs of cancer for a ground of general classification (see p. 328).

Among the different forms of cancer, I have already said (p. 605) that there appear to be unequal degrees of difference, which may be expressed by speaking of three forms—namely, the scirrhous, medullary, and epithelial—as species, and of the remainder as varieties, of cancer. All that has just been said of the want of circumscription for the so-called genus will, I need hardly say, be applicable to these smaller groups. But here is the chief point, at which, while avoiding too much precision, we must also guard against indifference; for, as it has been wisely said, truth is more likely to emerge from error than from confusion. The species and varieties of cancer, as of other diseases, do not correspond with those of living creatures; yet the differences of the groups thus named are inconsistent with the theory of a single unchanging disease: and I believe the future study of the grounds of these differences will prove very fruitful both in knowledge and in practical utility.

As yet we can only speculate on them in questions. Do they imply so many essentially and originally different morbid materials? or is there one material for cancer, one carcinogen, which, like an organic radical, may form different, yet closely allied compounds, in its combinations with the various substances provided by different bloods, or different parts? Is not this hypothesis more appropriate than the first for the less usual phenomena of transformation, such as I have described as occurring in the progress, succession, and hereditary transmission of the cancerous constitution? Is it inconsistent with the gradual fusion of the characters of typical cancer in those of other diseases?

LECTURE XXXV.

TUBERCLE.

One often speaks of cancerous and other tubercles, meaning only small knots or knotted masses of the specified morbid growth; and of tubercular cutaneous eruptions, meaning small circumscribed flattened elevations or thickenings of the cutis. But when "tubercles," without any specific designation, are spoken of, the word is always understood to refer to little masses of a peculiar product of disease, the type of which is found in the lungs as the essential anatomical constituent of pulmonary consumption or phthisis. The same material as composes the pulmonary tubercles is found in many different forms and organs, and, wherever it occurs, is described as "tubercle," or "tuberculous matter;" and "tuberculous disease," or "tuberculosis," is the usual designation of the specific diseases, of which the essential feature is the production of this peculiar matter.

Tubercle or tuberculous matter may be formed in distinct isolable masses, round which the adjacent tissues are extended. These, which are most frequent in the brain, and, I believe, in the subcutaneous tissue, may be like tumors, except in that they are not vascular, and, probably, have no inherent capacity of increase. But the most frequent formations of tuberculous matter are in infiltrations of the natural tissues, which infiltrations may be circumscribed, having definite, though generally irregular, outlines, or diffuse, i. e. wide-spread and indefinite.*

In the lungs (to which, on account of its exceeding frequency, we are bound to look for its type) tuberculous matter appears, as Rokitansky says, in two chief varieties, or in forms combining, or intermediate between them. These are generally distinguished as the "gray" and the

* The name, tuberculous infiltration, is commonly given to this diffuse form alone; but in the miliary and other tubercles, even in the lungs, the peculiar materials are equally infiltrated among the natural tissues; only, in these the infiltration occupies a defined area.

"yellow" tubercles; or the gray tuberculous granulations, and the crude tubercles. It may also appear as a diffuse tuberculous infiltration, either alone, or, more frequently, associated with the preceding forms, or the changes consequent on them.

The gray tubercles appear as masses about as large, on an average, as millet-seeds (whence their name of milliary tubercles), imbedded in the substance of the lungs. They are usually from a quarter of a line to a line in diameter; and when the lung is cut through, so that its elastic tissue can recoil and subside, they appear slightly raised on its cut surface, and the finger may feel them as little firm resisting bodies set in the lung. They look round or oval; but their borders are very irregular, with short outrunning processes. They are gray, semi-transparent, and moderately bright; or, sometimes are very glistening, with a greenish-gray "cat's-eye" tint. In the latter case, they may look like little vesicles; but they are always solid. They may be discrete, i. e. placed singly, and with distinct, though small, intervals in the lung, or collected in groups. They occupy and involve in their substance the tissues of the lung, and are so connected, that portions of these tissues always adhere to them when we try to separate them. They may be easily broken or crushed, and, when thus treated, they yield but little fluid.

The yellow tubercles in the lungs have the same general forms and relations as the preceding, but are commonly larger and less firm, and are more often grouped so closely that, by fusion, they make up nearly uniform tubercular masses half an inch or more in diameter. They are usually pale yellow, or, yellowish-white, opaque, friable, dry, cheesy, smearing the surface on which they are crushed. Very often, their color is varied with a smoky gray tint, partly due to intrinsic change, and partly derived from the pigment of the lung involved by them.

It has been generally considered that the two varieties of pulmonary tubercle here described represent two stages of the same disease; the gray substance being, after a time, changed into yellow. Rokitansky, however, holds that they are always different substances; and that, though they may be found, side by side, in the same lung, or may be mingled even in the same tubercle, yet the transformation of the gray into the yellow substance never takes place. His names of "simple fibrinous" applied to the gray tubercle, and "croupo-fibrinous" to the yellow, may imply that both the differences and the affinities between the two forms are comparable with those between the two chief varieties of inflammatory lymph (p. 217, &c.).

The minute structures of both the forms of tubercle are essentially similar; and their distinctive characters-(in the state in which they appear to persist longest) are, the absence of blood-vessels (except of such as are involved in the deposit and not yet wasted), and the defectively developed or aborted state of the blastema and the corpuscles.

The blastema, or basis-substance of a tubercle appears, usually, a fragments or flakes of a moderately firm, clear, or dimly molecular substance, swelling and made clearer by acetic acid. It is most abundant in the gray tubercle, most molecular or dotted in the yellow. It has no filamentous appearance, no trace of developing nuclei or fibres.

The corpuscles held together by this substance are (a) abundant minutest molecules, granules, and oil particles of various but usually small size: all these being extremely predominant in the yellow tubercle; (b) nuclei or cytoblasts, of various shapes and apparent structure, but all degenerate or defective; some glittering, hard-edged, wrinkled, and withered; others granular, few or none with distinct nucleoli; (c) nucleated cells, similarly misshapen, withered, or granular; (d) certain compound cells described on the next page.

Mingled with these, and varying according to the situation and circumstances of the tubercles, numerous other, but accidental, substances are often found; namely, (a) the involving and disintegrating structures of the lung; membrane or elastic fibres, degenerate epithelial cells of the air-vesicles or minute bronchi; (b) various and usually degenerate products of inflammation from the adjacent parts, granule-cells and masses, pus-cells, &c.: (c) molecules of calcareous matter, or of pigment, and crystals, especially of cholestearine.

Such are the ordinary constituents of pulmonary tubercle, and the shriveled nuclei and imperfect cells, being usually the most abundant and distinct, are called tubercle-corpuscles. Similar materials are found composing the tuberculous matter in other parts. In the lungs, according to Virchow* and Schroeder van der Kolk,† their origin may, in an earlier stage, be traced in changes of the epithelial cells of the air-vesicles.

Fig. 115.‡

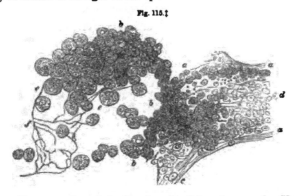

The adjacent copies of the drawings by Schroeder van der Kolk may, with his description of them, suffice to explain the process.

* Würzburg Verhandlungen, i. 81.

† Over den Oorsprong en de Vorming van Tubercula Pulmonum: Nederlandsch Lancet, 1852.

‡ Fig. 115. Very thin section of a portion of tuberculous lung, described in the text. Magnified 420 times.

The margin of an air-vesicle, from which most of the tubercle-cells are removed, is shown at *a a a ;* that of another adjacent vesicle, nearly filled with tubercle-cells, at *b b b ;* and that of a portion of a third vesicle, clear of tubercle-cells, at *c.*   At *d* the still unaffected wall of the air-vesicle is shown covered with epithelial cells of various sizes and containing nuclei, oil-drops, and granular matter.   In the middle and at the end of the same vesicle are some cells of darker tint; they are no longer flat, but filled with some material, and thereby more or less swollen and spherical; they are epithelial cells more or less distended with fluid, and detached, and, as the series of them shows, they constantly enlarge.   In the next vesicle, *b*, these cells have become much larger, and more closely adherent. It is observable that the largest cells commonly lie in the middle of the cavity of the air-cell: the larger are mostly filled with many nuclei; in the smaller there is but one.''

"It is thus evident, that these cells, which fill the air-vesicles and make up the tubercles, are nothing else than epithelial cells, which swell by imbibition of plastic matter, enlarge, and are detached from the wall of the air-vesicle.   The cells which are placed in the middle of the vesicle are, thus, the oldest, *i. e.* the first removed from the walls, the longest

Fig. 116.*

exposed to the influence of the surrounding fluid, and therefore the largest.†   They are all filled with granular matter and minute oil-spherules, and in the larger, an increase of nuclei has taken place.

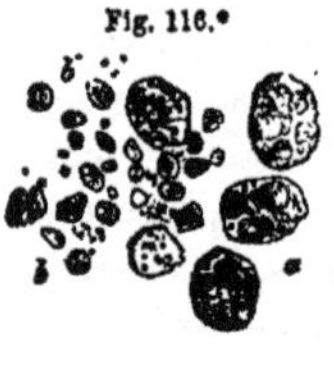

"If tubercles be examined in a somewhat further advanced stage, when they show more tendency to softening, the larger cells just described are found in much less quantity, and in place of them the air-vesicle is filled with smaller cells [and nuclei].   Among these, however, some smaller cells appear (as in fig. 116, *a*), containing smaller cells or nuclei, which are completely like those that are free (*bb*); so that there can be no doubt but that, in this state, the larger corpuscles are dissolved or burst, and the smaller ones set free."   These smaller cells and nuclei set free are what have been generally described as the tubercle-corpuscles; and, as I have already said, the tuberculous deposits, after the earliest periods of their formation, may appear to contain no other formed corpuscles besides them.

Now the most peculiar character of tuberculous matter which these descriptions illustrate, is its early degeneration, its abortiveness; it is shown as a material which, after proceeding for a little way in the acquirement of organic structure, then stops in its course, recedes and degenerates.   This is evident, at once, in the shriveled or granular state

---

* Fig. 116. Tubercle-corpuscles: magnified 420 times and described in the text. Copied from Schroeder van der Kolk.

† In the College Museum, No. 297, is the lung of a Benturong (Arctictis Benturong), which shows, apparently very well, this progressive accumulation of tuberculous matter from the walls to the centres of the air-cells.

of the set-free nuclei and cells; and the latter changes are still further degenerative; all prove tuberculous matter to be not only very lowly developed but generally incapable of development.*

These latter changes may be again illustrated by the examples of pulmonary tubercles, and, according to Rokitansky, may, like the differences of the original deposits, be compared with the degenerations of the fibrinous and corpuscular or croupous varieties of inflammatory lymph (pp. 242, 245).

(a) The withering (obsolescence, or Verhornung of Rokitansky) is the peculiar degeneration of the gray tubercle in the lungs. It loses, herein, its lustre, becomes dry, dense, and hard, and shrivels into a shapeless, or indistinctly fibrous, little mass. The change is sometimes associated with a calcareous degeneration of the tubercles, and often with corresponding changes in the part of the lung in which they are imbedded, and which becomes dry, shriveled, and dark with pigment.

(b) The calcification, or calcareous degeneration, occurs in the yellow, and in the mixed, forms of tuberculous matter. When achieved, it may be taken as an indication, like the withering of the gray form, that the tubercles are not longer subject to change; that they are, generally, obsolete, and without influence on the tissues around them. It may occur both in recent yellow tubercles, and in such as are already softened; it is exactly comparable with the calcareous degeneration of inflammatory lymph and pus, and is usually associated with withering and pigmental degeneration of the surrounding substance of the lung.

(c) The softening or liquefaction of tuberculous matter is, also, observed only in the yellow and mixed forms. Though more studied in tubercle than in any other morbid product, it is not peculiar to it, but is probably analogous with many other liquefactive degenerations, and may be in all points compared with that of inflammatory lymph (p. 242). It constitutes the so-called tuberculous suppuration, and precedes the formation of tuberculous ulcers and cavities.

The process of softening usually commences at or near the centre of the tuberculous mass; in the part of it which, we may believe, being most remote from blood, is least able to maintain itself in even such low development as it may have reached. The central softening is that which is spontaneous and normal in a tubercle: it may be regarded as a natural degeneration of the morbid substance; but any collection of tuber-

---

* An exception to this statement must be made, for certain cases, in which one part of what seems to be a uniform exudation is developed into, or towards, false membrane, and another part passes through the degenerative changes of tubercle. Such an event may be seen, according to Rokitansky (p. 263), in the tuberculous disease of the peritoneum and other serous membranes, and is due, he says, to a mixture of the tuberculous exudation, and of that of ordinary inflammation. Schroeder van der Kolk represents (as in fig. 115, b), filaments of rudimental new-formed tissue, which, he says, are sometimes found among the cells of pulmonary tubercle. In tuberculosis peritonitis, the portion of material developed into false membrane may become vascular, and may make a seeming, though not a real, exception to the rule of the non-vascularity of tuberculous matter.

43

culous matter may always be softened, at its periphery, by the mingling of liquid products of inflammation in the adjacent tissues. The two processes of softening may appear similar, and may coincide, but they are essentially distinct : one is spontaneous, the other accidental ; in the one the liquid material is the very substance of the tubercle, in the other it is derived from without.

In the proper softening of a tubercle one sees its central part become, first, soft, so that, when cut across, it looks cracked and crumbling, and may be pressed away from the surrounding firmer part, leaving a little central cavity. In further stage of the degeneration, it becomes liquid, like thin pus, with flakes or grumous particles in a pale yellowish turbid fluid ; and as the change makes progress, the whole tuberculous mass may be reduced to the same liquid state.*

The liquefied tuberculous matter consists of the lowest of the corpuscular materials already enumerated (p. 671); but they float now in a liquid containing more abundant molecules and particles of oily and calcareous matter. The usual sequence of the liquefaction is the discharge of the liquid, by ulceration of the tissues enclosing it ; but if the liquid be retained, it may undergo further changes, which may be compared with those of the retained contents of chronic abscesses (page 254). The chief are, that its fluid parts are gradually absorbed, and its fatty and calcareous matters increase, till it becomes a dry, greasy, crumbling, or gradually hardening, mortar-like concretion.

The discharge of a quantity of liquefied tuberculous matter, by ulceration through an adjacent bronchus, or through the integuments of a subcutaneous tuberculous lymphatic gland (for example), leaves a cavity, vomica, or abscess ; when the discharge takes place from single small tubercles, such as form beneath the surface of the mucous membrane of the intestinal canal, an ulcer remains ; and these are, severally, sufficiently peculiar in their characters to be known as the tuberculous cavity, and tuberculous ulcer.

The ulceration effecting the discharge is usually the consequence of inflammation in the tissues over the tuberculous matter, and resembles that for the discharge of common pus. By similar inflammatory ulceration of its boundaries, the tuberculous cavity or ulcer may be enlarged: but more generally, and more normally, its enlargement is due to the formation and discharge of fresh tuberculous deposits adjacent to it. This may be best seen in tuberculous ulcers of the intestines ; but the same process occurs at the cavities in such parts as the lungs and lymphatic glands. At the borders and bases of the cavity or ulcer one may often find small secondary tubercles, which, following the same course as the primary, liquefy, and are discharged into the cavity, or on the surface of the ulcer, which they thus increase by adding their cavities to it.

* Such changes may be seen better, I think, in the tubercles in the spleen than in those in any other part: Mus. St. Bartholomew's, Ser. xxii. 2, 3.

Other tubercles, again, may succeed to these and pass through the same changes; and when many cavities and ulcers are thus simultaneously enlarging they come into collision, and two or more are fused into one of sometimes vast dimensions.

In these changes, the tissue involved in the tuberculous deposits (whether primary or later) soften, and are disintegrated and discharged with them. There is thus, always a loss of substance in the affected part, coextensive with the tuberculous cavity. But, the bordering tissues, if not tuberculous, may be infiltrated with organizable inflammatory lymph, which, in its development, may form a tough boundary to the cavity or ulcer, and, if fresh tuberculous matter be not deposited in it, may lead to complete healing.

Before illustrating the foregoing general account of tuberculous matter, and of its principal changes, by some of the instances which are chiefly interesting in surgical pathology, it may be well to speak of some affections which have an apparent or real affinity with it.

Degenerative changes, similar to those which ensue in the lowly developed materials of tubercle, may produce a similar appearance in other materials; especially in those which consist of cells, or rudiments of cells. Thus, it is common to find, in medullary cancers, and more rarely in others, portions of yellow, half-dry, crumbling, and cheesy substance, so like tubercle that, with the naked eye, they can hardly be distinguished from it. The cancers in which they occur have been described as mixtures of cancerous and tuberculous matters; but the microscope finds that the tuberculoid, or, as M. Lebert calls it, the phymatoid, material in them consists of cancer-corpuscles, withered, with fatty and calcareous degeneration, and mingled with molecular and granular matter. By similar degeneration, material like tubercles may be found in cartilaginous, rudimental fibro-cellular, and probably other, tumors. In all these instances, the microscope may usually insure a just diagnosis, and may prove that the tuberculous appearance is only due to a withering and a fatty degeneration of materials that have nothing but their degeneration in common with true tuberculous matter.*

Greater difficulty of diagnosis exists when, through similar degeneration, inflammatory lymph assumes the appearance of tuberculous matter. It does so, sometimes, in chronic inflammation, or, when acute inflammation has subsided, in lymphatic glands, in the testicle, and, I believe, in some other parts. So, too, if the pus of chronic abscesses or other suppurations is not discharged, it may gradually dry; and as its corpuscles

* Virchow (Würzburg Abhandl. B. i. ii. iii.) had proposed to speak of the change, in all these cases, as a "tubercular metamorphosis," or "tuberculisation," and was, of course, misunderstood as if he had implied that every material may become tuberculous matter. He suggests, now, that the change by which so many essentially different things may become "cheesy," should be called, "the cheesy metamorphose."

wither, with fatty and calcareous degeneration, it may assume an appearance very like that of tuberculous matter. And, in all these cases,
the resemblance may extend equally to the microscopic characters; so
that there are, I believe, no signs by which degenerate lymph or pus
may be, in all cases, distinguished from ordinary tuberculous matter.
When, as in the cases cited in Lecture XIV., p. 245, the lymph-cells
have been developed and elongated before their degeneration, they may
be known from any corpuscles of tubercle; and the many nucleated
cells in tuberculous disease may be distinguished from the ordinary products of inflammation; but neither of these forms may exist, and then
I believe that a distinction of degenerate lymph from tubercle may be
impossible. Certainly, it is often very difficult to say whether the yellow,
dry, and cheesy material, found in chronic enlargements or suppurations
of lymphatic glands, should be regarded as tuberculous matter, or as
withered and degenerate lymph or pus, produced by inflammation. The
same difficulty may exist in the similar affections of the testicles; but in
these, more than in the case of the lymphatic glands, we may be extremely doubtful of any material being really tuberculous, if it be found
in them alone, and not at the same time in other parts of the genital
apparatus, or in the lungs. Similar difficulties may exist in the diagnosis
between tubercle and some instances of chronic pneumonia.*

Thus, then, there are not a few cases in which materials like those of
tubercles are found as results of diseases that are not tuberculous; i. e.
that are neither coincident with, nor according to the type of, tuberculous disease in the lungs. And the difficulty hence arising is increased
by this; that both tuberculous products, and the varieties of degenerate
and withered lymph and pus, are especially frequent among persons of
the "scrofulous" or "strumous" constitution; so that the degenerate
lymph and pus are often described as "scrofulous matter;" and "scrofula" and "tuberculous disease" are often regarded as the same disease.

It is, I fear, impossible to clear the confusion arising from the inter-
changing uses of these terms, or to define exactly the cases to which they
should severally be applied; but where definition of terms is impossible,
the next best thing is an understanding of their meaning according to
general usage. "Scrofula" or "struma," then, is generally understood
as a state of constitution distinguished, in some measure, by peculiarities
of appearance even during health, but much more by peculiar liability to
certain diseases, including pulmonary phthisis. The chief of these "scrofulous" diseases are various swellings of lymphatic glands arising from
causes which would be inadequate to produce them in ordinary healthy
persons. The swellings are due, sometimes, to mere enlargement, as from
an increase of natural structure; sometimes to chronic inflammation:

* Virchow has written fully on this point; and a clear statement of his and others
opinions, respecting the different forms of pulmonary phthisis, is given by Dr. Jenner in
the Br. and For. Med. Chir. Review, Jan. 1853.

sometimes to more acute inflammation, or abscess; sometimes to tuberculous disease of the glands.   But, besides these, it is usual to reckon as "scrofulous" affections certain chronic inflammations of joints; slowly progressive "carious" ulcerations of bones; chronic and frequent ulcers of the cornea; ophthalmia attended with extreme intolerance of light, but with little if any of the ordinary consequences of inflammation; frequent chronic abscesses; pustular cutaneous eruptions frequently appearing upon slight affection of the health, or local irritation; habitual swelling and catarrh of the mucous membrane of the nose; habitual swelling of the upper-lip.

Now these, and many more diseases of the like kinds, are, amongst us both in medical and in general language, called scrofulous, or strumous; but, though many of them are often coincident, yet it is very difficult to say what all have in common, so as to justify their common appellation. Certainly they are not all tuberculous diseases.   Little more can be said of them than that, as contrasted with other diseases of the same forms and parts, the scrofulous diseases are usually distinguished by mildness and tenacity of symptoms; they arise from apparently trivial local causes, and produce, in proportion to their duration, slight effects : they are frequent, but not active.   The general state on which they depend may be produced by defective food, with ill-ventilation, dampness, darkness, and other depressing influences: and this general state of constitution, whether natural or artificially generated, is fairly expressed by such terms as "delicacy of constitution," "general debility," "defective vital power," "irritability without strength."   Such terms, however, do not explain the state that they express, for they all assume that there are, in human bodies, different degrees of vital power, independent of differences of material ; which is at least not proved.

Such is the vagueness of "scrofula," and of the terms derived from it, as commonly used in this country.   They include some diseases which are, and many which are not, distinguished by the production of tuberculous matter.   It has been proposed, but I doubt whether it be practicable, to make "scrofulous" and "tuberculous" commensurate terms : as at present generally employed, the former has a much larger import than the latter.   The relation between the two is, that the "scrofulous" constitution implies a peculiar liability to the tuberculous diseases; and that they often co-exist.   Their differences are evident in that many instances of scrofula (in the ordinary meaning of the word) exist with intense and long-continued disease, but without tuberculous deposit ; that as many instances of tuberculous disease may be found without any of the non-tuberculous affections of scrofula ; that, as Mr. Simon has proved, while the diseases of "defective power" may be experimentally produced in animals by insufficient nutriment and other debilitating influences, the tuberculous diseases are hardly artificially producible ; that nearly all other diseases may co-exist with the scrofulous, but some are nearly incompatible with the tuberculous.

Now, whether we disuse, or still use in its vagueness, the term scrofula, we may make a group of the "tuberculous" diseases, defined by the peculiar morbid product, of which I have described the chief characters. Only, at present, we must be content, I believe, to be sometimes in doubt whether the substance found in lymphatic glands, and commonly known as scrofulous matter, be truly tuberculous matter, or degenerate lymph or pus.

The LYMPHATIC GLANDS, among the parts specially studied in surgical pathology, hold the first place in liability to tuberculous disease. In children, they are, even more often than the lungs, primarily affected; in adults, they are next to the lungs in the order of frequency; and in all ages, whatever part becomes tuberculous, the lymphatic glands in relation with it are apt to be similarly affected.

The glands most often primarily tuberculous are the bronichal, mesenteric, cervical, and lumbar. Their state, previous to the tubercular formation may seem healthy; or they may be simply enlarged; or signs of inflammation may precede and accompany the deposit. Rokitansky says that, in some cases, the tuberculous matter, as in the gray pulmonary tubercles, appears in small round masses of grayish substance. But its far more frequent appearance in the glands is, like the yellow, pulmonary tuberculous matter, in the form of roundish or irregular deposits of yellowish, opaque, half-dry, cheesy, crumbling substance. Such deposits are infiltrated among the proper textures of the glands. At first discrete, and contrasting strongly, both in substance and in color, with the unaffected portions of the gland, they gradually increase, till they may completely displace the natural structure, with its blood-vessels, or leave only a thin outer layer of it, enclosing the yellow mass which they form. By the increase of the tuberculous matter, as well as by the swelling of their proper textures, the glands are usually enlarged; they may acquire even an enormous volume, and, when whole series of them are affected, may construct great lobed and nodular swellings. In all cases, however, the several glands maintain a kind of independence; so that one may enlarge while others diminish, and one or more may inflame or suppurate, while, in others, the tuberculous matter remains stationary or retrogrades.

The minute structures in tubercle of the lymphatic glands are essentially similar to those described from examples in the lungs: and Virchow[*] has found that, in the first stage of the process, there is an endogenous increase of nuclei within the elementary structures, similar to that which I have described after Schroeder van der Kolk. The same softening and liquefaction, also, as in the lungs, is prone to ensue in the lymphatic glands.

The softening is usually central, and thence extending may affect the

[*] Würzburg Verhandlungen, i. 84.

whole morbid substance. The result of the change is not a homogeneous liquid; but, rather, a mixture of thin, turbid, yellowish-white liquid, and portions of soft, curd-like, cheesy substance, like fragments of tubercle softened by imbibed fluid. To these are commonly added the liquid products of the inflammation of whatever remains of the gland-substance, or its capsule, and the surrounding parts. The mixture constitutes the tuberculous, or, as it is generally called, scrofulous pus, of which the chief characters, as distinguished from those of ordinary inflammatory pus, are, that it has an abundant thin, yellowish, and slightly turbid liquid, with white, curdy flakes, that quickly subside when it is left at rest.

The liquefaction of the tuberculous matter in the glands usually leads to its discharge; and this is effected, in the case of the cervical and other similarly placid glands, by ulceration, which differs from that for the opening of common abscesses, chiefly, in being slower, and attended with less vivid and less concentrated inflammation. There is, therefore, less disposition to *point :* the skin is, proportionally, more widely undermined, more extensively thinned. Thus gradually, by thinning and inflammation, deprived of blood, the inflamed skin over the tuberculous gland whose contents are liquefied, may perish, and form a dry parchment-like slough, very slowly to be detached. More commonly, however, one or more small ulcerated apertures form in the skin, and let out the fluid. If the undermined skin be freely cut, its loose edges are apt to ulcerate widely; if it be only punctured and allowed to subside gradually, it usually contracts and recovers its healthy state.

The cavity left by the discharge of the liquefied tuberculous matter, and of the fluids mingled with it, may heal up like that of an ordinary abscess, but it does so slowly, and often imperfectly, enclosing portions of tuberculous matter, which soften at some later, and often at some distant, period, and lead to a renewal of the process for discharge. However, such retained portions of tubercle, or even the whole of what has been formed, and perhaps liquefied, in a lymphatic gland, instead of being discharged, may degenerate further, and be absorbed; or may wither and dry up into a fatty and calcareous concretion. Such chalky masses, even of large size, are frequently found in bronchial and mesenteric glands, that have been seats of tuberculous disease in childhood; and similar material, but usually in small fragments, is often discharged from healing tuberculous abscesses in the neck.

Whether by healing after discharge, or by calcification of the retained tuberculous matter, the recovery from the primary tuberculous disease of the lymphatic glands is often complete and permanent. The original substance of the gland may be wholly destroyed; or portions of it may remain indurated and fixed closely to the scar or the calcareous concretion.

I am not aware that tubercle is ever seen, primarily, in lymphatic vessels; but it may be often traced in those of the intestines and mesentery that are in relation with tuberculous ulcers involving the muscular and superitoneal tissues.

I am not aware that tubercular deposits have been proved to be the origin of the so-called scrofulous ulcers of the integument; but that they are so is highly probable, seeing that such ulcers sometimes supervene at the openings for discharge of liquefied tubercle from lymphatic glands, and that, in many characters, they remarkably resemble the tuberculous ulcers of the mucous membrane of the intestines.

The ulcers for which we may suspect a truly tuberculous origin are most frequent in the neck, at the sides of the face, at the upper part of the chest, and on the arms. They are sometimes preceded by the formation of one or more small oval masses of firm substance in the subcutaneous tissue: these, passing through the usual changes of suppurating tuberculous glands, discharge themselves; and the ulceration extends from the aperture of discharge. But, more often, the ulcers commence in patches of skin which, with the subcutaneous tissue, have appeared, for some days or weeks, inflamed, thickened, and slightly indurated. Central softening and liquefaction ensue in these; the cutis is gradually undermined, and then ulcerates, letting out a small quantity of thin, flaky, and turbid fluid, like that of liquefied tubercle. The ulcers thus formed have generally destroyed the thickness of the cutis. They are of various shapes; most often elongated oval, but sometimes round, or sinuous; more rarely annular or crescentic; very rarely quite regular in shape. Their margins are usually (if they are not quickly extending) undermined, rounded, thickened, and unequal. The skin upon and around their margins is pale rose-pink; or tends, according to the activity or torpor of the disease, towards florid redness, or a pale livid hue. Their bases are unequal, often nodular, or tuberculated, pale, with unequal or succulent granulations; they yield a thin, turbid, whey-like fluid, which may concrete in scabs, and sometimes irritates the parts on which it lies. They have no proneness to extend much in depth: neither do they extend widely, unless acute inflammation supervene at their boundaries; rather, their tendency is to remain long stationary, or partially healing; or, while some are healing, others may be progressive.

The scar formed in the healing of these ulcers is peculiar, resembling that of the healed tuberculous ulcers of the mucous membrane of the intestines. It is formed of very tough tissue, which remains long fixed to the subjacent structures, and of which the surface is generally colored with vascular congestion, seen through the thin covering of new cuticle. But, chiefly, the surfaces of such scars are deeply seamed and wrinkled; or have prominent hard ridges that tend towards their centres, or across their axes. The cutis that surrounds the ulcers is very much contracted in the formation of the scars: and both in this respect, and the abundant tough tissue constructing them, they may be likened to the scars following burns.

Among the Bones, tuberculous disease affects most frequently those of spongy cancellous tissue; such as the tarsal and carpal, the vertebræ, the phalanges, and the expanded articular portions of larger bones, especially of the femur, tibia, humerus, and ulna. When it affects bones that are arranged in a group or series, it is usually found in many of them at once. Thus, several vertebræ, or several carpal or tarsal bones, are commonly at the same time tuberculous; yet not often so equally, but that one of them appears first and chiefly diseased; while, in those gradually more distant from it on either side, the tuberculous deposits are gradually less abundant. In like manner, the parts of bones that act together in a joint are, usually, at the same time tuberculous.

Rokitansky says that gray tuberculous matter may be found, about tuberculous suppurations in bone, in the form of granulations seated in the medullary membrane. The usual appearance is that of yellow, soft, cheesy deposits, or infiltrations of tubercle. The infiltration may be either circumscribed or diffuse: and, in these differences, generally corresponds with the similar varieties in the lungs; especially in that, usually, the circumscribed infiltrations take place with scarcely any signs of inflammatory disease, while the diffuse are preceded and accompanied by all the signs and effects of slowly progressive inflammation of the bone.

In the circumscribed infiltrations, the tuberculous matter usually forms round, or oval masses, which are imbedded in cavities in the interior of the bones. At these cavities, several of which may exist near together, the normal textures of the bone appear to be disintegrated or absorbed, just as those of the lung are during the infiltration of the tuberculous matter among them. When the liquefaction of the tubercle takes place, a similar imitation of the formation of cavities in the lungs is noticeable. The usual thin puriform fluid is produced, and is often mixed with little fragments of bone. The bony cavity including it commonly becomes lined by a thin, smooth, closely adherent membrane—the product, apparently, of ordinary inflammation. Appearances are thus attained, especially in the bodies of vertebræ, like those of numerous small chronic abscesses in bones: and similar cavities may be found between the bone and periosteum, when the tuberculous matter has been formed between them, or has included the surface of the bone in its infiltration. The liquid contents of the cavities may be discharged through narrow apertures in the walls of the bone or other surrounding parts; but commonly, a more diffuse inflammatory or tuberculous formation ensues, destroying both the walls of the cavities and their boundaries.

The diffuse infiltration of tuberculous matter in bone may be the form assumed from the first, or it may supervene on the preceding.* The deposits observe no definite shape; they fill the cancellous spaces in the

* The two forms are illustrated in the College Museum, No. 854-5; and in that of St. Bartholomew's in Series I. 37, 38, 39, 70, 103, &c.

bone, displacing the medulla, and either leaving the osseous tissue entire, or softening and disintegrating it, so that small fragments, or larger sequestra, appear mixed with the crumbling tubercle. The abundant deposit of tubercle, and the fulness of the vessels of the inflamed and softening bone, making the swelling in this form more considerable than in the preceding; yet it is rarely, if ever, great. The liquefaction is attended with larger and more destructive, though slow, ulceration of the bone; and is followed by discharge of the fluid, together with products of inflammation, through many apertures, or from a widely ulcerated surface. The bone bounding such ulceration is, moreover, commonly inflamed, if not tuberculous; and thus the ulceration may constantly make progress in depth and width, imitating the types of tuberculous ulceration already described, in that the destruction is of two-fold character: due partly to secondary formations and liquefactions of tubercle, and partly to continued bordering inflammation.

The changes produced by circumscribed tuberculous deposits in bone are, comparatively, seldom seen; for the disease is of slow progress, and rarely leads to death, or amputation, before the more diffuse ulceration has supervened and destroyed its characteristic features. The diffuse disease is therefore that which has been most studied, and which has supplied most of the examples of "scrofulous caries," "Pott's disease of the spine," "Pædarthrocace," &c. It is this, also, which is chiefly attended with suppurations, or, perhaps tuberculous deposits, in the neighborhood of the diseased bone.

The tuberculous diseases of bone are, comparatively, rarely healed. Mr. Stanley has well shown that the completely curable cases of "scrofulous" disease in bone are those in which "the changes have not passed beyond those of simple inflammation:" i. e. of such inflammation as commonly precedes the diffuse deposit of tubercle. When tubercle is deposited in bone, its usual course is, as in other parts, only degenerative: it may liquefy, or calcify: it is, probably, never organized or absorbed. Calcareous concretions, that had their origin in tuberculous matter, may be found imbedded in or upon bone, enclosed in indurated osseous or periosteal tissue; but they are, I believe, extremely rare. Healing of tuberculous cavities and ulcers in bone is less rare. No new bone may be formed; but the membrane lining a cavity may become thick and tough: its contents may become denser and dryer; and the bone for a short distance around it may be hardened and solidified; and all the morbid process may cease. Or, the surface of an ulcer may gradually heal; compact hard bone forming on it, and combining with the thick and scarred periosteum and superjacent tissues. Or, lastly, though rarely after tuberculous disease, when two ulcerated surfaces of bone come into contact, they may unite and coalesce: as in the anchylosis which may ensue after the tuberculous ulceration of the articular portions of bones, or between vertebræ, in some of the cases of tuberculous disease of the spine,

or among the bones of the carpus or tarsus. In all these instances, it
may be generally observed that, as inflammation of the bone preceded
and bordered the tuberculous deposits and ulcers, so, when healing
ensues, the bone adjacent to the scar or cavity is hardened, pale yellowish white, less vascular than in health, and made heavier and more
nearly solid by the thickening of its cancelli.

The instances of tuberculous disease which have now been described
may suffice, I hope, for all that I can have in view; namely, the illustration of the general characters of the disease, and the principal facts
on which to form an opinion concerning its nature and affinities.

On first thought, there may seem little right to assume such a relation
between tubercles and tumors, as is implied by their inclusion in this
volume: yet the features of resemblance are not few or inconsiderable.
The question, broadly stated, is whether tuberculous diseases have nearest
likeness to inflammations, or to cancers.* It is a very difficult one to
answer, for there are apparently good arguments on both sides. On the
whole, I am disposed to think that the really tuberculous diseases are
more, and in more significant things, like the cancerous than they are
like any others. Therefore, I have spoken of them here, and have
arranged the illustrations of them in a corresponding place in the College Museum. But I will now state both sides of the question.

I. The likeness between the tuberculous diseases and the inflammations, with lymph products that are least capable of development, seems
to be shown in these things:—

(1) The likeness between tubercle and such lymph-products is often
too great for diagnosis: they have been, and are, often confounded: and
the withered and degenerate nuclei and other particles of which tubercles are chiefly composed are, at least, as much like those of degenerate
inflammatory lymph as they are like any other morbid products.

(2) Inflammation, indicated by all its signs, is a common precedent
and attendant of tuberculous deposit. It evidently exists in nearly all
cases of the acute, and in many of the chronic, tuberculous affections of
the glands, lungs, and other parts ; and inflammatory lymph capable of
complete development is sometimes mingled with tuberculous matter.

(3) The degenerations of tuberculous matter are, in all essential points,
parallel with those of inflammatory lymph: and so are the processes preceding and following the discharge of the liquefied product.

* The observations of Virchow and Schroeder van der Kolk, respecting the formation of
tuberculous matter in epithelial cells and other natural tissue-elements, are not opposed to
this mode of stating the question. It may be said that there are many points of resemblance
between tuberculous diseases and the degenerations of parts; but it would be a very far,
and, I think, a very injudicious, extension of our ideas of degenerations, to include the process for the formation of tubercles among them. The differences between the tuberculous
disease and all the natural processes of merely defective nutrition separate it widely from
all degenerations properly so-called. The tuberculous material naturally degenerates; but
its production cannot be reasonably called a process of degeneration in any normal part.

(4) The same constitutional peculiarities (so far as they can be observed) precede and attend the tuberculous diseases and the so-called scrofulous inflammations, which are not productive of tuberculous deposits.

Whether, therefore, we consider the local or the constitutional parts of the process, there may seem no boundary-line, no mark indicating essential dissimilarity, between the tuberculous diseases and the inflammations producing lymph nearly incapable of development. The conclusion, therefore, might be, that the local disease is a specific inflammation, dependent on a peculiar diathesis or constitution of the blood, and to be studied according to its analogies with gout, rheumatism, syphilis, and the constitutional affections that are manifested by local inflammations.

On the other side, it may be said,—(1) that the likeness between tubercle and degenerated lymph is only that into which a large number of both normal and morbid products merge in similar degenerations; (2) that the coincidence of inflammation and tuberculous deposit is accidental and inconstant, and that the mingling of the developing products of the one, with the degenerating material of the other, proves their essential difference; (3) that the same methods of degeneration, and of disposal of liquefied materials, which are observed in tubercle and aplastic lymph, may be noticed in other products,—for instance, in cancerous and other growths with ill-developed structure; and (4) that the similarity of the constitutional states only justifies the expression, that "scrofulous" persons are peculiarly liable to tuberculous, as well as to inactive inflammatory, diseases.

II. The chief grounds for regarding tubercle and cancer as diseases of the same order are the following :—

(1) Tubercles sometimes appear as distinct masses, like tumors, in the brain, and in other instances of so-called encysted tubercle. And the dissimilarity between these and tumors, in that they neither grow by inherent power, nor are vascular, is only because their elementary structures abort, and very early become degenerate; it is only the same dissimilarity as exists between a degenerate, and a growing, mass of cancer.

(2) The general characters of malignant tumors, as deduced from cancers (p. 824), are also observed in tuberculous diseases: namely, the elementary tuberculous structures are heterologous; they are usually infiltrated, and, at length, exclude, and occupy the place of, the natural textures; they have a peculiar tendency to induce ulceration after softening; the walls of the ulcer are commonly occupied by tuberculous deposits like those which preceded it, and, while thus occupied, have no disposition to heal; the tuberculous deposits apparently multiply in all the same manners as the cancerous do (compare p. 660, e. s.); and, whether in their extension or in their multiplication, there is scarcely an organ or tissue which they may not affect, though, like cancers, the primary tuberculous diseases have their "seats of election," and different seats at different periods of life.

(3) The tuberculous diathesis, the constitutional state which precedes the formation of tubercle, is scarcely producible by any external agencies, except climate; but it is frequently hereditary: and in both these respects it resembles the cancerous, and differs from the merely debilitated state in which the aplastic inflammations occur.

(4) The cancerous and the tuberculous diathesis appear to be incompatible and mutually exclusive: the production of tubercles is extremely rare, but that of lowly organized inflammatory products is frequent, in cancerous patients. Such incompatibility implies that cancer and tubercle are equally, and in the same sense, constitutional diseases; very different, yet of the same order in pathology.

(5) The tuberculous diathesis, like the cancerous, regularly increases, and is attended with cachexia, which is often disproportionate to the local disease. It is true that tuberculous disease frequently ceases in a part, and allows its healing; yet if we look to its enormous mortality as the index of its natural course, we must see in it a law of increase, like that exemplified with fewer exceptions in cancers. And such a law is not usually exemplified in the specific inflammatory diseases; for they generally tend to subside with lapse of time.

If, now, I leave the reader to consider for himself the question that may thus be argued, I shall but fulfil a purpose kept in view in all the lectures—the purpose, namely, of offering materials for thought upon subjects of which I have not knowledge. It will be within the same scope if I suggest a contemplation of the seeming opposition between the chief subjects of the first twenty, and the remaining lectures in this volume.

In all the affections considered in the former, we may trace purpose and design for the maintenance and recovery of the body's health. The strengthening against resistance, the reaction after injury, the turbid activity of repair, the collection and removal of inflammatory products, the casting of sloughs, the discharge of morbid materials from the blood, —all these are examples of the manifold good designs of disease; and they evince such strength and width of adaptation to the emergencies of life, that we might think the body was designed never to succumb before the due time of its natural decay.

But in the diseases considered in the latter, we trace no fulfilment of design for the well-being of the body: they seem all purposeless or hurtful: and if our thoughts concerning purpose were bounded by this life, or were only lighted by the rays of an intellectual hope, we could not discover the signs of benificence in violences against nature, or in early deaths, such as I have here described. But, in these seeming oppositions, faith can trace the Divine purposes, consistent and continuous, stretching far beyond the horizon of this life; and among the certainties of the future, can see fulfilled the intention of the discipline of sufferings that only death might mitigate. And, if we cannot always tell what is designed, for themselves, in either the agony or the calm through which we see men pass from this world, and cannot guess why, for their own sakes, some are withdrawn in the very sunrise of their life, and others left to abide till night; yet, always, GOD's purpose, for our own good, may be clearly read in the warning, that untimely deaths should make us timely wise.

INDEX.

A.

Abernethy, Mr., on classification of tumors, 332; on pancreatic tumors, 467.

Abscess, formation of, 249–255; opening of, 264; in bone, 261.

Absorption; preceded by transformation, 50; of bone, 170; of degenerate parts, 50; of blood, 123; of bloodvessels, 263; of cancer, 663; of dead tissues, 302; of inflamed parts, 261, 270; of inflammatory lymph, 244, 246.

Adhesion, primary, 134; secondary, 137.

Adhesions, formation of, 233.

Adhesive inflammation, 135, 218.

Adipose tissue, increased formation of, 33: and see Fat.

Adipose tumor: see Fatty tumor.

Affinity, elective, in parts, 52, 55.

Age, as affecting repair, 109; general relation to cancer, 642: and see Cancer.

Air, cysts containing, 339.

Albuminous sarcoma, 416.

Allocation of cancers, &c., 545, 647.

Alveolar cancer: see Colloid.

Amputation, healing after, 137, 158.

Anchylosis, followed by atrophy, 96.

Aneurism, of bone, 486; by anastomosis, 478; effects of pressure by, 71; Hunter's operation for, 38.

Antlers, growth of, after castration, 35.

Antrum, osseous growths of the, 463; polypi in the, 380; teeth in the, 378.

Aplastic lymph, 243, 675, e. s.

Apoplexy, with degenerate cerebral and pulmonary vessels, 102.

Arachnoid, organization of blood-clots in the, 121.

Arcus senilis, 105.

Arrests of development, 18.

Arterial vascular tumor, 482.

Arteries, contraction of, 182; degeneration of, 100; healing of injured, 181; obstruction of, inducing mortification, 38, e. s. 292; inducing degeneration in cancers, 664; ulceration of, in progress of cancer, 577: and see Bloodvessels.

Artery, femoral, traversing a tumor, 440, note.

Ascites, fibrine, exuded in, 281.

Assimilation, 19; of blood, 26; in diseased parts, 46; by cancer, 659.

Assimilative force, 51.

Asteriæ, repair in, 111.

Atheromatous affection of arteries, 100.

Atrophy, 72, e. s., from pressure, 70; modes of, 72: see Degeneration; of cancerous parts, 653; distinguished from inflammation, 279.

Auditory passage, polypi in, 380.

Auricle, cysts fasciculated like an, 348.

Autogenous cysts, 335.

B.

Baly, Dr., on ulceration, 272.

Barky warts, 594.

Barlow, Mr. W. F., on paralyzed muscles, 89; on fatty degeneration, 82.

Bats, circulation in the wings of, 197; their temperature, 197; rythmical contractions of veins, 198.

Baum, Prof., on teeth in the antrum, 373; on aural polypi, 381.

Bell, John, on aneurism by anastomosis, 478.

Bell, Sir C., on cancerous cachexia, 522.

Bennett, Dr. J. H., on fibro-nucleated tumors, 419; on cancroid disease, 564; on inflammation, 289; on blood in inflamed parts, 206.

Birkett, Mr., on mammary cysts, 343; on mammary glandular tumors, 468.

Bites, &c., venomous, 312.

Blastema, extension of disease along, 660.

Blastema, nucleated, its development, 128: see also Nucleated Blastema.

Bleeding: see Hemorrhage.

Blisters, different fluids in, 220.

Blood, absorption of extravasated, 123; accumulation inducing growth, 59; assimilation by, 26; in cancerous persons, 634; initiating inflammation, 283; death of, in dead parts, 300; defect and disease of, inducing mortification, 292, 296; effusion in inflammation, 215; effused, supposed origin of tumors, 529; extravasated, in wounds, its disposal, 120, 122; in inflammations, 205; influence on inflammatory products, 219; in vessels of inflamed parts, 194; life of, 27; maintenance of morbid state of, 47; materials of, determining formation, 33; morbid materials in, 27, e. s.; organization of, 120, e. s.; in tied arteries, 184; regular supply for nutrition, 37; right state of, for nutrition, 26, 27; clots, softening of, 243; stagnant after injuries, 139; transference of cancers, &c., by, 662.

Blood-cells, length, &c., of life, 25; development of, 51; in inflammation, 205; white, on wounds, 137.

Blood-scabs, 152.

Blood-vessels, absorption of, 263; adaptation to atrophy, 87; atrophy of, 100; initiating inflammation, 281; of cancers, 533, 656; enclosed by cancers, 532, 558; cancerous ulceration of, 577; contraction on stimulus 499; in granulations, 450; enlarged in growing parts, 359; in inflamed parts, 194; formation of new, 144, e. s. 238, 656, obstruction of: see Arteries; office of, in nutrition, 40; relation to organization, 149; growth of, in tumors, 485; supplying tumors, 375, 656; in erectile tumors, 480.

Boils, sloughs in, 296.

THE END.

CPSIA information can be obtained
at www.ICGtesting.com
Printed in the USA
LVHW011244200219
608165LV00009B/599/P